# *Clinical*
# *Nursing Skills*

# *Clinical*
# *Nursing Skills*

## *Presented in the Nursing Process*

### *Basic to Advanced Skills*

Sandra Smith, RN, MS
Donna Duell, RN, MS

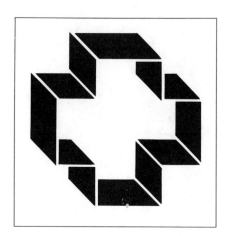

**NATIONAL NURSING REVIEW**
Los Altos, California

**Project Director:** Karen Hoxeng, RN
**Design:** R. Kharibian
**Photography:** Ronald W. May
**Illustrations:** Stephen M. Chapot
**Composition:** Vera Allen Composition
**Printing and Binding:** Kingsport Press

**Library of Congress Cataloging in Publication Data**

Smith, Sandra Fucci.
    Clinical nursing skills.

    Bibliography: p.
    Includes index.
    1.   Nursing.   I.   Duell, Donna J., 1938–
II.   Title.
                610.73          84-62493
ISBN 0-917010-14-0

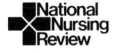 342 State Street, Suite #6
Los Altos, CA 94022

In the writing of this text, the authors and publisher have made every attempt
to follow current nursing practice and to ensure that suggested diets, drug selection and dosages, and nursing procedures are up-to-date and conform with
current recommendations and practices at time of publication. However, in view
of new research conclusions, technological advancements, and government regulations, it is the responsibility of the nurse to be aware of any changes which
may alter suggested drug and diet therapies or nursing protocols. The authors
recommend that nurses and nursing students be aware of hospital and school
policies regarding their role and responsibilities in performing nursing actions.

# Contributors

Joan N. Althaus, RN, MSN, CCRN
Medical Electronics Clinical Specialist
Hewlett-Packard, Dallas

Abby S. Bloch, MS, RD
Head Clinical Diet/Nutrition Specialist
Memorial Sloan Kettering
    Cancer Center

Barbara Devine Bode, RN, MN
Doctoral Program
University of Illinois

Christine Bolwell, RN, MSN, CCRN
Clinical Specialist
Sacramento, CA

Randy Caine, RN, MS
Assistant Professor
California State University,
    Long Beach

Janet W. Cook, RN, MS
Assistant Professor
University of North Carolina

Lou Ann Emerson, RN, MSN
Assistant Professor
University of Cincinnati

Marsha Heims, RN, MS
Assistant Professor
Oregon Health Sciences University

Nancy Meyer Holloway, RN, MSN,
    CCRN, CEN
Clinical Specialist and Consultant
Orinda, CA

Jill D. Holmes, RN, MS
Clinical Specialist
Scripps Clinic and Research
    Foundation

Kathleen Kaplan, RN, MSN, CNM
Associate in Nursing
Columbia University

Sue Kelly, RN, MS
Supervising Public Health Nurse
County of Santa Clara

Patricia A. Kynes, RN, ET
Enterostomal Therapist
Mobile, AL

Terry W. Miller, RN, MS
Assistant Professor
San Jose State University

Susan D. North, RN, MS
Clinical Specialist
Johns Hopkins Medical Center

Fay Alger O'Brien, RN, MA
Instructor
De Anza College, California

Sharon Dennis Raj, RN, MSN
Kaiser-Permanente Medical Center
Santa Clara, California

Judith A. Yanda, RN, MS
Inservice Education
Santa Teresa Hospital, San Jose

Mary G. Yarbrough, RN, MS
Associate Administrator /
    Director of Nursing Services
City of Hope, Duarte

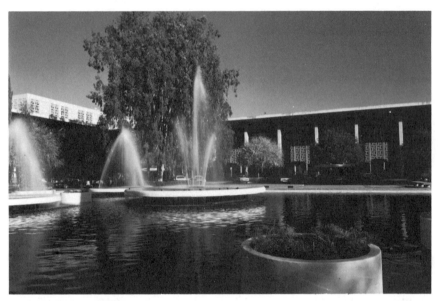

Stanford University Hospital

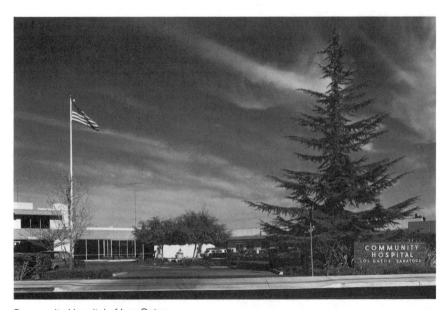

Community Hospital of Los Gatos

# *Preface*

CLINICAL NURSING SKILLS is designed for nursing students in bacca-
laureate, associate degree and diploma nursing programs. The objectives
of this text are twofold—to assist student nurses to learn basic and advanced
nursing procedures in the clinical setting and to present these skills in a
format adaptable to any curriculum. To accomplish these goals, the authors
present the skills not as rote memorization but as a combination of theory
and practical application in the nursing process framework.

During the past decade, health care has experienced startling developments
in technology and innovative changes in delivery systems and treatment
modalities. These advancements, along with changes in the design and focus
of nursing curricula, provide the rationale from which this book evolved.
At a fundamentals level, this is a skills book; at a basic textbook level, it is a
blend of theory and practice. At a learning level, the nursing process provides
the framework for the text, and clinical knowledge establishes the basis for
the nursing skills.

The authors believe that an effective nursing skills textbook must be
current, innovative, and relevant to enable nursing students to master the
many skills necessary to provide quality nursing care. This book answers
the need for a contemporary approach to teaching nursing skills. It is sufficiently comprehensive to be used by students for both initial learning and for
future reference.

To utilize this book in the most effective way, it is important that the reader
understands how the material is organized. From the most basic level of
mastery to the more complex skills, this book focuses on presenting nursing
procedures in a way that students will find easy to understand and to
apply directly in the clinical area.

In general, the text first describes basic concepts and then applies them to
clinical situations. The chapters include *learning objectives*, an *introduction*
(which provides the theoretical basis for skill performance), and *nursing diagnoses*. The clinical content follows next in a series of units and is presented
in terms of the nursing process—*assessment, planning, implementation* (which
specifies the skills included in the unit), and *evaluation*. This approach
enables the student, after being assigned to perform a specific skill, to learn
how to assess the patient, formulate goals, perform the procedure and, finally,
evaluate the results. Each procedure includes the equipment, the preparation,
and the step-by-step performance necessary to master the skill. The student
can easily access this material for immediate reference in the clinical area.
Illustrations and photographs within each unit will assist the student to
visually relate to the concepts presented. Finally, the unit is completed with a
section on *charting* and *clinical problem-solving*.

The problem-solving material was specifically developed to enable the
student to learn the problem-solving process. Nursing skills should not be

performed without considering the individual patient. This section encourages the student to consider potential problems that may arise while performing skills. It also presents suggestions for problem resolution. Rather than providing the student with answers to the potential problems, the student is encouraged to thoroughly consider each skill, its potential problems, and to individualize patient care.

While the nursing process provides the framework for this textbook, additional learning aids have been included to help the student assimilate the immense amount of nursing content. *Rationale* for specific nursing actions helps the student understand why a certain action is performed. *Clinical alerts* call the student's attention to a critical situation or action. *Boxed information* emphasizes specific aspects of patient care and the additional knowledge necessary for mastery of a particular skill. Finally, *patient teaching principles* are included as appropriate.

In order to assist both students and faculty, the publisher offers a separate booklet that includes individual checklists for all of the skills and post-test questions for each chapter. The checklists will enable both the student and the teacher to assess the student's performance and level of mastery for each skill. The post-test will evaluate the student's proficiency in the more traditional mode of a written exam.

The authors are confident that students will find CLINICAL NURSING SKILLS relevant, useful, and adaptable to their learning needs. Furthermore, the authors hope that faculty will find this textbook a valuable teaching tool and an important reference source for the students enrolled in the skills component of their nursing curricula.

## *Acknowledgements*

We would like to express our appreciation to the many people who assisted us during the production of CLINICAL NURSING SKILLS. Without them, the task of writing and editing the manuscript, as well as producing the illustrations, would have been monumental.

Through the assistance and generosity of Stanford University Hospital and Community Hospital of Los Gatos-Saratoga, we were able to conduct extensive photography in the appropriate clinical environment. We extend our thanks to the administrators and staff at these two hospitals for their aid in coordinating our photography sessions.

We also wish to express our gratitude to the other individuals who assisted in the creation and production of this text. Without their assistance, this book could not have been published: our associates and models, Ellen Troyer, Elizabeth Anderson, Carol Thoryk, Joan Althaus, and Sally Talley, as well as the many patients who consented to be photographed for the benefit of the students utilizing this text.

The never-ending task of editing and proofreading was expertly handled by Vi Sidre and Fay O'Brien. Their patience and fortitude in wading through mountains of pages was much appreciated. We would also like to thank our special consultants who painstakingly read the manuscript and provided clinical expertise for the book: Joan Althaus, Elizabeth Anderson, Barbara Pratley, and Sally Talley.

Last, but by no means least, we would like to thank our friends and families for their encouragement and support during this busy time.

Sandra F. Smith, RN,MS
Donna J. Duell, RN,MS

# Contents

Chapter *20*
*Bowel Elimination*                                                  509

Chapter **28**
*Pain Management*                                  *813*

Chapter **29**
*Diagnostic Tests*                                  *825*

## Chapter *30*
### *Operative Care*   851

## Chapter *31*
### *Crisis and the Dying Patient*   879

Chapter *1*

# Role of the Nurse

Professional Role of the Nurse
Legal Aspects of Nursing
Patient Rights
Clinical Practice
Medical Asepsis Principles
Protocol for Procedures

## LEARNING OBJECTIVES

Discuss what is meant by the concept "professional role of the nurse."

Define the term accountable.

List three ways you can assist the patient to assume and adapt to the patient role.

Identify the guidelines that will assist you to convey nursing competence to your patients.

Describe the Nurse Practice Act.

Define the term nurse licensure.

State four functions that the Board of Registered Nursing performs.

Discuss four grounds for licensure revocation for professional misconduct.

Explain the legal issues of drug administration.

Describe what is meant by "patient's rights."

List four actions or guidelines that you need to complete in order to prepare for daily patient care.

Describe the steps of planning for patient care.

State the components of the patient record.

Discuss the term asepsis.

List four principles that relate to preventing the spread of microorganisms.

## PROFESSIONAL ROLE

As you enter the profession of nursing, you will experience some of the most frustrating and some of the most rewarding situations of your life. In order to decrease the frustrations and increase the positive experiences, this chapter introduces you to the role of the nurse. Emphasis is placed on those procedures that will assist you to become a functioning member of the health team, even with limited experience.

The information in this chapter will help you through the first few critical days of your clinical experience. In addition, legal aspects of the nursing profession are discussed to make you aware of the far-reaching consequences of nursing actions. Patients' rights and the Nurse Practice Act are also presented for your information.

As a nurse you will be held accountable and responsible for your actions. What does all this mean? To be accountable means that you are answerable for all your activities surrounding patient care. Accountability can be observed and measured by a variety of factors. Nursing actions are evaluated against a set of standards, frequently referred to as standards of performance. In this evaluation the nurse is judged according to predetermined factors in which all nurses should be competent.

Responsibility means that the nurse is conscientious and honest in all her professional activities. A good example of responsibility deals with not betraying confidential information concerning patients in the hospital. In addition, a responsible nurse respects the rights of her patients and abides by the Patient's Bill of Rights.

Nurses must function within the Nurses' Code of Ethics. The code of ethics is a set of formal guidelines for governing professional action. It assists the nurse to problem-solve where judgment is required. More emphasis is now being placed on the professional organizations to uphold the code of ethics and to admonish those nurses who violate the code.

**Assuming the Patient Role**    Assisting the patient to adapt to hospitalization is one of the primary functions of the nurse. The less resistive the patient is toward receiving treatment during hospitalization, the more open he is to curative methods. The nurse can assist in adaptation by understanding that all patients have individual needs, concerns, and perceptions that require discussion and planning as they take on the role of patient in the health care setting. You must accept the patient's perceptions of his new surroundings. Be aware that anxiety is a natural reaction to an unfamiliar setting, to new procedures, and to new people. If, for example, a patient is extremely fatigued or overwhelmed by traveling to the hospital and the admission procedure, you can help the patient adapt to the surroundings, regain a sense of control and identity, and accept the changed circumstances.

Another way to assist the patient to retain his identity and uniqueness is to communicate with the patient as an individual. Ask questions and observe verbal responses as well as nonverbal cues. Provide ways to care for a patient's personal possessions, clothing, and physical comfort so that the patient adapts more easily to the change in environment and feels more secure and in control.

Be aware that the medical condition is only one part of the patient's life and that the changes that have led up to admission affect other areas of the patient's well-being. Patients may have concerns about new routines, financial matters, their families, or their future. By responding to a patient's total needs at the time of admission, you can help the patient establish a positive attitude toward the total care he will receive.

Acknowledge and accept any statements or behavior the patient uses to adapt to his new surroundings. Even though various cultures and groups differ in their response to illness, and some responses may differ from your personal beliefs, acknowledge the patient's individuality. Support the patient's beliefs and behavior as long as they do not increase the risk of injury or illness. Be sensitive to any past health care experiences that may influence the patient's feelings at the time of admission. A prior experience in the hospital may determine how a patient responds to the current environment.

**Assuming the Nursing Role**    Your actions, both verbal and nonverbal, will influence the patient's feelings and ideas regarding your level of competence, the role of nursing in administering care, and the patient's overall adaptation to hospitalization. Assuming a professional role means that you behave as a professional person. Following the guidelines below will assist you to convey nursing competence, not only to patients but also to your peers and other nursing staff.

☐ Always dress neatly in appropriate, clean attire, and follow the dress code of your school or facility.

☐ Speak in correct English without slang or inappropriate language.

☐ Relate to the patients as worthwhile individuals who deserve respect and consideration. Call the patient by his surname and do not use nicknames or first names.

☐ Do not "talk down" or patronize the patient. Remember that the patient knows more about his own body, symptoms, feelings, and responses than anyone else. Listen and pay attention to what the patient says about himself.

☐ Remain in a professional role at all times. Do not socialize with the patients. They need to view you as a knowledgeable professional who brings healing, caring, and teaching roles to the relationship.

☐ Use yourself as a therapeutic tool to convey caring and healing. Use body language to reinforce honest and direct verbalization, not to contradict it.

☐ Be accountable and answerable for your behavior and nursing actions and the nursing care you are expected to provide. If you do not understand what is expected, seek assistance from a staff member. Your responsibility is to remain reliable, honest, and trustworthy in administering nursing care.

## LEGAL ASPECTS

Legal issues and regulations play a dominant role in nursing practice today. The law provides a framework for establishing nursing actions in the care of patients. Laws determine and set boundaries and maintain a standard of nursing practice.

The Nurse Practice Act defines professional nursing and recommends those actions which the nurse can practice independently and those actions which require a physician's order before completion.

Each state has the authority to regulate and administrate health care professionals. While the provisions of the Nurse Practice Acts are quite similar from state to state, it is imperative that the nurse know the licensing requirements and the grounds for license revocation as defined by the state in which she works.

Legal and ethical standards for nurses are complicated by a myriad of federal and state statutes and the continually changing interpretation of them by the courts of law. Nurses are faced today with the threat of legal action based on negligence, malpractice, invasion of privacy, and other grounds. This chapter covers the basic legal issues and topics, from patients' rights and nurses' liability to drugs and grounds for professional misconduct proceedings.

**The Nurse Practice Act** The Nurse Practice Act is a series of statutes enacted by a state to regulate the practice of nursing in that state. Subjects covered by the Nurse Practice Acts include definition of the scope of practice, education, licensure and grounds for disciplinary actions. Nurse Practice Acts are quite similar throughout the United States, but the professional nurse is held legally responsible for the specific requirements for licensure and regulations of practice as defined by the state in which she works.

The responsibilities of the professional nurse involve a level of performance for a defined range of health care services. These services include assessment, implementation, and evaluation of nursing action, as well as teaching and related services, such as counseling. A summary of the skills and functions that professional nurses perform in daily practice is in the following list.

☐ Provide direct and indirect patient care services

☐ Perform and deliver basic health care services

☐ Implement testing and prevention procedures

☐ Observe signs and symptoms of illness

☐ Administer treatments per physician's order

- □ Observe treatment reactions and responses
- □ Administer medications per physician's order
- □ Observe medication responses and/or side effects
- □ Observe general physical and mental conditions of individual patients
- □ Document nursing care
- □ Supervise allied nursing personnel
- □ Coordinate members of the health team

**Nurse Licensure**    The authorization to practice nursing is defined legally as the right to practice nursing by an individual who holds an active license issued by the state in which she intends to work. The licensing process is administered by the state board of registration, frequently called the BRN. This board may also grant endorsement or reciprocity to an applicant who holds a current license in another state. The applicant for RN licensure must have attended an accredited school of nursing, be a qualified nursing professional or paraprofessional, or have met specific prerequisites if licensed in a foreign country.

*Board of Registered Nursing Functions*

- □ Establishes and oversees educational standards
- □ Establishes professional standards
- □ Conducts examinations for licensure (NCLEX)
- □ Registers and renews licenses
- □ Conducts investigations of violations of the statutes and regulations
- □ Issues citations
- □ Holds disciplinary hearings for possible suspension or revocation of the license
- □ Imposes penalties following disciplinary hearings

**Liability and Legal Issues**    Grounds for professional misconduct are defined and regulated by the individual state. The practicing nurse should know how her state defines professional misconduct although many states have similar standards. Any one of the following actions would constitute grounds for professional misconduct.

- □ Obtaining an RN license through fraudulent methods
- □ Practicing in an incompetent and/or negligent manner
- □ Practicing when ability to practice is severely impaired
- □ Being habitually drunk or dependent on drugs
- □ Being convicted of or committing an act constituting a crime under federal or state law
- □ Refusing to provide health care services on the grounds of race, color, creed, or national origin
- □ Permitting or aiding an unlicensed person to perform activities requiring a license
- □ Practicing nursing while license is suspended
- □ Practicing medicine without a license

The penalties for professional misconduct include probation, censure and reprimand, suspension of the license, or revocation of the license. The state's Board of Registered Nursing has the authority to impose any of the above penalties for professional misconduct.

**Drugs and the Nurse** In their daily work, most nurses handle a wide variety of drugs. Failure to give the correct medication or improper handling of drugs may result in serious problems for the nurse due to strict federal and state statutes relating to drugs. The Comprehensive Drug Abuse Prevention Act of 1970 provides the fundamental federal regulations for compounding, selling, and dispensing narcotics, stimulants, depressants, and other controlled items. Each state has a similar set of regulations for the same purpose.

Noncompliance with federal or state drug regulations can result in liability. Violation of the state drug regulations or licensing laws are grounds for the board of nurse registration to initiate disciplinary action.

---

*Legal Issues in Drug Administration*

Nurses must not administer a specific drug unless allowed to do so by the particular state's Nurse Practice Act.

Nurses are to take every safety precaution in whatever she is doing.

Nurses are to be certain that employer's policy allows her to administer a specific drug.

A drug may not lawfully be administered unless all the above items are in effect.

General rules for drug dispensing:

- Never leave tray with prepared medicines unattended.
- Always report errors immediately.
- Send labeled bottles that are unintelligible back to pharmacist for relabeling.
- Store internal and external medicines separately if possible.

---

**The Elements of Liability** The nature of the law is such that if the basic rules of human conduct are violated, the elements of liability exist. Nursing liability would involve either federal or state violation and result in either a civil or criminal proceeding. The end result of a civil proceeding would be a charge of negligence; the result of a criminal proceeding would be assault and battery, homicide, murder, or manslaughter. Certain elements of liability must exist for such a court proceeding to take place. First, there must be a legal basis, such as a statutory law, for finding liability. There must exist a causal relationship between harm to the patient and the act or omission to act by the nurse. Finally, there must be some damage or harm sustained by the patient.

| *Civil Law* | *Criminal Law* |
| --- | --- |
| Contract | Assault and Battery |
| Unintentional Tort | Homicide |
| Intentional Tort | Murder |
| Negligence | Manslaughter |

You should clearly understand several legal terms. One term is *negligence*— a breach of duty that is the cause of a compensatory injury to the patient when it is understood that the duty of the professional nurse is to provide patients with due care. *Malpractice,* or negligence, is classified as criminal, civil, or ethical. *Liability* occurs when the legal obligation to provide a standard of patient care is not met in terms of reasonable expectation. Professional nurses are held responsible (liable) for harm that results from their negligent acts or omissions to act.

**Classifications of Law**
**Related to Nursing**

| Classification | Example |
| --- | --- |
| Constitutional | Patients' rights to equal treatment |
| Administrative | Licensure and the state BRN |
| Labor Relations | Union negotiations |
| Contract | Relationship with employer |
| Criminal | Handling of narcotics |
| Tort | |
|    Medical Malpractice | Reasonable and prudent patient care |
|    Product Liability | Warranty on medical equipment |

Legal doctrine holds that an employer is also liable for negligent acts of employees in the course and scope of employment. Physicians, hospitals, clinics, and other employers may be held liable for negligent acts of their employees. This doctrine does not support acts of gross negligence or acts that are outside the scope of employment.

## PATIENT RIGHTS

In the United States all but ten states have some provision for the rights of patients. A right of the claim may be moral and/or legal; a legal right can be enforced in a court of law. It is important to remember that within a health care system all patients retain their basic constitutional rights, such as freedom of expression, due process of law, freedom from cruel and inhumane punishment, equal protection, and so forth.

Because patients' rights may conflict with the nursing function, you should be familiar with the key elements of these rights. Rights include consent, confidentiality, and involuntary commitment. In considering these rights, however, remember that they may be modified by the patient's mental or physical condition.

**Consent to Receive Health Services**   Consent is the patient's approval to have his body touched by specific individuals, such as doctors, nurses, laboratory technicians, etc. Informed consent refers to the process of informing the patient prior to granting a consent regarding treatment, tests, surgery, etc., and must be understood by the patient in terms of the intended outcome and the potential harmful results. The patient may rescind a prior consent verbally or in writing.

The authority to sign a consent must be given by a mentally competent adult. Court-authorized persons may give consent for mentally incompetent adults. In emergency situations, if the patient is in immediate danger of serious harm or death, action may be taken to preserve life without the patient's consent.

The nurse's liability in terms of consent is to ensure that the patient is fully informed before being asked to sign a consent form. The physician, nurse, or other health personnel must inform the patient of potentially harmful effects of the treatment. If this is not done, it may result in the nurse's being held personally liable. The nurse must respect the right of a mentally competent adult patient to refuse health care; however, a life-threatening situation may alter the patient's right to refuse treatment.

**Patients' Rights**   Patients are protected by law (invasion of privacy) against unauthorized release of personal clinical data, such as symptoms, diagnoses, and treatments. Nurses, as well as other health care personnel, may be held personally liable for invasion of privacy, should litigation arise from the unauthorized release of patient data. Confidential information, however, may be released by consent of the patient. Information release is mandatory when ordered by a court or when state statutes require reporting child abuse, communicable diseases, or other incidents. Nurses have a legal and ethical responsibility to become familiar with their employers' policies and procedures regarding protection of patient's information.

Medical records are the key written account of such patient information as signs and symptoms, diagnosis, treatment, responses to treatment, etc. Not only do these records document care given to patients, but they also provide effective means of communication among health care personnel. These records contain important data for insurance and other expense claims, as well as being utilized in court in the event of litigation.

Health professionals are becoming more aware of the implications of patients' rights, as society in general becomes more aware of every human being's basic rights. While there are still gaps in the legal process, many states are beginning to grapple with the status of laws applicable to patients who are hospitalized. It is essential that nurses be aware of the particular state's laws and statutes affecting patients and themselves. Nurses as well as physicians are accountable for their actions and the threat of liability is becoming more prevalent.

## CLINICAL PRACTICE

Before your first clinical experience, you will want to review the most essential components of patient care to enable you to practice safe and efficient nursing care. Guidelines for clinical practice, the parts of a patient chart, communication techniques, principles of medical asepsis, a basic nursing assessment, and protocols for nursing care procedures are presented to give you confidence and background information in order to provide nursing care.

**Guidelines for Clinical Practice**   Before attempting to provide patient care, you need to familiarize yourself with all aspects of care the patient will require. The following guidelines will assist you in this preparation. Usually, the preparation is completed the night before you go to the clinical setting. If this is not possible, you need to identify those aspects of preparation which will render you a safe practitioner.

☐ Obtain the clinical assignment in sufficient time to be able to prepare for safe practice.

☐ Read the patient's chart and obtain all the data necessary to assist you in patient care. This usually encompasses the following items: history and physical, physician's progress notes, graphic sheet, medication record, laboratory findings, nurses' notes and/or flow sheets, admissions data base, Patient Care Plan, Kardex card, and physician's orders. Each of these documents will be illustrated later in this chapter.

☐ Review all procedures that you will provide for the patient. Use your skills and fundamentals books for your review.

☐ Research the diagnosis so you are more aware of signs and symptoms the patient will exhibit. Identify alterations from normal such as altered lab values, vital signs, etc.

☐ Research all medications you will administer to the patient. Many instructors require medication cards be completed on all medications to be administered.

☐ Plan your day's experience by developing a time plan to help keep you organized and to enable you to complete patient care in a timely manner.

☐ Practice charting the procedures you will be administering so that you can identify appropriate vocabulary and include necessary information. Pertinent charting information is included with each procedure described in this text.

**Providing Patient Care**   You have prepared for this clinical practice before coming to the nursing unit. Now you will receive an update on the patient's condition, and a team leader will go over nursing procedures you will be completing. This will be accomplished during a report period. Each hospital has a method for presenting the report. Some facilities tape a report from the off-going shift which is listened to by the on-coming staff. Other nursing units give a verbal report in which they review the information obtained by the previous shift. Facilities where primary nursing is practiced will have a one-to-one report between the on-coming nurse and the off-going nurse for a specific group of patients. At this time a work sheet will be completed which lists times for treatments and medications. Following the report, the team leader or your preceptor nurse will go over all aspects of the care you will deliver for the patient. This is the time to ask any questions you may have regarding policy or procedure for the nursing unit or the patient. Your medication cards or unit dose sheet is checked at this time to ensure that you have all necessary medications and equipment to prepare and administer the drugs.

The following outline of patient care will assist you in planning your nursing care for the day.

1. Wash your hands.

2. Gather equipment, such as a stethoscope, sphygmomanometer, thermometer, and linen.

3. Check the patient's identaband. Introduce yourself to the patient and explain the nursing care you will be giving.

4. Check if the patient has any preference for the order in which the care will be given.

5. Complete a nursing assessment. You may use the basic nursing assessment outlined in this chapter as a guide if your instructor does not have one she prefers you to use.

6. Document your findings as you are completing the physical assessment and enter it in the nurses' notes section of the chart.

7. Take vital signs if it is the policy of the unit.

8. Complete all nursing interventions, and document the findings immediately after completion.

9. Administer all medications. Document medication administration in the appropriate place, and observe for signs of side effects or unusual findings.

10. During your nursing care, practice good communication technqiues.

11. Complete all charting.

12. Terminate the relationship with the patient.

13. Report off to the appropriate person.

14. Wash your hands before leaving the nursing unit.

**Patient's Records**   The following documents are those you will be using most often in clinical practice. Become familiar with each form, its placement in the chart, and the information that it contains. Examples are on page 15.

*KARDEX:*   The Kardex card represents the "hub" for all patient activities. Physician's orders are transcribed on the card. Lab tests, medications, and activity levels are just a few items documented in designated areas of the Kardex.

*CARE PLAN:*   The care plan identifies the patient's usual or potential problems, expected outcomes, and nursing actions. Discharge criteria is also an integral part of the care plan.

**Patient's Chart**   The chart itself contains several forms which are important to your preparation and administration of nursing care.

*NURSES' NOTES:*   Nurses' notes do not necessarily have a particular or specific format as do graphic records or physician's orders. One type of narrative nurses' notes is illustrated here. Clinical observations and nursing interventions are documented in nurses' notes. Flow sheets are becoming more popular, especially in critical care units.

*MEDICATION RECORDS:*   Medication records are usually similar to the one illustrated here. All medications should be documented on a medication record. Some facilities chart routine medications on one medication sheet and PRN and one-time only medications on another sheet. Check the institution's policy for each record's use.

*GRAPHIC RECORDS:*   Temperature, pulse, and respirations are graphed on the graphic sheet. Blood pressure readings, intake and output records, and dietary intake are also recorded on this form.

*PHYSICIAN'S ORDERS:*   Physician's orders are written on forms with carbon copies attached. This form allows copies of the orders to be sent to the pharmacy or CSR for supplies. Each facility dictates where each sheet is sent.

*PHYSICIAN'S PROGRESS NOTES:*   Physician's progress notes contain daily observations and thoughts regarding treatments, signs and symptoms experienced by the patient, operative risks explained to the patient, and the patient's responses to therapy.

*HISTORY AND PHYSICAL:*   The physician's report of his assessment is written on a special form. Most hospitals type the history and physical from dictated notes by the physician. When this occurs, it may be several days before this information is available.

   *LABORATORY FORMS:*   Laboratory results are sent back to the unit on the original laboratory order form. The information from each form may be transcribed to a laboratory data flow sheet. This sheet provides a valuable overview of all lab results.

**Communicating with the Patient**   The foundation of the person's perception of himself and the world is the result of communicated messages received from significant others. Communication is a basic human need, and since we live in a social society, everyone has a need to in some way communicate with others in his world. A basic proposition of communication is that a person cannot *not* communicate. Everything you observe in another person is a form of communication: the way one stands and moves, the gestures, total body position, and all the nuances of speech like tone, pace and choice of words. The communication process includes both verbal and nonverbal expressions. It is affected by the experience of the individuals, the relationship between them, and the context in which the communication takes place. It is also affected by the purpose of the sender in sending the message, the content of the message, the manner in which the message is sent, and, finally, the effect on the receiver. As you can see, the communication process can be very complex. As a beginning practitioner, however, the most important factor to remember is that *what* you say and *how* you say it has a very great impact on your patient.

   One of the most important skills you must master is to be able to talk therapeutically to patients and to be able to listen to them. Nurse-patient communication is an intimate process of providing nursing care. In fact, the initial step in the nursing process—assessment—is comprised of observation, interview, and examination. The interview involves talking and listening to the patient. Initially, it may be difficult for you to concentrate on both talking and listening, for you have not yet mastered the basic skills, such as a bedbath or backrub. As you gain experience, however, these skills will be more familiar and you can focus on the communication–interaction process with the patient.

   Learning to talk with patients and listening to them is the beginning of a nurse-patient relationship. Some of you will come to nursing with many of these basic communication skills already mastered. Others will experience shyness, hesitancy, and awkwardness in relating to patients. Try to keep in mind that you are being educated to be a professional person—a nurse— and as such you have a great deal to give to your patients. They will learn to respect your skill, value your presence, and depend upon you when they are ill. One of the most rewarding aspects to nursing is experiencing a communication between you and your patient. If you do feel shy or hesitant, remember that communication skills can be learned. Begin by practicing or role-playing with your classmates until you feel comfortable in the initial phases of a relationship.

   In establishing nurse-patient communication, there are some basic guidelines to remember.

☐  Accept the patient as a valued and worthwhile individual, for this acceptance is a prerequisite for a nurse-patient relationship.

☐  Be aware of the total patient, not just his physical needs. The patient's social, emotional, and spiritual needs are also important.

□ Understand your own needs, feelings, and reactions so that they do not interfere with the therapeutic process with the patient.

□ Be prepared to feel some degree of emotional involvement with your patient, evidencing caring and concern for his welfare. At the same time, however, it is necessary to maintain objectivity.

□ Remember that the nurse-patient interaction is a professional one. As such, there is a nurse who possesses the skills, abilities, and resources to relieve another's pain and discomfort, and a patient who is seeking comfort and assistance for alleviation of some existing problem.

□ A nurse-patient relationship does not require a long-term agreement or formal meetings between nurse and patient to be effective. You may still meet the objectives of such a relationship in a short clinical experience.

**Basic Nursing Assessment**   Each nurse develops her own routine for completing a basic nursing assessment. There is no right or wrong way, although it should be consistent and complete. The following outline for basic assessment is a simple approach to the assessment and one you may wish to adopt until you have established a good system for yourself.

The basic assessment is completed at the beginning and end of each shift. The assessment should take no longer than five to ten minutes to complete. You should concentrate on the specific system that correlates with the patient's diagnosis. For a more in-depth discussion of each system in the assessment, see the chapter on physical assessment.

The following outline will assist you in completing a basic physical assessment.

1. Vital signs.
   a. Temperature (method dictated by condition).
   b. Radial pulse: rate, volume, and rhythm.
   c. Respirations: rate, depth, and rhythm.
   d. Blood pressure: Korotkoff's sounds.
2. State of comfort: location and intensity of pain; response to medications if given.
3. Emotional responses: patient behavior, reactions and demeanor; general mood (crying, depression).
4. Skin: presence or absence of abrasions, contusions, erythema, decubitus ulcers, incision line, color, turgor, temperature.
5. Musculoskeletal: activity level, general mobility, gait, range of motion.
6. Neurological: pupils (size, response, equality); hand grips; strength and sensation of all extremities; ability to follow commands; level of consciousness.
7. Respiratory: breath sounds; sputum color and consistency; cough (productive or nonproductive).
8. Cardiovascular: heart sounds; presence of pulses; edema; presence of hair on extremities.
9. Gastrointestinal: bowel pattern and sounds; presence of nausea or vomiting; abdominal distention; consumption of diet.
10. Genitourinary: voiding; color, odor, and consistency of urine; dysuria; vaginal drainage or discomfort; penile discharge.

If any unusual findings are assessed, complete a more in-depth assessment of the particular system affected. Throughout the day, continue to assess changes in the patient's condition by paying particular attention to the alterations from normal that you identified in the initial assessment. At the end of the shift, make a notation of any changes in the patient's condition.

Microorganisms are found everywhere in nature. Pathogenic microorganisms or pathogens cause disease; nonpathogenic microorganisms or nonpathogens do not cause disease. Some microorganisms are nonpathogens in their normal body environment. An example of this is E.Coli which is normally present in the intestinal tract and does not cause a problem until it inhabits another environment such as the urinary tract.

## MEDICAL ASEPSIS PRINCIPLES

The spread of microorganisms is prevented by the use of two forms of asepsis: medical asepsis and surgical asepsis. Medical asepsis occurs when there is an absence of pathogens. Surgical asepsis occurs when there is an absence of all organisms. Medical asepsis is often referred to as "clean technique" whereas surgical asepsis is termed "sterile technique." A discussion of surgical asepsis can be found later in this book. This chapter will discuss medical asepsis as it affects nursing care.

Principles of medical asepsis are utilized in all aspects of patient care. In fact, the use of medical asepsis begins before you report to the nursing unit. To ensure protection for the patient, you begin practicing medical asepsis by limiting jewelry to only a wedding band and perhaps small earrings for pierced ears when administering patient care. Fingernails are short and in good repair. Your hair is off your collar and under control to prevent contaminating sterile fields and falling into patient's food or wounds.

While providing patient care, the following principles should be kept in mind.

- Linen rooms are considered clean; therefore, linen not used for patient care cannot be returned.

- Utility rooms are designated as areas for clean and dirty supplies. Cross-contamination must be avoided by not placing articles in the wrong area.

- Linen and articles are carried away from your uniform and are not held close to your body.

- Articles dropped on the floor are considered contaminated and must be discarded appropriately. If linen is accidentally dropped on the floor, it is placed in a soiled linen hamper. Patients are to wear slippers or shoes when out of bed.

- Patients have their own supplies and equipment, which are not used by other patients. Sterilization or disinfection is carried out between use.

- If you are not feeling well, you should not report for clinical experience. If you are running a temperature or have a cold and runny nose, call the appropriate person and report that you are ill.

- Paper handkerchiefs are utilized for removing patient's secretions. Discard the handkerchief in the trash basket.

- Equipment is cleaned and rinsed with cold water to remove secretions or substances before being returned to the central supply area. Heat will coagulate the substances and make it more difficult to remove.

□ Soap and water are considered the best cleansers because they help break down soil so it can be more readily removed. Detergents may be more effective in hard or cold water; however, tissue damage can result from their use. Germicides may be added to soap or detergent and increase the effectiveness of the cleansing agent.

□ Friction is used to facilitate soil removal. A brush, sponge, or cloth may be used to produce the friction.

□ When aseptic technique is utilized, cleaning is conducted from the cleanest to the least clean area. For example, always clean the incision area from the center of the incision to the periphery of the skin.

**Handwashing**   The single, most effective medical aseptic practice is handwashing. When you first arrive at the nursing unit and before beginning nursing practice, you will need to complete a medical handwashing procedure. The important concept to remember is that you soap and rinse your hands twice before providing any nursing care to the patient. Hands are washed before all procedures and in-between patients. The specific step-by-step handwashing procedure is covered in Chapter 9, "Basic Care."

Unsterile gloves may be used with unsterile procedures, such as enemas or cleaning excreta, to prevent contamination of the nurse's hands. The use of gloves decreases cross-contamination between patients. Patients frequently feel "unclean" when gloves are used in patient care; therefore, gloves should be used only when necessary. When gloves are no longer needed, dispose of them in the utility room, not in the patient unit.

## PROTOCOL FOR PROCEDURES

Each procedure in this text book follows a basic protocol. In order to save space and prevent repetition, all steps in the protocol are frequently not outlined in detail for each procedure. Remember, however, that these steps are important and must be followed if complete and responsible nursing care is to be delivered to the patient.

Check physician's orders.
Check Patient Care Plan and/or Kardex.
Identify patient.
Introduce yourself to the patient.
Explain procedure to be done.
Wash your hands.
Gather equipment and fill out charge slips.
Take all of the required equipment to the room.
Provide privacy for the patient—draw curtain or screen around bed.
Raise bed to HIGH position.
Lower side rail nearest nurse.
Drape patient (if appropriate).
Perform procedure according to protocol.
Clean patient as necessary.
Remove drape and position patient for comfort.
Raise side rail to UP position.
Lower bed.
Replace call bell.
Pull back curtain or remove screen.
Remove equipment and clean, dispose, and disperse used equipment.
Document or chart finding.

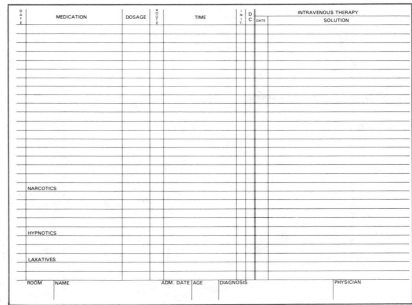

**COMMUNITY HOSPITAL**

| ACTIVITIES | HYGIENE | DIET | BLADDER/BOWEL | | LABORATORY | DATE SENT |
|---|---|---|---|---|---|---|

ACTIVITIES: Complete Bedrest, BR c̄ Commode, BR c̄ BRP, Amb c̄ help, Amb ad lib, Up in chair, Other, Vital Signs, Neuro Signs, S & A, WEIGHT

HYGIENE: Complete bed bath, Partial bath, Shower Tub, Oral Care, Dentures

THERAPY: PT, OT, Isolation

DIET: NPO, Clear Liq., Full Liq., Soft, Regular, Nourishments, Assist Feed, Tube Feeding

SAFETY: Restraints, Wrist, Rails up, Rails down, Side rail release

INTAKE AND OUTPUT

BLADDER/BOWEL: Peri-Care, date last BM, days, prn, nocs, Push Fluids, Special, Ostomy Care

RESPIRATORY: IPPB, Incentive Spirometer, O₂ cannula ___ mask ___

STROKE PROGRAM

LABORATORY: ADMIT CBC - VDRL - UA

TREATMENTS
DATE

X-RAY/OTHER
ADMIT CHEST

ALLERGIES | SURGICAL PROCEDURE | OLD CHART REQUESTED ___ RECEIVED ___

ROOM | NAME | ADM. DATE | AGE | DIAGNOSIS | PHYSICIAN

Kardex Card—ADL Information

| DATE | MEDICATION | DOSAGE | ROUTE | TIME | INIT | D/C | INTRAVENOUS THERAPY | |
|---|---|---|---|---|---|---|---|---|
| | | | | | | | DATE | SOLUTION |

NARCOTICS

HYPNOTICS

LAXATIVES

ROOM | NAME | ADM. DATE | AGE | DIAGNOSIS | PHYSICIAN

Kardex Card—Medication Section

**KARDEX/RAND PATIENT CARE PLAN**

| PATIENT EDUCATION PROGRAM | DISCHARGE CRITERIA | DISCHARGE PLAN | Addressograph |
|---|---|---|---|

PATIENT EDUCATION PROGRAM
DATE: Start | Finish
Diabetic ___
Coronary ___
Other ___

DISCHARGE CRITERIA
PLAN:
Stroke Rehab Eval ___
Cardiac Rehab Eval ___
SOCIAL SERVICE
Date Involved ___
Comment:

DISCHARGE PLAN
Discharge Coordinator
Date Involved ___
Home ___
ECF ___
OTHER ___

| Date | Patient Problem | Deadline Date | Expected Outcome | Health Team Action |
|---|---|---|---|---|

Discharge and Teaching Plan

**Nurses' Notes**

COMMUNITY HOSPITAL

NURSES' NOTES

Patient Information

| Time | Medications/Treatment | Observations | Signature |
|------|----------------------|--------------|-----------|
| | | | |

**Medication Record**

COMMUNITY HOSPITAL — ROUTINE

PRESS HARD

| MEDICATION DOSAGE ROUTE | SHIFT | / /19 | / /19 | / /19 | / /19 |
|---|---|---|---|---|---|

Shifts: 2300-0700, 0700-1500, 1500-2300 (repeated)

SITE CODE:
① – RUOQ ⑤ – R LOWER ABD
② – LUOQ ⑥ – L LOWER ABD
③ – R THIGH ⑦ – R DELTOID
④ – L THIGH ⑧ – L DELTOID

FORM 300114 (1-83)

CHART COPY

**Graphic Record**

COMMUNITY HOSPITAL

CLINICAL RECORD

| DATE | | | |
| HOSP DAY/POSTOP DAY | | | |
| TIME | 0200 0600 1000 1400 1800 2200 | 0200 0600 1000 1400 1800 2200 | 0200 0600 1000 1400 1800 2200 |

| KEY | PULSE | TEMP C / F |
|---|---|---|
| | 140 | 40.6 / 105 |
| | 130 | 40.0 / 104 |
| | 120 | 39.4 / 103 |
| | 110 | 38.8 / 102 |
| | 100 | 38.3 / 101 |
| | 90 | 37.7 / 100 |
| | 80 | 37.2 / 99 |
| | 70 | 36.6 / 98 |
| | 60 | 36.1 / 97 |
| | 50 | 35.5 / 96 |

BLACK – PULSE & RESPIRATIONS
RED – TEMPERATURE

RESPIRATIONS
BLOOD PRESSURE

HEIGHT | WEIGHT | WEIGHT | WEIGHT

| | BREAKFAST | LUNCH | DINNER | BREAKFAST | LUNCH | DINNER | BREAKFAST | LUNCH | DINNER |
|---|---|---|---|---|---|---|---|---|---|
| DIET – TYPE | | | | | | | | | |
| % CONSUMED | | | | | | | | | |

INTAKE & OUTPUT

| INTAKE | HOURS | 0600-1400 | 1400-2200 | 2200-0600 | 0600-1400 | 1400-2200 | 2200-0600 | 0600-1400 | 1400-2200 | 2200-0600 |
|---|---|---|---|---|---|---|---|---|---|---|
| Oral | | | | | | | | | | |
| IV | | | | | | | | | | |
| Blood - Plasma | | | | | | | | | | |
| Other | | | | | | | | | | |
| 8 Hr. Total | | | | | | | | | | |

Output
| Urine | | | | | | | | | | |
| Emesis | | | | | | | | | | |
| Stools | | | | | | | | | | |
| GI Suction | | | | | | | | | | |
| 8 Hr. Total | | | | | | | | | | |

24 Hr. Intake
24 Hr. Output

SIGNATURE
DATE:

CLINICAL RECORD

**COMMUNITY HOSPITAL**

**COMMUNITY HOSPITAL**
**HISTORY and PHYSICAL EXAMINATION**
Record all positive and all important negative findings in the following order:

| Chief Complaint | Family History | Lungs | Vascular/system |
| History of P.I. | System Review | Breasts | Extremities |
| Past History | Physical Examination | Heart | Locomotor |
| Illness | General | Abdomen | Neurological |
| Operations | Skin | Rectal | Provisional Diagnosis |
| Injuries | EENT | Pelvic | |

Name _____    Adm. No. _____

Last          First          Initial

Date _____

**M.D.**
**HISTORY AND PHYSICAL EXAMINATION**

Physician's History and Physical Record

**COMMUNITY HOSPITAL**

PROGRESS NOTES

Patient Information

| Date | Note progress of case, complications, change in diagnosis, condition on discharge |
|------|-----------------------------------------------------------------------------------|
|      |                                                                                   |
|      |                                                                                   |
|      |                                                                                   |
|      |                                                                                   |
|      |                                                                                   |
|      |                                                                                   |
|      |                                                                                   |
|      |                                                                                   |
|      |                                                                                   |
|      |                                                                                   |
|      |                                                                                   |
|      |                                                                                   |

Physician's Progress Notes

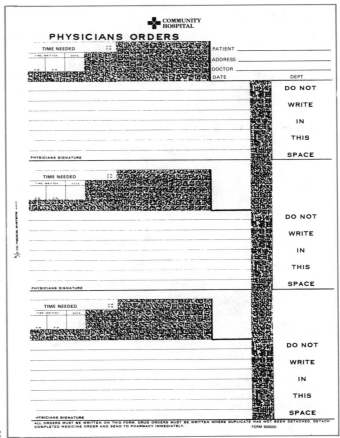

Physician's Order Sheet

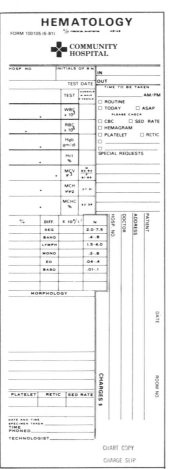

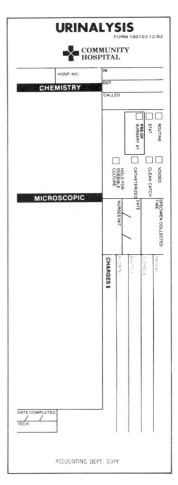

Laboratory Order Forms

## Laboratory Results Flow Sheet

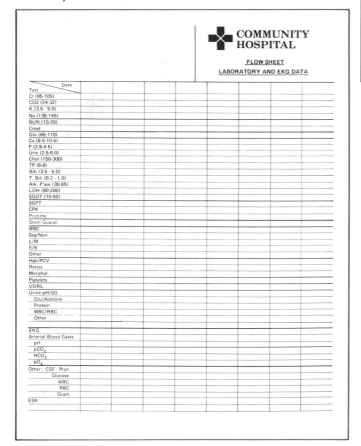

Chapter **2**

# Nursing Process and Nursing Diagnosis

## LEARNING OBJECTIVES

Define the term "nursing process."

Describe how the nursing process relates to nursing.

Discuss the term assessment and describe how it influences the nursing process.

List the components of the assessment step.

Describe the primary purpose of the analysis phase of the nursing process.

Define planning and give an example of this step in the nursing process.

Define what is meant by the implementation phase of nursing process.

Explain evaluation and include your understanding of why it is an important step in the nursing process.

Define the term nursing diagnosis.

Differentiate nursing diagnosis from medical diagnosis.

State two examples of nursing diagnoses.

Describe how etiology and defining characteristics relate to a nursing diagnosis.

## NURSING PROCESS

*Nursing process* is a familiar term in nursing and is utilized as a way of organizing nursing actions in health care delivery. By definition, the term *process* refers to a series of actions that lead toward a particular result. When attached to nursing, the term *nursing process* becomes a general description of a nursing care plan: assessment, analysis, planning, implementation, and evaluation. While the five steps can be described separately and in logical order, in practice the steps will overlap and events may not always occur in the order listed above. For purposes of understanding this process, however, it is appropriate to work through each phase in logical progression.

The five steps of the nursing process will be presented, defined, and illustrated to assist you to understand the importance of integrating this framework in your beginning mastery of nursing content. A model of each step will enable you to visualize how the individual components can be translated into direct nursing actions or behaviors.

**Assessment**  Assessment, the first step in the nursing process, refers to the establishment of a data base for a specific patient. Assessment requires skilled observation, reasoning, and a theoretical knowledge base to gather and differentiate data, verify data, organize it, and document the findings. The nurse gathers information relevant to the patient from a variety of sources and then assigns meaning to this data. Assessment is a critical phase because all the other steps in the process depend on the accuracy and reliability of the assessment.

A model of the assessment phase is on the following page.

| | |
|---|---|
| *Assessment* | *Observe—Interview—Examine* |
| Gather data | Identify patient needs |
|    Objective data | Be aware of staff reactions to patient |
|    Subjective data | Assess sources of data |
| Verify data |    Patient history |
| Confirm observations |    Data from family |
| Organize data |    Patient status—physical/emotional |
| Communicate data |    Signs and symptoms |
| |    Test results and findings |
| | Recall stored knowledge |

Assessment is based on concepts of physiology, pathophysiology, psychology, and social adjustment.

**Analysis**   The analysis phase focuses on comprehension and interpretation of data collected during the assessment of the patient. The purpose of this phase is to determine nursing diagnoses and formulate goals. It includes identifying patient needs, setting goals, and developing a plan of action for goal achievement. Goals are patient-centered statements of expected outcomes. Goals should be observable, realistic, and appropriate to other integrated therapies and to the total treatment plan. Analysis focuses on the understanding or the interpretation of data necessary to formulate a nursing diagnosis and to build a patient care plan.

A model of the analysis phase follows.

| | |
|---|---|
| *Analysis* | |
| Comprehend data | Identify patient's total needs: |
| Interpret data |    physical, emotional, social |
| Identify patient needs | State real or potential problem |
| Determine goals of care | Formulate patient goals, separating |
| Determine nursing |    observable, realistic long- and short-term |
|    diagnoses |    goals |
| | Prioritize patient goals |
| | Set time and deadlines of expected outcomes |

Analysis is based on data collected during the assessment phase. This includes interaction with the patient, family, and significant others, as well as the nurse's interpretation of the patient's needs and goals. This data will assist the nurse to formulate a nursing diagnosis.

**Planning**   The planning phase refers to the identification of nursing actions that are strategies to achieve the goals or the desired outcome of nursing care. This planning phase should be directly related to solving or alleviating the problems identified in the nursing diagnosis. It includes a plan, goals, strategies for goal outcome, and nursing measures for the delivery of care. Patients should be involved in the planning phase to ensure that the patient's and the health team members' goals are congruent. If they are not, goal achievement can be impaired. Planning focuses on the development of a plan of care individualized for a specific patient.

A model of the planning phase appears below.

| *Planning*<br>Develop a plan based on goals<br>Specify deadlines for completion of plan<br>Identify strategies for delivery of care<br>Record relevant information | Develop a plan of care including a teaching plan<br>Consider contingencies for modifying plan<br>Design strategies to achieve goals<br>Anticipate needs of patient and family based on priorities<br>Select nursing behaviors needed to accomplish goals<br>Coordinate care and community resources |
|---|---|
| Planning is based on patient's health care needs, selected goals, and strategies directed toward goal achievement. It is a plan of care where the appropriate nursing actions and patient's desires are considered and chosen to achieve a goal. ||

**Implementation**  The fourth phase in the nursing process is the implementation or intervention phase. This phase refers to the priority nursing actions or interventions performed to accomplish a specified goal. It explicitly describes the action component of the nursing process. This phase involves initiating and completing those nursing actions necessary to accomplish the identified patient goals. Nursing actions must be appropriate, individualized for the patient, and based on safe nursing practice; they should be formulated on scientific principles and derived from the problem-solving process. Finally, the interventions must be congruent with the total medical as well as nursing treatment plan. Implementation of the plan involves giving direct care to the patient to accomplish the specified goal.

A model of the implementation phase is illustrated below.

| *Implementation*<br>Implement patient care plan by giving direct care based on goals<br>Initiate nursing actions<br>Complete nursing actions<br>Record data<br>Continue assessment process | Perform actions and procedures in accordance with patient needs<br>Counsel and teach patients and/or family<br>Utilize preventive, palliative, or emergency measures for patient's welfare<br>Encourage independence and self-care<br>Motivate and maintain optimum wellness<br>Communicate to patient's family and allied staff<br>Supervise work of staff for whom nurse is responsible |
|---|---|
| Implementation is based on accurate and complete assessment, interpretation of data, identified patient needs, goals, nursing diagnosis and strategies to achieve goals. ||

**Evaluation**   The final phase of the nursing process is evaluation. Evaluation is the examination of the outcome of nursing actions or the extent to which the expected outcomes or goals were achieved. Was the goal achieved? What parts of the goal were not achieved? Was patient behavior modified? Evaluation is a necessary phase in order to complete the nursing process. It allows the nurse to continue to identify goals in the overall treatment plan and to alter the current plan to the patient's needs.

A model of the evaluation phase appears below.

| *Evaluation* | |
|---|---|
| Evaluate outcomes | Determine effects of nursing actions |
| Determine extent to which goals were achieved | Examine appropriateness of nursing actions |
| | Determine whether outcomes were expected or unexpected |
| Reassess care plan– judge if goal modification is necessary | Consider alternative nursing actions |
| | Investigate impact and degree of compliance for patient and family |
| Identify patient compliance | |
| Record patient responses | |

Evaluation is based on the previous phases of the nursing process (assessment, analysis, planning and implementation). The evaluation phase completes the process and examines the outcome.

The nursing process has provided the framework for the immense amount of nursing content that is contained in this textbook. The rationale for choosing this framework is that it provides a way to organize and present nursing knowledge as well as being an essential component of providing quality patient care.

## NURSING DIAGNOSIS

Nursing diagnosis is an integral component of the nursing process. Following the assessment step of the nursing process and during the analysis phase, the formulation of a nursing diagnosis is made. Nursing diagnosis is the statement of a patient problem derived from the systematic collection of data and its analysis. It is a clinical judgment about a designated patient, family, or community that provides the basis for completion of the nursing process. Nursing diagnosis includes the etiology, when known, and relates directly to the defining characteristics. Nursing diagnosis provides the foundation for each individual patient's therapeutic plan of care, and once it is established, the nurse is accountable for actions that occur within the scope of this nursing diagnosis framework.

An important implication of nursing diagnosis is that it refers to a health problem or condition that nurses are legally licensed to treat. The establishment and acceptance of this diagnostic category demonstrate recognition and legal sanction of nursing as a profession with its own body of knowledge, education, and experience.

The term *nursing diagnosis* is not comparable to or the same as medical diagnosis. Nursing diagnosis is derived from the assessment phase of the nursing process and is based on both subjective and objective data. As the data base evolves, patterns of health problems emerge, and alterations from normal health states are identified. A nursing diagnosis is a statement of an actual health problem or a potential one within the patient's biological, social, or personal system. The specific problem identified implies that the nurse is qualified and prepared to intervene and treat that condition. The nurse is not legally able to intervene and treat a medical diagnosis without specific physician's orders. Thus, the terms *potential atelectasis* or *pneumonia* are medical diagnoses while *potential ineffective breathing patterns* is a nursing diagnosis.

Components of the nursing diagnosis are divided into three major categories: the diagnosis of a patient's condition as potential or actual, the etiology to which the condition is related, and the defining characteristics that support the etiology. Thus, in practice, the patient's nursing diagnosis is stated: Skin Integrity, Impairment of: *related to.* This statement is followed by the etiology, if known, and the defining characteristics.

The rationale for specifying whether a diagnosis is actual or potential is that this judgment gives direction to the nursing interventions and enables the nurse to evaluate them on a realistic basis. Since there are many possible causes of any condition, the term *related to* gives direction to the etiology. And, since there are also various different interventions possible for different etiologies, the statement needs to be specific to individualize patient care. Finally, the third component of nursing diagnosis includes the defining characteristics or the observable signs and symptoms that directly relate to the etiology and, in turn, to the actual or potential nursing diagnosis.

Since the steps of the nursing process are based on formulating a nursing diagnosis, it is a critical component of providing high level professional nursing care. To ensure that the nursing terms used in diagnosis are standardized throughout the nursing profession, the National Conference Group Classification of Nursing Diagnosis established a list of accepted nursing diagnoses. This list standardized diagnostic terms in order to clearly communicate a patient's problems and needs. The accepted nursing diagnoses are listed at the end of this chapter.

The standardized list assists nurses to define and classify the scope of nursing practice. This classification system will assist the profession to expand its body of knowledge based on a firm scientific foundation.

Following is a more complete definition of the components of a nursing diagnosis:

*Diagnostic Category:* The specific nursing diagnosis identified according to the approved list of nursing diagnoses. The nursing diagnosis is a specific statement of the actual or potential health status or problem of an individual patient derived from a data base assessment that directs nursing interventions toward specific outcomes.

*Etiology:* The physiological, psychological, situational, or developmental factors that cause or are the source of the health problem or that influence its evolution.

*Defining Characteristic:* The specific, observable signs and symptoms that are manifested in relation to the identified health problem.

To illustrate the concept of nursing diagnosis, let us examine the nursing diagnosis of "Skin Integrity, Impairment of: Potential and Actual."

**Nursing Diagnosis: Skin Integrity, Impairment of:**

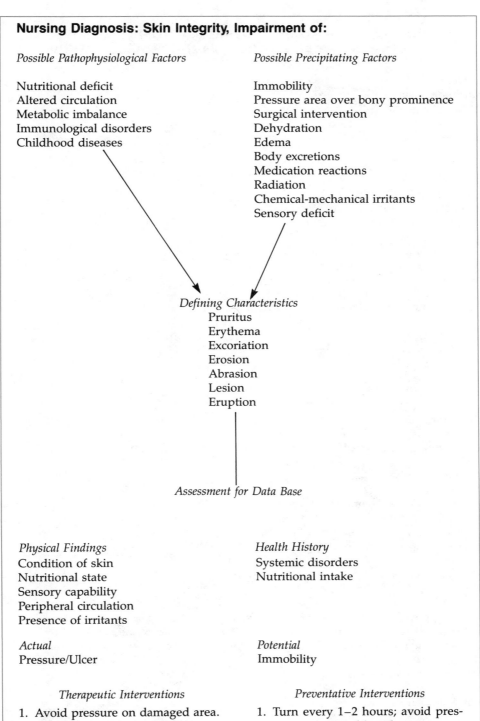

*Possible Pathophysiological Factors*

Nutritional deficit
Altered circulation
Metabolic imbalance
Immunological disorders
Childhood diseases

*Possible Precipitating Factors*

Immobility
Pressure area over bony prominence
Surgical intervention
Dehydration
Edema
Body excretions
Medication reactions
Radiation
Chemical-mechanical irritants
Sensory deficit

*Defining Characteristics*
Pruritus
Erythema
Excoriation
Erosion
Abrasion
Lesion
Eruption

*Assessment for Data Base*

*Physical Findings*
Condition of skin
Nutritional state
Sensory capability
Peripheral circulation
Presence of irritants

*Health History*
Systemic disorders
Nutritional intake

*Actual*
Pressure/Ulcer

*Potential*
Immobility

*Therapeutic Interventions*

1. Avoid pressure on damaged area.
2. Provide III or IV decubitus care.
3. Force fluids.
4. Increase protein intake.
5. Increase vitamin intake for skin repair.

*Preventative Interventions*

1. Turn every 1–2 hours; avoid pressure on any reddened area.
2. Increase protein intake.
3. Increase fluid intake.
4. Massage bony prominences every 2–4 hours with lotion or alcohol.
5. Request pressure sensitive mattress.

## Appendix I APPROVED NURSING DIAGNOSES, April, 1984
## NORTH AMERICAN NURSING DIAGNOSIS ASSOCIATION

Activity intolerance
Activity intolerance, potential
Airway clearance, ineffective
Anxiety
Bowel elimination, alteration in: constipation
Bowel elimination, alteration in: diarrhea
Bowel elimination, alteration in: incontinence
Breathing pattern, ineffective
Cardiac output, alteration in: decreased
Comfort, alteration in: pain
Communication, impaired: verbal
Coping, family: potential for growth
Coping, ineffective family: compromised
Coping, ineffective family: disabling
Coping, ineffective individual
Diversional activity, deficit
Family process, alteration in (formerly Family dynamics)
Fear
Fluid volume alteration in excess
Fluid volume deficit, actual
Fluid volume deficit, potential
Gas exchange, impaired
Grieving, anticipatory
Grieving, dysfunctional
Health maintenance, alteration in
Home maintenance management, impaired
Injury, potential for: (poisoning, potential for; suffocation, potential for; trauma, potential for)
Knowledge deficit (specify)
Mobility, impaired physical
Noncompliance (specify)
Nutrition, alteration in: less than body requirements
Nutrition, alteration in: more than body requirements
Nutrition, alteration in: potential for more than body requirements
Oral mucous membrane, alteration in
Parenting, alteration in: actual
Parenting, alteration in: potential
Powerlessness
Rape trauma syndrome
Self-care deficit: feeding, bathing/hygiene, dressing/grooming, toileting
Self-Concept, disturbance in: body image, self-esteem, role performance, personal identity
Sensory-perceptual alteration: visual, auditory, kinesthetic, gustatory, tactile, olfactory
Sexual dysfunction
Skin integrity, impairment of: actual
Skin integrity, impairment of: potential
Sleep pattern disturbance
Social Isolation
Spiritual distress (distress of the human spirit)
Thought processes, alteration in
Tissue perfusion, alteration in: cerebral, cardiopulmonary, renal, gastrointestinal, peripheral
Urinary elimination, alteration in patterns
Violence, potential for: self-directed or directed at others

# Chapter 3

# Patient Care Planning

## LEARNING OBJECTIVES

Describe the components of the patient care plan.

State the two types of patient care plan.

Explain the method for individualizing the care plan when a standard care plan is used.

Compare and contrast the initiation of a standard and individualized care plan.

Define term patient problem or need.

State the most important reason for using nursing diagnosis in care planning.

Describe the relationship between expected outcomes or goals and patient care.

Define the use of deadlines and check points in the patient care plan.

Describe the relationship between long-term goals and discharge criteria.

State how the patient care plan and nurses' notes relate to each other.

Discuss the relationship between patient care conferences and patient care plans.

Describe how information from the patient care plan is relayed to the nursing staff and other health team members.

**CARE PLANS**    Patient care plans are an integral part of providing nursing care. Without patient care plans, quality and consistency of patient care may not be obtained. Patient care plans provide a means of communication among nurses and other health care providers. The plan should serve as a focal point for patient care assignments and reporting.

Regardless of the type of care plan used, the following information should be included: patient's needs or problems stated as nursing diagnoses, expected outcomes or short-term goals, nursing interventions or actions, and discharge criteria or long-term goals.

Once the goals of patient care are established, they are formulated in a care plan. Each step in meeting these goals is detailed, including specific observations and how often the observations are made. Step-by-step directions are included for difficult problems, such as lengthy and involved dressing changes. Individualized patient teaching programs are described on the care plan. As is evident, all of this information is essential in providing continuity of patient care.

**Format**    Patient care plans are available in several formats. The patient's plan of care may be outlined on the Kardex (Figure 1), on a specific hospital form placed in the patient's chart (Figures 2 and 4), or on individual printed cards which are placed in the Kardex (Figure 3). The latter may be used many times as these cards do not become a permanent part of the patient's record.

**Types**    Patient care plans consist of two types—an individualized care plan completely written by the nurse for each specific patient and a standard patient care plan. Because of the large amount of time necessary to write

**KARDEX/RAND PATIENT CARE PLAN**

| PATIENT EDUCATION PROGRAM | | | DISCHARGE CRITERIA | DISCHARGE PLAN | Addressograph |
|---|---|---|---|---|---|
| | DATE | | PLAN: | | |
| | Start | Finish | Stroke Rehab Eval _____ | Discharge Coordinator | |
| Diabetic _____ | | | Cardiac Rehab Eval _____ | Date Involved _____ | |
| Coronary _____ | | | SOCIAL SERVICE | Home _____ | |
| Other _____ | | | Date Involved _____ | ECF _____ | |
| _____ | | | Comment: | OTHER _____ | |

| Date | Patient Problem | Deadline Date | Expected Outcome | Health Team Action |
|---|---|---|---|---|
| | | | | |
| | | | | |

Figure 1: Kardex Card form is not retained as a permanent part of the medical record.

**COMMUNITY HOSPITAL**

**PATIENT CARE PLAN**
Individualized

Patient Information

Discharge Criteria
1) Verbalizes understanding of discharge meds
2) States available resource agencies
3)
4)

Admitting Diagnosis:

Relevant Info:

| Date | Problem/Need | Expected Outcome/Goal | CP | DL | Nursing Interventions | Update / DC | Initial |
|---|---|---|---|---|---|---|---|
| 1/26/85 | 1. Knowledge deficit R/t discharge meds. | Verbalizes understanding of discharge meds. States s/s of side effects. | c̄ shift | Prior to disch | 1. a) Instruct in actions of and times for administration of each drug. b) Ask patient to recite s/s of side effects of meds. | | |
| | 2. Coping, ineffective individual | Able to demonstrate effective coping | c̄ shift | Prior to disch. | 2. a) Determine level of understanding of diagnosis and prognosis. | | |

Figure 2: Individualized Patient Care Plan is a permanent part of the medical record.

**NURSING CARE PLAN**

Nasal Surgery

| Date | Usual Problems | Expected Outcomes | Dead-Lines | Nursing Orders |
|---|---|---|---|---|
| | 1. Skin integrity, impairment of: R/t swelling and dis-coloration of eyes. | Gradual reduction of swelling and discolora-tion. | Day of Discharge | 1.a. Keep ice gloves on nose for 24 hrs. b. Keep head of bed ↑ 45°. |
| | 2. Airway clearance ineffective R/t edema from surgical site. | Absence of respiratory problems. | 24 h p̄ surgery | 2.a. Observe frequently for s/s airway obstruction. |

Figure 3: Pre-printed Patient Care Plan card is used repeatedly and is not retained in the chart.

individualized care plans, hospital nursing departments are developing preprinted standard care plans based on the most frequent hospital admission diagnoses for the hospital. The standard care plan outlines the usual problems or needs that occur with a specific diagnosis. It contains a list of usual nursing actions or interventions and the standard expected outcomes for each problem.

**Individualizing Care Plans** All patients must have an individualized plan of care even though the standard care plan is used. In order to individualize the care plan, there is generally space provided at the end of the preprinted form to allow the nurse to identify unusual problems or needs. Standard care plans can also be individualized by activating only those problems that pertain to a particular patient. For example, Figure 4 illustrates a standard care plan that has been individualized. Items 1 and 3 have been activated by circling, dating, and initialing the item number. The nurse may add another problem to the bottom of the form to further individualize the care plan.

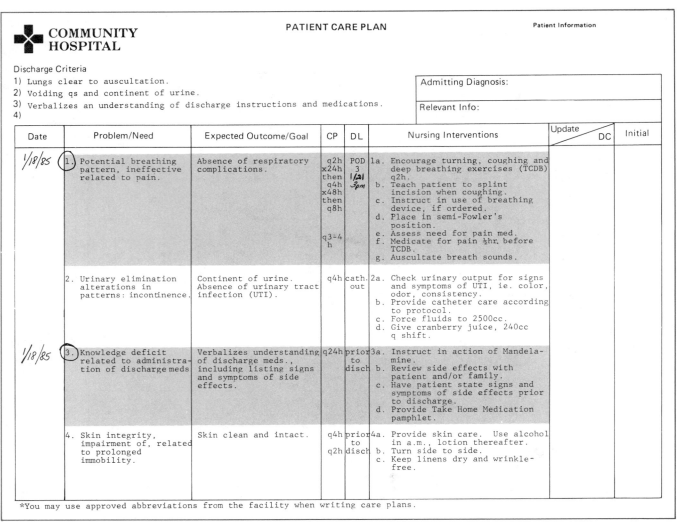

| | | | **PATIENT CARE PLAN** | | | | **Patient Information** | |

**COMMUNITY HOSPITAL**

**Discharge Criteria**
1) Lungs clear to auscultation.
2) Voiding qs and continent of urine.
3) Verbalizes an understanding of discharge instructions and medications.
4)

Admitting Diagnosis:

Relevant Info:

| Date | Problem/Need | Expected Outcome/Goal | CP | DL | Nursing Interventions | Update / DC | Initial |
|------|-------------|----------------------|-----|-----|----------------------|-------------|---------|
| 1/18/85 | ①. Potential breathing pattern, ineffective related to pain. | Absence of respiratory complications. | q2h x24h then q4h x48h then q8h<br><br>q3-4 h | POD 3 1/21 3pm | 1a. Encourage turning, coughing and deep breathing exercises (TCDB) q2h.<br>b. Teach patient to splint incision when coughing.<br>c. Instruct in use of breathing device, if ordered.<br>d. Place in semi-Fowler's position.<br>e. Assess need for pain med.<br>f. Medicate for pain ½hr. before TCDB.<br>g. Auscultate breath sounds. | | |
| | 2. Urinary elimination alterations in patterns: incontinence. | Continent of urine. Absence of urinary tract infection (UTI). | q4h | cath. out | 2a. Check urinary output for signs and symptoms of UTI, ie. color, odor, consistency.<br>b. Provide catheter care according to protocol.<br>c. Force fluids to 2500cc.<br>d. Give cranberry juice, 240cc q shift. | | |
| 1/18/85 | ③. Knowledge deficit related to administration of discharge meds | Verbalizes understanding of discharge meds., including listing signs and symptoms of side effects. | q24h | prior to disch | 3a. Instruct in action of Mandelamine.<br>b. Review side effects with patient and/or family.<br>c. Have patient state signs and symptoms of side effects prior to discharge.<br>d. Provide Take Home Medication pamphlet. | | |
| | 4. Skin integrity, impairment of, related to prolonged immobility. | Skin clean and intact. | q4h<br>q2h | prior to disch | 4a. Provide skin care. Use alcohol in a.m., lotion thereafter.<br>b. Turn side to side.<br>c. Keep linens dry and wrinkle-free. | | |

*You may use approved abbreviations from the facility when writing care plans.

Figure 4: Pre-printed Standardized Patient Care Plan utilizing Nursing Diagnosis format.

**Initiating the Plan**   The patient care plan is formulated after the assessment phase of the nursing process. The nurse, after completing the nursing history and assessment, determines if a standard care plan is available for the patient's medical diagnosis or if an individualized care plan must be written. If a standard care plan is available, the nurse need only circle, date, and initial the needs that are relevant for that patient. When an individualized care plan is being written, the nurse translates the patient's needs or problems into nursing diagnoses and writes them on the care plan. Nursing diagnoses are the acceptable terminology for use on patient care plans throughout the country. The terminology was established by the National Conference on Classification of Nursing Diagnosis.

**Patient Problems/Needs**   A patient problem or need is a condition that requires assistance or intervention from a health team member in order to return the patient to a healthy state. The patient problem is identified as any unmet need. It can be as basic as the need for adequate comfort or nourishment to the more complex psychosocial needs.

On many care plans problems are identified as either actual or potential. An actual problem is one that exists at that time. Interventions are planned to resolve or alter the problem. A potential problem describes a condition that frequently occurs with the patient's diagnosis or health problem. An actual problem, for example, is a reddened coccyx related to urinary incontinence. Interventions are developed to treat the reddened area to prevent further breakdown or decubitus ulcer formation. A potential problem, such as "Breathing patterns, ineffective, *related to* anesthesia" following gallbladder surgery, could affect any patient with that condition. Interventions are planned to prevent the problem. Some potential problems are identified in order to more carefully assess for them. For example, a debilitated patient with poor nutrition would be assessed for possible wound infection.

**Nursing Diagnosis**   Using a nursing diagnosis to state the patient's real or potential problems takes the problem out of the realm of a medical diagnosis. The nursing diagnosis does not focus on a problem or disease state but rather on a physical, psychological, or behavioral response. Nursing diagnosis can change frequently as the patient's health status changes and potential health problems become actual health problems. The nursing diagnosis approach, unlike the medical model or systems approach to care planning, allows for this flexibility in focus.

The use of nursing diagnosis in care planning is a universal method of communication to all health team members. When the diagnosis "Skin integrity, impairment of: actual" is written, the entire health team knows that the patient has a broken area on the skin with destruction of skin layers. The relationship of skin impairment to cause is usually stated as "Skin integrity, impairment of: *related to* prolonged immobility."

**Expected Outcomes/Goals**   After the problems have been identified, the nurse sets goals or expected outcomes for patient care which are congruent with the patient and/or significant other's goals. Patient-centered goals should be concise and identify specific observable and measurable behaviors. Expected outcomes or goals should indicate what is to be expected when the goal is achieved, by whom, when, and to what degree of accuracy. Figure 5 shows several examples of a patient-centered goal and the nursing interventions necessary to attain each goal.

| | COMMUNITY HOSPITAL | | | PATIENT CARE PLAN | | Patient Information | | | |

Discharge Criteria
1) Lungs clear to auscultation.
2) Voiding qs and continent of urine.
3) Verbalizes an understanding of discharge instructions and medications.
4)

Admitting Diagnosis:

Relevant Info:

| Date | Problem/Need | Expected Outcome/Goal | CP | DL | Nursing Interventions | Update DC | Initial |
|------|--------------|-----------------------|----|----|-----------------------|-----------|---------|
| 1/18/85 | 1. Potential breathing pattern, ineffective related to pain. | Absence of respiratory complications. | q2h x24h then q4h x48h then q8h | POD 3 1/21 3pm | 1a. Encourage turning, coughing and deep breathing exercises (TCDB) q2h. | | |
| | | | | | b. Teach patient to splint incision when coughing. | | |
| | | | | | c. Instruct in use of breathing device, if ordered. | | |
| | | | | | d. Place in semi-Fowler's position. | | |
| | | | q3-4 h | | e. Assess need for pain med. | | |
| | | | | | f. Medicate for pain ½hr. before TCDB. | | |
| | | | | | g. Auscultate breath sounds. | | |
| | 2. Urinary elimination alterations in patterns: incontinence. | Continent of urine. Absence of urinary tract infection (UTI). | q4h | cath. out | 2a. Check urinary output for signs and symptoms of UTI, ie. color, odor, consistency. | | |
| | | | | | b. Provide catheter care according to protocol. | | |
| | | | | | c. Force fluids to 2500cc. | | |
| | | | | | d. Give cranberry juice, 240cc q shift. | | |
| 1/18/85 | 3. Knowledge deficit related to administration of discharge meds | Verbalizes understanding of discharge meds., including listing signs and symptoms of side effects. | q24h | prior to disch | 3a. Instruct in action of Mandelamine. | | |
| | | | | | b. Review side effects with patient and/or family. | | |
| | | | | | c. Have patient state signs and symptoms of side effects prior to discharge. | | |
| | | | | | d. Provide Take Home Medication pamphlet. | | |
| | 4. Skin integrity, impairment of, related to prolonged immobility. | Skin clean and intact. | q4h q2h | prior to disch | 4a. Provide skin care. Use alcohol in a.m., lotion thereafter. | | |
| | | | | | b. Turn side to side. | | |
| | | | | | c. Keep linens dry and wrinkle-free. | | |

*You may use approved abbreviations from the facility when writing care plans.

Figure 5: Expected outcomes and nursing interventions.

**Interventions**   After problems and expected outcomes are written on the care plan, the nurse determines appropriate nursing interventions that will meet the goals of care. Interventions, if written properly, will specify the exact nursing actions to be carried out or provide explicit instructions on how care is to be delivered. Time and frequency of the intervention should also be provided. (Figure 5)

**Check Points and Deadlines**   The standard care plan illustrated in this text includes check point (CP) and deadline (DL) columns (see Figure 6). The check point indicates how often the action or intervention should be checked, observed, or carried out, and, therefore, how often it should be charted. The deadline column indicates the time when the goal should be met or the action is no longer necessary. It is important to document the exact time and date when the nursing action should be completed in order to communicate this information to the entire nursing staff. In the example, you will notice that item 1—Breathing patterns ineffective–should be alleviated by the third

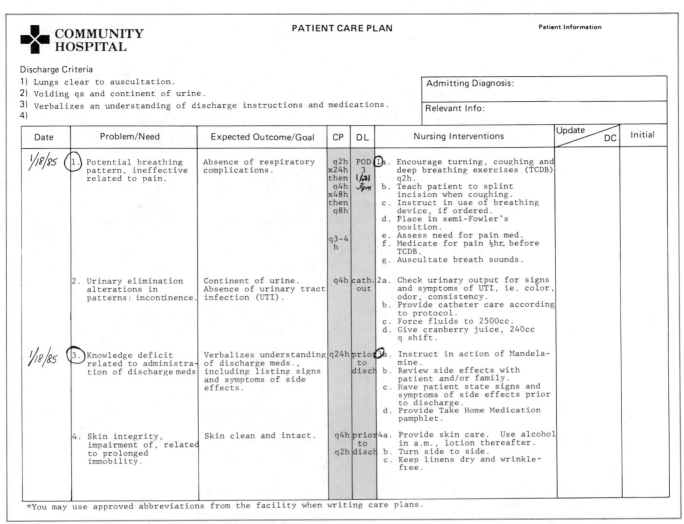

Figure 6: Check points, deadlines, and discharge criteria.

postoperative day, in this case, January 21 at 3:00 PM. The check points are listed in sequence to meet the goal. For the first 24 hours the nursing interventions (1a through 1d) should be completed every two hours and then advanced to every four hours for the next 48 hours.

**Short- and Long-Term Goals**   Patient care plans must include both short- and long-term goals. Long-term goals are frequently stated as discharge criteria and as such should be met prior to discharge, if possible. Short-term goals usually appear in the form of expected outcomes for each problem. They are designed as stepping stones to assist the patient to meet discharge criteria or long-term goals. Some hospitals, particularly rehabilitation facilities, use short-term goals differently. They frequently set weekly steps or phases in the rehabilitative process that patients meet before the final expected outcome is achieved. For example, to meet the long-term goal of ambulation without use of devices, a short-term goal would be to ambulate with a walker without assistance. These types of goals are prioritized and updated regularly.

**Updating Care Plans**  To ensure that patient care plans are current and relevant, they should be reviewed on a daily basis and updated at least every 24 to 48 hours. There are several ways to update a care plan. Some facilities have spaces designated on the nursing Kardex or nurses' notes. In Figure 7, the update column is used when the original deadline is reached but the problem persists. A new deadline must then be established. If the ineffective breathing pattern exists beyond the third postoperative day, a new time frame for goal achievement is determined and documented in the update column. As the example shows, the fourth postoperative day is determined to be the new time frame. The update would then read 1/21 @ 3p.m.

**Activating Care Plans**  When standard care plans are used, a systematic approach to activation and deactivation must be understood by all nursing personnel. As already stated, a common approach is to circle, date, and initial problems that are relevant for the individual patient. Any problem that is not circled remains inactivated and should not be assessed, treated, or documented. From the example, you can see that the patient has two of the problems listed, a potential ineffective breathing pattern and a knowledge deficit regarding discharge medication. Items 1 and 3 are circled. In the date column, date, time, and initials of the nurse activating the problem are entered. The second problem is not activated; therefore, a circle is not placed around the number.

**Inactivating Care Plans**  To inactivate the problem, a single line through the problem and/or intervention with a black pen can be made. In the update/dc column the date, time, and nurse's initials should be placed next to the crossed out, inactivated information. If only one of the interventions is not necessary, a line is drawn through that intervention and initials placed next to it in the initial column. The other interventions are left current and active.

**COMMUNICATION**

**Documentation**  Documentation of findings in the nurses' notes should closely parallel the intervention column for all activated problems. When a problem is assessed every two hours, it should be documented appropriately in the patient's chart every two hours. If breath sounds are auscultated every four hours, they are documented on a flow sheet or in the nurses' notes every four hours. If a chart audit were done on the patient's chart, the quality assurance auditor should be able to find each activated problem identified in the chart with appropriate interventions documented.

**Report**  A shift-to-shift report should be given not only from the Kardex but from the patient care plan. There is no need to review particular procedures for such activities as dressing changes when they are outlined on the care plan. A simple statement to the effect that the procedure is listed on the care plan is all that is necessary. This decreases both time and repetition of information.

To avoid confusion from shift-to-shift, specific times for treatments and for activities of daily living (ADLs) are indicated. For example, it is noted on the patient care plan that the patient prefers his bath before 8:00 AM to avoid having to ask the patient every day when he wants his bath. This consistency promotes a feeling of confidence in the nursing staff and alleviates fear.

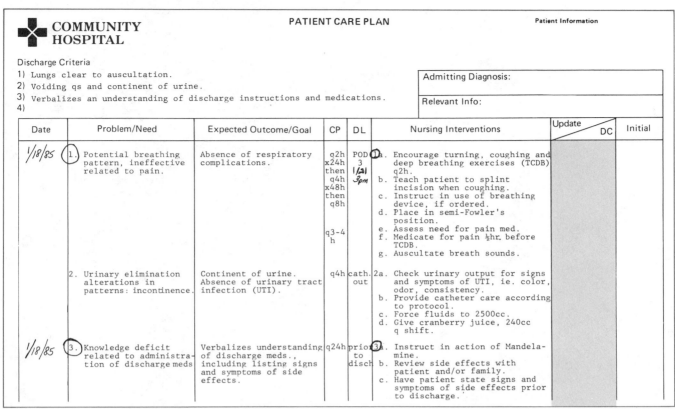

Figure 7: Updating and inactivating of care plan.

**Care Conferences**  Patient care conferences and patient care plans play an integral role in planning and delivering health care for difficult or unusual patient problems. The patient care conference can focus on developing the patient care plan or identifying difficult problems. A conference can then be scheduled to plan appropriate interventions and to inform all health team members of the goals for that patient's care.

**Patient Assignments**  Patient care assignments should be based on careful analysis of each patient's needs and goals of care. The patient care plan can be consulted for an effective utilization of health team members to their best advantage as well as for the patient's welfare. A patient requiring extensive sterile dressing changes, frequent assessments, and IV medications would be more appropriately assigned to a professional nurse. A patient who is convalescing following a stroke and requires mainly bathing and ambulation assistance can usually be assigned to another member of the health team such as a nursing assistant.

**Evaluation**  The evaluation of how well the patient care plan was individualized to meet the needs of the patient is tested at discharge. If the care plan was appropriate, the discharge criteria is met. The nursing interventions and problems would be inactivated or discontinued. Frequently, there are patients who, on discharge, have not met the discharge criteria for various reasons. The documentation in the chart should reflect those problems that still exist, the extent to which the problem is being resolved, and additional information to indicate what plans were formulated for goal achievement.

# Chapter 4

# Charting and Reporting

## LEARNING OBJECTIVES

Define the term charting.

Explain at least three purposes of charting.

Describe at least three major components for accurate charting.

Differentiate between the advantages and disadvantages of the three charting systems: source-oriented, problem-oriented, and computer-assisted charting.

Explain the importance of relating the nursing process to charting.

Complete a charting exercise in all three charting systems utilizing a simulated situation.

Describe the rationale for using flow sheets.

List the four items that should be charted for every patient.

Discuss the relationship between the nursing assessment data base, nursing problem list, and problem-oriented medical records.

Define the terms subjective and objective data, assessment, and plan when referring to SOAP notes.

Explain the information contained in a discharge summary when using POMR charting.

Discuss the purpose of completing an incident report.

Describe the legal ramifications for completing incident reports.

Discuss specific patient activities requiring consent forms.

## CHARTING

Next to direct patient care, charting is one of the nurse's most important functions. Charting, the process of recording vital information, serves many important purposes:

Charting communicates facts, figures, observations, etc., to other members of the patient's health care team.

Charting assists supervisory personnel to evaluate the staff's performance on a day-by-day basis for specific patients.

Charting provides a permanent record for future reference which may become a legal document in the event of litigation or prosecution.

**Charting—A Method of Communication**   In communicating your observations and actions, charting helps to ensure both quality and continuity of health care for your patients. Information recorded by you becomes a valuable data base for nurses on subsequent shifts. Then, when you reassume responsibility for the patient, you can determine what events occurred during prior time periods. In addition to the patient's attending physician, other personnel interested in the chart may include the infection control nurse, discharge coordinator, utilization review personnel, or other hospital staff specialists who are checking on the patient's progress or lack of positive reaction to treatment.

The patient, as an individual, should receive individualized attention which focuses on his or her specific needs. As these needs are identified by each member of the health care team, they can be communicated to the others. Since nurses have the greatest amount of direct patient contact, it is appropriate for the nurse to coordinate the important function of charting.

Charting provides one means for assessing the quality and effectiveness of nursing care. Head nurses, team leaders, and supervisors use nurses' notes as a basis for staff evaluations. Because charts are documented descriptions of nursing actions, the quality of nursing care may be evaluated on the basis of the quality of charting notes.

Complete and accurate charting is essential to protect both the patient and the nurse. Since charting describes nursing interventions and their outcomes, other health care personnel can determine if subsequent treatment should be changed. Frequently, a patient's reaction time is nearly as important as the reaction itself; therefore, accuracy of time observations becomes an integral part of the charting process.

A patient's record includes all charting and becomes part of a legal document. Should a patient's hospital record be introduced in court, the notes become a legal record of the care provided by each health care provider. Legally, care that is not recorded is considered to be care that was not provided. It is necessary, therefore, to chart all care that you *do* provide, as well as any care that you *do not* provide.

The legal requirement for charting is found in state laws and/or professional requirements. For example, Title 22 of the California Administrative Code states, "Each inpatient medical record shall consist of at least the following items: nurses' notes which shall include but not be limited to the following: concise and accurate record of nursing care administered, record of pertinent observations including psychosocial and physical manifestations as well as incidents and unusual occurrences, and relevant nursing interpretation of such observations, name, dosage and time of administration of medications and treatment. Route of administration and site of injection shall be recorded if other than by oral administration, record of type of restraint and time of application and removal. The time of application and removal shall not be required for soft tie restraints used for support and protection of the patient."

The Manual of the Joint Commission for Accreditation of Hospitals states, "The plan of care must be documented and should reflect current standards of nursing practice . . . Documentation of nursing care shall be pertinent and concise, and shall reflect the patient's needs, problems, capabilities and limitations . . . Nursing interventions and patient response must be noted."

**The Charting Process**   The format of the chart varies from hospital to hospital. Most important is the content of the notes. First, your notes should describe the assessment that you completed at the beginning of your shift. This information provides a baseline for changes that may occur later in the patient's condition. If there are no such changes, this fact should be entered as the final note. Some hospitals require that all parts of the assessment be documented; others require that only abnormalities be documented.

As your shift progresses, you should always include certain items in your notes, including changes in the patient's medical, mental, or emotional condition. Nurses are well attuned to medical changes, such as shock, hemorrhage, or a change in level of consciousness; however, the nurse may overlook subtle emotional changes. Anger, depression, or joy should also be documented, because these emotions often are indications of the patient's response to his or her illness. Recording these changes is absolutely necessary if other nurses are to act appropriately during subsequent shifts. You should also chart if *no* changes occurred in the patient's condition so that treatments can be modified as necessary. Normal aspects of the patient's condition should be noted also.

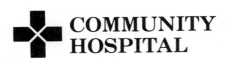

**COMMUNITY HOSPITAL**

Patient Information

NURSES' NOTES

| Time | Medications/Treatment | Observations | Signature |
|------|----------------------|--------------|-----------|
| 7 p.m. | | c/o ROQ abdominal incisional pain | |
| | | p̄ ambulating. Drsg dry and intact. | |
| | Demerol 50 mgm IM LOQ | for pain. | A.Head RN |
| 8 p.m. | | States pain is relieved. | A.Head RN |
| | | | |
| | | | |
| | | | |
| | | | |
| | | | |
| | | | |
| | | | |
| | | | |

Nurses' Notes

Reactions to any unscheduled or p.r.n. medications must be recorded. Because each medication is given to meet a specified need, the patient's response or lack of response must be recorded to document whether the need was met. To complete this part of the entry, note the time the medication was given, the problem for which the medication was given, and the expected solution. For example: "7 p.m. c/o ROQ abdominal incisional pain after ambulation. Demerol, 50 mg, LOQ IM for pain." When the effects of the medication are known, write another note: "8 p.m. States pain has been relieved."

Finally, it is important to record the patient's response to teaching. These notes may describe return demonstrations, verbalization of learning, or resistance to instruction. Because most teaching takes place over a period of days, record both what you taught and how the patient responded. Then, other nurses will know whether to repeat the previous instructions, reinforce them, or start a new topic.

Frequently, repetitive aspects of nursing care, such as vital signs and intake and output, are recorded on flow sheets. If flow sheets are used, you need not repeat the same information in your notes. An exception would be an abnormal measurement that is a part of a larger assessment. For example: "c/o sharp abd. pain. BP-78/50. P-136. Skin cold & diaphoretic. NG tube draining bright red bloody fluid c̄ small clots. Reported to Dr. Jones."

**COMMUNITY HOSPITAL**

**PATIENT CARE PLAN**

Patient Information

Discharge Criteria
1) Lungs clear to auscultation.
2) Voiding qs and continent of urine.
3) Verbalizes an understanding of discharge instructions and medications.
4)

Admitting Diagnosis:

Relevant Info:

| Date | Problem/Need | Expected Outcome/Goal | CP | DL | Nursing Interventions | Update | DC | Initial |
|------|-------------|----------------------|-----|-----|----------------------|--------|-----|---------|
| 1/18/85 | 1. Potential breathing pattern, ineffective related to pain. | Absence of respiratory complications. | q2h x24h then q4h x48h then q8h / q3-4 h | POD 3 1/21 3pm | 1a. Encourage turning, coughing and deep breathing exercises (TCDB) q2h. b. Teach patient to splint incision when coughing. c. Instruct in use of breathing device, if ordered. d. Place in semi-Fowler's position. e. Assess need for pain med. f. Medicate for pain ½hr. before TCDB. g. Auscultate breath sounds. | | | |
| | 2. Urinary elimination alterations in patterns: incontinence. | Continent of urine. Absence of urinary tract infection (UTI). | q4h | cath. out | 2a. Check urinary output for signs and symptoms of UTI, ie. color, odor, consistency. b. Provide catheter care according to protocol. c. Force fluids to 2500cc. d. Give cranberry juice, 240cc q shift. | | | |
| 1/18/85 | 3. Knowledge deficit related to administration of discharge meds | Verbalizes understanding of discharge meds., including listing signs and symptoms of side effects. | q24h | prior to disch | 3a. Instruct in action of Mandelamine. b. Review side effects with patient and/or family. c. Have patient state signs and symptoms of side effects prior to discharge. d. Provide Take Home Medication pamphlet. | | | |

**COMMUNITY HOSPITAL**

**PATIENT CARE PLAN**
**Individualized**

Patient Information

Discharge Criteria
1) Wound healing progressing satisfactorily
2) Verbalizes ability to care for wound at home
3) Verbalizes understanding of discharge instructions
4)

Admitting Diagnosis:

Relevant Info:

| Date | Problem/Need | Expected Outcome/Goal | CP | DL | Nursing Interventions | Update | DC | Initial |
|------|-------------|----------------------|-----|-----|----------------------|--------|-----|---------|
| 1/18/85 | 4. Skin integrity, impairment of: actual | Wound healing c̄ complications | q4h | prior to Discharge | 4. a. Place on Lt. side c̄ chux under hips & abd. Gently move into this position. Do not rush c̄ move. b. Note drainage, location, quantity, color & odor. c. Irrig. wound c̄ 50cc. equal parts NSS & H₂O. Use asepto syringe. Catch solution in emesis basin. d. Gently pack area in distal | | | |

Individualized Patient Care Plan

**Charting and the Nursing Process** The nursing process provides the framework for decision-making throughout all phases of nursing care. The components of the nursing process are assessment, planning, implementation (or intervention), and evaluation. This cycle is applied by the nurse both to routine situations and critical care emergencies.

It is important to relate the nursing process to charting because, for experienced nurses, the process may become only a mental exercise. The nurse "thinks through" the situation, makes decisions, takes action, and then observes the results. Unless the entire process is recorded on the patient care plan and documented in the chart, the next nurse who encounters a similar situation with the same patient is deprived of important and potentially valuable background data. The second nurse, without knowing the full background, may repeat the entire process resulting in a loss of valuable time and an increase in patient discomfort. When similar nursing interventions completed by different nurses have the same positive results, the patient will experience a feeling of reassurance that may not be achieved if each nurse attempts a totally different set of interventions to reach the same objective.

The patient, in a strange environment with unknown people doing unfamiliar and often uncomfortable things, often tries to find reassurance in any type of routine. The patient soon expects a certain procedure to be done by the same person in the same way and at a predictable hour. Changes in the procedure are often upsetting to the patient. It is imperative that the steps of any procedure, especially those that are complicated or personalized to the patient, be documented in detail on the patient care plan so that each nurse will do it the same way. However, the detailed description of how to perform a dressing change is written in the patient's care plan, not in the nurses' notes.

The nurses' notes would describe the amount, color, consistency, and odor of the drainage. In addition, the amount and type of irrigating solution and type of abdominal dressing would be noted. It is important to add a statement as to the patient's tolerance of the procedure.

**Types of Charting** The three main charting systems are source-oriented, problem-oriented, and computer-assisted charting. The most common system is the source-oriented chart, so named because the information is organized and presented according to its source. For example, there are separate sections for doctors' progress notes, nurses' notes, respiratory therapy notes, etc. To obtain a complete "picture" of the patient, one must read through all sections and piece together the separate bits of data. This may be a time-consuming process and the result may not produce an accurate or complete assessment of the patient.

A second system for chart organization is the problem-oriented medical record. In this system the chart is based on the problem list—all problems, present or potential, identified with that patient. Using the problems as reference points, each person giving care charts progress notes on the same sheets. In this way assessment of a specific incident by everyone concerned (MD, RN, dietitian, enterostomal therapist, etc.) is in the same location and the patient's overall picture can be easily seen.

The third and newest type of organizing data is computer-assisted charting. This type of charting constantly updates information from many sources. For example, physiological measurements are recorded and updated on the computer terminal at least hourly.

The information is easily retrievable by the nursing personnel as questions

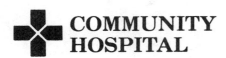

**COMMUNITY HOSPITAL**

Patient Information

**NURSES' NOTES**

| Time | Medications/Treatment | Observations | Signature |
|------|----------------------|--------------|-----------|
| 1/29/85 7³⁰ AM | | Awake and ready for breakfast. | |
| 8 AM | | Ate 100%. | |
| 8¹⁵ AM | | Assessment completed: Neuro: Oriented x 3, PERL, strength equal bilaterally. Moves all extremities, negative Babinski. Cardio: Rate 84, reg. HT sounds WNL, o rubs, murmurs. Resp: Rales in lower bases bilaterally. Exp. & Insp. excursion equal c̄ WNL. Resp. labored @ 18/min. Renal: Voiding q.s. Urine clear, straw colored s̄ sediment or odor. GI: abd. distended, non-tender. B.S. present but sluggish. Passing flatus. Musc-skel: Lt. leg maintained in proper alignment. | A. Mead RN |

Nurses' Notes Using Systems Charting

arise. Reference material for common nursing problems ensures quick reference and easily retrieved information in order to provide safe nursing care.

**Source-Oriented Systems Charting**   Systems charting is a common and efficient way of organizing patient information in source-oriented nurses' notes. An outline of the systems to be reviewed, and sometimes specific subheadings for each, is established. Medical units may use one type of systems nurses' notes, while critical care may use another.

At the beginning of the shift the nurse performs a physical assessment on each patient to determine the patient's current status. This information becomes the initial systems charting. When changes occur, they are noted with the time under the appropriate system. If no changes occur during the shift, no other charting of this type may be necessary.

To record all pertinent patient information, several flow sheets are used in conjunction with the systems form. One flow sheet is the vital signs sheet,

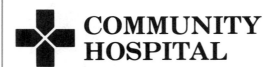

# COMMUNITY HOSPITAL

## ICU NEURO/SPINAL FLOW CHART

| Date: 1/25/85 | | Time: | 8AM | | |
|---|---|---|---|---|---|
| | | Right: size | 4mm | | |
| | | Reaction | S | | |
| Pupils | | Left: Size | 4mm | | |
| | | Reaction | S | | |
| | | Visual Acuity | C | | |
| Mental Status | | | | | |
| C O M A | Eyes Open | Spontaneously | | | |
| | | To Speech | | | |
| | | To Pain | + | | |
| | | Never | | | |
| S C A L E | Verbal Response | Clear | | | |
| | | Confused | | | |
| | | Inappropriate | + | | |
| | | Incomprehensible | | | |
| | | None | | | |
| M O V E M E N T | Arms | Normal Power | | | |
| | | Weakness | + | | |
| | | Flexion | | | |
| | | Extension | | | |
| | | No Response | | | |
| | Legs | Normal Power | | | |
| | | Weakness | + | | |
| | | Flexion | | | |
| | | Extension | | | |
| | | No Response | | | |
| Reflexes | | Gag/Cough | 0 | | |
| | | Corneal | + | | |
| | | Babinski R/L | +/+ | | |
| | | Oculocephalic | 0 | | |
| Respiratory | | Pattern | REG. | | |
| | | Rate | 28 | | |
| Seizures | | Type | 0 | | |
| | | Duration | | | |
| Fluid Drainage from Ears or | | | 0 | | |
| | | Nose | 0 | | |

Signature ___Head, RN___

Neurological Flow Sheet

## COMMUNITY HOSPITAL

DIABETIC RECORD

| DIRECTION: Test second voiding whenever possible. |
|---|

| DATE | | | 1/25/85 | | | | | | | | | | | | | |
|---|---|---|---|---|---|---|---|---|---|---|---|---|---|---|---|---|
| TIME | 1st void / 2nd void | | 6 AM / 6 AM | 11 AM / 11:30 AM | 4:15 PM / 4:30 PM | | | | | | | | | | | |
| VOLUME | 1st void / 2nd void | | 200cc / 60cc | 150cc / 45cc | 350cc / 25cc | | | | | | | | | | | |
| SUGAR | | | 1+ | Neg | 2+ | | | | | | | | | | | |
| ACETONE | | | Neg | Neg | Neg | | | | | | | | | | | |
| INSULIN | TYPE | | REG | -o- | REG | | | | | | | | | | | |
| | DOSE | | 5u | | 10u | | | | | | | | | | | |
| | TIME | | 6:30 AM | | 4:45 PM | | | | | | | | | | | |
| | ROUTE | | SQ | | SQ | | | | | | | | | | | |
| | SITE | | R U Arm | | L U Arm | | | | | | | | | | | |
| SIGNATURE | | | J Mead RN | | J Mead RN | | | | | | | | | | | |

Diabetic Flow Sheet

which contains information such as temperature, pulse, blood pressure, respiration, urine output, hemodynamic monitoring values, infusion rates of vasoactive drugs, and daily weights. Other flow sheets may include a medication and an intake and output record. Special sheets such as neurological monitoring sheets and diabetic sheets are used as necessary. Flow sheets eliminate the need to write excessive notes and avoid duplication of information. Flow sheets do not negate the need for narrative descriptions.

Refer back to the Patient Care Plan to ensure that all problems have been assessed and documentation completed. It is a good idea to check the care plan several times a day.

**Source-Oriented Narrative Charting** Narrative charting is based upon chronology rather than systems. Information is charted in chronological order regardless of the subject of the note. For example, the nurses' notes for a patient could appear as follows:

| | |
|---|---|
| 0735 | c/o dull aching pain in RLQ inc. area. |
| 0745 | Demerol 50 mg IM, ROQ for pain. |
| 0820 | States pain relieved. |
| 0845 | RLQ dressing changed. Inc. area clean, s̄ edema or erythema. Scant serous drainage on drsg. |
| 0930 | Amb. in hall s̄ assistance. |

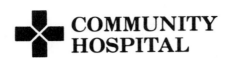

## COMMUNITY HOSPITAL

**Patient Information**

### NURSES' NOTES

| Time | Medications/Treatment | Observations | Signature |
|---|---|---|---|
| 1/25/85 7³⁵/AM | | c/o dull aching pain in RLQ incisional area. | |
| 7⁴⁵/AM | Demerol 50 mgm. IM RUQ | for incisional pain. | A.Mead RN |
| 8²⁰/AM | | States pain relieved. | |
| 8⁴⁵/AM | Dressing change | Inc. area clean s̄ edema or erythema. Scant serous drainage on dressing. | |
| 9³⁰/AM | | Amb. in hall s̄ assistance. | A.Mead RN |
| 12¹⁵/PM | | Dr. Peter visited. | A.Mead RN |
| | | | |
| | | | |
| | | | |
| | | | |
| | | | |
| | | | |
| | | | |

Nurses' Notes Using Source-Oriented Charting

Hospitals usually have maximum time requirements for this type of note, with common parameters being every two or three hours. While there may be a requirement for frequency of charting, there usually is not one for charting content. This leads to the primary deficiency of narrative charting; it is very easy to chart without specifying why the patient is in the hospital or what is the patient's overall condition. Note the example above. Why is the patient in the hospital? What is the patient's general condition? How is the patient progressing?

When using narrative charting, an assessment should be performed at the beginning of the shift and as needed thereafter. When assessment is the initial entry in narrative charting, subsequent entries are more relevant and understandable. This combination of assessment and narrative charting is the best technique to ensure that adequate information about the patient is recorded for all personnel who utilize nurses' notes.

In that the patient's chart is considered a legal document, it is important that nurses chart relevant, accurate, and appropriate information in a timely manner. The following rules for charting narrative notes will assist you to maintain an acceptable chart.

1. Use ink, not felt pen or pencil. Black ink microfilms best.

2. Correct errors by drawing a single line through the error, write the word *error* above it, and then initial the error. The error must be readable. Ink eradication, erasures, or use of occlusive materials are not acceptable.

3. Sign each entry with your first initial, last name, and status, e.g., SN for student nurse, LVN for licensed vocational nurse, or RN for registered nurse. Script, not printing, is used for the signature. Each signature should appear at the right hand margin of the nurses' notes.

4. Notes should appear on each succeeding line. Lines should not be omitted in the nurses' notes. A horizontal line is drawn to "fill-up" a partial line. Continuous charting is done for each entry unless a time change occurs. You do not need a new line for each new idea or statement.

5. Entries should be concise. Complete sentences are not required. Start each entry with a capital letter and end the entry with a period even if the entry is a single word or phrase.

6. The date is entered in the date column on the first line of every page of nurses' notes and whenever the date changes.

7. Time is entered in the time column whenever a new time entry occurs. Do not put time changes in the text of the nurses' notes. If only one time is entered for block charting, enter the last time you were with the patient.

8. Chart objective facts, not your interpretations. For example, *Chart: ate 100%,* not *good appetite.* If the patient offers complaints, place the complaint in quotation marks to indicate that it is his statement. For example, "c/o chest pain radiating down left arm."

9. Objective data is to be charted as well. In addition to the statement offered by the patient, the nurse should chart her observations: *Skin cold and clammy. Diaphoretic. Vital signs stable.*

10. Refusal of medications and treatments must be documented. A circle is placed around the time the medication or treatment is to be given in the appropriate area of the chart. An explanation as to the reason medication was not given is entered in the nurses' notes.

11. Sign each entry before it is replaced in the chart rack. An entry is not to be left unsigned. If all the charting is completed for the shift at one time, a single signature is placed at the end of the charting.

12. Accuracy is important. Describe behaviors rather than feelings. This allows other health team members to determine the actual problems of the patient.

13. Chart only those abbreviations and symbols approved by the facility. Information can be misinterpreted or misleading when unfamiliar abbreviations are used.

14. Spell correctly, using proper terminology and grammar.

15. Write legibly. If writing is not legible, then print.

16. Only chart what you personally have done or observed. An exception to this rule is when you are responsible for charting for nonprofessional personnel.

17. Do not use the word "patient" or "pt" in the chart. The chart belongs to that patient.

**NURSING ASSESSMENT DATA BASE**

## COMMUNITY HOSPITAL

| Date | Time | Room # | Admit by: | ambulatory _____ guerney _____ |
|------|------|--------|-----------|-----------------------------------|
| 1/25/85 | 4 p.m. | 110A | | W/C ✓ ambulance _____ |

| T.P.R. | B/P RT | B/P LT | Height | Weight |
|--------|--------|--------|--------|--------|
| 99⁸-110-24 | 160/90 | 164/94 | 5'6" | 200# |

**Instructed in use of:** — **Articles at bedside (describe item)**

| Yes | No | |
|-----|-----|---|
| ✓ | ☐ | Telephone |
| ✓ | ☐ | Bed-Controls |
| ✓ | ☐ | Lights |
| ✓ | ☐ | Nurse call System |
| ✓ | ☐ | Visiting hours |

| | Article | | |
|---|---------|---|---|
| ✓ | Ring | Yellow Metal | |
| ☐ | Watch | | |
| ✓ | Money (amt.) | $10.50 | |
| ✓ | Eyeglasses | | |
| ☐ | Hearing Aid | | |

| | |
|---|---|
| ☐ Contact Lenses _____ |
| Dentures: Upper ✓ |
| Lower ✓ |
| ☐ Other _____ |

Reason for No: _____    Other _____

**Tests completed on admission**

| ☐ | Lab Work | ✓ | X-ray | CHEST |
| ✓ | UA | ☐ | Other | _____ |

Above information obtained by: K. Mead, RN

| Previous illness | Meds taken @ home on routine basis | Meds taken today state time | Meds brought to hospital | Allergies: |
|------------------|-----------------------------------|----------------------------|--------------------------|------------|
| ☐ Diabetes | Lasix 40 mgm. P.O. | | None | ✓ FOOD Shellfish, Citrus fruits |
| ✓ Hypertension | Digoxin 0.25 mgm PO | | | |
| ✓ Heart Disease | | | | |
| ☐ Lung Disease | | | | ✓ DRUGS ASA, Codeine |
| ☐ Other | | | | |
| | | | **Disposition of Meds** | |
| | | | ☐ Home | ☐ None Known |
| | | | ☐ Pharmacy | |

Data Base Record

18. Do not double-chart. If something appears on a flow sheet, it does not need to appear on the nurses' narrative record unless there is an alteration from normal.

19. Do not squeeze information into a space because you forgot to chart it earlier. Add the information on the first available line. Write in the time the event occurred, not the time you entered the information.

20. The following information should be charted.
    a. Physician's visits.
    b. Times patient leaves and returns to the unit, mode of transportation, and destination.
    c. Medications (chart immediately after given). Include dosage, route of administration, if parenteral where given, whether pain was relieved (if pain medication), and side effects.
    d. Treatments (chart immediately after given).

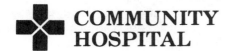

## COMMUNITY HOSPITAL

### NURSING PROBLEM LIST

| Date Problem Began | Prob. # | Problem | Date Resolved | Date Recurred |
|---|---|---|---|---|
| 1/25/85 | 1 | Urinary elimination, alteration in voiding, R/t incontinence | 1/30/85 | |
| 1/25/85 | 2 | Self-care deficit R/t right sided weakness. | | |
| 1/25/85 | 3 | Nutrition, alteration in: less than body requirement R/t refusal to eat. | | |
| 1/27/85 | 4 | Skin integrity impaired: R/t reddened coccyx. | 2/4/85 | |
| | | | | |

Problem List

**Problem-Oriented Medical Records** The second major type of charting is the problem-oriented medical records, or POMR. This system differs from source-oriented narrative charting, not only in format but in philosophy. Problem-oriented medical records focus on the patient's status rather than on the source of the information, i.e., department or member of the health care team who is originating the information. Narrative charting typically consists of doctors' progress notes, physical therapy progress notes, nurses' notes, respiratory therapy progress notes, etc. With POMR, only one set of progress notes is used, and all personnel caring for the patient record their data on this set.

In its purest form, a POMR consists of five distinct parts: the data base (initial assessment), problem list, initial plan, progress notes, and discharge summary. The data base is made up of information from and about the patient that is used to develop the problem list. Because the POMR system is systematic and well-defined, the data base consists of specific types of data, including the chief complaint (why patient came to the hospital), personal and family medical history, allergies and reactions, medications taken at home, physical assessment, mental and emotional assessment, and lifestyle.

Development of a complete data base requires skill and practice. Basic features of patient interviewing and physical assessment are covered in other sections of this text, but a few tips and reminders may help to sharpen your skills. First, select a time mutually acceptable to both you and the patient. Know how much time you have for the interview and whether the patient has scheduled appointments or tests. Be aware of the patient's physical and emotional comfort, the physical environment of the interview location, and pending meal times. Second, consider how your questions might affect the patient. Phrase questions that will cause the patient to explain and answer—a "yes" or "no" is not sufficiently informative. Do not make the patient defensive by being judgmental about his actions. Patients who believe you do not approve of their actions often will withhold potentially important information. Third, avoid leading statements. Many patients try to respond in an agreeable manner. For example, "You don't . . ." statements may be answered by "No, of course not." Also, avoid using medical jargon unfamiliar to the patient. Some words you use daily may be unknown to your patient. The patient will answer what he *thinks* you asked to avoid showing his ignorance. This situation may result in an invalid data base because the data is incorrect.

After completing the data base, the nurse next defines the patient problems for the problem list. A "problem" is any difficulty that the patient cannot handle by himself—the patient needs assistance from someone on the health care team. The difficulty may be a physical symptom, such as pain or infection; an emotional problem caused by fear of impending surgery or worry about a family member; or a social problem, such as loss of job and income or inability to live independently at home. Problems are usually defined as active (acute or chronic) or inactive (resolved). Active problems may also be potential—not yet present but likely to occur. Examine the following list of problems and see if you can determine how to categorize them.

| | |
|---|---|
| Upper GI bleeding, 3 days' duration | Active |
| Children, 2 and 5 years old, at home with father | Active |
| Possible skin breakdown | Active-Potential |
| Appendectomy 1954 | Resolved |
| Asthma since childhood | Active-Chronic |

Medical diagnoses are included on the problem list if they are definite. If they are only tentative, the patient's symptoms should be put on the list until the actual diagnosis is made. Of course, many of the symptoms may qualify as nursing diagnosis since they can be defined as interfering with the patient's sense of well-being. For example, anxiety related to one's medical diagnosis would be a nursing diagnosis.

The categories of the POMR closely approximate the steps in the nursing process. The data base and problem list equate to assessment; the initial plan equates to planning; the progress notes discuss intervention; and the discharge summary is an evaluation.

After you complete the data base and start the problem list, you then formulate the Patient Care Plan (PCP). For each major problem or group of problems, the PCP should include the following information: date, problem, expected outcome, check point, deadline, and nursing actions.

In the POMR system, one set of progress notes is used by everyone. This means that all members of the health care team write their observations on the same part of the chart. The entries on the problem list are always numbered, so when the nurse, physician, and the respiratory therapist all refer to problem 3 in their progress notes, everyone knows that they are referring to Airway clearance, ineffective, *related to* pain.

Within the well-organized POMR system, progress notes have a specific format, usually called SOAP or SOAPIER. These acronyms translate as:

*Subjective:* patient's symptoms and own description of problem.
*Objective:* clinical findings; include observations and factual data, e.g., intake and output, vital signs, drainage, presence of rash, etc.

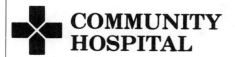

## COMMUNITY HOSPITAL

Patient Information

### PROGRESS NOTES

| Date | Note progress of case, complications, change in diagnosis, condition on discharge |
|------|-----------------------------------------------------------------------------------|
| 1/25/85 | Problem #3 |
| | S Refuses to eat. States "I'm afraid to swallow because I choke sometimes." |
| | O Has difficulty swallowing fluids. Chokes if not sitting upright. |
| | A Swallowing difficulty—probably related to CVA. |
| | P Contact dietitian to see pt. |
| | Place in high-Fowler's position when feeding. |
| | Feed slowly and reassure pt. often. |
| | K. Mead, RN |

Progress Notes Using SOAP Charting

*Assessment:* your conclusions about the problem based on subjective and objective data. Nursing diagnoses may be written here.
*Plan:* what you decide to do about the problem.
*Implementation:* your nursing interventions.
*Evaluation:* how the implementation worked.
*Revision:* how you plan to change the PCP if improvement is needed.

When writing progress notes, remember that a separate SOAP note is needed for each problem. You should not combine problems. It is not always necessary to include the I, E, and R portions of the note; however, always include the S, O, A, and P parts, even if the patient does not supply subjective statements. The I, E, and R can be included under the P section.

The discharge summary, the final step in the POMR system as well as all forms of charting, includes both a summary of the patient's hospitalization and documentation of patient teaching. SOAPIER notes are again used as the charting format, and a summary should be written for each problem on the problem list. If the problem is fully resolved during hospitalization, that fact and the date it occurred (from the progress notes) are all that is necessary. The discharge summary is not a day-by-day account of the patient's stay, but a short review. It is beneficial to include specific highlights such as the highest serum glucose level or the highest temperature, but all the values need not

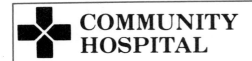

# COMMUNITY HOSPITAL

## PROGRESS NOTES

| Date | Note progress of case, complications, change in diagnosis, condition on discharge |
|------|---|
| 1/28/85 | Mrs. Dannard was admitted to the Rehab Unit 11/10/84. Major problems were inability to swallow, Lt. sided weakness, aphasia, reddened coccyx, and requiring assistance with ADL's. Laboratory values have consistently been WNL except for 2 episodes of urinary tract infection, the most recent occurring 12/20/84. Problem #1, inability to swallow, resolved 11/30/84; Problem #4, reddened coccyx resolved 11/21/84; Problem #2, Lt. sided weakness continues. Walks with tripod cane, slightly unsteady gait. Problem #3, aphasia, persists. Able to communicate in simple terms, slow, hesitant speech. Problem #5, needs assistance with ADL's. Unable to bathe and dress self without assistance. Referral made to Visiting Nurse Assoc. for assistance ē ADL's. Daughter and granddaughter have been instructed in the care of Mrs. Dannard and will assist when able. Patient and family have been instructed on safety factors at home, personal hygiene care, discharge medications including Lasix, Digoxin, Inderol. Necessity for return visits to O.P. Rehab Clinic. Dietitian instructed in low sodium, low cholesterol diet. |
| | Psychosocially, Mrs. Dannard is eager for discharge and looking forward to continuing therapy on O.P. basis. |
| | K. Mead, RN |

Discharge Summary in POMR System

be included. Remember, a separate SOAPIER note should be written for each problem that is not fully resolved at the time of the discharge.

All invasive procedures, surgical interventions, and major diagnostic tests should be listed and the results outlined. Braces, equipment, and supplies (for dressing changes, catheterizations, etc.) should be included in the summary. If the equipment or braces are difficult to use or apply, it is helpful if pictures or diagrams are included. Patient teaching completed, discharge medications, and specific teaching regarding the medications should also be documented.

Referrals to other health care services should be identified with the name of the agency and the contact person listed on the chart. If patients are being discharged to other health care facilities or to a visiting nurse, it is helpful if they receive not only a copy of the discharge summary, but a copy of the last patient care plan. This provides for a smooth transition of care from one health care setting to another.

Because of the many changes necessary when implementing POMR, hospitals often use only part of it, or are changing to it in stages; therefore, it is common to find situations in which parts of several systems are in use. For example, SOAP nursing notes may be used while the remainder of the chart is source oriented, or doctors may use the problem list and SOAP progress notes while nurses use systems charting for nurses' notes. Although progress is rather slow, it appears that many more hospitals will adopt the POMR system, not only for its format and ease of use, but also for its completeness on documenting patient care.

*Examples of SOAP charting:*

Problem #1  Fluid volume, alterations in, excess, *related to* poor compliance to medication administration.
    S  "My rings are tight and my shoes don't fit."
    O  Fingers are edematous. 3+ pitting edema of both ankles.
    A  Due to fluid overload as a result of refusing diuretics.
    P  Elevate feet. Explain necessity for diuretics. Administer drug, obtain order for IM med if nec. Observe dietary intake of $Na^+$ to determine if compliant to diet.

Problem #2  Airway Clearance ineffective, *related to* pain.
    S  "I'm having difficulty bringing up mucus."
    O  Lungs sound congested, rales present bilaterally in lower bases.
    A  Unable to deep breathe and cough due to high abdominal incision.
    P  Elevate HOB 45 degrees. Enc. coughing and deep breathing. Medicate for pain q 3 hrs. Splint inc. when coughing.

**Computer-Assisted Charting**  Computers have become a valuable tool in documenting patient care. One common system focuses on the patient's physiological parameters. With input from various monitoring devices such as an arterial line and a Swan-Ganz catheter, the computer can automatically determine and frequently update many pieces of data, including hematology and chemistry tests, ABGs, cardiac output, and DE, VS, CVP, and PA pressures to name only a few. These results can be viewed on a VMT (video matrix terminal similar to a TV screen) or printed out on paper. The VS and hemodynamic data are continually updated, and many of the lab tests can be updated at least every hour.

```
MATRIX NO.3201        HOSP. NO.01      01/05/82
DYNAMIC MATRIX

          GENERAL ADMIT NOTES                        01
                                                     02
 *CLIENT ADM:        /GUERNEY                         03
    AMB   /WC   /AMBULANCE   FROM EMERG RM            04
            FROM--                                    05
                                          **         06
 (PRIMARY LANGUAGE OTHER THAN ENGLISH)               07
 CLIENT SPEAKS--                          **         08
 (CLIENT HAS:) (LOCATED AT:) (HOME) (HOSP)           09
    GLASSES                    **      **            10
    CONT LENSES                **      **            11
    HEARING AID                **      **            12
    CANE                       **      **            13
    CRUTCHES                   **      **            14
    WALKER                     **      **            15
    DENTURES                   **      **            16
    PROSTHESIS                 **      **            17
    --              (HOME) UPPER  U&L                18
    --              (HOSP) LOWER  PARTIAL            19
                         *ADMIT VITAL SIGNS          20
```

```
MATRIX NO.1347        HOSP. NO.01      01/05/82
DYNAMIC MATRIX

       NSG MASTER GUIDE - GENERAL                    01
 RN/LVN-------------------------------               02
 *VS-RESULTS,OBSV        *GEN REPORTING              03
 *VS-OBSV ONLY           *GEN RPTG-SURG              04
 *DIET,FLD BAL                                       05
 *UNIT TESTS/EXAMS       *IMMED POST-OP:             06
 *HYG,ACTIV,SAFETY       *ADMIT NOTES                07
 *PROCEDURES                                         08
                         *MISC DATA                  09
 *BASIC CARE NEEDS                                   10
 *PHYSICAL ASSESS        *SPECIAL OBSV               11
 *TEACH/DISCH PLANS                                  12
                         *READY FOR THE OR           13
 *UNSCHED,MISC MED       *TO THE OR                  14
 *MED FOLLOW-UP                                      15
                         *NSG DISCH SUMMARY          16
 *IV,BLD BEGIN           *NSG TRANS SUMMARY          17
 *IV,BLD END             *EXC CHARTING               18
 *IV,BLD GEN OBSV                                    19
 *IV,NO.0---             *CHANGE SPECIALTY           20
```

General Admission Notes Matrix          General Nursing Master Guide

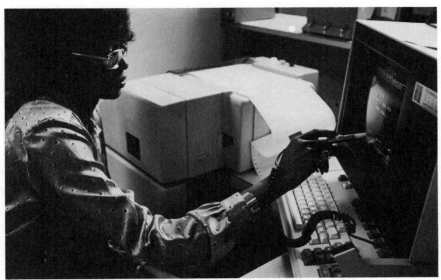

Printed record is sent to nursing unit and placed on chart.

Another type of computer system records, stores, and retrieves many pieces of data about the patient that must be communicated throughout the hospital in order for the patient to receive optimal care. For example, when a patient is admitted and the physician enters orders into the computer, many things automatically happen. The dietary department is notified of the diet needs, pharmacy is notified of medications and IVs that are ordered, CSR is notified of special equipment needs, and the laboratory is notified of required tests. It is no longer necessary for the nurse to make out and deliver requests to all these departments and then arrange for delivery or pick-up of the desired items. This has been a basic and broad overview of some of the functions of the Technicon Medical Information System (MIS), which is gaining popularity throughout the country.

At each nursing station in a hospital using this system, there are several computer terminals. These consist of VMT, a keyboard, and a light pen. The VMT shows a matrix-like TV picture, which the nurse can select using the light pen. These matrices are grouped together in a logical order so that general categories of information can be recorded. The nurse records the information by pointing the light pen at the proper word/phrase and pressing a button on the pen. With three quick taps on the button, the nurse can record "Patient admitted ambulatory from the emergency room." If the patient speaks only Spanish, she would tap "Patient speaks" and then type in "Spanish" using the keyboard just below the VMT. All the pertinent information obtained while admitting the patient and doing the initial physical assessment can easily and quickly be recorded using only the light pen and typing in data such as how the patient feels about hospitalization. The admitting sheets the nurse takes to the bedside correlate to the information on the matrices, so that the data is easy to transfer and nothing is omitted.

Hospitals usually have programs that contain special matrices such as "The Nursing Master Guide." This is an example of a matrix that only lists other matrices that may be needed. Much of the routine care a nurse gives can be charted rapidly and completely in a matter of seconds using this and associated matrices.

When the nurse has completed the charting, she taps "Review" and the VMT automatically displays all the data. At this time, the nurse can make

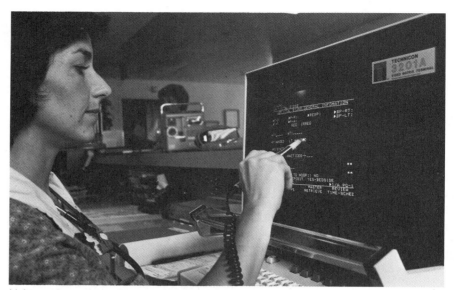

Light pen is used to select appropriate information.

corrections, additions, or deletions using only the light pen and the keyboard. If the data displayed is correct, the nurse taps "Enter" (not shown), the data becomes a permanent part of the computer record for that patient, and a hard copy is printed out to be put in the chart. There are also ways of retrieving and changing mistakes. Also, it is easy to see the logical progression of the charting process. The matrix titles act as gentle reminders of what needs to be charted.

When the patient is to be discharged, the nursing discharge summary is completed. This shows not only the patient's physical condition but also the status of patient teaching and follow-up plans. Again, it is simply punched or tapped on the terminal and the data is displayed.

In addition to making the charting of patient care and the communication between departments much simpler and less time-consuming, the computer provides reference material for common nursing problems. For example, a matrix may show the signs and symptoms associated with diabetes mellitus. If the nurse is unsure of the signs and symptoms of the different forms of this disease, he or she can easily find them in the computer, and, if needed, this information can be printed out and put in the chart. In this way, the nurse can quickly update him or herself about the patient's condition and thereby provide optimal care.

As in many professions, use of the computer in nursing and medicine has become more common and its possible uses are rapidly expanding. If learning the skills of computer use is viewed as a challenge and the reward is more efficient nursing care and less time spent on paperwork, the learning time will have been well spent.

**REPORTING**

**Intrashift Reports**  Reporting your observations and interventions to other health team members is as essential as documenting them on the patient's chart. Intrashift reports are usually verbal reports relayed to team members, team leaders or charge nurses to keep them informed of changes in patient's conditions. Examples of findings which need to be communicated to other health team members include significant changes in vital signs, unusual responses to treatments, medications, or changes in the patient's physical or emotional condition.

**Intershift Reports** Intershift reports disseminate patient information between shifts. It may be accomplished through a verbal report or by tape recording the information. The intershift report should include the following data: patient's name, room number, physician's name, diagnosis and date of surgery when appropriate. In addition, report unusual findings based on the nursing assessment, response to treatments or medications, unusual occurrences, lab results, lab studies, tests to be completed on the next shift and any physical or psychosocial problems that exist.

Physicians should be notified whenever treatment or nursing care parameters are exceeded, there are significant alterations in physical assessment findings, or abnormal lab findings and test results are obtained.

**PHYSICIAN NOTIFICATION**

Before calling the physician, have all data available to allow you to answer questions: current vital signs, lab results, when medications were given last, etc. It is a good idea to have the entire chart with you.

When calling the physician, identify yourself by name, your status (RN or SN), nursing unit, and the patient's name. State the exact reason you are calling. Give pertinent and succinct information.

Written documentation of findings will be placed in the Patient Care Plan. This process is described in detail in Chapter 3.

**DOCUMENTATION**

Written or verbal reports are given to nursing supervisors or clinical coordinators during each shift. The report includes information on all critically ill patients, those with unusual occurrences or complications and difficult-to-manage patients. It is also a good idea to alert the supervisor to problems with families, physicians or other health disciplines in order that she can assist you in problem-solving.

**Incident Reports (IR)** Incident reports serve three main purposes: to help in documenting quality of care, to identify areas in which in-service education is needed, and to record the details of an incident for possible legal use.

With some staff nurses IRs have a poor reputation and, perhaps, with some justification. When something goes wrong, and a nurse is told to "make out an IR," many nurses assume that IRs are a form of punishment for real or alleged misdeeds.

Although IRs should be completed regularly with any unusual occurrence and may, on occasion, be used as a form of reprimand, they are no more nor less than what their title suggests: a report of an incident.

As a tool for documenting quality of care, IRs inform the quality assurance coordinator and the head nurse of areas of practice on the unit that need improvement. For example, there may be an increase in the number of patients who fell out of bed. Further research may show that, because the census is up, the staff is very busy and is forgetting to reposition patients' overbed tables. In their attempts to get water, kleenex, etc., more patients are falling out of bed. The solution to the problem may be to speak with the staff regarding the consequences of this action and, as a group, find a mutually acceptable way of preventing this type of incident from recurring.

IRs also suggest and document the need for in-service education. For example, when an unusual number of IRs are written regarding a new piece of equipment, the head nurse may conclude that the staff, especially those on evening and night shifts, needs instruction on operating this equipment

# INCIDENT REPORT

COMPLETE IMMEDIATELY FOR EVERY
INCIDENT AND SEND TO ADMINISTRATOR

_____
**HOSPITAL NAME**

_____
CITY

ADMINISTRATOR:
Please forward to
Hospital Attorney

_____
**FOR ADDRESSOGRAPH PLATE**

CONFIDENTIAL REPORT OF INCIDENT (NOT A PART OF MEDICAL RECORD)

PATIENT_____ AGE _____ SEX _____ ROOM _____
　　　　　　(LAST NAME)　　　　　　　(FIRST NAME)　　　　　　　　　　　　(M OR F)

ADMITTING DIAGNOSIS _____ DATE OF ADMISSION _____

ATTENDING PHYSICIAN _____ DATE OF INCIDENT _____ TIME ____ M

WERE BED RAILS UP? _____ WAS SAFETY BELT IN USE? _____

WAS PATIENT RATIONAL _____ HI LO BED POSITION _____

SEDATIVES _____ DOSE _____ TIME _____ ⎰ GIVEN WITHIN 12
　　　　　　　　　　　　　　　　　　　　　　　　　　　　　　　　　⎱ HOURS PREVIOUS

NARCOTICS _____ DOSE _____ TIME _____ ⎱ TO INCIDENT

TIME DOCTOR WAS CALLED _____ A.M. _____ P.M. TIME RESPONDED _____ A.M. _____ P.M.
　　　　　　　　　(I.E., HOUSE PHYSICIAN-RESIDENT-INTERN-ETC.)

I NOTIFIED DR. _____ TIME _____ M　　BY _____

NURSE'S ACCOUNT OF THE INCIDENT (INCLUDE EXACT LOCATION)

_____

_____

_____

_____

_____

_____

LIST PERSONS FAMILIAR WITH DETAILS OF INCIDENT - AND OTHER PATIENTS IN THE SAME ROOM

NAME _____ ADDRESS _____

NAME _____ ADDRESS _____

NAME _____ ADDRESS _____

HISTORY OF INCIDENT AS RELATED BY PATIENT _____

_____

_____

_____

_____

_____

DATE OF REPORT _____ _____
　　　　　　　　　　　　　　　　　　　　　　　SIGNATURE OF NURSE OR SUPERVISOR REPORTING

_____

DOCTOR'S REPORT OF PATIENTS CONDITION (FROM PROGRESS REPORT) _____

_____

_____

_____

_____

**ORIGINAL TO HOSPITAL ATTORNEY**

properly and effectively. Another example would be an increase in IRs regarding IVs that are behind or ahead of schedule. This might indicate that the nurses do not know how to apply and regulate the IV pump correctly. A solution to this problem would be to conduct a series of classes for all shifts in which the operation of the IV pump is discussed and hands-on practice is given. Such classes could be given by someone in the hospital's in-service education department or by a representative of the manufacturer of the IV pumps.

Incident reports may also record the details of an occurrence for possible legal use. In some hospitals incident reports are called unusual occurrences and cover any situation that prevented the patient from having a normal recovery. These incidents could include non-nursing actions such as returning to surgery for control of bleeding or having chest tubes inserted for a pneumothorax. In most situations, though, IRs pertain to nurse/patient activities.

When completing an IR with possible legal implications, it is doubly important to record all details of the incident. It is not easy to recall details of the care you gave a patient one or two months ago. Frequently, lawsuits are not filed for months or even years after an incident, so it is essential that you record important details promptly.

Information to record on the IR includes general details of the incident, the patient's response, your action or reaction to the incident, and a list of other personnel who were aware of the details of the incident. Often there is space on the IR in which to record the physician's report of the patient's condition following the incident. To fill in the section regarding the physician's report, the nurse later copies the doctor's progress notes from the chart onto the IR. At no time is the incident report given to the physician. This is a written document between the hospital and its insurance carrier, not the physician.

Upon completion, IRs are forwarded to the unit head nurse and then to nursing administration. Information from the report of interest to in-service education or quality assurance departments can be obtained at this time. Ultimately, the IR will be passed along to the hospital's legal department to be retained indefinitely in the event that legal action is later initiated on behalf of the patient.

**Consent Forms**    When an individual enters a hospital, some of the person's basic legal rights are affected. In order that these rights are not violated, the patient must give permission (consent) for all treatment. If consent is not obtained, the hospital, doctor, and/or nurse may be charged with committing "battery" against the patient. Battery, as defined by law, is an "offensive touching" of the patient. This could include injection or any breaking of the skin's surface, x-rays, insertion of tubes, etc.

Before you panic and attempt to get a consent signed for the patient's next blood pressure, you should know that routine nursing care is "consented to" when the patient signs the "Conditions of Admissions." Also, certain procedures such as injections, intubations, dressings, etc., are treatments ordered by the physician and agreed to by the patient. If the patient has listened to the explanation of a specific procedure and agreed to allow the procedure to be carried out, he or she is giving implied consent; however, the patient has the right to refuse any treatment. In that case the physician must be contacted regarding alternative actions.

When discussing the formal written or explicit consents, the two key activities are obtaining and witnessing consent. Obtaining consent is not

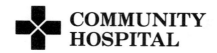 **COMMUNITY HOSPITAL**

Client Information

## AUTHORIZATION FOR AND CONSENT TO SURGERY, ADMINISTRATION OF ANESTHETICS, SPECIAL DIAGNOSTIC OR THERAPEUTIC PROCEDURES

Date _____ Time _____

Your admitting physician is _____, M. D.

Your surgeon is _____, M. D.

1.  The hospital staff and facilities assist your physicians and surgeons in the performance of various surgical operations and other diagnostic and therapeutic procedures. These surgical operations and special diagnostic or therapeutic procedures all may involve calculated risks of complications, injury or even death, from both known and unknown causes and no warranty or guarantee has been made as to result or cure. Except in a case of emergency or exceptional circumstances, these operations and procedures are not performed upon clients unless and until the client has had an opportunity to discuss them with his/her physician. Each client has the right to consent to or refuse any proposed operation or special procedure (based upon the description or explanation received).

2.  Your physicians and surgeons have determined that the operations or special procedures listed below may be beneficial in the diagnosis or treatment of your condition. Upon your authorization and consent, the operations or special procedures will be performed by your physicians and surgeons and their staff. The persons in attendance for the purpose of administering anesthesia or performing other specialized professional services, such as radiology, pathology and the like, are not the agents, servants or employees of the hospital or your physician or surgeon, but are independent contractors performing specialized services on your behalf and, as such, are your agents, servants, or employees. Any tissue or member severed in any operation will be disposed of in the discretion of the pathologist, except _____ and those body parts specified as donor organs.

3.  Your signature opposite the operations or special procedures listed below constitutes your acknowledgement (a) that you have read and agreed to the foregoing, (b) that the operations or special procedures have been adequately explained to you by your attending physicians or surgeons and that you have all of the information that you desire, and (c) that you authorize and consent to the performance of the operations or special procedures.

*Operation or Procedure*

_____

_____

Signature _____  Signature _____
                        Client                                                    Witness

(If client is a minor or unable to sign, complete the following): Client is a minor, is unable to sign because

_____

_____

_____                    _____
            Father                                                       Guardian

_____                    _____
            Mother                                              Other person and relationship

a nursing function because it includes the explanation of what will be done, the risks of the procedure to that patient, alternative procedures, and probable outcomes. This information should be given by the doctor.

The nurse's role is to witness the signing of the consent. When the consent form is presented to the patient, it should be explained and the patient should be encouraged to read it thoroughly before signing. Occasionally, a nurse is asked to explain or expand the physician's presentation. Acceptable practice is for the nurse to clarify, define a medical term, or add more details to the physician's initial information. If the nurse feels that the patient does not really understand what is going to occur, it is the nurse's responsibility to notify the doctor to give further explanation before the patient signs the consent. An easy way to determine what the patient understands is to ask the patient to repeat back the physician's explanation. Under ordinary circumstances, only one witness to signing the consent is necessary. The witness does not have to be an RN, just someone over the age of eighteen.

There are many rules and regulations governing consents. If you have questions about them, consult the consent manual for your hospital, or a supervisory person. There are several important situations in which more information may be needed. One relates to the competency of the patient. Generally, the patient must sign personally, and spouses are unable to sign for the patient. Permanent incompetence usually involves legal action to assign someone else as conservator. Temporary incompetence may be the result of hospital treatments such as drugs or anesthetics. When a narcotic or sedative has been given, at least four hours lapsed time is recommended before the patient is considered competent to sign a consent. A second situation concerns the patient who is a minor. The age of consent varies according to state and also according to specific situations such as emancipation (being away from the family and supporting self) and the type of medical problem (reportable diseases or pregnancy). An associated problem may arise when deciding who can legally sign for a minor.

## TERMINOLOGY

**Care Plan, Patient:** a plan of care, usually written, that meets the special needs of each patient.

**Charting:** process of recording information about a patient concerning the progress of his disease and treatment.

**Computer-assisted charting:** patient information is entered into the computer for storage and retrieval at a later time.

**Flow sheets:** patient data is recorded and/or graphed in order to show patterns or alterations in findings.

**Incident report:** recording of an unusual happening or event, which could affect patient or staff safety.

**Kardex:** a convenient and readily accessible file of cards containing current patient information.

**Nursing process:** a set of actions that includes as-sessment, planning, intervention, and evaluation.

**Problem oriented medical record (POMR):** a patient record that is organized according to the person's specific health problems.

**Report:** to give an account of something that has been seen, heard, done, or considered.

**SOAP notes:** nursing notes organized consistently by what the patient feels "Subjectively"; what the nurse observes "Objectively"; how the nurse "Assesses" the situation; and what the nurse "Plans."

**Source-oriented charting:** information in the chart is organized according to its source, e.g., doctor's progress notes, nurses' notes.

**Systems charting:** charting or documentation relative to the assessment data obtained during the physical assessment of the patient.

## WORD ROOTS, PREFIXES AND SUFFIXES

**a, an:** without, not
**ab:** away from
**abd:** abdominal
**a.c.:** before meals
**acro:** extreme, top, extremity
**acu:** sharp
**ad, al:** to toward
**adeno:** gland
**adip:** fat
**ad lib.:** freely, as desired
**-aemia:** blood
**aero:** air; gas
**-aesthesia:** sensation
**-al:** action, process
**alg:** pain
**-algesia, algia:** suffering pain
**amb.:** ambulatory, walking
**amput:** cut away, cut off
**amt.:** amount
**ante:** before
**anti:** against, opposed to
**ap, apo:** away from
**arteri:** artery
**arthro:** joint
**-ase:** enzyme
**aur:** ear
**auto:** self
**bacill:** rod
**bacter:** rod
**bi:** double, two
**b.i.d.:** twice each day
**bile:** bile
**bio:** life
**blephar:** eyelid
**B.M.:** bowel movement.
**brachi:** arm
**brady:** slow
**B.R.P.:** bathroom privileges
**bucc:** cheek
**c̄:** with
**cale:** stone
**capit:** head
**cardi, cardio:** heart
**cathart:** cleansing
**caud:** tail
**cav:** hollow
**cec:** blind
**cent:** hundred
**-chem, -chemo:** chemical
**chole:** bile
**chron:** time

**cid:** kill
**-cide:** causing death
**cili:** eyelid
**circum:** ring, circle
**C/O:** complains of
**cogni:** know
**colo:** colon
**com, con:** with, together
**crani:** skull
**cry:** cold
**cut:** skin
**cyan:** blue
**cyst:** bladder
**cyt:** cell
**-cyte:** cell
**DC:** discontinue
**demi:** half
**dent:** tooth
**derm:** skin
**di, dis:** double, separation, reversal
**dors:** back
**dur:** hard
**dy:** two
**-dynia:** pain
**dys:** abnormal, different
**e, ec:** out from
**-ectomy:** cutting out
**em, en:** in, within
**embol:** inserted a wedge
**-emesis:** vomiting
**-emia:** blood
**emulsi:** milk out, exhaust
**endo:** within
**entero:** intestinal
**epi:** upon
**erythro:** red
**eso:** inside
**-esthesia:** sensation
**et:** and
**eu:** normal
**ex:** out of
**exo:** the outside, beyond
**fore:** before, in front of
**gastro:** stomach
**genito:** genital
**-gens, -gent:** clan, tribe
**glosso:** relating to the tongue
**glyco:** sugar
**-gram:** tracing, a mark
**-graphy:** a writing, a record

**grav:** heavy
**gyn:** woman
**H₂O:** water
**heme:** one-half
**hemi:** half
**hemo:** blood
**hepar, hepatio:** liver
**hisc:** open
**homeo:** same, similar
**HS:** bedtime
**hydro:** related to water
**hyper:** above, beyond
**hypo:** under, below
**I&O:** intake and output
**-iasis:** condition, pathological state
**ile, ilo:** intestine
**in:** not, within, into
**in.:** inch
**incont:** incontinent
**infra:** below
**inter:** between
**intra:** inside
**is:** equal
**isch, ischo:** hold, suppress
**-ism:** condition, theory
**itis:** inflammation
**juxta:** next to
**latero:** side
**lb or #:** pound
**leuko:** white
**lip:** fat
**lith:** stone
**ly:** loose, dissolve
**-lysis:** dissolving, decomposition
**macro:** large, big
**mal:** bad, poor
**mamm:** breast
**man:** hand
**mani:** mental alterations
**megaly:** large
**meta:** beyond
**metra, metro:** uterus
**micro:** small
**nebul:** cloud, mist
**ne:** young, new
**nebul:** cloud, mist
**necr, necro:** dead
**neo:** new
**neuro:** nerve
**noct:** night
**-nos, -noso:** disease

**n.p.o.:** nothing by mouth
**nucleo:** nucleus
**nutri:** nourish
**ob:** against
**oc:** occlude
**olig:** few, small
**oob:** out of bed
**opisth:** backward
**-opsy:** examination
**opthalm:** eye
**-orrhaphy:** repair of
**ortho:** straight, normal
**-osis:** process, condition
**oss, ost:** bone
**-ostomy:** creation of an opening
**-otomy:** opening into
**palp:** touch, feel
**pan:** all, entire
**para:** beside, beyond
**paten, patent:** spreading open
**path:** disease, sickness
**p.c.:** after meals
**ped, pedi, pedo:** foot
**ped, pedo:** child
**pen:** lack of
**per:** by, through
**peri:** around
**pet:** tend toward
**pha:** speak
**phag:** eat
**phleb:** vein
**phon:** sound
**phot:** light
**phthi:** waste away
**-phylaxis:** protection

**-plasm:** to mold
**-plasty:** formed or repaired by plastic surgery
**platy:** broad, flat
**-plegia:** paralysis
**pleur:** rib
**plur:** more
**pne:** breathing
**-pnea:** respiration, respiratory condition
**pneumo:** air, gas, lung
**post:** after, behind
**pre:** before
**p.r.n.:** whenever necessary
**pro:** before
**pruri:** itch
**pseud, pseudo:** false
**psych:** the soul, mind
**-ptosis:** a lowered position of an organ
**pulmo:** lung
**pur:** pus
**pyo:** pus
**pyro:** fire
**q.d.:** every day
**q.h.:** every hour
**q.i.d.:** four times each day
**q.s.:** as much as required
**q2h:** every two hours
**q3h:** every three hours
**q4h:** every four hours
**ren:** kidneys
**retro:** backwards
**-rhage, -rhagia:** hemorrhage, excessive flow or discharge

**s̄:** without
**-sclerosis:** dryness, hardness
**-scopy:** to see
**sedat:** soothed, calm
**semi:** half
**sens:** sense
**sept:** wall off
**socio:** social
**som:** sleep
**spiro:** breathe
**stasis:** stoppage, slowing
**stat:** immediately
**steat:** fat
**sub, sup:** under, below
**super:** over, above, higher
**syn:** with, together
**tach:** fast
**therm:** heat
**therapeu:** serve, treatment
**thromb:** clot
**t.i.d.:** three times each day
**-tomy:** cut
**top:** place
**toxic:** poisonous
**troch:** wheel
**trop:** turn, change
**-trophy:** nutrition, nourishment
**ultra:** beyond, excessively
**un:** one
**-uria:** a specific condition of, or related to urine
**vaso:** vessel
**veno:** vein
**ventro:** abdomen
**°:** degree

Chapter **5**

# Communication Skills

## LEARNING OBJECTIVES

Define the term communication.

Explain why communication is such an important concept in nursing.

Describe what is meant by the communication process.

Discuss four factors that affect communication.

List five examples of therapeutic communication.

List five examples of blocks to communication.

Demonstrate the steps for beginning a patient interaction.

Explain why it is therapeutic to encourage the patient to express feelings and thoughts.

State two nursing diagnoses that relate to communication with patients.

**COMMUNICATION**    Communication is the process of sending and receiving messages by means of symbols, words, signs, gestures, or other actions. It is a multilevel process consisting of the content or information part of the message and the part that defines the meaning of the message. Messages sent and received define the relationship between people. From the point of view of a learned skill, communication is intended to accomplish a defined goal. It is the transmission of facts, feelings, and meaning through the communication process.

The communication process forms one of the primary bases for administering all skills. Without clear communication the nurse cannot assess, administer, or evaluate his actions in performing the skill. The principles of therapeutic communication form a basis for interviewing and counseling skills.

Communication is a vital element in nursing. Everything that occurs within the nurse-patient interaction involves some form or mode of communication, whether it be listening to an upset family member, assisting a patient in health teaching, or performing a nursing procedure. Without communication there would be no nursing.

The communication process includes both verbal and nonverbal expressions and is affected by the intrapersonal framework of the person, the relationship between the participants and the purpose of the sender. The content of the message and the context also influence the communication process. The manner in which the message is sent and the effect on the receiver also play a role in the eventual outcome of the communication process.

Five factors have been identified that influence effective communication.

☐ One cannot *not* communicate. This idea is basic to communication. We have an inherent need to communicate whether it be verbal or nonverbal. Even silence is a form of communication.

☐ There is a content or informational value to messages sent and received that explains what the message is about and expresses how the sender regards the receiver.

☐ The message sent is not necessarily the message received.

☐ Messages contain overt and covert meanings. The sender is aware of the overt, or direct, message, and may or may not be aware of the hidden, or covert, meaning.

☐ Communication becomes dysfunctional when a person does not assume responsibility for his communication. Dysfunctional communications result from failing to learn to communicate properly and leaving the responsibility for communicating to others.

When you are communicating with a patient, there are some useful guidelines that will assist you to become a more therapeutic and effective communicator.

☐ Take an active role and guide the conversation if the patient is overly hesitant. For example, "I'm here to listen to any concerns you might have, Mr. Smith. You were mentioning having trouble understanding. . . . . ."

☐ Give broad opening statements and ask open-ended questions to help the patient describe what is happening to him. Pick up cues and follow through with the subject that the patient introduces to provide continuity.

☐ Use body language to convey empathy, interest and encouragement to facilitate communication.

☐ Use silence as a therapeutic tool, as it allows the patient to pace and direct his own communications. Long periods of silence, however, may increase the patient's anxiety level so use this technique wisely .

## THERAPEUTIC COMMUNICATION TECHNIQUES

Communication includes the totality of the human person and reflects what is happening within and outside of us. Body sensations, thoughts, feelings, emotions, ideas, perceptions, judgments, previous experiences, and memories are all part of how and what we communicate. Effective, functional communication only occurs when what is happening within is congruent with what we share with the outside. It is important to be a therapeutic as well as a functional communicator and not to disturb the communication process by using nontherapeutic techniques or blocks to communication.

Therapeutic communication techniques assist the flow of communication and always focus on the patient. Nontherapeutic communication techniques block or hinder communication and generally focus on the nurse and meet the nurse's needs. The major therapeutic and nontherapeutic techniques are listed below.

*Acknowledgement*

Acknowledge the patient without inserting your own values or judgments. Acknowledgement may be simple and with or without understanding, verbal or nonverbal.

*Example:*
In the response "I hear what you're saying," the person acknowledges a statement without agreeing with it.

| | |
|---|---|
| *Clarification* | Clarify the patient's message. Check out or make clear either the intent or hidden meaning of the message or determine if the message sent was the message received.<br><br>*Example:*<br> "You said it was hot in here. Would you like to open the window?" |
| *Feedback* | Use feedback to relay to the patient the effect of his words. This method helps keep the patient on course or alters the course. It involves acknowledging, validating, clarifying, extending, and altering.<br><br>*Example:*<br> "You did that well." |
| *Focus* | Focus or refocus on patient's statement. Pick up on central topics or "cues" given by the patient.<br><br>*Example:*<br> "You were telling me how hard it was to talk to your mother." |
| *Incomplete Sentences* | Encouraging the patient to continue.<br><br>*Example:*<br> "Then your life is . . ." |
| *Listening* | The process of consciously receiving another person's message.<br><br>*Example:*<br> Listening eagerly, actively, responsively, and seriously. |
| *Minimum Verbal Activity* | Keeping your own verbalization minimal and letting the patient lead the conversation.<br><br>*Example:*<br> "You feel . . .?" |
| *Mutual Fit or Congruence* | Harmony of verbal and nonverbal messages.<br><br>*Example:*<br> A patient is crying, and the nurse says, "I want to help," and puts her hand on the patient's shoulder. Or, a patient tells the nurse he feels fine but his body language indicates that he feels down, depressed, and not fine. |
| *Neutral Response* | Showing interest and involvement without attaching a value to it or saying anything else.<br><br>*Example:*<br> "Yes . . ." "Uh hm . . ." |

Using body language to communicate interest, attention, understanding, support, caring, and/ or listening in order to promote data gathering.

*Nonverbal Encouragement*

*Example:*
Nods appropriately as someone talks.

Asking questions that cannot be answered "Yes" or "No" or "Maybe," generally requiring an answer of several words in order to broaden conversational opportunities and to help the patient communicate.

*Open-ended Questions*

*Example:*
"How did your weekend pass go?" rather than "Did you have a good weekend?"

Rewording or summarizing what has been said.

*Paraphrase*

*Example:*
"You mean you're unhappy."

Identifying and sending back a message acknowledging the feeling or repeating the last few words the patient said. (Conveys acceptance and great understanding.)

*Reflection*

*Example:*
". . . distrust your doctor?"

Repeating the patient's statement as encouragement for the patient to continue.

*Restatement*

*Example:*
"You said that you hear voices."

The process of verifying the accuracy of the sender's message.

*Validation*

*Example:*
"Yes, it is confusing with so many people around."

Introducing new topics inappropriately, a pattern that may indicate anxiety.

*Changing the Subject*

**BLOCKS TO COMMUNICATION**

*Example:*
The patient is crying and discussing her fear of surgery when the nurse asks, "How many children do you have?"

Using cliches, pat answers, "cheery" words, advice, and "comforting" statements as an attempt

*False Reassurance*

to reassure the patient. Most of what is called "reassurance" is really false reassurance.

*Example:*
   "It's going to be all right."

*Giving Advice*

Telling the patient what to do. Giving your opinion, or making decisions for the patient implies he cannot handle his own life decisions and that you are accepting responsibility for him.

*Example:*
   "If I were you . . ."

*Incongruence*

Sending verbal and nonverbal messages that contradict one another; two or more messages, sent via different levels seriously contradicting one another. The contradiction may be between the content, verbal, nonverbal, and/or content (time, space).

*Example:*
   Patient: "I like your dress." Nurse: Annoyed, frowns and looks disgusted.

*Making Assumptions*

Making an assumption about the meaning of someone else's behavior that is not validated by the other person.

*Example:*
   The nurse finds the suicidal patient smiling and joking and tells the staff he's in a cheerful mood and much better.

*Invalidation*

Ignoring or denying another person's presence, thoughts, or feelings.

*Example:*
   Patient: "Hi, how are you?" Nurse: "I can't talk now, I'm on my way to lunch."

*Overloading*

Talking rapidly, changing subjects, and giving more information than can be absorbed at one time.

*Example:*
   "What's your name? I see you're forty-eight years old and that you like sports. Where do you come from?"

*Social Response*

Responding in a way that focuses attention on the nurse instead of the patient.

*Example:*
   "This sunshine is good for my roses. I have a beautiful rose garden."

Remaining silent and unresponsive, not picking up cues, and failing to give feedback.

*Underloading*

*Example:*
"What's your name?" Nurse: Smiles and walks away.

Giving one's own opinion, moralizing or implying one's own values by using words such as "nice," "good," "bad," "right," "wrong," "should," and "ought."

*Value Judgments*

*Example:*
"I think he's a very good doctor."

The following nursing diagnoses may be appropriate to include in a Patient Care Plan when the components are related to establishing and maintaining therapeutic communication with your patient.

**NURSING DIAGNOSES**

| **Nursing Diagnosis** (Potential) | **Defining Characteristic; Etiology** (Examples) |
|---|---|
| ☐ Communication, Impaired: Verbal, *related to* | Inability to verbalize needs or desires, e.g., speaks a foreign language; dysarthria. |
| ☐ Social Isolation, *related to* | Insufficient interactions or communication, e.g., hospitalization. |
| ☐ Thought Processes, Alteration in, *related to* | Confusion or disorientation, e.g., sensory overload, sleep deficit. |

## UNIT ONE   THERAPEUTIC COMMUNICATION

### NURSING PROCESS DATA

**ASSESSMENT**   *Data Base*

Determine individual's ability to process information at the cognitive level.

Evaluate mental status data to establish baseline for intervention.

Evaluate ability of patient to communicate on a verbal level.

Observe what is happening with the patient here and now.

Identify developmental level of patient so interaction expectations will be realistic.

Determine whether patient exhibits primarily verbal or nonverbal behavior so you can relate to patient on the appropriate level.

Assess anxiety level of patient as anxiety will interfere with communication.

**PLANNING**   *Objectives*

To assist patient to meet own needs.

To assist patient to experience the feeling of being accepted.

To increase self-esteem of the patient.

To provide a supportive environment for change.

To institute therapeutic rather than casual or nongoal-oriented communication.

To affect or influence the patient's physical, emotional, and social environment.

### IMPLEMENTATION   *Procedures*

Introducing Self to a Patient

Beginning a Patient Interaction

Assisting a Patient to Describe Personal Experiences

Encouraging a Patient to Express Feelings and Needs

Utilizing Communication to Increase Patient's Sense of Self-Worth

### EVALUATION   *Expected Outcomes*

Patient develops the ability to assess and meet own needs.

Communication becomes clearer, more explicit, and centered on problem areas.

A supportive environment is created so that patient can reduce anxiety level and experience change.

## INTRODUCING SELF TO A PATIENT

### Procedure

1. Obtain patient assignment.
2. Read chart and review physician's orders.
3. Check Patient Care Plan.
4. Clarify any questions about patient assignment.
5. Proceed to patient's room and check room number.
6. Introduce self to patient (Example: "Good morning, Mr. Jones. My name is Miss Barnes. I am a student nurse from the Beaver School of Nursing and I will be caring for you today.")
7. If patient is blind, introduce self as you come in the door: tell exactly what you are doing and when you are leaving. **Rationale:** Blind patients become anxious when they hear someone enter room who does not speak.
8. Begin to establish a nurse-patient relationship using clear, open communication.

## BEGINNING A PATIENT INTERACTION

### Procedure

1. Following introduction, (where you call the patient by name and tell the patient your name,) relate purpose of interaction.
2. Tell patient specifically what you will be doing in terms of his care.
3. Ask if the patient understands or has any questions.
4. Encourage patient to describe how he is feeling at the time.
5. Encourage patient to participate in his care—verbally and nonverbally.
6. Pay attention to communication as well as the procedure you are administering. **Rationale:** Often, your best data base is drawn from observation.
7. Complete communication by asking patient for feedback.

8. Complete interaction by telling patient when you will return.

9. Follow through on agreed upon meeting time to build patient trust.

## ASSISTING A PATIENT TO DESCRIBE PERSONAL EXPERIENCE

### Procedure

1. Encourage patient to describe his perceptions and feelings.

2. Focus on communication but use an indirect approach.

3. Use minimal verbal activity. **Rationale:** The less you say, the more it will encourage spontaneity and verbalization from the patient.

4. Assist patient to clarify feelings.

5. Maintain an accepting, nonjudgmental attitude. **Rationale:** Making value judgments, even nonverbal ones, will destroy a nurse-patient relationship.

6. Give broad opening statements and ask open-ended questions. **Rationale:** This open approach enables the patient to describe what is happening.

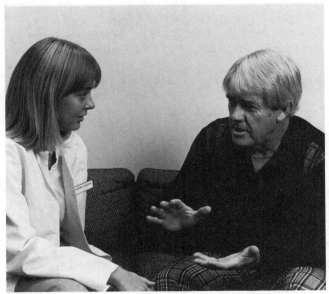

Establish a nurse-patient relationship in a safe environment before encouraging patient to describe concerns, thoughts, and feelings.

## ENCOURAGING A PATIENT TO EXPRESS NEEDS, FEELINGS, AND THOUGHTS

### Procedure

1. Focus on feelings during interactions.

2. Assist patient to identify thoughts and feelings.

3. Pick up on verbal cues, leads, and signals from the patient.

4. Convey attitude of acceptance and empathy toward the patient. **Rationale:** Being aware of your own feelings and attitudes and separating them from the patient's contributes to acceptance.

5. Note what is said as well as what is not said.

6. Assist the patient to become aware of differences between behavior, feelings, and thoughts.

7. Give honest, nonjudgmental feedback to the patient.

## UTILIZING COMMUNICATION TO INCREASE THE PATIENT'S SENSE OF SELF-WORTH

### Procedure

1. Use body language as well as verbal communication to convey empathy. **Rationale:** Sitting down at the patient's bedside or not acting as if you are in a hurry will encourage communication.

2. Respect the patient's personal "space."

3. Encourage the patient to apply the problem-solving approach to different situations.

4. Be nonjudgmental.

5. Mutually identify goals to meet the patient's individual needs.

6. Keep all agreements with the patient.

7. Be the patient's advocate.

### CHARTING *for Therapeutic Communication*

☐ Identification of patient needs

☐ Explicit goals of interaction

☐ Communication patterns of patient

☐ Emotional state of patient

☐ Expressed feelings and/or thoughts if relevant

## CLINICAL PROBLEM SOLVING

| Potential Problems | Suggested Solutions |
|---|---|
| Therapeutic communication is not achieved. | ☐ Eliminate blocks to communication from interaction style. If a block does occur, recognize it. Move to correct communication by utilizing therapeutic modes of communication.<br>☐ Evaluate own process of communication during as well as after interaction.<br>☐ If patient needs to verbalize and you cannot help him do so, contact another nurse or the social worker. |
| Patient's demanding behavior interferes with the therapeutic communication process. | ☐ Do not ignore demands; they will only increase in intensity.<br>☐ Attempt to determine causal factors of behavior, e.g., high anxiety level.<br>☐ Set limits to response patterns when patient is demanding. Control own feelings of anger and irritation.<br>☐ Teach alternative means to getting needs met. |

## TERMINOLOGY

**Acceptance:** favorable reception; basic acknowledgement.

**Agitation:** excessive restlessness and increased mental and especially physical activity.

**Anxiety:** a state of uneasiness and distress; diffuse apprehension.

**Apprehension:** a fearful or uneasy anticipation of the future; dread.

**Assistance:** aiding, helping, or giving support.

**Ataraxia:** a state of complete mental calm and tranquility.

**Attitude:** a state of mind or feeling with regard to some matter; disposition.

**Behavior:** the actions or reactions of persons under specified circumstances.

**Clarify:** to make clear or easier to understand.

**Cliché:** stereotyped response; a trite or overused expression or idea.

**Cognition:** the mental process or faculty by which knowledge is acquired.

**Communication:** the exchange of thoughts, information, or messages.

**Confusion:** disorder; jumble; distraction; bewilderment.

**Congruence:** agreement; conformity.

**Consent:** to agree; to be of the same mind.

**Convey:** to communicate or make known; to impart.

**Coping mechanism:** a means by which to adjust or adapt to disequilibrium; defense mechanism against anxiety.

**Counseling:** to give support or to provide guidance.

**Emotion:** any strong feeling, as of joy, hate, sorrow, love.

**Empathy:** ability to readily comprehend the feelings, thoughts, and motives of another person.

**Esteem:** to consider as of a certain value; regard; respect.

**Evaluate:** to examine and judge; appraise.

**Expression:** to manifest or communicate; make known.

**Helping relationship:** an interaction of individuals that sets the climate for movement of the participants toward common goals.

**Perception:** the process of receiving and interrupting sensory impressions.

**Rapport:** a feeling of mutual trust experienced by persons in a satisfactory relationship.

**Refer:**  to send or direct someone for action or help.

**Relationship:**  an interaction of individuals over a period of time.

**Self-esteem:**  a sense of pride in oneself or self-love.

**Social:**  involvement with communities and other persons.

**Support:**  to lend strength or give assistance to.

**Therapeutic:**  having medicinal or healing properties; a healing agent.

**Touch:**  a tactile sense.

**Understanding:**  to perceive and comprehend the nature and significance of; to know.

**Unique:**  being the only one of its kind.

**Validate:**  to substantiate or verify.

# Chapter *6*

# Environment and Patient Safety

## LEARNING OBJECTIVES

Define the term adaptation.

Describe three characteristics that influence adaptation.

Outline four sociocultural dimensions of environmental adaptation.

State two nursing diagnoses which could be used for maintaining a safe environment.

Outline the objectives for providing a safe environment.

List and briefly describe at least four guidelines for using restraints to prevent mechanical injuries.

Explain four methods of preventing drug injuries.

List the guidelines for providing safety when patients are receiving radioactive materials.

Demonstrate the application of wrist restraints.

Demonstrate the application of a posey restraint.

Identify at least five actions that will maintain a safe environment for infants.

List the components that should be included when charting for application of restraints.

## ORIENTATION TO THE PATIENT ENVIRONMENT

**Maintaining Homeostasis**   As a nurse, one of your primary responsibilities is to make sure your patients have a safe and comfortable health care environment. It is your responsibility to help patients adapt to this environment in addition to health care in general.

From a holistic or total view, the term "environment" can generally be explained as the total of all the conditions and influences, both external and internal, that affect the life and development of an organism. As human beings we are constantly exposed to changing physical, biological, and social conditions. In order to survive, we continually assess our relationship to our changing surroundings. We also learn how to make adjustments that help us control and improve our environment. This complex process is called "adaptation."

Adaptation includes adjustments in all conscious and unconscious forms. People in most situations are able to control or adapt to their immediate surroundings. Usually the individual knows best how to adapt to the conditions that are specifically affecting him. Although no two people will respond to the environment in exactly the same way, common principles related to adaptation can be found in all human beings:

☐ All adaptations are attempts to maintain optimum physical and chemical states or homeostasis.

☐ Individuals retain their own identity and uniqueness regardless of the degree of adaptation required.

☐ Adaptation affects all aspects of human existence.

☐ Human beings have limits in the process and degree of adaptation.

☐ Adaptation is measured in relationship to time.

☐ Adaptive responses to the environment may or may not be adequate or appropriate.

☐ Adaptive attempts may be stressful.

☐ The degree and process of adaptation varies from individual to individual.

☐ Adaptation is an ongoing and continuous process about which the individual may be consciously or unconsciously aware.

Each of us adjusts to our immediate environment in a way that is unique to us. When this environment changes suddenly, for instance when we are hospitalized, we may not be able to adapt independently to our immediate surroundings safely and comfortably. It is at this point that assistance must be provided.

The characteristics that make all people unique also provide information about the process of adaptation to the environment. These factors must be considered when assessing the patients' needs and ability to safely adjust to their immediate surroundings.

## CHARACTERISTICS THAT INFLUENCE ADAPTATION

**Age** A patient's age is a critical factor in the assessment process. Because terms such as "elderly" and "young" can be interpreted in many different ways, the nurse may need to look at the patient's developmental stage (physical and mental growth) rather than at the patient's chronological age.

As people develop, sensory receptors help process day-to-day events. Human beings learn how to protect themselves and how to adjust to changing needs through experiencing these events. During the learning process, young children may require entirely different precautions from teenagers. A thirty-year-old man who has learned through experience how to protect himself in a routine environment may not have adequate skills in an unfamiliar atmosphere.

The older adult often requires special assistance. Sensory impairments such as slowness of movement, poor vision or hearing, loss of balance, and even diminished acuity for taste and touch are not uncommon. When impairments occur, interpretation of sensory messages is altered. This can result in a decreased ability to sense harmful environmental stimuli. The older person may not see or hear an approaching car, detect the taste of spoiling food, or move quickly enough to avoid falling.

**Level of Consciousness** The ability to perceive and react to environmental stimuli is closely related to level of consciousness. Adapting to a new or different environment requires learning through experience and possessing an awareness of the immediate surroundings. Making adjustments in the environment requires stimuli to travel over the sensory pathways of nerves to the central nervous system. In order to respond to stimuli, such as avoiding a burn from a hot object, motor neurons carry impulses to muscles to cause an involuntary reflex action, such as withdrawing the hand from hot water. Sensory impulses traveling to the cerebral cortex of the brain inform the person that this stimuli is potentially harmful. Voluntary movement then provides additional adaptation.

Consciousness is the state in which individuals are aware of themselves and their relationship to their surroundings. Unconsciousness indicates a lack of response or awareness of the environment. Levels of consciousness range from fully conscious to comatose. Difficulty in adapting to the immediate environment due to varying levels of consciousness can manifest itself in a variety of ways:

☐ Disoriented patients often view their environment in a fearful, distorted way. This condition can lead to extreme behavioral changes, self injury, or combativeness.

☐ Neurologically injured patients may have decreased perceptions of stimuli such as heat, cold, pain, or friction. In extreme cases, they may have no perception of stimuli at all.

☐ Partial or total paralysis inhibits movement and is accompanied by a loss of position sense (dangling limbs or poor body alignment).

☐ Alterations in communication, sight, or hearing because of altered consciousness are barriers to sharing fears or concerns with others.

☐ Fluctuating levels of consciousness create difficulty in promoting self-care and self-image because of an inability to follow directions.

Continuous assessment of changes in the patient's level of consciousness is essential. Degree of awareness influences the type and amount of assistance the patient will need while in less than familiar surroundings.

**States of Illness**   Illness or injury causes a person to focus more intensely on himself. The very nature of disease or trauma requires the individual to use physical and mental energy to adapt to the situation and to become more egocentric. A patient often cannot perform even the simplest daily activity. Fatigue or pain may render patients helpless. Assistance with activities such as bathing, eating, skin care, and elimination may be necessary.

When medications are used, side effects such as drowsiness prevent the individual from adequately assessing the environment. Perceptions may be distorted, and the patient is more vulnerable to hazards.

Emotional stress and anxiety can occur in mild to acute degrees. While mild anxiety very often increases perceptual awareness, acute anxiety reduces perceptual awareness.

Because an individual is able to focus only on a specific amount of stimuli at one time, additional stimuli that may be equally important are not perceived. Potential environmental dangers are not processed. The patient whose energy is focused on pain may not even hear instructions from the nurse. Depressed patients will also require assistance. Depression often results in slower than normal responses to stimuli. Alcohol, a central nervous system depressant, also causes dull, slow reactions to stimuli.

When pain, anxiety, illness, injury, weakness, medications, or even lack of sleep cause a decrease in sensory acuity, awareness of potential hazards is altered. The patient may not be able to make the necessary biological, physical, or emotional adjustments to adapt to the immediate environment. Any of these conditions necessitates immediate assessment and action.

**PHYSICAL AND BIOLOGICAL DIMENSIONS**

The influences that make up an environment include the basic categories of biological and physical conditions. The biological dimensions of our environment that will be covered in this section include all living things, such as plants, animals, and microorganisms. Water, oxygen, sunlight, organic com-

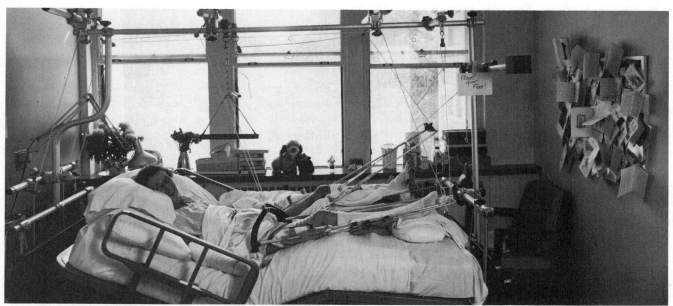

Provide a safe and comfortable environment with space for personal effects.

pounds, and other components in which living things exist and develop make up the physical dimensions of an environment.

As you become more aware of the factors that affect environmental adaptation, providing a safe and comfortable atmosphere for your patients becomes a greater challenge. As you assess your patients and help them adapt to the environment of a health care facility, you will want to consider the following essential elements: space, lighting, humidity, temperature, ventilation, sound levels, surfaces and equipment, safety, food and water and waste disposal.

**Adequate Space**   Everyone needs space in which to grow and develop. This space may consist of a room or an area as small as a shelf or corner. No matter what form space takes, individuals need to feel they have control over it—to be able to arrange it or decorate it to their liking.

Providing space for patients encourages stimulation and experimentation. Toddlers need the space of an area like a recreation room for discovery and motor skills, since playtime is their primary source of development. Adults often enjoy the social activities of a lounge, but may also require well-defined personal areas even if these areas are as simple as a bedside table or a bulletin board.

**Natural and Artificial Light**   Light, like space, is necessary for growth and development. The production of vitamin D, a critical component of bone structure, occurs from ultra-violet radiation on the skin. Natural light also helps wounds heal. In a hospital setting, natural light can be used to decrease feelings of isolation and to encourage patients to continue their normal routine.

Whether natural or artificial, adequate light is essential for the preservation of sight, for safety, and for accurate assessments and nursing care. Because eye strain, as well as nervousness and fatigue can result from improper lighting, care should be taken to avoid glare, sharp contrast, and flickering lights.

**Humidity and Temperature**   The ability to adapt to changes in humidity and/or temperature is directly related to comfort. Most people in this country are comfortable at a room temperature of 18.3° to 25° C (65° to 77° F) with the humidity at 30 to 60 percent. People in other cultures function equally well at lower or higher readings.

Conditions that may inhibit a person's ability to adjust to high temperatures include excessive physical work, dehydration, extremes in age (the very young and very old), decreased physical fitness, and inappropriate clothing. An individual who has difficulty adapting to high temperatures may experience a rapid rise in pulse rate, cramps, nausea, and vomiting. Severe inability to adapt to heat can result in heat stroke and death.

An individual who has difficulty adapting to lower temperatures may experience a change in behavior, depressed vital signs, and eventual unconsciousness. Hypothermia, an abnormally low body temperature, occurs when there is an imbalance between heat loss and heat production.

Extreme heat or extreme cold increases the incidence of infection and adds to discomfort. Temperatures in health care institutions can be regulated with air conditioners and dehumidifiers, although care should be taken to avoid drafts and excessive dryness.

**Ventilation**   Particular attention should be given to assessing the movement or air within a patient's immediate environment. An adequately ventilated room should contain a comfortable amount of moisture, be free of irritating pollutants, odors, or noxious fumes, and be at a tolerable temperature.

Adequate ventilation is especially important when more than one patient is in a room. Other areas requiring optimum ventilation are operating rooms, delivery rooms, nurseries, isolation rooms, and sterile supply rooms.

A properly functioning ventilation system reduces airborne contaminants by regulating the amount of air movement within an enclosed area. When ventilation cannot be maintained by using doors and windows, mechanical devices such as fans or air conditioners may be used.

**Comfortable Sound Levels**   Noise can be defined as any undesirable sound. The degree of noise that is comfortable is highly individual and related to past experiences. A businessman who lives on a busy street in a city may not adjust well to the absolute quiet he may experience at night in a hospital room. On the other hand, a farmer from a rural community may be disturbed by the slightest sound. Infants often sleep peacefully in an atmosphere of loud noise and activity.

"Decibel" is the term used to describe the intensity of noise, or the measurement of the sensation produced by sound on the human ear. At close range noise produced from heavy traffic, for example, has a decibel measure of 90, whereas a whisper at three feet has an intensity of 20 decibels.

At certain levels noise is considered hazardous. Temporary or permanent hearing loss or damage can occur when noise is present for a prolonged time at intensities over 90 decibels. Other effects of sustained loud noise are muscle tension, increased blood pressure, blood vessel constriction, pallor, increased secretion of the adrenal hormone, and nervous tension.

The pitch and quality of noise may also affect the patient's environment. Unwanted sounds produced by sirens, traffic, and aircraft are often beyond the control of the nurse. But noise within a hospital setting, especially loud talking, television, call systems, careless handling of dishes and other equipment, visitors, and excessive conversation at the nurses' station, can be controlled.

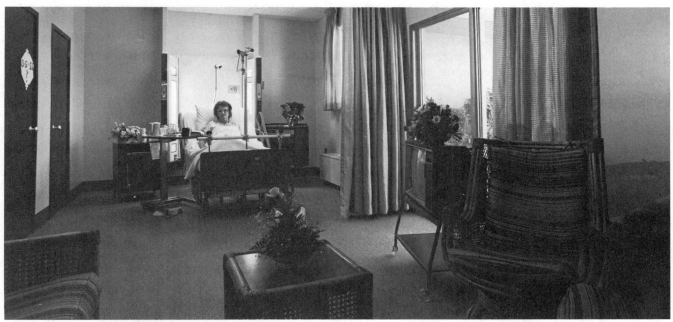

A pleasant environment promotes a feeling of well-being.

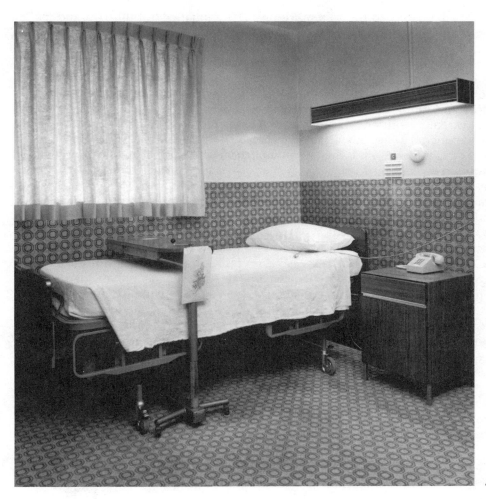

A typical basic room in the hospital.

Nursing personnel should always be aware of the noise level and its effects on the patient's well-being. Very ill individuals are often more sensitive to noise. Although too much noise can be a barrier to adapting to the immediate environment, absolute silence can be annoying and even frightening. Certain sounds can be reassuring because they represent activity or assistance to the patient.

**Furniture and Clean Surfaces**    Today, most health care facilities are designed to be attractive, orderly, efficient, and clean. Since a person's outlook is strongly influenced by the surroundings, careful attention to appearance and cleanliness can assist with adjustment to the health care environment. Although it is essential to assess the routines and standards of cleanliness of each patient, the nurse may also have to teach the patient how to organize and clean up. In some cases, instruction to the patient may be critical to maintain or improve a health care condition.

The standards and routine cleaning procedures of the hospital are generally not a nursing function now because hospital housekeeping has become a specialized occupation. Maintaining an organized, clean environment, however, requires coordination by all health care providers.

Furnishings should be arranged to be physically comfortable, safe, aesthetically appealing for the patient and easily cleaned. Adequate cleaning of the room should be done at a time of day that is coordinated with the patient's needs so that the resulting sense of security adds to the patient's ability to adapt adequately to the surroundings. The ambiance of the room and a sense of order contribute to the patient's sense of well-being.

The furniture in a typical patient unit should be comfortable, safe for the patient, and convenient for the staff. All furniture and equipment should be movable and easily cleaned. Hospital beds are usually adjustable in height from the floor; when the bed is in "LOW" position the patient can more easily and safely get in or out of it; when it is in "HIGH" position, the nursing staff can more efficiently render care. A step stool may be necessary to enable some patients to get in and out of bed safely. The head and knee areas of the bed can be elevated; this is accomplished by electric controls or by hand cranks. The cranks, if used, are at the foot of the bed with the "head" crank on the left and the "knee" crank on the right. Remember to replace the cranks under the bed when not in use. This placement prevents the hospital staff from running into them. The electric controls are found on either the foot or the side of the bed. When placed at the side, the patient can more easily control his own bed positions. Bed wheels should be equipped with locks. Adjustable side rails are placed on both sides of the patient's bed for safety and a sense of security. Hospital policy dictates the use of side rails, so remember to replace them in position when you have completed patient care.

The overbed table is adjustable in height and slides over the bed to provide space for self-care activities or additional working surface for the nurse. The overbed table may also be used when the patient sits in a chair. Small bed trays are sometimes convenient when the overbed table cannot be used.

The bedside table, similar to a nightstand, holds the patient's valuable or personal possessions in drawers. A cabinet section in the table can be used to store bathing or toiletry equipment, and the top provides space for the patient's familiar items such as pictures or books.

A chair with firm back and arm supports should always be a part of the patient's furnishing. Chairs should be made of durable, easily cleanable materials such as plastic or naugahyde. The patient should be instructed to avoid

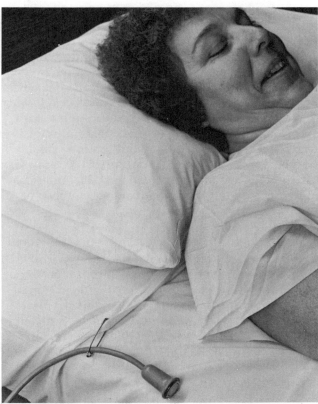

Attach call button within patient's reach and instruct how to use.

contact between skin surfaces and the chair when sitting in a chair. A small towel or blanket can be placed under the patient for this purpose.

A signaling system is also essential for the patient to call for assistance. A signaling system may be an intercom, buzzer, electric light, or handbell. Whatever device is available must be within a patient's reach and ability to use.

**Food and Water**   Fresh, healthful food and clean water, vital elements in an everyday routine, must be planned for and ensured in appropriate amounts in health care facilities. While a patient's well-being can be positively affected by the ingestion of the correct number of calories, fat, proteins, carbohydrates, minerals, vitamins, and water, it is well known that many people have nutritional habits that can negatively affect their well-being. A careful nutritional assessment is a critical step in helping the patient adjust to the environment.

**Waste Disposal**   All waste products, whether contaminated equipment, human body wastes, garbage, soiled dressings, or refuse, must be disposed of in a way that prevents the spread of microorganisms. Hospital wastes can be hazardous and highly infective. If wastes cannot be properly removed, the individual is at a risk and may not be able to adjust safely and comfortably to the surroundings.

Nurses must be aware of the potential dangers to themselves as well as to their patients when disposing of waste materials. Most health care agencies have specific guidelines regarding the removal of various types of contaminated materials. Many of these guidelines have been established by experts (epidemiologists) knowledgeable in the detection and spread of diseases. The U.S. Public Health Service Center for Disease Control, the American Hospital Association, and State Departments of Health are some of the agencies that prepare guidelines for the disposal of dangerous products.

In some health care facilities, a position of infection control nurse has been created to gather data on the type and frequency of various infections found in the hospital. Data about infections helps the infection control nurse to locate the source of the problem, to predict its spread, and to identify the best method of prevention to decrease its recurrence. Many of the nosocomial, hospital-originated disease states, can be traced to inappropriate or careless disposal of wastes. Each nurse plays a significant role in establishing a safe environment for the patient by carrying out the recommended methods of waste disposal.

## SOCIOCULTURAL DIMENSIONS

The first two dimensions of the environment, the biological and physical or ecosystem, refer to all living and nonliving elements. The third dimension of an environment is sociocultural, which includes both past and present influences from the people and the culture surrounding the individual. Customs, religious and legal systems, and economic and political beliefs are all part of this environment. *See* chapter seven "Religious Guidelines for Patient Care." This dimension also involves responses and adjustments to the ideals, concepts, beliefs, activities, and pressure of various groups such as social clubs, peer groups, or colleagues.

**Organization of Time**    How patients perceive and deal with time and the passing of time depend on their age, immediate situation, culture, and past experiences as well as their present physical and emotional condition. To a mother waiting for her child to return from surgery, hours seem like days. Small children generally do not have a well-developed sense of time. A three-year-old may act out feelings of abandonment when separated from a parent for just a few minutes. In an intensive care unit, time can be severely disrupted since health care activities continue around the clock. The ability to organize time is a critical element in adaptation. Helping patients assess and plan their time is one of the most important ways you can help them cope with their new surroundings.

**Privacy**    Many people who enter a health care facility fear exposure and loss of identity. Providing privacy for a patient is more than a luxury or a desirable condition. It is necessary and vitally important to the individual's attitude toward health care.

Patients should be given as much privacy as possible. Most individuals will give clues to the nurse about the degree of privacy that is comfortable. The patient's culture, past experience, values, and age should all be considered when planning for privacy.

Hospital routines should be planned to promote privacy. If an embarrassing or upsetting situation occurs, the feelings of the patient must be protected. People require time and space to think, organize, and reflect. Privacy is necessary for human development even at home. In the hospital, privacy is critical to the patient's attitude and well-being.

Privacy can be promoted by drawing curtains or screens. Doors and window shades may also be used. Signs posted on room entrances give the patient a sense of security from disturbances. This is especially important

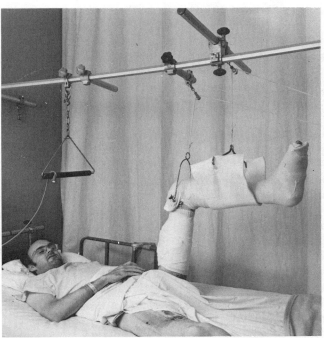

When giving individualized care, ensure privacy by closing curtains.

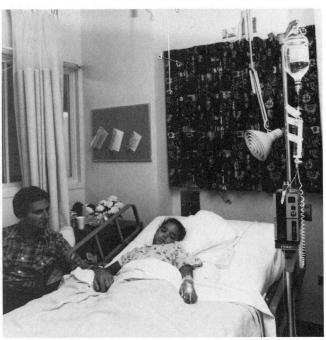

Encourage family visits to reduce stress and maintain contact.

during physical exams, personal care, or emotional upset. Knocking or asking for permission to enter the patient's room or area promotes mutual respect and enhances a sense of emotional space.

Privacy also extends beyond the physical need of the individual. Health status, conversation, and records are privileged information. A more trusting, therapeutic relationship will evolve if the patient understands that the confidences the patient shares with nurses will be used appropriately for his well-being.

**Individualized Care**    Providing an environment that is comfortable, safe, and individualized to meet the specific needs of a patient is a challenging task. The patient's adaptation to the immediate environment can either improve or interfere with the patient's well-being. In order to assist the patient in adjusting to the environment, a careful assessment of the situation should always include the person's usual routines, self-care abilities, cultural beliefs, and past experiences. To promote the best adaptation to a different environment, encourage as much independence as possible with each patient. You may be required to use your resourcefulness, imagination, and ingenuity to assist the patient through less than desirable periods. Open communication processes from patient to staff is essential if positive adaptation is to occur.

Hospitalized patients also need emotional space. This form of space is that psychological area where the person can experience a sense of self. This is particularly difficult to achieve in a hospital setting when caretakers exercise control over many of the activities of daily living. It is important that the staff be aware of this element of space so that they can provide adequate privacy, quiet, and freedom of choice over all of the areas that the patient can control. The staff must also be aware that the patient never need relinquish total responsibility for his care.

**Information and Teaching**    The amount of information the patient has about the environment and immediate situation directly affects the patient's ability to safely and comfortably adjust. When the individual is given information and explanation about strange equipment, diagnostic procedures, or unfamiliar health care personnel, fears and feelings of helplessness can be reduced and a shared sense of responsibility enhanced. The patient becomes more capable of asking questions and expressing concerns if prepared for unfamiliar occurrences.

Providing the patient and the patient's family, if appropriate, with information about the patient's environment is the responsibility of the nurse. As more people assume the role of consumers of health care, there is more demand for knowledge about aspects of health care. Including the patient in planning and caring for himself promotes a sense of responsibility, independence, and self-respect.

Teaching the patient about various aspects of health care is one method of information-sharing. Over the years, the focus has changed from the professional staff doing everything for the patient to helping the patient be more independent. This change enables the patient to adapt to the environment with guided assistance from nurses. As the patient learns about his own health care and becomes involved in meeting his particular needs, a sense of trust, responsibility, and usefulness develops.

## A SAFE ENVIRONMENT

Providing a safe environment involves a number of people, including the patient, visitors, and health care providers. Providing protection from hazardous situations and education about safety precautions is one of your most important responsibilities as a nurse.

Patients who are moved from their usual environment into one that is unfamiliar and often frightening may act in ways that are very different from their usual behavior. A threatening situation can interfere with the individual's adaptation to the immediate surroundings.

The design and decor of the patient's room must satisfy two needs: patient comfort and patient safety. Tasteful, unobtrusive color helps to normalize the hospital room. Interesting color combinations and patterns generally appeal more to the senses than do the traditional white or green choices. Pictures, flowers, cards, colorful linens, and curtains can add variety and familiarity to a room.

**Safety Precautions**    The age of the patient influences the specific safety precautions that need to be taken to provide a safe environment. For example, infants require constant supervision since they may attempt to put anything in their mouths or up their noses.

Preschool age children can be taught more detailed aspects of safety. Fire precautions and guidelines for bathing should be stressed.

Elementary school age children can usually protect themselves from hazards. They will require instruction on how to operate mechanical equipment, as well as information about fires and emergency exits.

Teenagers, adolescents, and adults should be given instruction about smoking, fire exits, and the use of special equipment. In addition, general information regarding their safety during hospitalization should be explained.

Elderly adults are especially susceptible to injury from falls. Poor vision, decreased balance and stability, disorientation, or chronic physical problems such as arthritis contribute to the high incidence of falls among the elderly. Safety precautions for the elderly include the following:

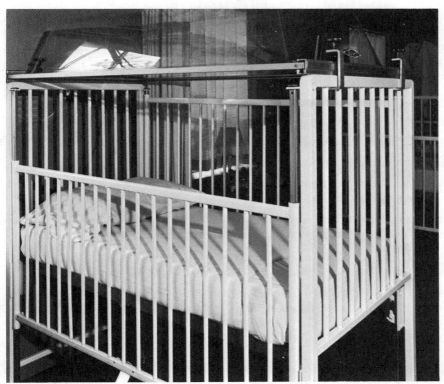

Hood prevents child from climbing out of bed.

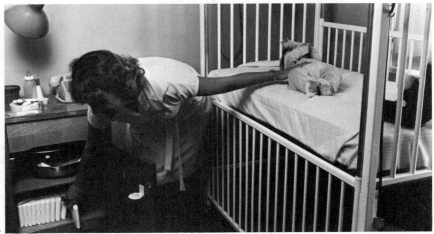

Always provide patient with a safe environment.

□ Keep hallways clear of toys, scatter rugs, lamp cords, etc.

□ Provide adequate lighting.

□ Put necessary articles for personal hygiene and activities of daily living within easy reach.

□ Provide nonslip mats and handrails in bath tubs and showers.

□ Provide handrails in hallways and near toilets.

**Preventing Injury Using Restraints**  Restraints may be ordered to prevent injury to the patient or to promote safety when the patient is in bed or in a chair. A physician's order is usually required when soft restraints are used.

The most common type of soft restraints is often referred to as a "posey," since most soft restraints are made by the Posey Company. In some facilities the physician's order will read "Posey prn." In other facilities the order may read "supportive/restrictive garment for patient's protection prn."

If restraints are necessary these guidelines should be followed.

☐ Use restraints for the patient's protection, not for your convenience.

☐ Review hospital policy or doctor's orders for the use of restraints.

☐ Allow patient as much freedom of movement as possible.

☐ Always explain the purpose of the restraint to patient.

☐ Remember that restraints can cause increased anxiety and a feeling of decreasing self-image.

☐ Remember that circulation and skin integrity can be affected by restraints. Frequently observe areas around the restraint for circulatory impairment or broken skin.

☐ Pad bony prominences, i.e., wrists and ankles, beneath a restraint.

☐ Attempt to make restraints as inconspicuous as possible for the patient's sake as well as relatives and friends, who may be upset by seeing restraints.

## NURSING DIAGNOSES

The following nursing diagnoses may be appropriate to include in a Patient Care Plan when the components are related to maintaining a safe environment.

| Nursing Diagnosis (Potential) | Defining Characteristic; Etiology (Examples) |
|---|---|
| ☐ Injury, Potential for, *related to* | Impaired judgment, muscle weakness, e.g., age and/or disease process. |
| ☐ Sensory-Perceptual Alteration, *related to* | Disorientation, confusion, e.g., altered sleep pattern, environmental factors. |
| | Hearing loss, cataracts, e.g., age and/or disease process. |
| ☐ Thought Processes, Alteration in, *related to* | Altered perception of reality, e.g., psychosocial, emotional or chemical factors (drugs). |

## UNIT ONE   A SAFE ENVIRONMENT

### NURSING PROCESS DATA

#### ASSESSMENT   *Data Base*

Identify patient's age, previous or chronic sensory impairments, previous level of mobility, ambulatory aids used, and general health history.

Observe and record patient's present level of consciousness, orientation, mobility, and restrictions.

Identify any impending loss of sensory or motor abilities due to illness or injury.

Evaluate patient's ability to comprehend instruction about how to use potentially dangerous equipment.

Assess need for specific devices to promote a safe environment.

Assess type of fire extinguisher needed for specific types of fires.

Assess the need for protection while administering care to patients with radioactive implant.

Evaluate patient's ability to make judgments.

Assess the patient's reliability as an accurate health historian.

## PLANNING   *Objectives*

To assist patient to interpret environmental stimuli relevant to his or her safety.

To provide protection when states of illness decrease the individual's ability to receive and interpret environmental stimuli.

To enhance degrees of mobility in a safe environment.

To determine that all electrical equipment is intact and operated safely.

To place all personal articles and call light within easy reach of patient.

To determine safety equipment necessary to promote a safe environment.

To determine the protective devices needed when caring for patients receiving radioactive material.

## IMPLEMENTATION   *Procedures*

Preventing Mechanical Injuries

Preventing Thermal Injuries

Providing Safety for Patients During a Fire

Providing Safety for Patients Receiving Radioactive Materials

## EVALUATION   *Expected Outcomes*

Patient receives information regarding mechanical, chemical, and thermal safety precautions appropriate to his or her needs.

Patient's immediate environment is safe from potential mechanical, chemical, and thermal hazards.

Patients who smoke do so according to hospital policy.

All electrical equipment is intact and operated safely.

If oxygen is used, appropriate safety measures are in effect.

All personal articles and call light are within easy reach of the patient.

Personnel are protected from radioactive material.

## PREVENTING MECHANICAL INJURIES

### Equipment

Side rails

Restraints

Locks for movable equipment such as wheelchairs and guerneys

### Procedure

1. Put bed in low position when you are not in patient's room.

2. Tell patients who are weak, in pain, or who have had surgery to ask for assistance before getting out of bed.

3. Make sure floors are free of debris that might cause patients to slip and fall. Spilled liquids should be wiped up immediately. Encourage housekeepers to use signs for slippery areas.

4. Check to see that patient's unit and hallway are neat and free of hazardous equipment such as foot stools, electrical cords, shoes, etc.

5. Place articles such as call light, cups, etc., within the patient's reach.

6. Remind patient and hospital personnel to lock wheelchairs and guerneys and to release the lock only after patient is secure.

7. Keep side rails up for all confused, elderly, seizure and surgical patients.

8. Soft restraints should be ordered and applied to any patient in danger of falling from bed or wheelchair.

## PREVENTING THERMAL INJURIES

### Equipment

Fire extinguishers

Covers for heat and cold application devices

Oxygen-In-Use signs

No smoking signs

### Procedure

1. Make sure that all electrical appliances are routinely checked and maintained.

2. Have all electrical appliances brought to the hospital by patient (radios, electric razors, etc.) checked by the hospital maintenance staff.

3. When hot-water bottles, heating pads, baths, hot compresses, and heat lamps are used, check the patient frequently for redness.

4. When oxygen sources are used, post "No Smoking" signs and explain the combustible nature of oxygen to patients and families.

5. If smoking is allowed where oxygen is not in use, provide non-tip ashtrays. Inform patients and visitors about hospital's smoking regulations. Do not allow confused, sedated, or severely incapacitated patient to smoke without direct supervision.

6. Store all combustible materials securely to prevent spontaneous combustion.

7. Make sure that all staff and employees participate in and understand fire prevention measures such as extinguishing fires and evacuating patients.

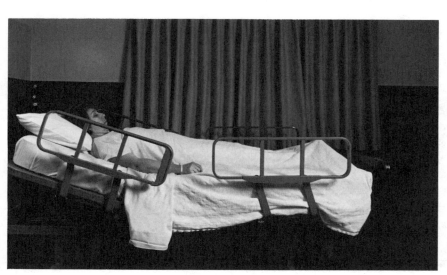

Side rails are up for the patient's safety.

## PROVIDING SAFETY FOR PATIENTS DURING A FIRE

### Equipment

Appropriate extinguisher for fire:

Water type

Soda-acid type

Foam type

Dry chemical type

Carbon dioxide type

### Procedure

1. Remove all patients from the immediate area to a safe place.

2. Follow hospital policy and procedure for type of fire prevention program and ringing the fire alarm to summon help.

3. Secure the burning area by closing all doors.

4. Shut off all possible oxygen sources and electrical appliances in the fire area.

5. If possible, employ the appropriate extinguishing method without endangering yourself.

6. Be familiar with the different types of fire extinguishers.

   *Class A*
   a. Water type or soda-acid type.
   b. Used on cloth, wood, paper, plastic, rubber, leather.
   c. Never used on electrical or chemical fires due to danger of shock.

   *Class B*
   a. Foam, dry chemical, carbon dioxide types.
   b. Used on fires such as alcohol, acetone, oil, grease, paint thinner and remover.
   c. Class A extinguisher is never used on class B fires.

   *Class C*
   a. Dry chemical or carbon dioxide types.
   b. Used on electrical wiring, electrical equipment, or motors.
   c. Class A or class B extinguishers are never used on a class C fire.

7. Clear all fire exits.

8. To safely remove a patient from the fire, use carrying method that is most comfortable for you and safe for the patient.

## PROVIDING SAFETY FOR PATIENTS RECEIVING RADIOACTIVE MATERIALS

### Equipment

Protective shields for x-ray

Lead shielded container if required

Film badge if required

### Procedure

1. Review these guidelines:
   a. Increased time in the presence of a radioactive source increases exposure to radiation.
   b. Shields, such as lead walls or lead aprons, are used as a protective source.
   c. Exposure is greater the closer you are to the radioactive source.
   d. When not in use, radioactive material must be stored in lead-shielded containers.

2. If you or a family member are assisting with a radioactive procedure, put on a shield.

3. If a radioactive implant is used in a patient, make sure all nurses and visitors are protected with a shield. Limit their exposure with the patient.

4. Keep track of how much time you spend in the presence of radioactive material. Request film badge if in area where ionizing radiation is used frequently.

5. Dispose of excreta carefully, according to hospital policy. Wear rubber gloves when handling bedpans, urinals, drainage bags and specimens for specified period following nuclear medicine procedures.

6. Determine the type and amount of radiation used and its side effects and hazards.

7. Constantly assess and support patients who are undergoing radiation therapy. Bed rest, isolation, and unpleasant side effects are sometimes common.

### CHARTING *for Providing a Safe Environment*

☐ Assessment notes

☐ Actual incidents involving mechanical, chemical, or thermal trauma

☐ Patient education given

☐ Safety devices used

## CLINICAL PROBLEM SOLVING

| **Potential Problems** | **Suggested Solutions** |
|---|---|
| The patient, nurse, or visitor experiences an accident or injury related to mechanical, chemical, or thermal trauma. | ☐ Provide immediate first aid or care.<br>☐ Assess vital signs and notify physician.<br>☐ Report the incident according to hospital procedure. Incident reports are used to protect the injured individual as well as the nurse and the hospital.<br>☐ Review safety procedures to ensure a safe environment.<br>☐ Report all malfunctioning equipment immediately to the proper department. |
| Unfamiliarity with hospital and/or fire and disaster protocol results in poor performance. | ☐ Review protocols frequently to update knowledge base.<br>☐ Participate in fire and disaster drills to become familiar with protocols. |
| Radium implant becomes dislodged and falls out. | ☐ Put on lead gloves and pick up radium with forceps and place in lead-shielded container.<br>☐ Notify physician immediately. |

# UNIT TWO   RESTRAINTS

## NURSING PROCESS DATA

### ASSESSMENT   *Data Base*

Assess need for restraints.

Identify appropriate type of restraint needed.

Assess area under and surrounding a restraint to ensure it is not restrictive.

Evaluate the affected extremity for circulation, sensation and movement.

### PLANNING   *Objectives*

To identify patients who are at risk for injury.

To prevent a patient from injuring himself in a fall.

To apply restraints safely and effectively.

To restrain a child's elbow to prevent the child from reaching an incision.

To promote patient safety when ambulating or sitting in a chair.

To obtain physician's order for restraints.

### IMPLEMENTATION   *Procedures*

Using Wrist Restraints

Using Mitt Restraints

Using Elbow Restraints

Applying a Safety Belt

Applying a Posey Restraint

Applying Mummy Restraints

**EVALUATION** *Expected Outcomes*

Restraints are applied appropriately.

Injuries to surrounding tissue are avoided when restraints are applied.

Patient is prevented from falling and injuring himself.

Child is prevented from reaching the incisional site.

## USING WRIST RESTRAINTS

### Equipment

Kerlix gauze

Cloth restraints with flannel padding

Ace bandages of appropriate size for area to be immobilized

Call bell for communication

### Procedure

1. Check physician's order for soft restraints if required.

2. Obtain Kerlix gauze or cloth restraint with flannel padding.

3. When using Kerlix gauze, make a clove hitch to place over wrist or ankle and secure under bed.

4. When using cloth restraint, place padded section over the wrist or ankle, wrap restraint around the wrist, and slide the strap through the slit in the wrist area. Tighten the strap securely but maintain adequate circulation. Fasten strap under the bed frame using a square knot.

5. Check limbs every two hours for circulation and skin condition.

6. Change patient's position every two hours.

7. Release restraints every two hours and administer skin care.

8. Put extremities through range of motion every two hours.

9. Document use of wrist restraints in nurses' notes.

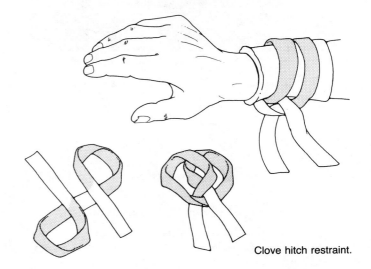

Clove hitch restraint.

If using leather restraints as wrist restraints, keep the key in patient's room taped to the wall or top of bed. It must be in sight and have easy access in case of emergency.

## USING MITT RESTRAINTS

### Equipment

Mitt restraint

Gauze padding

Call bell for communication

### Procedure

1. Check physician's order or unit policy for soft restraint.

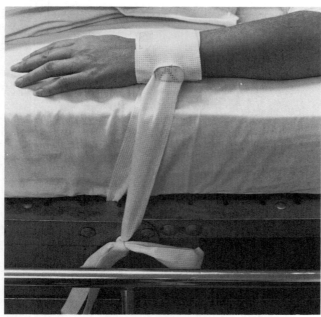

Tie soft wrist restraints firmly on bed frame, not on side rail.

2. Check nursing care plan or Kardex for specifics.
3. Wash hands.
4. Obtain mitt restraint and gauze padding, if needed.
5. Identify the patient by checking identaband.
6. Explain steps and purpose of procedure to patient (to gain his/her cooperation) if patient is able to understand.
7. Raise bed to high position.
8. Lower side rail.
9. Check condition of skin and circulation in involved extremity.
10. Wrap fingers with gauze to absorb moisture and prevent abrasion, if necessary.
11. Apply mitt; secure wrist ties snugly, but maintain circulation.
12. For hand control, tie restraints to moveable part of bed frame, not to side rail.
13. Place call-light within easy reach for patient.
14. Remove mitt every two hours to check adequacy of circulation and skin condition.
15. Put extremity through range of motion.
16. Reposition patient for comfort and reapply mitt.
17. Raise bedrail and lower bed.

18. Wash hands.
19. Chart on nurses' notes: patient behavior necessitating restraint; condition of skin and adequacy of circulation of involved extremity; time and site of mitt application; time of release and reaction of patient.

## USING ELBOW RESTRAINTS

### Equipment

Elbow restraint

Soft padding

### Procedure

1. Check physician's order and Patient Care Plan for elbow restraints.
2. Obtain elbow restraints (many types are available).
3. Explain necessity of restraints to parents of child.
4. Place restraints over elbow of both arms. You may need to insert tongue blades into pockets of restraint.
5. Wrap restraints snugly around the arm. Secure by tying the restraints at the top. Many restraints have ties long enough to cross under the child's back and tie under the opposite arm.
6. For small infants and children, tie or pin restraints to their shirts.
7. Release the restraints every two hours to allow joint mobility.
8. Assess position of restraints, circulation, skin condition and sensation every hour.
9. Provide diversionary activity for small child.
10. Encourage parents or hospital personnel to hold child to promote a feeling of security.
11. Document use of restraints in nurses' notes.

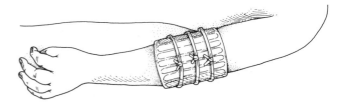

Elbow restraints prevent children from reaching equipment.

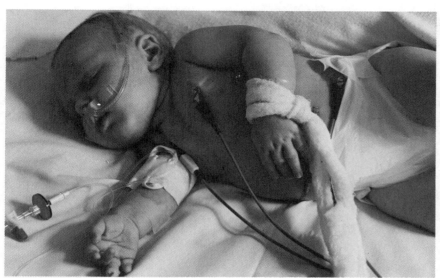

Soft restraints protect infant from injury.

## APPLYING A SAFETY BELT

### Equipment

Safety belt

### Procedure

1. Check physician's order and Patient Care Plan for safety belt restraint.
2. Obtain safety belt. (Belts usually have a buckle to prevent slipping and to provide a snug fit.)
3. Explain necessity for safety belt to patient.
4. Apply safety belt as follows:
   a. If patient is ambulating, place belt around patient's waist.
   b. If patient is on a guerney, CircOlectric bed, or Stryker frame, fasten belt around patient's abdomen.
   c. If patient is in a wheelchair, place belt around patient's abdomen and under arm rests, and secure in back.
5. If strap does not have a buckle, tie the belt in a square knot to allow for quick removal in an emergency.
6. Document use of safety belt in nurses' notes.

## APPLYING A POSEY RESTRAINT

### Equipment

Posey jacket

Call bell for communication

### Procedure

1. Check physician's order and Patient Care Plan for restraint if required.
2. Explain necessity for restraint to patient and family.
3. Place front part of jacket over patient's chest, and instruct patient to lean forward slightly.
4. Cross the lower and upper straps and tie the straps to frame of bed or behind wheelchair.
5. If jacket has slits in the side, pass the straps through the slits and then secure them to the bed frame or the wheelchair.
6. Observe patient frequently to ensure proper fit of the jacket.
7. Document use of restraints in nurses' notes.

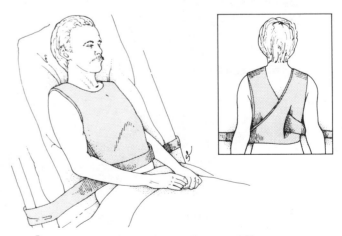

Posey restraints are most often used for the safety of the patient.

# APPLYING MUMMY RESTRAINTS

## Equipment

Blanket

## Procedure

1. Place the blanket on a secure surface.
2. Fold down one corner of the blanket until the tip reaches the middle of the blanket.
3. Place the baby in a diagonal position with the head halfway off the folded edge of the blanket.
4. Bring one side of the blanket over the infant's arm and trunk and tuck it under his other arm and around his back.
5. Tuck the bottom part of the blanket up onto the abdomen of the infant.
6. Fold the second side over the infant and tuck it snugly around his body.

> Mummy boards with Velcro straps are used more often in the hospital setting. A diaper or chux is placed on the board, the infant is placed in the board and secured with the Velcro straps.

## CHARTING  *for Applying Restraints*

☐ Time and type of restraint applied

☐ Rationale for applying restraints

☐ Condition of extremity following application: skin color and temperature

☐ Time of removal and reapplication of restraint

☐ Effectiveness of restraint

☐ Patient's tolerance of restraint

---

## CLINICAL PROBLEM SOLVING

### Potential Problems

Skin abrasion, maceration or rash occurs following application of restraints.

### Suggested Solutions

☐ Reassess application method if problem is caused by improperly applied restraints.

☐ Increase padding of soft restraints before application.

☐ Keep restraints off as much as possible and have family member or staff stay with patient when restrained.

Impaired circulation and/or edema evidenced by change in color, sensation, movement and blanching of nail beds.

☐ Upon observation of signs of neurovascular changes, immediately release restraints.

☐ Massage area gently to increase circulation.

☐ If extremity is edematous, elevate extremity above level of heart.

☐ Request order for different type of restraint.

Patient unties restraints while in wheelchair.

☐ If a half-bow was used to secure the restraint, retie in a square knot.
Tie one end of a restraint (not the one used for patient) to the arm of the wheelchair and the other end to a railing or immovable equipment and allow the patient to untie the knot on the pseudo restraint. For confused or head-injured patients it is useful to divert attention from the restraint knot.

Child is able to reach incisional site even with elbow restraints in place.

☐ Make sure the elbow restraints are tight enough and extend over the elbow.

□ Tie the one elbow restraint to the opposite elbow restraint by placing the tie under the child's back and securing the tie with the upper tie on the opposite restraint.

□ Check that the restraint is large enough to completely immobilize the elbow. If not, obtain a larger size or use two restraints and tie them together securely.

Patient successfully gets out of the posey restraint.

□ Put one posey restraint on frontwards and one posey restraint on backwards. Secure both of the restraints under the bed frame.

## ━━━━ TERMINOLOGY ━━━━

**Adaptation:**  ability of an organism to adjust to a change in environment.

**Ambiance:**  the pervading atmosphere of the surrounding environment.

**Ambulation:**  to move from place to place by walking.

**Aseptic:**  sterile; a condition free from bacteria and infection.

**Assessment:**  critical evaluation of information; the first step in the nursing process.

**Behavior:**  a person's total activity—actions or reactions; especially conduct that can be observed.

**Comprehensive health care:**  a total system of health care that takes the whole person into account.

**Contaminated waste:**  radioactive waste which, if improperly disposed of, may be harmful or cause a radiation hazard.

**Decibel:**  a unit used to express a difference in power, as with acoustic signals; a unit of intensity and volume of sound.

**Ecosystem:**  the biological and physical dimensions of the environment that refer to all living and non-living elements.

**Epidemiologist:**  one who studies the causes, distribution and frequency of disease outbreaks in a human community.

**Homeostasis:**  a state of equilibrium of the internal environment.

**Hygiene:**  pertinent to a state of health and its preservation.

**Limitation:**  the state of being limited or restricted.

**Maladaptation:**  inability of an organism to adjust to a change in environment.

**Nosocomial:**  infection or disease originating in a hospital.

**Physiological:**  in accord with or characteristic of the normal functioning of a living organism.

**Psycho:**  indicates the mind of mental processes of an individual.

**Psychosocial:**  a term that refers both to psychological and social factors.

**Restraint:**  containment of a person in a chair or bed to promote safety.

**Sociocultural:**  a term that refers both to society and culture.

**Stress:**  pressure, strain, or force sufficient to throw an individual out of balance.

**Supervise:**  to direct or inspect performance; to oversee.

**Therapeutic:**  having healing or curative powers.

**Thermal:**  pertaining to using, producing, or caused by heat.

# Chapter 7

# Admission and Discharge

## LEARNING OBJECTIVES

Explain the steps of admitting a patient to a health care unit.

Describe the patient assessment that is completed at the time of admission.

List the data that is included in charting when admitting a patient to the health care environment.

Describe the disposition process for patients' valuables when hospitalized.

Outline the steps in transferring a patient within the hospital environment.

Describe two suggested solutions for patients who are unable to adapt to the hospital environment.

Discuss the discharge procedures when a patient leaves the health care unit.

Identify three suggested solutions for a patient leaving the hospital against medical advice.

Describe the expected outcomes for patients being discharged from the hospital.

Complete discharge charting on a patient record utilizing specific criteria.

**ADMISSION TRANSFER AND DISCHARGE**

The admission procedure for patients can be a negative experience if it is impersonal, mechanized, or impolite. It can be a positive step in health care if handled with attention and care. The impressions formed by the patient during the admission process have a strong effect on his attitude toward the total care the patient will receive. Because the admission procedure can be the initial introduction into the health care system, the nurses should consider this process a key step in patient care.

**Admission to the Hospital**    The process of admitting a patient to a health care facility will vary in institutions such as nursing homes, clinics, and hospitals. Regardless of the size or type of facility, the admission process is vitally important in order to provide safe, adequate care. Because the nurse-patient relationship begins with admission, you should have a thorough understanding of the standard admission process.

If a patient enters the hospital in an emergency situation, he may feel insecure or fearful because he has had little time to make plans concerning family, travel, finances, or employment.

When the patient arrives at the hospital, the first contact is usually with the admitting receptionist, who assigns a hospital number and interviews the patient. If preadmission material was mailed to the patient, it will be verified by the receptionist at this time; otherwise, the patient must answer questions about age, address, financial or insurance status, next of kin, religion, employment, and consent for treatment. If the patient cannot answer these questions due to age or condition, a relative usually gives the information. A parent or guardian must do this for a child.

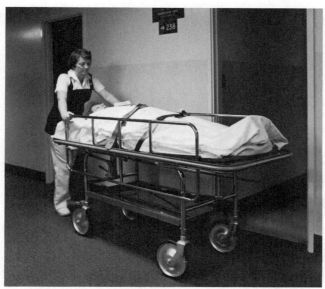

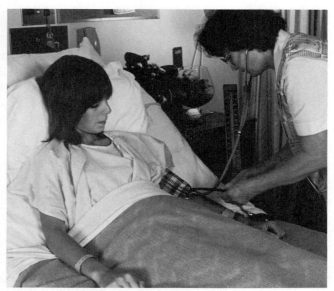

Patients are often admitted on a guerney in emergency situations.

Vital signs are obtained during the initial admission procedure.

During admission, patients should be requested to place valuables in the hospital safe or to send them home with their family. Valuables include jewelry, money, credit cards and blank checks. Patients also receive identification bracelets/identabands at this time.

Unless laboratory procedures are carried out in the patient's room, the patient will be directed or escorted to the clinical laboratory for baseline values on hemoglobin, hematocrit, complete blood count, differential, and serological screening for syphilis. Depending on the policy of the facility, the patient may then proceed to the electrocardiographic laboratory and to radiology to obtain a chest x-ray.

These procedures sometimes take several hours. Delays often result in physical and emotional strain for the patient. When an alternative is offered, such as having laboratory procedures performed the day before admission, the patient should be encouraged to use these options to decrease emotional and physical fatigue. More time can then be allowed on the actual admission day for adapting to the hospital environment.

**Admission to the Nursing Unit**    When admission to the hospital is complete, the patient is either directed to the nursing unit or escorted by a volunteer. The patient may be met by a staff nurse assigned to admissions for that day or by the nurse who will be working with the patient during the patient's stay in the hospital. It is at this time that you must begin to assess your patient's needs and to plan for their care.

When you meet a patient, introduce yourself and any other personnel who will provide care including the ward clerk. Explain your role and functions to the patient. Your initial contact will leave a lasting impression on the patient, so try to present information in an uninterrupted, organized, and friendly manner. If there are other patients in the room, introduce them to the new patient.

Tell the patient about mealtimes, visiting hours, telephone use, requests for clergy, recreational and lounge use, physicians' visits, and other schedules.

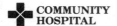 **COMMUNITY HOSPITAL**

## LIST OF PATIENT RIGHTS IN CALIFORNIA

In accordance with section 70707 of the California Administrative Code, the hospital and medical staff have adopted the following list of patient rights. Each patient has the right to:

1. Exercise these rights without regard to sex or cultural, economic. educational, or religious background or the source of payment for his care.

2. Considerate and respectful care.

3. Knowledge of the name of the physician who has primary responsibility for coordinating his care and the names and professional relationships of other physicians who will see him.

4. Receive information from his physician about his illness, his course of treatment, and his prospects for recovery in terms that he can understand.

5. Receive as much information about any proposed treatment or procedure as he may need in order to give informed consent or to refuse this course of treatment. Except in emergencies, this information shall include a description of the procedure or treatment, the medically significant risks involved in this treatment, alternate course of treatment or nontreatment and the risks involved in each, and to know the name of the person who will carry out the procedure or treatment.

6. Participate actively in decisions regarding his medical care. To the extent permitted by law, this includes the right to refuse treatment.

7. Full consideration of privacy concerning his medical care program. Case discussion, consultation, examination, and treatment are confidential and should be conducted discreetly. The patient has the right to be advised as to the reason for the presence of any individual.

8. Confidential treatment of all communications and records pertaining to his care and his stay in the hospital. His written permission shall be obtained before his medical records can be made available to anyone not directly concerned with his care.

9. Reasonable responses to any reasonable requests he may make for service.

10. Leave the hospital even against the advice of his physicians.

11. Reasonable continuity of care and to know in advance the time and location of appointment as well as the physician providing the care.

12. Be advised if hospital/personal physician proposes to engage in or perform human experimentation affecting his care or treatment. The patient has the right to refuse to participate in such research projects.

13. Be informed by his physician or a delegate of his physician of his continuing health care requirements following his discharge from the hospital.

14. Examine and receive an explanation of his bill regardless of source of payment.

15. Know which hospital rules and policies apply to his conduct as a patient.

16. Have all patients' rights apply to the person who may have legal responsibility to make decisions regarding medical care on behalf of the patient.

Drugs may *not* be kept at the bedside without a physician's order. Some hospitals have printed booklets describing this information. The more information your patient receives, the more control he has over the environment.

Help the patient become familiar with his immediate physical space by showing the location and the operation of the intercom system or call bell, the location of the bathroom, and the operation of the call system inside the bathroom. If electric beds are used, show the patient how to operate bed controls. You may also want to show the patient how to operate the television and the radio set. Explain the cost and availability if not included with the room.

Because patients may not be sure of their role while in the hospital, many hospitals have adopted versions of the American Hospital Association's *Patient's Bill of Rights*. This Bill includes the following rights: to obtain information about the patient's illness or injury, to refuse medication or treatment, to participate in his own care, to know the rationale and/or risks of the treatment, and to receive courteous care. Make sure your patients understand their rights. Clear, uncomplicated explanations help them adapt to their new environment.

Once you have completed introductions and the environmental orientation, you may begin the nursing history and assessment to establish baseline data about the patient's general condition. (See Chapter 17, Physical Assessment.) After completing the assessment, you may begin providing other care.

**Transfer Unit to Unit**    Patients are frequently transferred from one unit to another as their condition fluctuates. When a patient is moved, all of the records, charts, drugs, belongings and personal hygiene and special equipment are transferred with him. After accompanying the patient to a new unit, introduce him to new roommates, the charge nurse and the nurse who will be responsible for his care. Assist him to get settled in the new room. Make a complete report to the nursing staff utilizing the Patient Care Plan.

**Discharge from a Unit**    When a patient is discharged from a health care unit, preparations must be made to help the patient transfer from a dependent role to a more independent role. Discharge from the hospital can be a welcome relief for the patient, but it can also be a time of anxiety and fear. During this transition, the nursing staff can facilitate the process by being aware of individual patient needs.

During the discharge process, you must take into consideration the physical, emotional, and psychosocial needs of the patient and family. Your responsibilities for the discharge process will include assessing the patient's post-hospitalization needs and planning with the patient and family to meet discharge needs. It is also important to communicate with appropriate health team members and community agencies. The final responsibilities of the discharge process will be terminating the nurse-patient relationship and evaluating the discharge process.

The following nursing diagnoses may be appropriate to include in a Patient Care Plan when the components are related to Admission, Transfer and Discharge of a patient.

**NURSING DIAGNOSES**

| Nursing Diagnosis (Potential) | Defining Characteristic; Etiology (Examples) |
|---|---|
| ☐ Anxiety, *related to* | Fear of unknown outcome, e.g., admission to the hospital, undiagnosed symptoms. |
| | Apprehension, uncertainty, e.g., transfer between health care settings. |
| ☐ Comfort, Alteration in: Pain, *related to* | Immobility, tissue damage, e.g., trauma or disease conditions. |
| ☐ Grieving, Anticipatory, *related to* | Feelings of loss or isolation, e.g., change in health status. |
| | Loss of body part or capability, e.g., amputation, debilitating or degenerating disease. |
| ☐ Health Maintenance, Alteration in, *related to* | Cognitive or physical limitations, e.g., mental or physical disease state. |
| ☐ Social Isolation, *related to* | Decreased social interaction, e.g., family and/or peers unable to visit. |

## UNIT ONE   ADMISSION AND TRANSFER

### NURSING PROCESS DATA

#### ASSESSMENT   *Data Base*

Observe and record patient's physical, emotional, and intellectual status.

Observe and record patient's ability to adapt to the environment of a hospital unit. Observe for disabilities or limitations.

Observe patient's condition and ability to orient to the nursing unit.

Assess the patient's level of comfort or discomfort.

Determine patient's understanding of his disease and its limitations.

Assess condition prior to transfer.

#### PLANNING   *Objectives*

To assist patient to adapt to hospital environment with minimal distress.

To encourage the patient to participate in his own plan of care.

To provide a comfortable and esthetically pleasing environment for the patient.

To provide the patient with some control over the patient's immediate environment.

To provide the patient with an opportunity to verbalize his or her feelings about hospitalization.

To facilitate transfer if required.

#### IMPLEMENTATION   *Procedures*

Admitting a Patient

Transferring a Patient

## ADMITTING A PATIENT

### Equipment

Admission kit for personal hygiene

Thermometer

Blood pressure cuff and stethoscope

Urine container

Kardex card and Patient Care Plan

Patient's chart

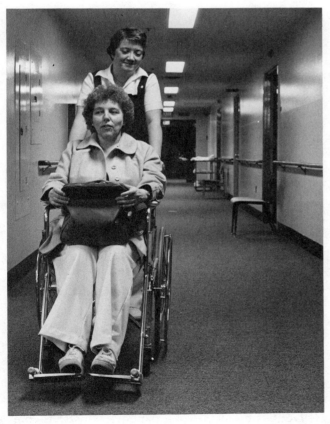

Hospital policy may require ambulatory patients be admitted by wheelchair.

### Procedure

1. Introduce yourself to the patient and begin to establish a therapeutic nurse-patient relationship.
2. Introduce the patient to staff and to roommate if present.
3. Explain equipment and hospital routines.
4. Obtain the patient's health history and complete a nursing assessment.
5. Obtain the patient's weight and height.
6. Obtain urine specimen and vital signs.
7. Inform laboratory that patient is available for chest x-ray and routine blood work if not obtained earlier.
8. Identify patient's problem areas and needs.
9. Notify physician that the patient has been admitted and obtain orders if policy permits.
10. Reassess patient's level of comfort and ability to adapt to hospitalization.
11. Complete patient teaching for all unfamiliar procedures or interventions.
12. Fill out Kardex card and Patient Care Plan.
13. Document information on appropriate forms in chart.

## TRANSFERRING A PATIENT

### Equipment

Wheelchair or guerney

Warm covering for guerney

Patient's records, chart and Patient Care Plan

Medications and med cards

Personal hygiene equipment

Special equipment (e.g., sheepskin)

Personal belongings

Valuables receipt

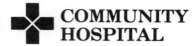

| Admission Questionnaire | Addressograph Plate |
|---|---|
| **COMMUNITY HOSPITAL** | |

Please answer the following questions so that we may plan your nursing care more efficiently and your discharge when it occurs. If you do not understand a question, please ask for help.

1. What health problem was responsible for admission to the Hospital at this time?

   _____

2. How long have you had this problem? _____

3. Briefly state what your understanding is of your present problem? _____

   _____

   _____

4. If known, what are your doctor's plans for you? _____

   _____

5. How long do you expect to be in the Hospital? _____

6. List any other health problems you are aware of besides the one other than hospitalized for: _____

   _____

7. List any major health problems, illnesses, surgeries, or hospitalizations you have had in the past, including the date of each:

   _____
   (Date)

   _____
   (Date)

8. Do you have any food allergies or restrictions?    ☐ YES    ☐ NO

   If yes, explain _____

   _____

## Procedure

1. Obtain physician's order if needed. **Rationale:** Physicians order transfers from and to critical care unit. They do not always order transfer within departments.

2. Contact admitting office to arrange for transfer.

3. Communicate with transfer unit to determine the best time for moving the patient.

4. Inform and talk to patient of impending transfer. **Rationale:** Discussing the rationale for transfer and eliciting the patient's feelings facilitate adjustment to the transfer unit.

5. Gather equipment, belongings and records.

6. Wash hands to prevent transfer of microorganisms to new unit.

7. Obtain necessary staff assistance for smooth transfer.

8. Transfer patient to wheelchair or guerney unless patient is remaining in bed for the transfer.

9. Cover patient to provide warmth and avoid exposure during transfer.

10. Notify head nurse when you arrive on the new unit.

11. Introduce and acquaint patient with new roommates.

12. Introduce patient to new staff, especially the nurse who will be caring for the patient that day.

13. Give a complete report to staff, using the Patient Care Plan and Kardex. Give information concerning individualized care needs, patient problems, progress, when next medications or treatments are due, etc.

14. Notify physician when patient's transfer is completed.

**NURSING ASSESSMENT DATA BASE**

## COMMUNITY HOSPITAL

| Date | Time | Room # | Admit by: | ambulatory _____ guerney _____ |
|------|------|--------|-----------|-----------------------------------|
|      |      |        |           | W/C _____ ambulance _____ |

| T.P.R. | B/P RT | B/P LT | Height | Weight |
|--------|--------|--------|--------|--------|

**Instructed in use of:**

Yes  No

☐ ☐ Telephone
☐ ☐ Bed-Controls
☐ ☐ Lights
☐ ☐ Nurse call System
☐ ☐ Visiting hours

**Articles at bedside**
(describe item)

☐ Ring _____
☐ Watch _____
☐ Money (amt.) _____
☐ Eyeglasses _____
☐ Hearing Aid _____

☐ Contact Lenses _____
☐ Dentures: Upper _____
       Lower _____
☐ Other _____

Reason for No: _____          Other _____
_____
_____

**Tests completed on admission**

☐ Lab Work
☐ UA
☐ X-ray _____
☐ Other _____

Above information obtained by: _____

| Previous illness | Meds taken @ home on routine basis | Meds taken today state time | Meds brought to hospital | Allergies: |
|------------------|-----------------------------------|-----------------------------|--------------------------|------------|
| ☐ Diabetes ☐ Hypertension ☐ Heart Disease ☐ Lung Disease ☐ Other | | | | ☐ FOOD _____ |
| | | | | _____ |
| | | | | ☐ DRUGS _____ |
| | | | **Disposition of Meds** ☐ Home ☐ Pharmacy | _____ ☐ None Known |

15. Notify the switchboard and admitting office when transfer is completed. A written transfer slip must be sent to the appropriate departments.

16. Notify dietary department, x-ray and the laboratory if tests were scheduled or results pending.

17. Determine that valuables receipt is either with patient or on chart.

### CHARTING *for Admitting and Transferring*

☐ Admission procedures

☐ Adaptation to hospitalization

☐ Admission assessment data: height, weight, vital signs, physical assessment findings

☐ Laboratory specimens obtained and sent

☐ Types of x-rays

☐ Transfer, time of arrival to new unit, method of transfer and condition of the patient.

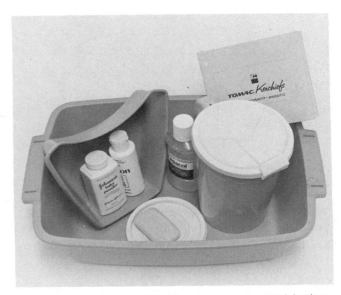

The admission kit usually contains necessary personal hygiene items including lotion and mouth wash.

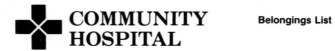

**COMMUNITY HOSPITAL**

**Belongings List**

Patient's Name _____

Date _____

Male ☐ Female ☐

Admitting Unit _____

☐ Discharged

☐ Deceased

☐ Transferred

Unit and Rm # From _____

Unit and Rm # To _____

| CLOTHING LIST | | | | MISCELLANEOUS | |
| --- | --- | --- | --- | --- | --- |
| PLEASE DESCRIBE | NUMBER | PLEASE DESCRIBE | NUMBER | PLEASE DESCRIBE | NUMBER |
| Bathrobe | | Shoes | | Cane | |
| Belt | | Slacks/Shorts | | Crutches | |
| Blouse | | Slippers | | Dentures ☐ Upper ☐ Lower ☐ Partial | |
| Coat | | Skirts | | | |
| Dress | | Sweater | | Flowers or Plants | |
| Gloves | | Tie | | Glasses or Contact Lens | |
| Gown | | Underclothes | | Jewelry Remaining with Pt. | |
| Hat | | | | | |
| Helmet | | | | | |
| Hose/Socks/Pantihose | | | | Luggage | |
| Jacket | | | | Radio | |
| Pajamas | | | | Wallet/Purse | |
| Shirt | | | | Watch | |
| | | | | Wig | |

Signature of Person Listing _____

Signature of Personnel Handling Belongings _____

Signature of Receiving Personnel or Relative _____

If Relative:    Address _____    Phone _____

## CLINICAL PROBLEM SOLVING

| Potential Problems | Suggested Solutions |
|---|---|
| Patient is unable to adapt to hospital environment. | ☐ Assess physiological and/or emotional basis for maladaptation. Request consultation with nurse manager, patient advocate, physician, etc. |
| Patient resists transfer. | ☐ Allow opportunity to ventilate feelings. |
| | ☐ If possible, allow some choice (room, bed, number of roommates, etc.) in new unit. |
| Following transfer, patient's personal belongings are lost. | ☐ Return to previous unit and check with staff. |
| | ☐ Ascertain that belongings were in fact at the hospital. |
| | ☐ Check the clothing list for actual articles brought to hospital. |

# UNIT TWO   HEIGHT AND WEIGHT

## NURSING PROCESS DATA

### ASSESSMENT   *Data Base*

Check the need for daily or weekly body weight measurements.

Determine appropriate method for obtaining patient's weight (bedside scale, bed scale).

Determine ability to stand for height measurement.

### PLANNING   *Objectives*

To establish baseline data to check against total body fluid balance.

To identify excess or deficits of fluid balance.

To establish baseline data for diagnostic tests that involve dye and radioactive material injections.

To determine drug dosage.

### IMPLEMENTATION   *Procedure*

Obtaining Height and Weight

### EVALUATION   *Expected Outcomes*

Patient's weight, depending on status, disease state, and therapy, shows expected losses, gains, or stabilization.

Weight is obtained and recorded as ordered by the physician.

Height is obtained and recorded in admission form.

## OBTAINING HEIGHT AND WEIGHT

### Equipment

Balance beam scale (for patients who are able to stand without assistance)

Bed scale (for patients who are confined to bed or who are unable to stand)

Bed scale that is built into the bed

Floor scale (for patients in wheelchairs) with height bar

### Preparation

1. Ask patient to void before weighing.
2. Weigh patient in the morning before breakfast.
3. Use the same scale each time you weigh the patient. **Rationale:** For consistency in weight from day to day, keep as many variables the same as possible.
4. Make sure the patient wears the same type of clothing (e.g., gown or robe) for each weighing.
5. If the patient is bedridden, weigh linens used for covering the patient each time the patient is weighed.
6. Change wet gowns or heavily saturated dressings before weighing the patient.

### Procedure

1. Transport patient to scale or bring scale to bedside.
2. Balance scale so that weight will be accurate.
3. Place a clean paper towel on scale and ask patient to remove shoes.
4. Assist patient to stand with back towards balancing bar.
5. Move weights until the weight bar is level or balanced.
6. Record weight on appropriate record.
7. Place height bar level on top of the person's head.
8. Read patient's height as measured.
9. Record height on appropriate record.
10. Throw away paper towel on scale and assist patient back to room.

### CHARTING  *for Height and Weight*

□ Patient's weight and height recorded in weight book or on graphic sheet

□ Type of scale used for weighing

□ Bed linens, gowns, and/or equipment weighed (record on care plan or on Kardex)

---

## CLINICAL PROBLEM SOLVING

### Potential Problems

Weight varies excessively from one day to the next.

Patient is too critically ill to be weighed accurately because of mechanical devices used to sustain life.

### Suggested Solutions

□ Check if same scale was used for both weighings.
□ Check what clothing or linen was on the patient when he or she was weighed on both days.
□ Check that scale was balanced appropriately.
□ Reweigh the patient to determine if an error was made in the weight.

□ Estimate weight loss and gain by assessing other factors, e.g., skin turgor, output, presence of edema.
□ Weigh the patient on a bed scale and make a notation of what equipment was used when patient was weighed.

# UNIT THREE  DISCHARGE

## NURSING PROCESS DATA

### ASSESSMENT  *Data Base*

Identify physical, emotional, and psychosocial information concerning patient's discharge.

Identify disabilities and limitations that will extend after discharge.

Observe patient's strengths.

Assess need for health care assistance in the home.

### PLANNING  *Objectives*

To prepare the patient for discharge.

To assist in the transfer of a patient whose condition necessitates care at another facility.

To allow the patient to verbalize his feelings about discharge and identify the patient's strengths and weaknesses.

To help the patient be aware of potential changes in environment and life-style due to his disability or limitation.

### IMPLEMENTATION  *Procedures*

Discharging a Patient

Discharging a Patient AMA

### EVALUATION  *Expected Outcomes*

Patient verbalizes his feelings about being discharged and identifies strengths and weaknesses.

Patient is aware of potential changes in environment and life-style due to his or her disability or limitations.

Patient and family discuss how they can work together to help the patient maximize his potential.

Patient knowledgeably discusses all points included in the nurse-patient teaching, including medication and self-care.

Home care assistance is arranged when needed.

## DISCHARGING A PATIENT

### Equipment

Educational pamphlets

Telephone numbers and information regarding clinic appointments or special groups

Specific equipment such as wheelchair or commode needed upon discharge

Medications

Materials for dressing changes (if indicated) or anti-embolic stockings

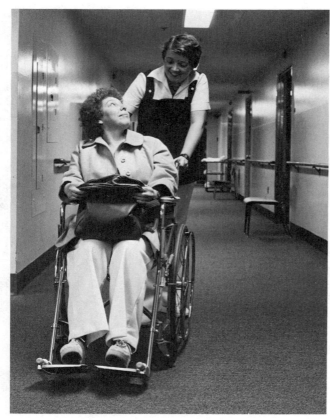

Patients are discharged in a wheelchair for their safety.

## Preparation

1. Determine that physician's discharge orders have been written.
2. Notify family or significant other to arrange transportation. If unavailable, notify discharge coordinator for arrangements.
3. Notify all hospital departments, admitting, cashier, dietary, etc.
4. Ensure that all lab work, x-rays, treatments and procedures are completed prior to discharge.
5. Provide opportunities for patient to discuss impending discharge.
6. Complete patient teaching if applicable.

## Procedure

1. Review details of discharge with patient.
2. Assist patient with hygiene, dressing, packing, etc.

3. Review instructions and answer questions about medications, physical care, and supplies.
4. Terminate relationship with the patient. Remember that each individual handles termination in his own way. **Rationale:** Providing an opportunity for the patient to express his feelings and impressions will contribute to a positive termination.
5. Follow your hospital's prescribed procedure for patient discharge, i.e., discharge time and method of leaving hospital unit. **Rationale:** Many hospitals insist that patients be transported by wheelchair to prevent falls and injury.
6. Document the patient's discharge on the chart.

## DISCHARGING PATIENT AMA

### Equipment

Form for discharge against medical advice

Pen

### Procedure

1. If patient insists on leaving the hospital, notify the physician.
2. Ascertain from the patient exactly why he wants to leave the hospital.
3. Explain and validate the physician's reasons that continued hospital care is necessary.
4. If patient insists on leaving, offer him the appropriate form and request that he sign it. **Rationale:** This form states that the hospital is relieved from responsibility for the patient's condition.
5. If patient refuses to sign the form, note this fact on the form and have it witnessed.
6. Put the copy of the form on the patient's chart.
7. Notify the appropriate people—the physician, nursing supervisor, administration—when the patient leaves.
8. Escort the patient to the door as you would any discharged patient. **Rationale:** The hospital is still responsible for the patient while he is on hospital property.

### CHARTING  *for Discharging a Patient*

☐ Day-to-day preparatory activities such as teaching, return demonstrations, discussion with dietician, etc.

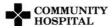 **COMMUNITY HOSPITAL**

## RELEASE FROM RESPONSIBILITY - I

### TREATMENT OF MISCARRIAGE OR PARTIAL ABORTION
**(Other Than Therapeutic)**

Date _____Time_____

I, the undersigned, a patient at the above named hospital, am advised by my doctor that I may be in a condition of abortion. I hereby declare that neither the physician nor any person employed by or connected with the said hospital has performed any act which may have contributed to the interruption of my pregnancy and do hereby absolve the said hospital and treating physician from any responsibility for my condition. My condition has been caused by the following facts occurring prior to the time of my admission to the hospital and treatment by my physician.

_____

Witness _____    Signature _____
                                                                            PATIENT

This form to be completed in the case of patients who are or MAY BE in a condition of abortion. Patient should state facts of her case in her own handwriting whenever possible.

### LEAVING HOSPITAL AGAINST ADVICE

Date _____Time_____

This is to certify that _____
a patient in the above named hospital, is leaving the hospital against the advice of the attending physician and the hospital administration. I acknowledge that I have been informed of the risk involved and hereby release the attending physician, and the hospital from all responsibility and any ill effects which may result from this action.

Witness _____    Signature _____
                                                                            PATIENT

### TEMPORARY ABSENCE RELEASE

Date _____Time_____

Having received permission from the attending physician to be absent from the above named hospital for my convenience from _____ m to _____ m, date _____ I assume all responsibility for myself or _____ patient, who is my _____ (specify relationship), during this temporary absence and hereby release the above named hospital, its employees and the attending physicians from all responsibility during this absence and for my or patient's condition as result thereof.

I understand that I am remaining an inpatient at the above named hospital. My accommodation is being held for me, and I am responsible for all the usual hospital charges that would be payable by me if I remained in the hospital.

Witness _____    Signature _____
                                                                   (PATIENT, PARENT OR LEGAL GUARDIAN)

### CONSENT TO PHOTOGRAPH

Date _____Time_____

The undersigned do hereby authorize the above named hospital, and the attending physician to photograph or permit other persons to photograph _____
while under the care of the above institution, and agree that they may use or permit other persons to use the negatives or prints prepared therefrom for such purposes and in such manner as may be deemed necessary.

Witness _____    Signature _____
                                                                   (PATIENT, PARENT OR LEGAL GUARDIAN)

### RELEASE OF SIDE RAILS

Date _____Time_____

Having been informed by the above named hospital that protective side rails should be placed on my bed and raised for my personal protection, I hereby instruct the hospital and its employees not to place or raise protective side rails on my bed and hereby assume all risks in connection therewith and fully release the said hospital, its employees and my physician from any and all liability for any injury or damage to me by reason of its failure to place or raise protective side rails on my bed.

Witness _____    Signature _____

FORM 300050 (7-83)

**TABLE 1**   RELIGIOUS GUIDELINES FOR PATIENT CARE

| RELIGIOUS GROUP | BAPTISM | DEATH RITUALS | HEALTH CRISIS | DIET |
|---|---|---|---|---|
| Adventist | Opposed to infant baptism | No last rites | Communion or baptism may be desirable | No alcohol, coffee, tea, or any narcotic |
| Baptist | Opposed to infant baptism | Clergy support and counsels | Some believe in healing and laying on of hands Some sects resist medical help | Condemn alcohol Some do not allow coffee and tea |
| Black Muslim | No baptism | Prescribed procedures for washing body and shrouding | No faith healing | Prohibit alcohol and pork |
| Buddhist | Rites are given after child is mature | Send for Buddhist priest Last rite chanting | Family should request priest to be notified | Usually no restrictions although some are vegetarian |
| Christian Scientist | No baptism | No last rites No autopsy | Deny the existence of health crises Many refuse all medical help, blood transfusions, or drugs | Alcohol, coffee, and tobacco viewed as drugs and not allowed |
| Episcopalian | Infant baptism mandatory | Last rites not essential for all members | Medical treatment acceptable | Some do not eat meat on Fridays |
| Jehovah's Witness | No infant baptism | No last rites | Opposed to blood transfusions | Do not eat anything to which blood has been added |
| Judaism | No baptism but ritual circumcision on eighth day | Ritual washing of body | All ill people seek medical care | Orthodox observe kosher dietary laws, which prohibit pork, shellfish, and the eating of meat and milk products at the same time |
| Methodist | Baptism encouraged | No last rites | Medical treatment acceptable | No restrictions |
| Mormon | Baptism eight years or older | Baptism of the dead very important | Do not prohibit medical treatment although they believe in divine healing | Do not allow alcohol, caffeine, tobacco, tea, and coffee |
| Roman Catholic | Infant baptism mandatory | No special requirements | Sacrament of the sick | Most ill people are exempt from fasting |

☐ If specific discharge forms or patient teaching sheets are used, record data using these forms

☐ Discharge data such as time, how discharged (ambulatory, wheelchair, ambulance, etc.), if accompanied by relative or nurse, and patient's physical and psychosocial condition

☐ Discharge medications, special equipment, and materials taken home by patient

☐ Discharge criteria that was not met and reason criteria was not met as identified on Patient Care Plan

## CLINICAL PROBLEM SOLVING

**Potential Problems**

Patient is discharged to an extended care facility (ECF).

Patient does not understand the discharge process.

Patient wants to leave the hospital against medical advice (AMA).

**Suggested Solutions**

☐ Reinforce physician's explanation as to why patient needs to go to an ECF.
☐ Provide time for patient and family to deal with the loss of the patient's independence and his previous role in the home setting.

☐ Repeat information as needed to help clarify unfamiliar terms or statements.
☐ Explain to the patient's relative the necessary care that will be required upon discharge.

☐ Attempt to identify patient's reasons for wanting to leave AMA.
☐ Provide alternatives to leaving the hospital.
☐ Do not force the adult patient to remain in the hospital but do encourage discussion about the situation.
☐ Notify the charge nurse or supervisor so that she can contact the patient advocate, a social worker, or the clergy to discuss the situation with the patient.
☐ If possible, consult your hospital's policies and procedures regarding AMA before releasing patient.
☐ Have patient sign AMA form, if possible.
☐ If patient will not sign AMA forms, have another nurse witness refusal and chart details of discharge.

## TERMINOLOGY

**Adaptation:**  ability of an organism to adjust to a change in environment.

**Admit:**  the process of getting a patient signed into the hospital.

**Ambulatory:**  able to walk, or not confined to bed.

**Antiembolic:**  a preventative measure, such as elastic hosiery, to avoid emboli.

**Aseptic:**  sterile; free from bacteria and infection.

**Assessment:**  critical evaluation of information; the first step in the nursing process.

**Behavior:**  a person's total activity—actions or reactions; especially, conduct that can be observed.

**Blood count:**  enumeration of the red corpuscles and leukocytes per cu mm. A blood count indicates the total number of cells.

**Cardio:**  prefix pertinent to the heart.

**Comfort:**  to ease physically; relieve, as of pain.

**Communication:**  to convey or transmit knowledge, information, or messages to another person.

**Comprehensive health care:**  a total system of health care that takes the whole person into account.

**Criteria:**  a standard, rule, or test on which a judgment or decision can be based.

**Diagnostic test:**  a test used to determine a diagnosis or to determine the cause and nature of a pathological condition.

**Disability:**  a disabled state or condition; incapacity; a handicap.

**Discharge:**  to let go, as in discharging a patient from the hospital; the flowing away of a secretion or excretion of pus, feces, urine, etc.

**Home care assistance:** nursing care actually given in the patient's home.

**Homeostasis:** state of equilibrium of the internal environment.

**Hygiene:** the study of health and observance of health rules.

**Hypoallergenic:** a substance deemed to cause very little, if any, allergic response.

**Hypotension:** decrease of systolic and diastolic blood pressure below normal.

**Identaband:** a band, usually worn on a patient's wrist, with the patient's name and medical record number.

**Kardex:** a system of cards that contains pertinent medical information about patients.

**Limitation:** the state of being limited or restricted.

**Maladaptation:** inability of an organism to adjust to a change in environment.

**Patient Care Plan:** a plan for care of a specific patient or one designed especially for one patient.

**Potential:** possible but not yet realized.

**Procedure:** a particular way of accomplishing a desired result.

**Radiology:** the branch of medicine concerned with radioactive substances.

**Regression:** a turning back or return to a former state.

**Serology:** the scientific study of serum.

**Serum:** any serous fluid, especially the fluid that moistens the surfaces of serous membranes; the watery portion of blood after coagulation.

**Specimen:** a part of a thing intended to show kind and quality of the whole, as a specimen of urine.

**Stress:** a state of agitation that throws the body out of balance.

**Supervise:** to direct or inspect performance; to oversee.

**Termination:** the spatial or temporal end of something; a limit or boundary.

**Therapeutic:** having healing or curative powers.

**Transfer:** to convey or shift from one person or place to another.

**Transition:** the process or an instance of changing from one form, state, activity or place to another.

**Verbalize:** to express in words.

**Void:** to urinate or to evacuate the bowels.

**Volunteer:** a person who performs or gives his services of his own free will.

# Chapter 8

# Body Mechanics and Positioning

## LEARNING OBJECTIVES

Discuss the primary function of the skeletal muscles, joints, and bones.

Describe nursing measures that will assist in preserving joints, bones, and skeletal muscles.

Describe a minimum of two principles of correct body mechanics.

State two expected outcomes of utilizing proper body mechanics.

Discuss the objectives for moving and turning patients.

Compare and contrast the methods used in moving patients up in bed for a single nurse and when assistants are available.

Demonstrate passive range-of-motion exercises using all muscle groups.

Explain the rationale of assisted ambulation for patients.

Demonstrate the procedures for moving a patient to the side of the bed and dangling a patient.

Outline the steps in logrolling a patient.

Demonstrate a three-man lift.

List the pertinent data that should be charted when moving a patient from the bed.

Write a patient care plan using at least three nursing diagnoses for a patient requiring moving and turning interventions.

## MUSCULOSKELETAL SYSTEM

The musculoskeletal system protects the body, provides a structural framework, and allows the body to move. The primary structures in this system are muscles, bones, and joints.

**Skeletal Muscles**  Skeletal muscles move the bones around the joints by contracting and relaxing so that movement can take place. Each muscle consists of a body, or belly, and tendons, which connect the muscle to another muscle or to bone.

When skeletal muscles contract, they cause two bones to move around the joint between them. One of these bones tends to remain stationary while the other bone moves. The end of the muscle that attaches to the stationary bone is called the origin. The end of the muscle that attaches to the movable bone is called the insertion.

Muscles are designated flexors or extensors according to whether they flex the joint (decrease the angle between the bones) or extend the joint (increase the angle between the bones). For example, when the deltoid muscle contracts, it abducts the arm and raises it laterally to the horizontal position. The anterior fibers aid in flexion of the arm, and the posterior fibers aid in extension of the arm.

**Joints**  Joints are the places where bones meet. Their primary function is to provide motion and flexibility. Although the internal structure of joints varies, most joints are composed of ligaments, which bind the bones together, and cartilage, or tissue, which covers and cushions the ends of the bones.

**Bones**   Bones provide the major support for all the body organs. Bone is composed of an organic matrix, deposits of calcium salts, and bone cells. The organic matrix provides the framework and tensile strength for the bone. The calcium salts, which are about 75 percent of the bone, provide compressional strength by filling in the matrix. As a result, it is very difficult to damage a bone by twisting it or by applying direct pressure.

Bone cells include osteoblasts, osteocytes, and osteoclasts. Osteoblasts deposit the organic matrix; osteocytes and osteoclasts reabsorb this matrix. Because this process is usually in equilibrium, bone is deposited where it is needed in the skeletal system. If increased stress is placed on a bone, such as the stress of continued athletic activity, more bone will be deposited. If there is no stress on a bone, as is often the case with patients on prolonged bedrest, part of the bone mass will be reabsorbed or lost.

Alterations in mobility can result from problems in the musculoskeletal system, the nervous system, and the skin. A primary cause for alterations in muscles is inactivity. With forceful activity muscles increase in size. With inactivity muscles decrease in size and strength. When patients are in casts or in traction, on prolonged bedrest, or unable to exercise, their muscles become weak and atrophied.

**SYSTEM ALTERATIONS**

Alterations in joints result when mobility is limited by changes in the adjacent tissues. When muscle movement decreases, the connective tissue in the joints, tendons, and ligaments becomes thickened and fibrotic.

Chronic flexion and hyperextension can also cause alterations in the joints. Chronic flexion can cause joints to become contracted in one position so that they are unmovable. Hyperextension occurs when joints are extended beyond their normal limits, which is usually 180 degrees. The results of hyperextension are pain and discomfort to the patient and abnormal stress on the ligaments and tendons of the joints.

Alterations in bone are caused by disease processes, decalcification and breaks caused by trauma, or twisting. Encouraging patients to stand and to walk is important because the body functions best when it is in a vertical position. When a person is horizontal, the abdominal organs press on the diaphragm and inhibit its movement, thus decreasing respiratory efficiency. Physical activity forces muscles to move and increases blood flow, which improves metabolism and facilitates such body functions as gastrointestinal peristalsis.

**Nursing Measures**   Nursing care measures to preserve the joints, bones and skeletal muscles should be carried out for all patients who require bedrest. Positions in which patients are placed, methods of moving and turning should all be based on the principles of maintaining the musculoskeletal system in proper alignment. The nurse must also utilize good body mechanics when moving and turning patients to preserve her own musculoskeletal system from injury.

Knowledge of a patient's body and how it moves is important. Knowledge of your own body and what happens to it when you care for patients with altered mobility is also important. Before you lift or move a patient, determine the causes and consequences of the patient's illness. This knowledge will enable you to move the patient without causing him additional discomfort. Before you begin, thoroughly explain the procedures you will be completing so that you obtain the patient's cooperation.

**BODY MECHANICS**

Trying to lift or move too much weight forces you to use your body incorrectly and frequently causes injuries. Incorrect lifting puts most of the pressure on the muscles of your lower back. Because these muscles are not strong enough to handle the stress, you can sustain severe injuries. If you do not follow guidelines for promoting proper body mechanics, you are putting yourself in jeopardy.

Proper use of body mechanics prevents injuries to patients and all members of the health team. Guidelines that underly the implementation of body mechanics appear below.

- Assume a proper stance before moving or turning patients.
- Distribute workload evenly before moving or turning patients.
- Establish a comfortable height when working with patients.
- Push and pull objects when moving them to conserve energy.
- Use large muscles for lifting and moving, not the back muscles.
- Avoid leaning and stretching.
- Request assistance from others when working with heavy patients to avoid strain.
- Avoid twisting the body.

**NURSING DIAGNOSES**

The following nursing diagnoses are appropriate to utilize on Patient Care Plans when the components are related to body mechanics.

| Nursing Diagnosis (Potential) | Defining Characteristic; Etiology (Examples) |
| --- | --- |
| Comfort, Alteration in: Pain, *related to* | Restricted movement or agility, e.g., recent surgery or cast application. |
| Injury, Potential for, *related to* | Footdrop or contractures, e.g., inaccurate positioning. |
| Mobility, Impaired Physical, *related to* | Joint contractures, e.g., improper body alignment, inadequate range of motion. |
| Sensory-Perceptual Alteration: Kinesthetic, Tactile, *related to* | Interruption of central nervous system, e.g., physical injury or disease process (spinal cord injury, CVA). |
| Skin Integrity, Impairment of, *related to* | Altered circulation and/or pressure on bony prominence, e.g., infrequent or improper positioning, inadequate skin care. |

## UNIT ONE   PROPER BODY MECHANICS

### NURSING PROCESS DATA

**ASSESSMENT** *Data Base*

Evaluate personnel's knowledge of the principles of body mechanics.

Evaluate personnel's knowledge of how to use correct muscle groups for specific activities.

Assess knowledge and correct any misinformation about body alignment and how to maintain it with each position.

Assess knowledge of physical science and application to balance and body alignment.

Assess the competency of spinal cord and associated musculature.

Assess the muscle mass of the long, thick, and strong muscles of the shoulders and thighs.

### PLANNING   *Objectives*

To promote proper body mechanics while caring for patients.

To maintain good posture, thereby promoting optimum musculoskeletal balance.

To provide knowledge of the musculoskeletal system, body alignment and balance in order to assist the nurse in caring for patients.

To correct body mechanics, promote health, enhance appearance, and assist body function.

### IMPLEMENTATION   *Procedures*

Establishing Body Alignment

Maintaining Proper Body Alignment

Utilizing Coordinated Movements

Utilizing Basic Principles

### EVALUATION   *Expected Outcomes*

Correct body mechanics are utilized in caring for patients.

Injuries are prevented to both the nurse and the patient.

Proper body mechanics facilitate patient care.

Coordinated movements prevent patient discomfort.

Center of gravity is maintained when lifting objects.

## ESTABLISHING BODY ALIGNMENT

### Procedure

1. Establish a firm base of support by placing both feet flat on the floor, with one foot slightly in front of the other.
2. Distribute weight evenly on both feet.
3. Slightly bend both knees.
4. Hold abdomen firm and tuck buttocks in so that spine is in alignment.
5. Hold head erect and secure firm stance.
6. Use this stance as the basis for all actions in moving, turning, and lifting patients.

## MAINTAINING PROPER BODY ALIGNMENT

### Procedure

1. Begin with the proper stance established in the previous intervention.
2. Evaluate working height necessary to achieve objective.
   a. Test parameters of possible heights, i.e., bed

moves within an approximate range of 18 inches from floor.

b. Establish a comfortable height in which to work; usual height is between waist and lower level of hip joint.

3. Test that this level minimizes muscle strain by extending your arms and checking that your body maintains proper alignment.

4. If you need to work at a lower level, flex your knees. Do not bend over at the waist as this results in back strain.

5. Make accommodations for working at high surface levels because reaching up may result in injury to the back through hyperextension of muscles.

6. Work close to your body so that your center of gravity is not misaligned and your muscles are not hyperextended.

7. Use your longest and strongest muscles (biceps, quadriceps, and gluteal) when moving and turning patients.

8. Whenever possible, roll, push, and pull objects instead of lifting.

## UTILIZING COORDINATED MOVEMENTS

### Procedure

1. Plan muscle movements to distribute workload before you actually begin turning, moving, or lifting patients.
   a. Establish a clear plan of action before you begin to move.
   b. Take a deep breath so oxygen is available for energy expenditure.
   c. Tense antagonistic muscles (abdomen) to those you will be using (diaphragm) in preparation for the movement.
   d. Release breath and mobilize major muscle groups (abdominal and gluteal) to do the work.

2. Move muscles in a smooth, coordinated manner to avoid putting strain on one muscle and to be more efficient.

3. Do not make jerky, uncoordinated movements as this may cause injury and/or frighten the patient.

4. When you are working with another staff member, coordinate plans and movements before implementing them.

## UTILIZING BASIC PRINCIPLES

### Procedure

1. Move an object by pushing and pulling to expend minimal energy.
   a. Stand close to the object.
   b. Place yourself in proper body alignment stance.
   c. Tense muscles and prepare for movement.
   d. Pull toward you by leaning away from the object and letting arms, hips, and thighs *(not back)* do the work.
   e. Push away from you by leaning toward object, utilizing body weight to add force.

2. When changing direction, use pivotal movement-moving muscles as a unit and in alignment, rather than rotating or twisting upper part of body.

3. When working at lower surface levels, do not stoop by bending over. Flex body at knees and, keeping back straight, use thigh and gluteal muscles to accomplish task.

4. Use the muscles of arms and upper torso in an extended, coordinated movement parallel to body stance when reaching to prevent twisting or hyperextension of muscles.

5. Lift or carry patients or objects with the maximum use of these body alignment principles:
   a. Determine that the movement is within your capability to perform without injury.
   b. Place yourself in proper body alignment stance.
   c. Stand close to and grasp the object or person near the center of gravity.
   d. Prepare muscles by taking a deep breath, and set muscles.
   e. Lift object with arms or by stooping and using leg and thigh muscles.
   f. Carry the object or person close to your body to prevent strain on your back.
   g. Take frequent rest periods to prevent additional strain.

### CHARTING  *for Body Mechanics*

☐  Injury to patient resulting from poor body mechanics

☐  Devices needed for turning and moving

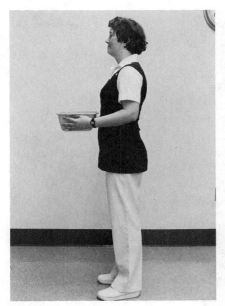

*Correct*
Place both feet flat on the floor and keep your back straight to prevent back injury.

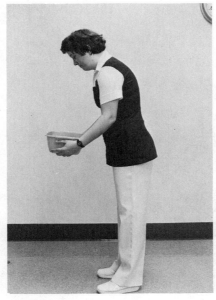

*Incorrect*
Improper body alignment places pressure on the spine and can lead to a back injury.

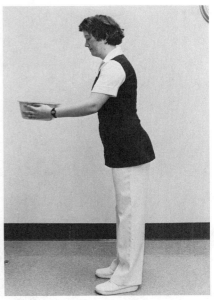

*Incorrect*
Hold objects close to the body to prevent muscle strain and possible back injury.

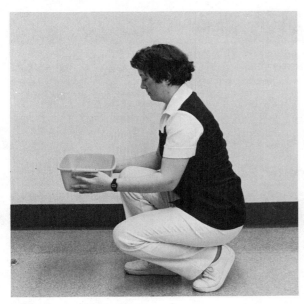

*Correct*
Keep body in proper alignment by bending your knees and keeping back straight when lifting objects to prevent injury.

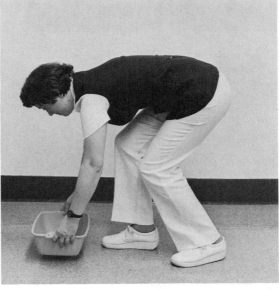

*Incorrect*
Prevent injury to back muscles; for proper alignment, bend at knees and use leg muscles.

☐ Number of personnel required for turning and moving

☐ Ways in which patient assists in moving

☐ Special requirements of patient for proper body alignment

☐ Special turning and moving requirements

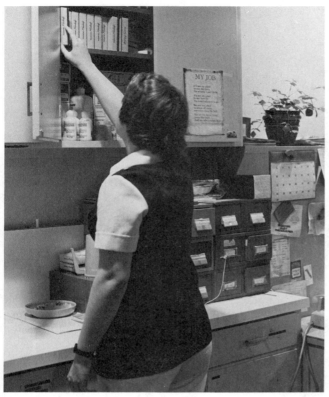

*Correct*
Keep body in correct alignment when turning and reaching for objects to prevent muscle strain or back injury.

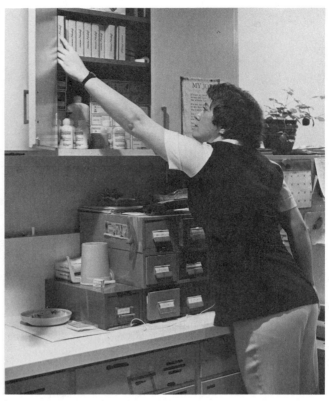

*Incorrect*
Do not use stretching or twisting movements when you reach for objects out of close proximity to your body.

## CLINICAL PROBLEM SOLVING

### Potential Problems

Incorrect body mechanics are used while giving patient care.

Nurse injures self while giving patient care.

### Suggested Solutions

☐ Identify areas of your body where you feel stress and strain.
☐ Evaluate the way you use body mechanics.
☐ Attend an in-service program on using body mechanics appropriately.
☐ Concentrate on how you are using your body when moving and turning patients.
☐ Position bed and equipment at a comfortable height and proximity to working area.
☐ Use your longest and strongest muscles to prevent injury.

☐ Report any back strain immediately to supervisor.
☐ Complete incident report.
☐ Go to health service or emergency room for evaluation and immediate care.
☐ Evaluate any activities that led to injury to determine incorrect use of body mechanics.

Nurse uses poor body mechanics and injures patient.

□ Prevent additional injury by obtaining assistance when needed.
□ Use devices such as turning sheets to assist in turning difficult patients.

□ Assess the extent of patient's injury.
□ Notify patient's physician.
□ Complete incident report.
□ Carry out physician's orders for follow-up treatment.

Due to staffing shortage, nurse is unable to obtain sufficient assistance with turning and moving patients.

□ Place turning sheets on all patients who are difficult to move.
□ Use principles of leverage in moving patients.
□ Until adequate staff is available, turn and position patient from side to side at least every two hours.
□ Use Hoyer lift.

## UNIT TWO   MOVING AND TURNING PATIENTS

### NURSING PROCESS DATA

**ASSESSMENT**   *Data Base*

Observe the patient and identify ways to improve the patient's position and alignment.

Determine the patient's physical ability to assist you with positioning.

Note the presence of tubes, incisions, etc., that will alter the positioning and alignment procedures.

**PLANNING**   *Objectives*

To provide increased comfort.

To provide optimal lung excursion and ventilation.

To prevent contractures due to constant joint flexion.

To promote optimal joint movement.

To help maintain intact skin.

To prevent injury due to improper movement.

**IMPLEMENTATION**   *Procedures*

Turning to Side-lying Position

Turning to a Prone Position

Moving the Patient Up in Bed

Moving the Patient with Assistance

Preparing to Move Patient From Bed

Dangling at the Bedside

Moving from Bed to Chair
Using a Hoyer Lift
Logrolling the Patient
Using a Footboard
Placing a Trochanter Roll

**EVALUATION**   *Expected Outcomes*

Patient's comfort is increased.

Skin remains intact without evidence of breaking down.

Breathing is adequate and unlabored.

Joint movement is maintained.

Foot drop is prevented.

Alignment is maintained.

**TABLE 1**   BED POSITIONS FOR PATIENT CARE

| Positions | Placement | Use |
|---|---|---|
| Fowler's | Head of bed 45-degree angle; hips may or may not be flexed | Postoperative, gastrointestinal conditions |
| Semi-Fowler's | Head of bed 30-degree angle | Cardiac, respiratory, neurosurgical conditions |
| High-Fowler's | Head of bed 60-degree angle | Thoracic surgery, severe respiratory conditions |
| Knee-gatch | Lower section of bed (under knees) slightly raised | For patient comfort; contraindicated for vascular disorders |
| Trendelenburg's | Head of bed lowered and foot raised | Spinal fluid leak following myelogram or laminectomy |

## TURNING TO SIDE-LYING POSITION

### Equipment

Pillows for positioning

Turning sheet

Drawsheet for trochanter roll

### Procedure

1. Identify the patient.

2. Explain the rationale for the procedure to the patient.

3. Lower the head of the bed completely or to a position that is as low as the patient can tolerate.

4. Elevate the bed to a comfortable working height.

5. Move the patient to your side of the bed. Put siderails up and move to other side of bed.

6. Flex the patient's knees.

7. Place one hand on patient's hip and one hand on the patient's shoulder; roll onto side.

8. Position pillow to maintain proper alignment.

9. Be sure to position the patient's arms so that they are not under the body.

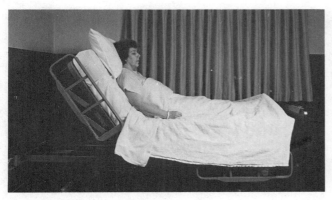

High-Fowler's position

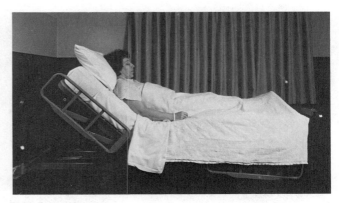

Fowler's position

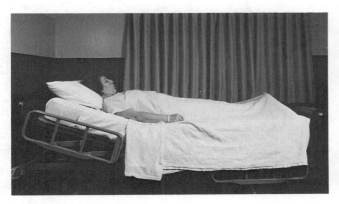

Low-Fowler's position

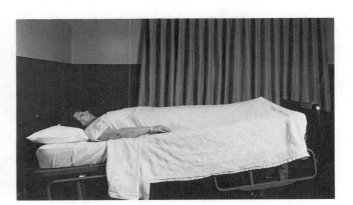

Trendelenburg's position

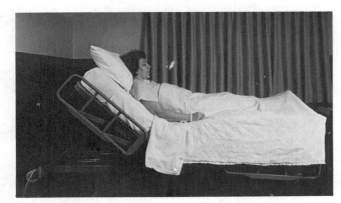

Knee-Gatch position

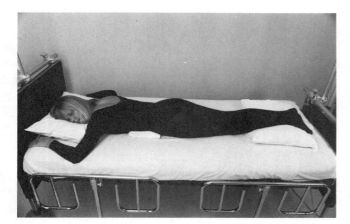

Prone position

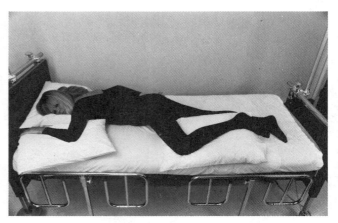

Sims' (semi-prone) position

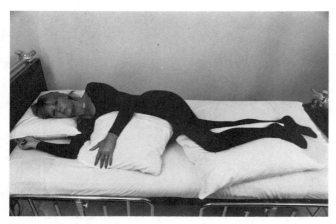

Lateral (side-lying) position

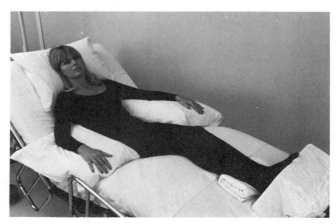

Semi-Fowler's position

## TURNING TO A PRONE POSITION

### Equipment

Pillows for positioning

Turning sheet

### Procedure

1. Identify the patient.

2. Explain the rationale for the procedure to the patient.

3. Lower the head of the bed completely or to a position that is as low as the patient can tolerate.

4. Elevate the bed to a comfortable working height.

5. Move the patient to the side of the bed away from the side where the patient will finally be positioned.

6. Position pillows on the side of the bed for the patient's head, thorax, and feet.

7. Roll the patient onto the pillows, making sure that the patient's arms are not under his body.

8. Reposition pillows as necessary for patient's comfort.

## MOVING THE PATIENT UP IN BED

### Procedure

1. Identify the patient.

2. Explain the rationale for the procedure to the patient.

3. Lower the head of the bed so that it is flat or as low as the patient can tolerate.

4. Raise the bed to a comfortable working height.

5. Remove the pillow and place it at the head of the bed to prevent striking the patient's head against the bed.

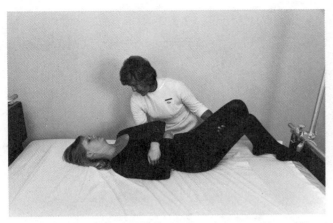

Assume proper body alignment when moving patient up in bed.

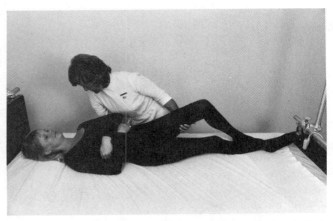

Use large leg muscles for leverage when moving patient up in bed.

6. Place one arm under the patient's shoulders and the other arm under the patient's thighs.

7. Instruct the patient to put his arms across the chest.

8. Instruct the patient to bend legs and to put feet flat on the bed.

9. Lift and pull the patient as he pushes with feet.

10. Position the patient comfortably, replacing the pillow and arranging bedding as necessary.

## MOVING THE PATIENT WITH ASSISTANCE

### Equipment

Drawsheet folded to use as lift sheet

### Procedure

1. Identify the patient.

2. Explain the rationale for the procedure to the patient.

3. Lower the head of the bed so that it is flat or as low as the patient can tolerate.

4. Raise the bed to a comfortable working height.

5. Remove the pillow and place it at the head of the bed.

6. Positioning with two nurses or staff members.
   a. First position: Position one nurse on each side of the patient. Each nurse should have one arm under the patient's shoulders and one arm under the patient's thighs.
   b. Alternate position: Position one nurse at the patient's upper body. The nurse's arm nearest

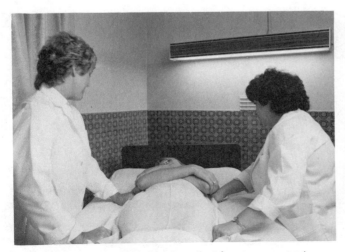

Hold drawsheet firmly and close to patient for proper support.

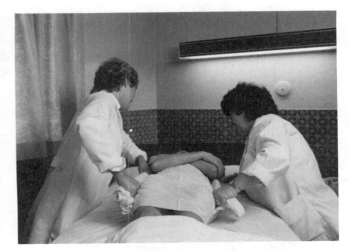

Shift weight from back to front leg when moving patient up in bed.

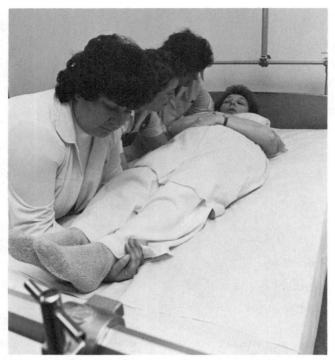

Position all staff at same side of bed when using the three-man lift.

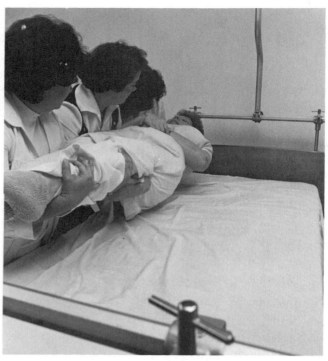

Move patient to the side of the bed before lifting to a guerney.

the head of the bed should be under the patient's head and opposite shoulder. The other arm should be under the patient's closest arm and shoulder. Position the other nurse at the patient's lower torso. The nurse's arms should be under the patient's lower back and thighs.

c. Alternate position: Place folded draw/turn sheet under patient's body extending from shoulder line to just below buttocks. Position one nurse on each side of bed. Roll up sides of lift sheet as close as possible to sides of patient. Assist patient to flex knees, if possible. Each nurse firmly grasps sheet at level of patient's upper back with one hand and at level of buttocks with other hand. Then with one firm, coordinated, rocking movement, lift patient toward head of bed.

7. Positioning with three staff members.
   a. Position two nurses so that each one is supporting the patient's shoulders as described above.
   b. Position the third nurse at the patient's lower torso.

8. Positioning with four staff members.
   a. Position two nurses, one on each side of the patient, so that each one is supporting the patient's shoulders.
   b. Position the other two nurses, one on each side of the patient's hips or legs.

9. Coordinate the movements of all nurses. **Rationale:** One nurse is responsible for stating when to move patient.

10. Place patient in a comfortable position.

## PREPARING TO MOVE PATIENT FROM BED

### Procedure

1. Elevate the bed to a comfortable working height.

2. Place the bed in a flat position. Lower the side rail on the side nearest you.

3. Position yourself at the head of the patient's bed on the side toward which the patient will move.

4. Place the patient's arms across his chest.

5. Place one foot in front of the other. **Rationale:** This stance gives you a broad base of support.

6. Flex your knees.

7. Place your arm closest to the head of the bed under the patient's head and shoulder farthest from you.

8. Place your other arm under the small of the patient's back.

9. Rocking backward and shifting your weight from the front foot to the back foot, pull the upper part of the body toward you.

10. Move your arms to the middle section of the patient. Place one arm under the patient's waist and the other arm under the thighs.

11. Repeat step number 9.

12. Move to the foot of the patient and place one arm under the thighs and the other arm under the calves.

13. Repeat step number 9.

14. Proceed as ordered: transfer patient to guerney by using three-man lift, or assist patient to dangle at bedside.

## DANGLING AT THE BEDSIDE

### Procedure

1. Identify the patient.

2. Lower the bed to the lowest position.

3. Raise the head of the bed until the patient is sitting upright.

4. Stand at the patient's waist with one of your arms under the patient's arm and around upper back. Put your other arm over the patient's legs.

5. Bend the patient's legs and grasp them at the knees.

6. In one motion, swing the legs over the side of the bed and pull the patient's torso upright. Use thigh muscles for leverage when pulling.

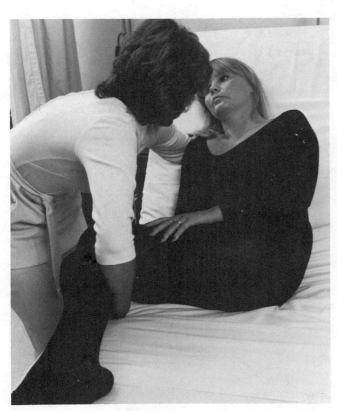

Place one arm around shoulders and grasp knees with the other.

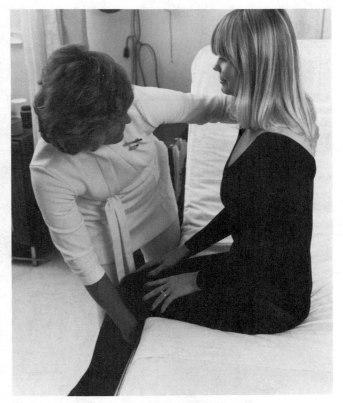

Swing patient's legs over bedside to sitting position.

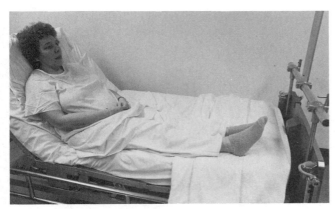

Move patient to the side of bed closest to the edge where the patient will be getting up.

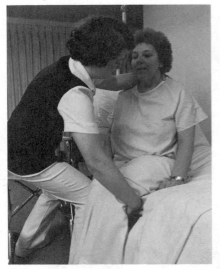

Raise head of bed to assist the patient in pivoting to the side of the bed.

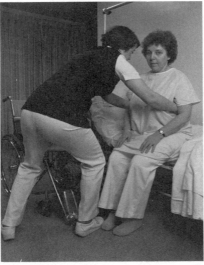

Move patient to edge of bed and place feet flat on floor.

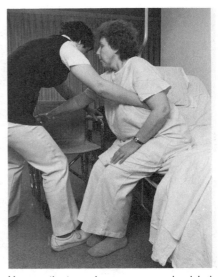

Have patient reach arm across wheelchair and grasp arm.

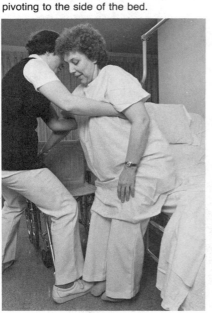

Stabilize patient by positioning your foot at the outside edge of her foot.

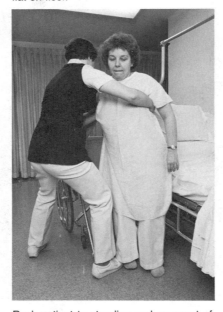

Rock patient to standing and on count of three, pivot patient into chair.

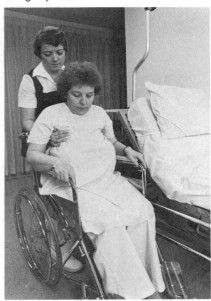

Position patient for maximum comfort and to prevent pressure areas.

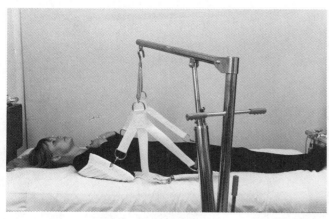

The Hoyer lift is a mechanical device used to move immobilized or difficult patients without strain on staff.

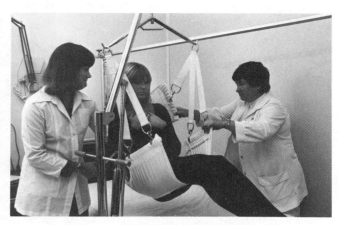

The Hoyer lift is used to move patients in and out of bed to prevent back strain for hospital personnel.

7. Stabilize the patient by pushing your knees against the patient's knees and grasping the torso under the patient's arms.

8. Assess the patient for dizziness or lightheadedness.

9. Dangle patient for a few minutes before transferring to a chair or ambulating.

## MOVING FROM BED TO CHAIR

### Equipment

Chair

Bath blanket

### Procedure

1. Identify the patient.

2. Lock the bed in place.

3. Place the chair at the head of the bed. Be sure to lock chair wheels or have someone hold the chair as you move the patient.

4. Dangle the patient until he is stable.

5. Give the patient nonslip shoes or slippers.

6. Have the patient reach across the chair and grasp the chair arm.

7. Place your hands under the patient's axilla.

8. Place your feet slightly to the side and in front of the patient.

9. Rock the patient and, on the count of three, pivot the patient into the chair.

10. Position the patient in the chair to prevent pressure areas.

## USING THE HOYER LIFT

### Equipment

Hoyer lift base

2 canvas pieces, 1 large, 1 small

2 sets of canvas straps

### Procedure

1. Check orders and Patient Care Plan. Determine that lift can safely move the weight of the patient.

2. Explain the procedure to the patient. **Rationale:** Patients may be frightened by the use of a mechanical device.

3. Wash your hands.

4. Bring Hoyer frame to bedside.

5. Provide privacy for patient.

6. Lock wheels of bed.

7. Place patient's chair by the bed. Allow adequate space to maneuver the lift.

8. Raise the bed to HIGH position and adjust head and knee gatch so that mattress is flat.

9. Keep side rail on opposite side in UP position.

10. Roll patient away from you.

11. Place the lower edge of the wide canvas piece under the patient's knees.

12. Place the upper edge of the narrow canvas piece under the patient's shoulders.

13. Raise side rail on your side of bed.

14. Move to opposite side of bed and lower side rail.

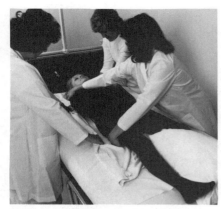

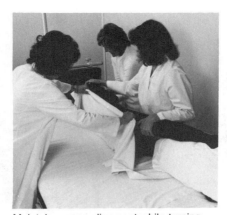

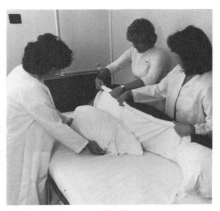

Position nurses on each side of patient. Maintain proper alignment while turning. Maintain position with pillow support.

15. Roll patient away from you to opposite side and straighten out canvas pieces. Turn patient to supine position.

16. Place U base of the frame under the bed on side where chair is positioned.

17. Lock wheels of frame. Lower side rail.

18. Attach canvas straps from swivel bar to each canvas piece using the hooks.

19. Be sure straps are evenly placed on canvas pieces.

20. Elevate head of bed.

21. Raise patient by turning release knob clockwise to close pressure valve.

22. Pump the lift handle until patient is lifted clear of the bed.

23. Maneuver the patient over the chair.

24. Lower the patient by turning release knob *slowly* counterclockwise.

25. Guide patient into the chair.

26. Align patient into chair.

27. Remove the straps from the bar and move the lift out of the way.

28. Check for patient's comfort in chair; place call bell close at hand.

29. Wash your hands.

30. Return patient to bed using the same method.

## LOGROLLING THE PATIENT

### Equipment

Pillows, towels, blankets for positioning

Turning sheet

### Procedure

1. Check order for logrolling patient.

2. Check Kardex and Patient Care Plan as to exactly why the patient needs to be logrolled.

3. Obtain sufficient assistance to complete the procedure with ease. Three nurses are preferable.

4. Before moving the patient, place a pillow between the patient's knees.

5. Position two nurses on side of the bed to which the patient will be turned. Position third nurse on the other side of the bed.

6. Designate the person at the head of the bed to be in charge of coordinating move.

7. Assume the correct position for patient move:
   a. Nurse at head: one arm supports patient's head, second arm supports shoulders and neck.
   b. Second nurse: one hand grasps patient's other shoulder, the other hand and arm around hip.
   c. Third nurse: on the opposite side of the bed, nurse holds drawsheet firmly to support torso in alignment.

8. Move the patient in one coordinated movement when the nurse at the head of bed signals. **Rationale:** To maintain proper alignment, all of the body parts must be moved at the same time. If not, injury to the patient's neck and spinal column may occur.

9. Maintain patient's position in alignment with pillows, towels, or folded blankets.

10. Change patient's position frequently (minimum 2 hours) according to physician's orders.

## USING A FOOTBOARD

### Equipment

Footboard

### Procedure

1. Assess patient's ability to place feet in dorsal flexion. If unable to do so, or plantar flexion is continuous, provide a footboard.

2. Cover footboard with a bath blanket to protect feet from rough surfaces.

3. Place footboard on the bed in a place where patient's feet can firmly rest on it without sliding down in bed.

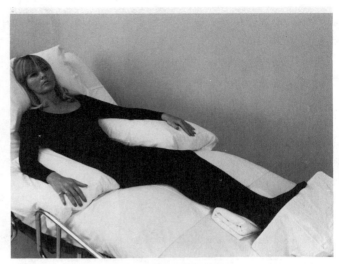

Footboards can be improvised if regular footboard is not available.

---

**Clinical Alert**

Footboards are utilized to prevent plantarflexion and/or external rotation of the hip. Ensure proper positioning to prevent footdrop.

---

4. Observe legs to ensure that they are not in a flexed position when feet are against the board.

5. Tuck top linen under mattress at foot of bed, and bring linen up over the footboard to the top of the bed. Do not drape top linen over footboard as it can easily be pulled off the bed.

6. Put feet and ankles through range-of-motion exercises every four hours for patients on prolonged bedrest.

7. Observe heels and ankles frequently for signs of breakdown.

## PLACING A TROCHANTER ROLL

### Equipment

Bath blanket

### Procedure

1. Place patient in supine or prone position.

2. Place folded bath blanket on bed next to patient.

3. Extend blanket from patient's waist to knee.

4. Place blanket edge under leg and buttocks to anchor.

5. Roll bath blanket toward patient by rolling it under.

6. Rotate affected leg to slight internal hip rotation. **Rationale:** The purpose is to prevent external rotation of the head of the femur in the acetabulum.

7. Tighten the roll by tucking the roll under the hip joint.

8. Allow affected leg to rest against trochanter roll. Hip should be in normal alignment, not internally or externally rotated. **Rationale:** This is used most commonly for patients who have a muscle weakness or paralysis of that side of the body.

### CHARTING  *for Moving and Turning Patients*

☐ How often patient turned or moved

☐ Condition of skin and joint movement

☐ Unexpected problems with moving or positioning patient and solutions to problems

☐ Patient's acceptance of and feelings about the procedure

☐ Number of staff needed to complete the procedure

☐ Transferred by Hoyer lift from bed to chair, if appropriate

☐ Time patient was in chair or dangling at bedside

☐ Use of a footboard or trochanter roll

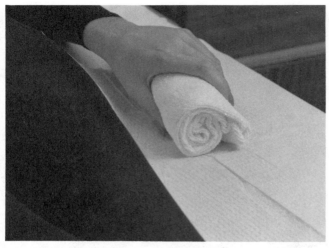

Use handrolls made from towels to position patient's hand and wrist. This will help to prevent contractures and immobility.

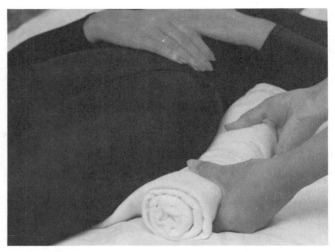

Use trochanter rolls made from bath blankets to align the patient's hips and keep them in internal rotation.

## CLINICAL PROBLEM SOLVING

| Potential Problems | Suggested Solutions |
|---|---|
| Patient unwilling to move due to fear of pain or discomfort. | ☐ Explain rationale and need for the procedure more thoroughly.<br>☐ If possible, check if patient can be medicated before the procedure.<br>☐ Obtain additional assistance to decrease patient's apprehension. |
| Patient unable to assist with movement. | ☐ Use a turn sheet to provide more support for patient.<br>☐ Obtain additional assistance to help with moving "dead" weight. |
| Patient unable to maintain any type of position without assistance. | ☐ Use trochanter roll to prevent external rotation of patient's hip.<br>☐ Use foam bolsters to maintain side-lying positions.<br>☐ Using folded towels, blankets, or small pillows, position patient's hands and arms to prevent dependent edema. |
| Skin begins to break down. | ☐ Keep patient off affected area until healed.<br>☐ Change patient's position every two hours.<br>☐ Check with physician for therapeutic mattress or medications for decubitus care. |

# TERMINOLOGY

**Alignment:**  referring to posture, the relationship of body parts to one another.

**Ambulate:**  walking; able to walk.

**Amphiarthrotic joint:**  a joint that has limited movement.

**Appendicular skeleton:**  composed of 126 bones which include the shoulder, girdle, arm bones, pelvic girdle and leg bones.

**Axial skeleton:**  includes the head and trunk which form the central axis to which the appendicular skeleton is attached.

**Base of support:**  surface area on which an object rests, e.g., for a patient lying in prone position, the base of support is the entire undersurface of the body.

**Body mechanics:**  movement of the body in a coordinated and efficient way so that proper balance, alignment and conservation of energy is maintained.

**Brachial plexus:**  network of spinal nerves supplying arm, forearm, and hand.

**Cartilage:**  bone-like tissue of the very young that is replaced by bone tissue through the process of ossification. In adults cartilage is found in such areas as the nose, ears, and knees.

**Center of gravity:**  midpoint or center of the body weight. In an adult it is the mid-pelvic cavity between the symphysis pubis and umbilicus.

**Compact bone layer:**  dense, hard layer of bone tissue.

**Dangle:**  to have a patient sit on the edge of the bed with feet in a dependent position.

**Diarthrotic joint:**  type of joint that allows for free movement; a cavity enclosed by a capsule lined with synovial membrane that secretes a lubricant.

**Dorsiflexion:**  flexion of the foot at the ankle joint; the act of turning the foot and toes upward, as in standing on the heel.

**Flexion:**  the act or condition of being bent.

**Footdrop:**  a falling or dragging of the foot from paralysis of the flexors of the ankle.

**Fowler's position:**  head of bed is at a 45-degree angle; patient's knees may or may not be flexed.

**Gravity:**  the force that pulls objects toward the earth's surface.

**High-Fowler's position:**  head of bed is at a 90-degree angle; often used to achieve maximum chest expansion.

**Hoyer lift:**  a mechanical device that enables one person to safely transfer a patient from bed to chair.

**Joint:**  the portion of the body where two or more bones join together.

**Leverage:**  the use of a lever to apply force.

**Ligament:**  a band or sheet of strong fibrous connective tissue connecting the articular ends of bones serving to bind them together and to facilitate or limit motion.

**Line of gravity:**  an imaginary line that goes from the center of gravity to the base of support.

**Marrow:**  soft tissue that is contained in the compact bone hollow.

**Mobility:**  state or quality of being mobile; facility of movement.

**Musculo:**  pertaining to muscles.

**Musculoskeletal:**  pertaining to the muscles and bones.

**Paralysis:**  temporary or permanent loss of function, especially loss of sensation or voluntary motion.

**Periosteum:**  the thin, tough membrane of fibrous tissue that forms the outer or exterior layer of bone.

**Posture:**  attitude or position of body.

**Prone:**  lying horizontal with face downward.

**Reverse Trendelenburg's position:**  mattress remains unbent, but head of bed is raised and foot is lowered.

**Semi-Fowler's position:**  head of bed is at a 30-degree angle; often used for patients with cardiac and respiratory problems.

**Skeletal system:**  system of separate bones (206) bound together by ligaments and responsible for supporting, moving and giving shape to the body.

**Sprain:**  injury caused by wrenching or twisting of a joint that results in tearing or stretching of the associated ligaments.

**Stable:**  when the center of gravity is close to the base of support.

**Strain:**  injury caused by excessive force or stretching of muscles or tendons around the joint.

**Synarthrotic joint:**  type of joint that is immovable and includes suture lines of the skull.

**Trendelenburg's position:**  mattress remains unbent but the head of the bed is lowered and the foot is raised. "Shock blocks" may be used under the legs of the bed to achieve this position.

**Trochanter:**  either of the two bony prominences below the neck of the femur.

# Chapter 9

# Bathing and Bedmaking

## LEARNING OBJECTIVES

Demonstrate handwashing technique maintaining medical asepsis.

Demonstrate donning and removing clean gloves according to gloving protocol.

Compare and contrast the steps in making an occupied, unoccupied, and surgical bed.

Demonstrate the skill of folding a mitered corner.

Outline the steps in bathing a bedridden adult patient.

Differentiate between bathing a bedridden patient and a critically ill patient.

Compare and contrast the differences in bathing an infant and an adult patient.

Describe the assessment modalities completed while bathing a patient.

Outline the steps in providing AM care.

Demonstrate the skill of placing a bedpan for a bedridden patient.

Describe briefly the components of evening care.

Define the three back care strokes and their use in back care.

Complete patient charting for evening care on nurses' notes.

Write three nursing diagnoses appropriate for providing basic hygienic care to patients.

## BASIC HEALTH CARE

Patients enter the hospital environment because of an accident or acute illness requiring immediate care, or because the physician has recommended diagnostic procedures or surgery. The latter is commonly referred to as an "elective admission." Regardless of the reason, the patient must rapidly alter everyday routines and activities of daily living. The patient may be concerned about his health and well-being and may experience varying degrees of anxiety as a reaction to unfamiliar procedures, hospital personnel, and the hospital environment.

After the patient has been admitted to the health care unit, many independent actions such as bathing, personal hygiene, and general care may be curtailed by the nature of the illness and confinement. The patient may require assistance with even the simplest of actions. Without therapeutic intervention, the total adaptation process may be put in jeopardy as additional physical problems occur.

Knowing when and how to intervene and performing skills such as bedmaking, bathing and personal hygiene will facilitate the process of adapting to the health care.

When the patient is confined to bed even for a short period of time, comfort is essential in order to promote rest and sleep. Beds must be kept clean, free of debris and wrinkles to prevent skin irritation and breakdown. The bed needs to be straightened frequently during the day to accomplish this. If the patient is to remain in bed for an extended length of time, all care and daily routines will be directed from bed. It will become the center of activity.

There are many different types of beds and related equipment available to meet the special health care needs of individual patients.

**Types of Beds**   The hospital bed is a standard twin size bed in a frame that allows for different positions to facilitate care and comfort for the patient. The height, head and foot positions in most beds are electrically operated to assist both the patient and the nursing staff.

The Stryker frame or Foster frame bed is generally used for individuals who are unable to move, such as those with spinal cord injuries, and for patients who must be placed in the prone position, such as those with decubitus ulcers. Canvas pieces are attached to a frame, which is placed over the patient. It is then secured to the lower section of the frame so the patient can be flipped over to the reverse position. The upper frame is then removed.

Another type of bed is the circular frame, an electrically operated bed that is attached to a circular frame. The patient can be placed in a variety of positions with the support of an upper frame. The patient can gradually be raised to a standing position or can be placed in the prone position. Circular beds can be operated by one person, although it is strongly advised to use two people.

The recovery room bed is an adaptation of the basic hospital bed. This bed has the same features as the basic bed but is usually nonelectric. It is generally narrower and has side rails all the way around the bed instead of a head and footboard. It is easily movable and is occasionally used in intensive care units, labor rooms, and emergency rooms.

Two other special types of beds are air and water beds. These beds are most commonly used for obstetrical patients and severe skin conditions such as decubitus ulcers or burns. Instead of the standard mattress, a specially designed heavy plastic casing is filled with water or air and serves as the mattress. They are used to create less pressure on weight-bearing areas of the body.

**Bathing**   Routine bathing is an essential component of daily care. It is essential to prevent body odor, as excessive perspiration interacts with bacteria to cause odor. Dead skin cells can lead to infection if impaired skin integrity occurs. Excessive bathing, on the other hand, can be dangerous to elderly patients. In the aged the skin may become dry and cracked which can lead to infection.

Bathing promotes a feeling of self-worth by improving the person's appearance. Relaxation and improved circulation are benefits of bathing and play a therapeutic role in the care of patients on bedrest. The apocrine glands, found in the axillae and pubic areas, produce sweat which leads to odor. Therefore, special bathing considerations should be given to these areas.

In addition to the therapeutic effects, the bath affords the nurse time to spend in communication and assessment. Assessment of skin conditions, mobility and self-care deficits can be detected while bathing the patient.

Bathing is accomplished in a variety of ways, according to the patient's needs, condition, and personal habits. Bathing is necessary to cleanse the skin and to promote circulation. Baths may also be used as a treatment to promote healing for a patient with burns. Various types of bathing include:

☐ Complete bed bath: The patient is bathed by the nurse due to physical and/or mental incapacity. The patient is encouraged to complete as much of his bath as possible.

☐ Partial bath: Face, axilla, hands, back and genital area are bathed. Partial bath may be completed by patient or nurse.

☐ Therapeutic bath: This bath is used as part of a treatment regime for specific conditions such as skin disorders, burns, high body temperature, and muscular injuries.

☐ Shower: Preferred method of bathing if patient is ambulatory or can be transported to use a shower chair.

☐ Tub bath: Utilized by ambulatory patients as well as those who must be assisted by a device such as the Hoyer lift.

**Skin Problems**    Skin types, colors, textures, and condition are as different as each person's unique individuality. The condition of a patient's skin will be determined by his health status, age, activity level, and environmental exposure. For example, the skin of an infant is often more sensitive and delicate than that of an adult because it has not been exposed to many of the elements of the environment. Most infants cannot tolerate strong soaps and lotions, and must be handled gently to avoid trauma. Adolescents are affected by acne and have areas of increased oil secretion. Adults may have drier skin, especially as they age. Older adults cannot always tolerate harsh soaps because their skin is more delicate. They require less frequent bathing and more lubrication with oil-rich creams and lotions.

Maintaining skin integrity is an integral part of providing nursing care; being aware of the patient's skin condition and alterations in the integrity is a critical aspect of providing total patient care.

## NURSING DIAGNOSES

The following nursing diagnoses may be appropriate to include in a Patient Care Plan when the components are related to Basic Care of the Patient.

| **Nursing Diagnosis** (Potential) | **Defining Characteristic; Etiology** (Examples) |
|---|---|
| ☐ Activity Intolerance, *related to* | Physiological or therapeutic limitations, e.g., surgical intervention, medications, respiratory or circulatory impairment (fatigue, SOB). |
| ☐ Health Maintenance, Alteration in, *related to* | Impaired mobility, e.g., motor skill or cognitive deficit. |
| ☐ Self-Care Deficit: Bathing/ Hygiene, *related to* | Dependence on others for assistance, e.g., complete bedrest, unavailable equipment. |
| ☐ Skin Integrity, Impairment of: Potential, *related to* | Skin irritation, e.g., incontinence or wound drainage. |

## UNIT ONE    BASIC MEDICAL ASEPSIS

### NURSING PROCESS DATA

**ASSESSMENT** *Data Base*

Assess need for handwashing.

Identify patients at risk for infection.

Assess availability of equipment for frequent handwashing.

Evaluate health status of the nurse.

Check agency policy for handwashing protocol.

Assess need for use of unsterile gloves.

## PLANNING   *Objectives*

To deliver patient care with pathogen-free hands.

To prevent pathogenic microorganisms from spreading from patient to patient.

To protect patients from cross-contamination.

To protect the nurse.

## IMPLEMENTATION   *Procedures*

Handwashing (Medical Asepsis)

Cleaning Washable Articles

Donning and Removing Clean Gloves

## EVALUATION   *Expected Outcomes*

Infection is prevented from spreading.

Cross-contamination is prevented.

Nurse is protected from infection.

## HANDWASHING (MEDICAL ASEPSIS)

### Equipment

Soap containing a germicide

Orangestick for cleaning nails

Running warm water

Paper towels

Trash basket

### Procedure

1. Stand in front of but away from sink. **Rationale:** Uniform should not touch sink to avoid contamination.

2. Crank towel out of holder before washing. **Rationale:** Crank is considered contaminated.

3. Turn on water faucet so that flow is adequate, but not splashing.

4. Adjust temperature to warm. **Rationale:** Cold does not facilitate sudsing/cleaning; hot is damaging to skin.

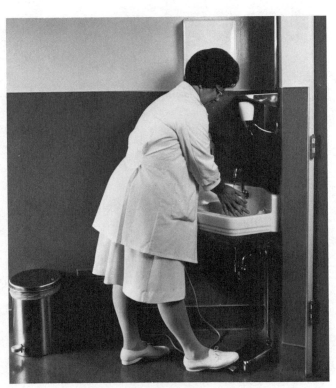

Use foot pedals when available to prevent contamination of hands.

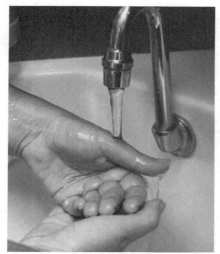

Wet hands thoroughly before applying soap to facilitate removal of pathogens.

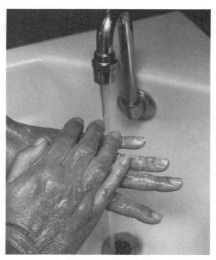

Use generous amount of soap and friction during hand washing procedure.

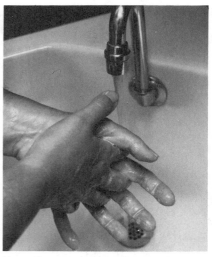

Keep fingers pointed down during hand-washing to prevent contamination of arms.

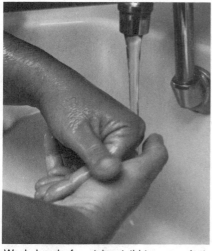

Wash hands for at least thirty seconds to remove pathogens.

> **Clinical Alert**
> Aseptic technique, especially handwashing, prevents the spread of infection in hospitalized patients.

11. Resoap your hands, rewash, and rerinse if heavily contaminated.
12. Dry hands thoroughly with a paper towel, while keeping hands positioned with fingers pointing up.
13. Turn off water faucet with paper towel used to dry hands.
14. Restart procedure at step 5 if your hands touch the sink any time between steps 5 and 14.

## CLEANING WASHABLE ARTICLES

### Equipment

Article to be washed

Soap

Running warm water

Paper towels

Trash basket

### Procedure

1. Rinse under cold running water.
2. Wash with warm, soapy water using friction.
3. Rinse well with clear water.
4. Dry thoroughly.

5. Wet hands under running water.
6. Place a small amount, one to two teaspoons, of liquid soap on hands.
7. Rub vigorously, using a firm, circular motion, while keeping your fingers pointed down, lower than wrists. Start with each finger, then between fingers, then palm and back of hand.
8. Wash your hands for at least 30 seconds.
9. Clean under your fingernails with an orangewood stick. (This should be done at least at start of day and if hands are heavily contaminated.)
10. Rinse your hands under running water, keeping fingers pointed downward.

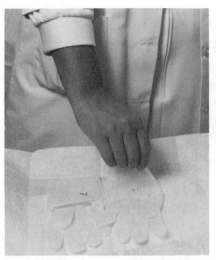

Pick up sterile glove by rolled edge. Be careful not to touch the outer surface.

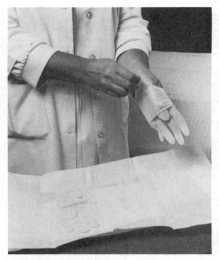

Lift glove up and away from sterile package to prevent contamination of gloves.

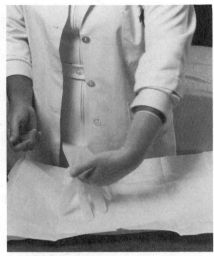

Place sterile gloved fingers under the cuff of the second glove and lift it up and away.

5. Return to proper place or prepare for sterilization or disinfection if indicated. Wash your hands.

## DONNING AND REMOVING CLEAN GLOVES

### Equipment

Unsterile gloves

Discard basket

### Procedure

1. Explain to the patient the reason for glove use if appropriate.
2. Pick up glove at wrist edge and slip fingers into openings. Pull glove up to wrist.
3. Repeat step 2 for second glove.
4. Remove glove by pulling off, touching only outside of glove at cuff, so that glove turns inside out. (Omit this step if only one glove is used.)
5. Remove second glove by slipping one finger under glove edge and pulling down and off so that glove turns inside out.

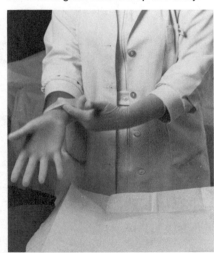

Maintain sterility while gloving by allowing only sterile surfaces to touch each other.

6. Dispose of gloves in proper container, not at bedside. Wash your hands.

### CHARTING  *for Basic Asepsis*

☐  Infection control measures utilized

☐  Clean gloves used for procedure

---

## CLINICAL PROBLEM SOLVING

### Potential Problems

Infection occurs in patient.

### Suggested Solutions

☐  Administer antibiotics specific to microorganism as ordered.
☐  Review hand washing technique.
☐  Attend in-service program on infection control procedures.

# UNIT TWO   BEDMAKING

## NURSING PROCESS DATA

### ASSESSMENT   *Data Base*

Assess the patient's need to have linen changed.

Determine if the patient's present condition will permit a change of bed linen.

Determine how many and what type of linens will be required.

Check patient's unit for available linens.

Determine patient's prescribed level of activity and any special precautions in movement.

Assess patient's ability to get out of bed during linen change.

### PLANNING   *Objectives*

To provide a clean, comfortable sleeping and resting environment for the patient.

To eliminate irritants to skin by providing wrinkle-free sheets and blankets.

To avoid patient exertion by making bed while occupied. (Do not move more than necessary.)

To enhance patient's self-image by providing a clean, neat, and comfortable bed.

To properly dispose of soiled linens and not promote cross-contamination.

To correctly align patients to assist in promoting a physically and emotionally safe and comfortable position.

To prevent stress to the nurse's back or limbs during procedure.

### IMPLEMENTATION   *Procedures*

Folding a Mitered Corner

Changing a Pillowcase

Making an Unoccupied Bed

Making a Surgical Bed

Changing an Occupied Bed

### EVALUATION   *Expected Outcomes*

Patient is rested during and after bedmaking procedure.

Bed remains clean, dry, free of wrinkles or other skin irritants, and at a comfortable temperature.

Skin remains free of irritation caused by contact with linens.

The nurse feels no stress to back or limbs during the procedure.

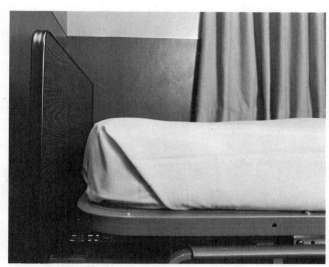

Miter corners to keep bed linens tight and wrinkle-free.

## FOLDING A MITERED CORNER

### Equipment

Same as for Unoccupied Bed

### Procedure

1. Tuck sheet tightly and smoothly under mattress at top of the bed.
2. Grasp edge of sheet with hand and bring sheet onto mattress so that edge forms a right angle.
3. Tuck lower edge of sheet under mattress.
4. Place finger on sheet where it meets mattress and lower top of sheet over finger. **Rationale:** This action makes the mitered corner neat and tight.
5. Remove finger without disturbing folds.
6. Tuck sheet securely under mattress.

## CHANGING A PILLOWCASE

### Equipment

Clean pillowcase

### Procedure

1. Pick up center of closed end of pillowcase.
2. Continue to firmly grip end of pillowcase; then with other hand gather pillowcase from open end and fold back (inside-out) over closed end.
3. Pick up center of one end of pillow with the hand holding the gathered pillowcase.

4. Pull pillowcase over pillow with other hand. Do not place pillow and/or case under arm, chin, or in teeth. **Rationale:** Contamination occurs from using these methods.
5. Adjust pillow corners in pillowcase by placing hand between case and pillow.

## MAKING AN UNOCCUPIED BED

### Equipment

Chair or table

Linen hamper

Linens (in order of use):
    Bath blanket
    Mattress pad
    Bottom sheet
    Drawsheet
    Incontinent pad, if needed
    Top sheet
    Blanket
    Bedspread
    Pillowcase

### Preparation

1. Gather linen and hamper and bring to room.
2. Explain need for patient to be out of bed during procedure.
3. Wash hands.
4. Assist patient out of bed and into chair.
5. Arrange chair and hamper conveniently for use.
6. Wipe chair off before placing linen on chair. **Rationale:** This action provides a clean surface and promotes infection control.
7. Place linen on chair.
8. Remove call signal from linen.
9. Adjust bed to a comfortable working height.

### Procedure

1. Lower both side rails.
2. Loosen linen on all sides, including head and foot of the bed.
3. Remove spread and blanket. If they are to be reused, fold them and place on the chair.
4. Remove top, draw, and bottom sheet and place in linen hamper. **Rationale:** Never place dirty linen on the floor as cross-contamination occurs from this action.

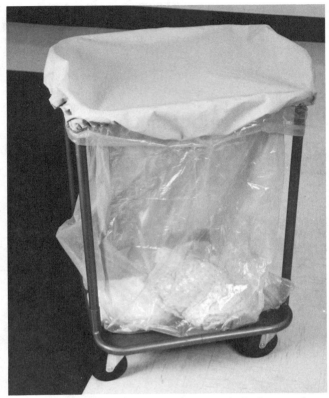

Keep linen hamper covered to prevent spread of microorganisms. This type of linen hamper can be taken into the patient's room.

5. Push mattress to head of bed. Center the mattress if necessary.

6. If mattress pad is not changed, smooth out wrinkles and recenter pad on the bed surface.

7. Make up one side of the bed, then move to the other side of bed and make it. **Rationale:** This step saves time and energy.

8. Place clean bottom sheet on mattress. Place the center fold of the sheet in the middle of the mattress with the end of the sheet even with the end of the mattress.

9. Unfold the bottom sheet and cover the mattress.

10. Tuck the top of the sheet under the head of the bed.

11. Miter the corner of the bottom sheet at the head of the bed. (See procedure for mitered corner.) **Rationale:** A mitered corner is tighter and less likely to come apart.

12. Tuck the remaining side of the bottom sheet well under the mattress.

13. If the patient needs a drawsheet, center the draw-sheet on the bed and open draw sheet top to opposite side. Tuck the sheet under the mattress. Smooth out wrinkles.

   a. If a pull sheet is needed, fold drawsheet in half or quarters. Position sheet in middle of bed. **Rationale:** Pull sheets are used with heavy or difficult-to-move patients.

   b. If absorbent pad is needed, center it on bed over draw or pull sheet.

14. Move to the other side of the bed. Pull linen toward you and straighten out linen.

15. Tuck the top of the sheet under the head of the bed.

16. Miter the corner of the bottom sheet at the head of the bed.

17. Tuck remaining bottom sheet well under the mattress. Gather sheet into your hand, lean away from the bed, and pull sheet downward. Tuck sheet under mattress.

18. If drawsheet is used, tighten and tuck the same as bottom sheet.

19. Straighten out absorbent pad and pull sheet if used.

20. Place top sheet, blanket, and spread full length on top of bed.

21. Leave a cuff of top sheet and spread at the head of the bed.

22. Tuck sheet, spread and blanket well under foot of mattress, one side at a time.

23. Miter corners at the foot of the bed, one side at a time.

24. Make a small pleat to allow room for patient's feet.

25. Fanfold linen to foot of bed.

26. Change pillowcase.

27. Return bed to lowest position. Reattach call signal to linens.

28. Pull side rail up on side furthest from patient.

29. If the unit is unassigned, leave top linen pulled up, covering the bed.

30. Dispose of soiled laundry.

31. Wash your hands.

## MAKING A SURGICAL BED

### Equipment

Same as for Unoccupied Bed

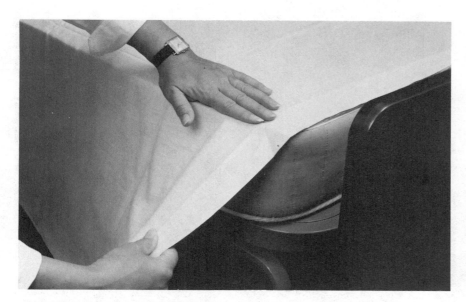

Place bottom sheet at mattress edge when contour sheet is not available.

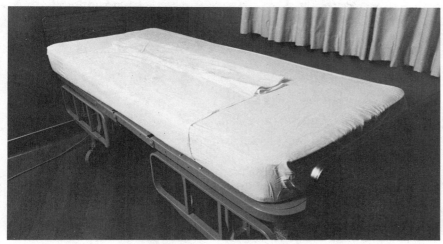

Tuck drawsheet in tightly. This assists in keeping the linen wrinkle-free.

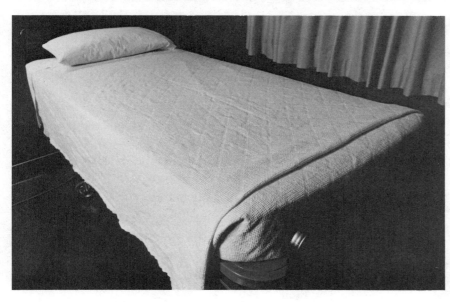

The top linen must be pleated to allow space for movement of the patient's feet.

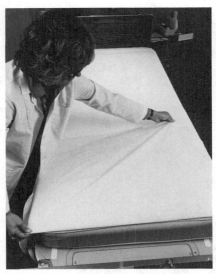

Fold back top linen from foot of bed until linen is flush with edge of mattress.

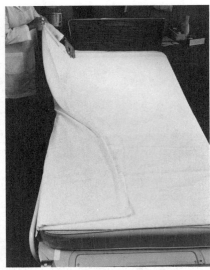

Fold back top linen from side of bed until linen is flush with side of mattress.

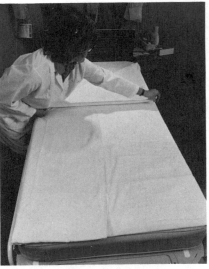

Pick up linen from top corner of bed near you and fold back to form triangle.

## Procedure

1. Wash your hands.

2. Bring linens to the room.

3. Arrange chair and linen hamper conveniently for use.

4. Wipe off chair before placing linen on it.

5. Raise bed to highest position.

6. Place the bottom sheet on the bed, using the same method for making an unoccupied bed.

7. Place a plastic and/or cloth drawsheet and absorbent pad on the bed.

8. Lay top sheet, blanket, and bedspread over top of bed.

9. Fold up linen from foot, head, and one side of the bed toward center of the bed.

10. Fold bottom and top edges nearest you to the opposite side, forming a triangle. Pick up center point of triangle.

11. Fanfold linen to side of bed. **Rationale:** Folding linen at side of the bed facilitates moving surgical patients into the bed.

12. Leave bed in HIGH position to facilitate easy transfer of surgical patient from guerney to bed.

13. Change pillowcase and leave on chair or at foot of bed.

14. Move all objects away from bedside area. **Rationale:** This allows surgical guerney to be placed close to bed for patient transfer.

## CHANGING AN OCCUPIED BED

### Equipment

Chair or table

Linen hamper

Linens (in order of use):
 Bath blanket
 Mattress pad
 Bottom sheet
 Plastic drawsheet, if needed
 Cloth drawsheet
 Incontinent pad, if needed
 Top sheet
 Blanket
 Bedspread
 Pillowcase

### Preparation

1. Talk with the patient and explain how he can be involved in the procedure.

2. Explain the sequence for the procedure.

3. Arrange furniture and equipment, e.g., linen hamper and chair for convenience of use.

4. Wipe chair or table before putting linen on it.

5. Wash your hands and collect the linen.

6. Place linen on chair or table after wiping it off.

7. Remove call signal from linens.

8. Pull curtain closed to provide privacy for the patient.

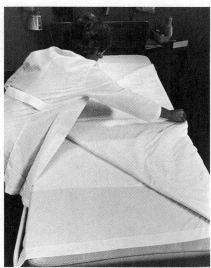

Pick up linen from bottom corner of bed near you and fold back to form triangle.

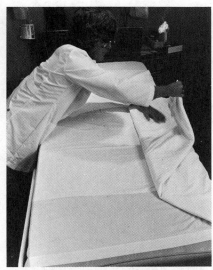

Fanfold linen to opposite side of bed to facilitate easy transfer of surgical patients.

9. Adjust the bed to a comfortable working height with side rails up. Help patient into a supine position.

**Procedure**

1. Lower side rail on your side of the bed but make sure side rail on opposite side is in UP position.

2. Loosen top linens.

3. Remove spread, sheet and blanket at the same time the bath blanket is pulled over patient. If they are to be reused, fold them and place on the chair.

4. Place top sheet in linen hamper.

5. Push mattress to head of bed. Center the mattress if necessary.

6. Assist patient to the side of the bed, place in side-lying position facing away from you as near the far side rail as possible.

7. Loosen bottom linens on your side of the bed.

8. Push dirty linen under or as close as possible to patient.

9. If mattress pad is not changed, smooth out wrinkles and recenter pad on the bed surface.

10. With patient on the opposite side of the bed, place clean bottom sheet on mattress. Place the center fold of the sheet in the middle of the mattress with the end of the sheet even with the end of the mattress.

11. Unfold the bottom sheet and cover the mattress.

Make sure the clean bottom sheet is underneath any used linen.

12. Tuck the top of the sheet under the head of the bed.

13. Miter the corner of the bottom sheet at the head of the bed.

14. Tuck the remaining bottom sheet well under the mattress from head to foot.

15. Center the plastic and/or cloth drawsheet on the bed, if the patient requires a drawsheet, and fanfold half of the sheet under the patient. Tuck side of the sheet under the mattress. Smooth out wrinkles.

    a. Fold cloth drawsheet in half or quarters if a pull sheet is needed. Position sheet in middle of bed. Fanfold half of the pull sheet under patient.

    b. Fanfold absorbent pad and center it on bed under patient's buttocks. Place the pad close to the patient for ease in pulling it through to the other side of the bed, absorbent side up and plastic side down.

16. Help the patient roll over to the other side of the bed.

17. Tell the patient why there is a hump of linen in the center of the bed. Make the patient comfortable.

18. Raise the side rail. Move to other side of bed.

19. Move linens to the other side of the bed, by gently pulling linens toward you.

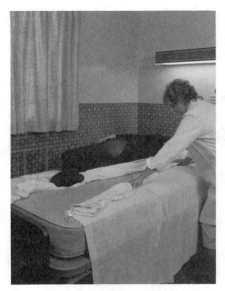

Place center fold of sheet in middle of bed.

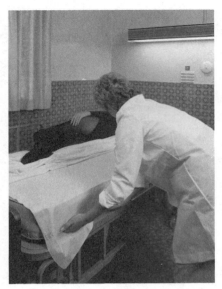

Tighten bottom sheet under mattress.

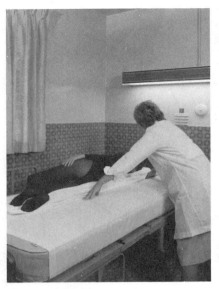

Place drawsheet in middle of bed.

20. Lower side rail and loosen bottom sheets.

21. Pull dirty linen to side of bed and roll into a bundle at the foot of the bed or place linen in linen hamper.

22. Never place dirty linen on the floor. **Rationale:** Cross-contamination occurs from this action.

23. Pull clean linen across mattress and straighten under patient.

24. Miter the top corner of the bottom sheet.

25. Gather bottom sheet into your hand, lean away from the bed and pull linens downward at an angle. Tuck remaining bottom sheet well under the mattress. If drawsheet is used, tighten and tuck it in the same way.

26. Help the patient into a supine position and adjust the pillow.

27. Place top sheet, blanket, and spread over the patient. Leave a 6 inch cuff of top sheet at the head of the bed.

28. Remove bath blanket and straighten top sheet and blanket.

29. Miter corners at foot of bed.

30. Pull up all layers of linen at patient's toes. Make a small pleat to allow room for patient's feet.

31. Raise side rail.

---

**PRINCIPLES OF MEDICAL ASEPSIS**

Place dirty linen in hamper.
Do not place dirty linen on floor.
Discard all unused linen from patient area.
Do not transfer linen from one patient area to another.
Do not allow dirty linen to touch uniform.

---

32. Remove pillow from bed and change pillowcase.

33. Return bed to lowest position. Reattach call signal to linens.

34. Position patient for comfort.

35. Dispose of soiled laundry.

36. Wash your hands.

**CHARTING** *for Bedmaking*

☐ Specific linens or equipment that cause discomfort for the patient

☐ Special requirements for linens, e.g., certain detergents or elimination of starch

☐ Use of pull sheets, incontinent pads, or specified ways to keep bed dry

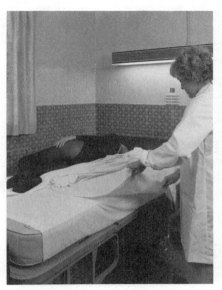

Tighten drawsheet under mattress.

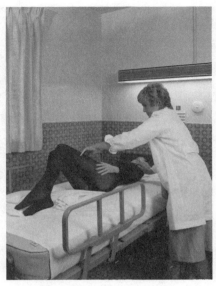

Put siderail up before moving patient.

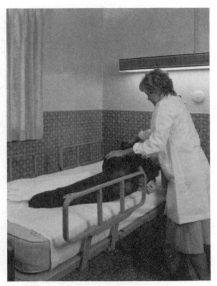

Instruct patient to roll over linen.

## CLINICAL PROBLEM SOLVING

**Potential Problems**

Patient refuses to have bed made.

Cross-contamination occurs from improper linen disposal.

Patient's skin becomes irritated from linen or begins to break down.

The nurse feels stress on back during bedmaking.

**Suggested Solutions**

☐ Assess reason for refusal. Patient may be in pain or does not want to be disturbed.
☐ Offer to make the bed at a later time.
☐ Change only the pillowcase and drawsheet, if patient allows.
☐ Beds do not need to be changed unless soiled or damp so allow patient's independence if possible.

☐ Provide adequate linen hampers for the nursing personnel.
☐ Attend inservice education programs on infection control.

☐ Obtain hypoallergenic linen.
☐ Place sheepskin under patient.
☐ Use eggcrate mattress.

☐ Make sure bed is positioned for comfort of the nurse.
☐ High position is generally used.
☐ If patient is heavy, ask for assistance with bedmaking, especially in moving side-to-side.
☐ Attend inservice classes on "preventing back strain."

# UNIT THREE   BATH CARE

## NURSING PROCESS DATA

### ASSESSMENT   *Data Base*

Assess patient's need for bathing and other personal hygiene activities.

Check patient's activity order. Note special precautions related to movement or exercise.

Assess patient's ability to perform his own care and determine how much assistance he will need.

Discuss patient's preferences for the bathing procedure, bath, and personal articles.

Check patient's room for availability of bathing articles and linens.

### PLANNING   *Objectives*

To decrease the possibility of infection by removing excessive debris, secretions, and perspiration from the skin.

To promote circulation.

To maintain muscle tone through active or passive movement during bathing.

To alternate points of pressure on the body by changing patient's position during the bath.

To provide comfort for the patient.

To assess the patient's overall status, skin condition, level of mobility, comfort.

### IMPLEMENTATION   *Procedures*

Folding a Washcloth Mitt

Providing AM Care

Bathing an Adult Patient

Bathing an Infant

Bathing the Critically Ill

### EVALUATION   *Expected Outcomes*

Patient's skin is free of excessive perspiration, debris, secretions, and offensive odors.

Body positions have been changed and muscles and joints have been exercised actively and/or passively during the bath.

Patient feels comfortable and does not complain of pain, fatigue, itching, irritated, or excessively dry skin.

Patient participates in bath procedure to the best of his ability.

The nurse has assessed the integrity and condition of the patient's skin and the level of mobility, comfort, or pain.

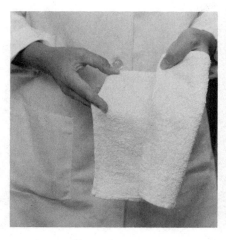
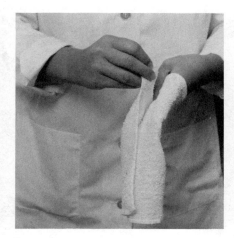
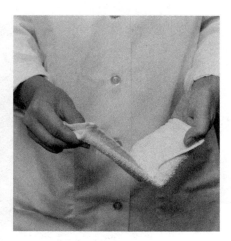

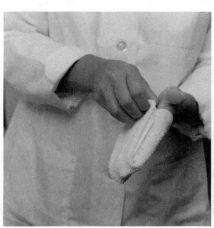
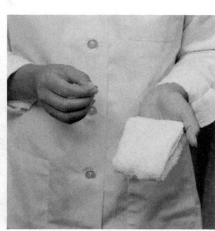

To easily form the washcloth into a mitt for bathing the patient, follow the five steps shown in the illustrations.

## FOLDING A WASHCLOTH MITT

### Procedure

1. Unfold the wash cloth.
2. Place one corner of cloth in the palm of your hand, just above your fingers.
3. Wrap one edge of the cloth around the palm and fingers.
4. Anchor cloth with your thumb.
5. Bring far edge of cloth up and tuck under edge in palm of hand.

## PROVIDING AM CARE

### Equipment

Basin of warm water

Soap

Towel and wash cloth

Emesis basin

Toothbrush and paste

Bedpan or urinal

Toilet tissue

### Preparation

1. Determine if patient wishes AM care. **Rationale:** AM care is provided to "freshen" the patient in preparation for breakfast, physicians' visits, and/ or procedures occurring prior to bathing.
2. Wash your hands. **Rationale:** When providing AM care to several patients, it is important to wash your hands between patients so that microorganisms are not transmitted from one patient to another.
3. Gather equipment and take it to patient's room.
4. Explain that early morning care is available while patient remains in bed. If patient is able, assist him to the bathroom. Provide privacy

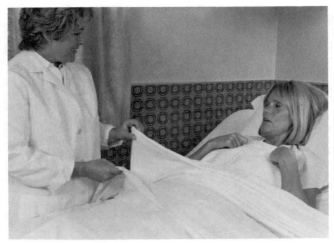

Remove top linen before bathing.

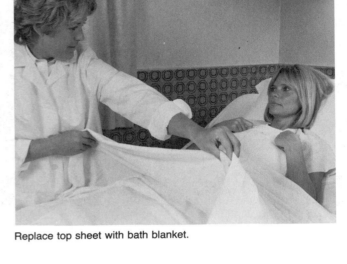

Replace top sheet with bath blanket.

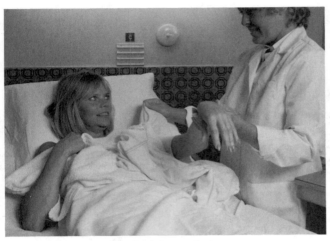

Take patient's gown off maintaining modesty.

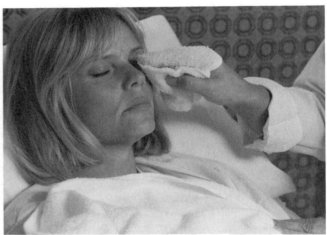

Wash eyes first, from inner to outer canthus.

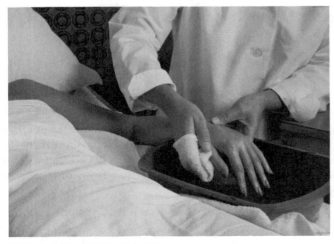

Wash hand by soaking in basin.

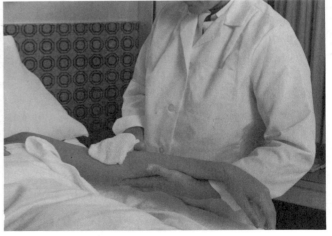

Hold wrist when washing arm.

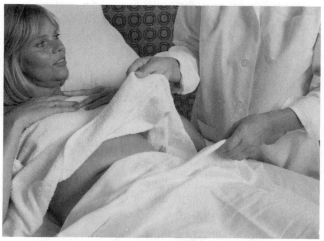

Keep patient covered with towel or bath blanket during the bath.

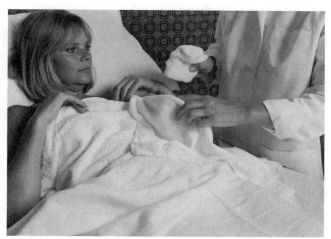

Maintain privacy by keeping towel in place while washing chest.

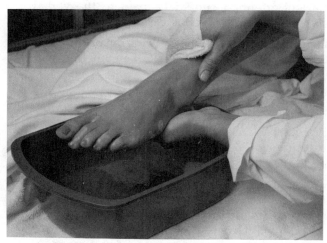

Placing patient's feet in basin while bathing promotes relaxation.

## Procedure

1. Offer bedpan or urinal and assist patient as needed.
2. Wash your hands.
3. Move bed to comfortable working height and lower side rail.
4. Put equipment on over-bed table within reach.
5. Wash patient's face and hands or assist as needed. Dry face and hands.
6. Offer oral hygiene. Assist as needed.
7. Hold emesis basin so patient can rinse after brushing teeth.
8. Assist patient to comfortable position.
9. Reposition bed and replace side rails.
10. Remove equipment and draw curtains.

## BATHING AN ADULT PATIENT

### Equipment

Basin or sink with warm water (110° to 115° F)

Soap and soap dish

Personal articles, i.e., deodorant, powder, lotions

Laundry hamper

Two to three towels

Washcloth

Bath blanket

Clean pajamas or hospital gown

Table for bathing equipment

Shaving equipment for male patients

### Preparation

1. Provide a comfortable room environment, i.e., comfortable temperature, lighting, etc.
2. Talk with patient about plan for bathing to meet personal care needs.
3. Encourage patient to bathe himself. This promotes exercise and a sense of self-worth.
4. Explain any unfamiliar methods or procedures regarding bathing.
5. Wash your hands.
6. Collect necessary equipment and place articles within reach on over-bed table.

7. Ask the patient if he needs to void or defecate before starting the bath. **Rationale:** Warm water of the bath and movement can stimulate the patient to void.

8. Position the bed at a comfortable working height.

9. Assure privacy.

**Procedure**

1. Place bath blanket over patient and over top linen. Loosen top linen at edges and foot of bed.
   a. Remove dirty top linen from under bath blanket, starting at patient's shoulders and rolling linen down toward the patient's feet.
   b. Ask patient to grasp and hold top edge of bath blanket to keep it in place while you pull linen to foot of bed.
   c. Place dirty linen in laundry hamper.

2. Help patient to the side of the bed closest to you. Keep the side rail on the far side of the bed in the UP position.

3. Remove patient's hospital gown. Keep patient covered with bath blanket. Place gown in laundry bag.

4. Remove pillow if patient can tolerate.

5. Place towel under patient's head.

6. Make a mitt with a washcloth. Fold washcloth around your hand as illustrated. **Rationale:** This prevents wet ends of cloth from annoying patient.

7. Bathe patient's face.
   a. Wash around patient's eyes, using clear water. With one edge of facecloth, wipe from the inner canthus toward the outer canthus. Using a different section of the washcloth, repeat procedure on other eye. Dry thoroughly.
   b. Wash, rinse, and dry patient's forehead, cheeks, nose, and area around lips. Use soap with patient's permission.
   c. Wash, rinse, and dry area behind and around the patient's ears.
   d. Wash, rinse, and dry patient's neck.

8. Remove towel from under patient's head.

9. Bathe patient's upper body and extremities. Place towel under area to be bathed.
   a. Wash both arms by elevating patient's arm and holding patient's wrist. Use gentle strokes from the wrist toward the shoulder, including the axillary area.
   b. Wash, rinse, and dry patient's axillae. Apply deodorant and/or powder if desired.
   c. Wash patient's hands by soaking them in the basin or with a washcloth. Nails can be cleaned now or after the bath.
   d. Keeping chest covered with the towel, wash, rinse, and thoroughly dry patient's chest, especially under breasts. Apply powder or cornstarch under breasts if desired.

10. Bathe patient's abdomen. Using a towel over chest area and bath blanket, cover areas you are not bathing. Wash, rinse, and dry abdomen and umbilicus. Replace bath blanket over patient's upper body and abdomen.

11. Bathe patient's legs and feet. Place towel under leg to be bathed. Drape other leg, hip, and genital area with the bath blanket.
    a. Carefully place bath basin on the towel near the patient's foot.
    b. With one arm under the patient's leg, grasp the patient's foot and bend knee. Place foot in basin of water.
    c. Bathe patient's leg, moving toward hip. Rinse and dry patient's leg.
    d. Wash patient's foot with washcloth. Rinse and dry foot and area between toes thoroughly.
    e. Carefully move basin to other side of bed and repeat procedure for patient's other leg and foot.

12. Change bath water. Raise side rails when refilling basin. Check the water temperature before continuing with the bath.

13. During the bath, you should continuously assess the patient's skin and musculoskeletal system. Careful attention should be paid to the verbal statements and nonverbal expressions.

14. Help patient turn to a side-lying or prone position. Place towel under area to be bathed. Cover patient with a bath blanket.

15. Wash, rinse, and dry patient's back, moving from the shoulders to the buttocks.

16. Provide back massage now or after completion of bath. (For procedure see Back Care).

17. Bathe patient's genital area. Cover all body parts except area to be bathed. Place towel under patient's hips.
    a. For a female patient: Bathe from front to back. Use a different section of the washcloth for each stroke. Wash, rinse, and dry thoroughly between all skin folds.

b. For a male patient: Carefully retract the foreskin on the uncircumcised penis. Wash, rinse, and dry gently and replace foreskin to its original position. Continue to wash, rinse, and dry penis, scrotum, and remaining skin folds.

18. Dress patient in a clean hospital gown.

19. Clean and store bath equipment. Dispose of dirty linen.

20. Proceed with any other personal hygiene activities as needed.

21. Replace call light, lower bed, and place side rails in UP position before leaving patient.

22. Wash your hands.

## BATHING AN INFANT

### Equipment

Tub or basin filled with warm water (100° F)

Two towels

Washcloth

Suction bulb

Soap or cleaning agent

Cotton balls

Blanket

Clean clothing

### Preparation

1. Provide a comfortable room environment, i.e., comfortable temperature, lighting, etc.

2. Wash your hands.

3. Collect necessary equipment and place articles within reach.

4. Position the bed at a comfortable working height.

5. Place towel, laid out in diamond fashion, on bed next to basin.

### Procedure

1. Test water temperature with your wrist or elbow.

2. Lift infant onto bed, using football hold.

3. Remove all clothing except shirt and diaper.

4. Cover infant with towel or blanket. Keep your hand on the infant at all times.

5. Clean infant's eyes, using a cotton ball moistended with water. Wipe from inner to outer canthus, using a new cotton ball for each eye. **Ra-**

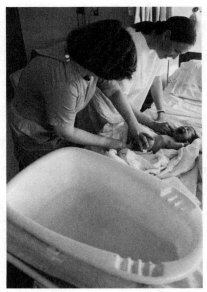
Bathing an infant.

> **Clinical Alert**
> Discharge is present for two to three days due to prophylactic eye drops administered at birth.

**tionale:** This procedure prevents water and particles from entering the lacrimal duct.

6. Make a mitt with the washcloth.

7. Wash infant's face with water.

8. Suction nose, if necessary, by compressing suction bulb prior to placing it in nostril. Release bulb after it is placed in nostril.

9. Wash infant's ears and neck, paying attention to folds; dry all areas thoroughly.

10. Use a football hold when washing an infant's head. Soap your own hands and wash infant's hair and scalp, using a circular motion. Rinse hair and scalp thoroughly. **Rationale:** Football hold is the most secure for active infants.

> **Infant Diapers**
> Most hospitals now use disposable rather than cloth diapers for the following reasons:
> Prevention of nosocomial infections
> Decreased skin irritation
> Safety of the infant (No pins for application)
> Simplified application and increased convenience

11. Place infant on a towel with head facing the top corner.

12. Use the corner of the towel to dry infant's head with gentle, yet firm, circular movements.

13. Remove shirt or gown.

14. Remove and place closed safety pins in a safe area away from child. Remove diaper by picking up infant's ankles in your hand. Wipe buttocks with diaper if necessary.

15. Pick up infant and place feet first into basin or tub. Immerse infant in tub of water only after umbilical cord stub has fallen off. Pick up infant by placing your hand and arm around infant, cradling the infant's head and neck in your elbow. Grasp the infant's thigh with your hand. **Rationale:** The umbilical cord is kept dry to prevent infection and encourage it to "fall off."

16. Wash and rinse the infant's body, especially the skin folds.

17. Carefully remove the infant from the water.

18. Dry infant's body gently but thoroughly.

19. Wash infant's genitalia.
    a. For a female infant: Separate labia and with a cotton ball moistened with soap and water, cleanse downward once on each side. Use a new piece of cotton on each side.
    b. For an uncircumcised male infant: Do not force foreskin back. If it can be retracted, gently cleanse glans penis with a cotton ball moistened with soap and water.
    c. For a circumcised male infant: Gently cleanse with plain water.

20. Replace infant's diaper and re-dress in a new gown or shirt.

21. Provide comfort by holding the infant for a period of time following the bath procedure.

22. Wash your hands.

# BATHING THE CRITICALLY ILL

## Equipment

Two bath blankets

Septi-soft soap

Wash basin

Washcloth

Towel

## Preparation

1. Provide a comfortable room environment, i.e., comfortable temperature, lighting, etc.

2. Talk with patient about plan for bathing to meet personal care needs if alert.

3. Encourage patient to bathe hands and face if able. **Rationale:** This promotes exercise and sense of self-worth.

4. Explain any unfamiliar methods or procedures regarding bathing.

5. Wash your hands and collect necessary equipment; place articles on overbed table within easy reach.

6. Position the bed at a comfortable working height, lower side rail nearest you.

## Procedure

1. Have patient wash own face and hands if able; otherwise, wash them before starting Septi-soft bath.

2. Place bath blanket in basin and soak bath blanket with very warm water.

3. Pour Septi-soft soap into bath blanket and work soap into bath blanket.

4. Wring out bath blanket.

5. Remove top covers from patient and place wet bath blanket over patient. Bath blanket extends from under patient's chin down to feet.

6. Keep patient covered with bath blanket while you rub anterior surfaces with your hands. Entire surfaces of legs and arms can be washed at this time. **Rationale:** This bath decreases the time it takes to bathe a patient. Critically ill patients are not exposed to the long ordeal of a bath or to changes in temperature for long periods of time.

7. After all body surfaces are washed, place dry bath blanket under patient's chin. As you pull dry bath blanket down over patient, remove wet blanket.

8. Dry patient thoroughly.

9. Turn patient on side.

10. Wash and dry back and buttocks with towel.

11. Give back rub.

12. Change bed linen.

13. Position for comfort, replace side rail to UP position.

**CHARTING** *for Bath Care*

☐ Patient's overall ability to participate in own care

☐ Type of bath given, i.e., complete or partial and by whom, e.g., patient, nurse, family member

☐ Condition of patient's skin and any interventions provided for the skin, e.g., lotion, massage

☐ Patient's educational needs regarding hygienic care

☐ Information shared with patient or family

---

## CLINICAL PROBLEM SOLVING

**Potential Problems**

Patient is unwilling to accept a complete bed bath.

**Suggested Solutions**

☐ Respect patient's wishes and take other opportunities for assessment.

☐ Have patient wash hands, face, and genitals. You should wash back and give back care.

☐ Reexplain the purpose of the bath to the patient and request patient participation.

Patient is too shy to allow bath.

☐ Respect patient's privacy and only wash areas patient wishes you to do.

☐ Give assistance so patient can bathe himself.

☐ Allow spouse or parent to give bath if this is more acceptable to patient.

Patient complains of dry, itching skin following the bath.

☐ Assess for cause of itching.

☐ Ask physician for an order for Alpha Keri lotion.

☐ Do not use soap for the bath.

---

# UNIT FOUR  BEDPAN AND URINAL

## NURSING PROCESS DATA

### ASSESSMENT  *Data Base*

Determine patient's usual voiding pattern.

Assess patient's ability to assist with the procedure.

### PLANNING  *Objectives*

To assist the patient to void when on bed rest or unable to urinate.

To help patient void 200 to 500 ml of urine without discomfort or difficulty.

### IMPLEMENTATION  *Procedure*

Using a Bedpan and Urinal

### EVALUATION  *Expected Outcomes*

Patient voids 200 to 500 ml of urine without discomfort or difficulty.

Bladder does not become distended.

Genitourinary system is free of infection.

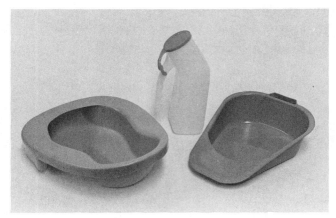

Standard bedpan, fracture pan, and urinal for bedridden patients.

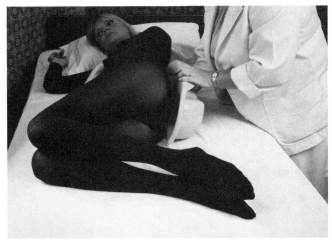

Turn patient on side, place bedpan, and assist patient to roll on back.

## USING A BEDPAN AND URINAL

### Equipment

Bedpan or urinal

Toilet tissues

Absorbent pad, if needed

### Procedure

1. Wash your hands.
2. Obtain bedpan or urinal and warm a metal bedpan or urinal by running warm water around the edges of the receptacle.
3. Provide privacy.
4. Elevate the head of the bed, or position patient on the edge of the bed or in a chair.
5. Instruct the patient to sit on the bedpan or urinal. If the patient needs assistance, follow these steps:

   *Using a bedpan*
   a. Place absorbent pad under hips, if needed.
   b. Raise the patient's hips and slip your arm under the patient or turn the patient on his side. Roll the patient onto the pan.
   c. Place a rolled towel or blanket under the patient's sacrum. **Rationale:** This provides comfort by padding the bony area.

   *Using a urinal*
   a. Place the base of the urinal flat on the bed between the patient's thighs.
   b. Position the patient's penis or vaginal opening over the urinal.

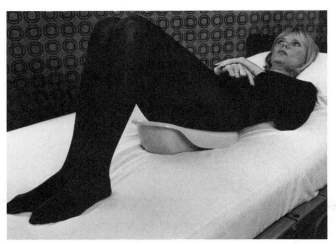

Ensure patient privacy and allow time to complete elimination.

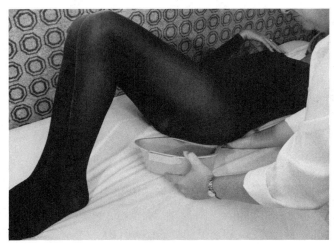

Use fracture badpan for patients requiring minimal movement.

6. Place the signal light and toilet tissue within easy reach.

7. When the patient has voided, remove the receptacle and assist with wiping as necessary.

8. Provide an opportunity for the patient to wash his or her hands.

9. Reposition the patient for comfort, pull back curtains.

10. Measure intake and output if required.

11. Empty bedpan or urinal, clean equipment, and return to proper area in patient's room.

12. Wash your hands.

### CHARTING   *for Bedpan and Urinal*

☐   Amount, color, appearance, and odor of urine

☐   Techniques effective in stimulating voiding

☐   Equipment used, e.g., commode, bedpan

---

## CLINICAL PROBLEM SOLVING

**Potential Problems**

Patient is unable to turn and has difficulty raising hips.

Patient is unable to void on bedpan.

**Suggested Solutions**

☐   Use a fracture pan rather than a bedpan. Powder the fracture pan.
☐   Insert the fracture pan with the flat side toward the head, under the patient's thighs.

☐   Run water in sink.
☐   Massage the lower abdomen.
☐   Place a hot washcloth on the abdomen.
☐   Pour warm water over the perineum with patient positioned on toilet or bedpan.
☐   Give patient a Sitz bath after obtaining an order.
☐   Put oil of wintergreen on a cotton ball in the bedpan or urinal.

---

## UNIT FIVE   SKIN INTEGRITY

### NURSING PROCESS DATA

#### ASSESSMENT   *Data Base*

Assess for signs of skin breakdown or the eruption of lesions.

Assess color of skin.

Assess color of mucous membranes.

Check for alterations in skin turgor.

Evaluate for complaints of itching, tingling or numbness.

Evaluate texture of skin.

Assess general hygienic state.

Observe skin for increased or decreased pigmentation and/or discoloration.

#### PLANNING   *Objectives*

To maintain skin intact without signs of ischemia, hyperemia, or necrosis.

To recognize a break in skin integrity.

To avoid introduction of pathogens through break in skin integrity.

To prevent skin breakdown from pressure points or strain.

To prevent excessive dryness, flaking, itching, or burning.

### IMPLEMENTATION  *Procedures*

Monitoring Skin Condition

Preventing Skin Breakdown

### EVALUATION  *Expected Outcomes*

Patient's skin remains intact without signs of ischemia, hyperemia, or necrosis.

Patient is able to change position without evidence of pressure areas.

Patient's skin does not show signs of dryness, flaking, itching, or burning.

## MONITORING SKIN CONDITION

### Equipment

Artificial light for observation if natural light is not available

Bath blanket

Alcohol

Lotion

### Procedure

1. Explain monitoring process to patient.

2. Provide privacy for patient and wash your hands.

3. Remove linens and gown if necessary. Cover patient with bath blanket.

4. Compare color of patient's skin with normal range of color within the individual's race. Observe for pallor (white color), flushing (red color), jaundice (yellow color), ashen (gray color), or cyanosis (blue color).

5. Place the back of your fingers or hand on patient's skin to check temperature. *Consider the temperature of the room and of your hands.* **Rationale:** The back of the hand is more sensitive to changes in temperature than the palm.

6. Correlate abnormalities in skin color with changes in skin temperature.

7. Observe for areas of excessive dryness, moisture, wrinkling, flaking, and general texture of skin.

8. Gently pick up a small section of the skin with your thumb and finger. Observe for ease of movement and speed of return to original position to check for skin turgor.

9. Press your finger firmly against patient's skin for several seconds (especially ankle area). After removing your finger, observe for lasting impression or indentation.

10. When checking skin temperature and texture of skin, note the patient's response to heat, cold, gentle touch, and pressure.

11. Observe the amount of oil, moisture, and dirt on the skin surface.

12. Note presence of strong body odors.

13. Use a disposable blunt-end probe such as a comb to detect small moving white specks. Lice or white specks may be present on head as well as in pubic area when body lice is present.

14. Observe for areas of broken skin (lesions) or ulcers. Check if lesions are present over entire body or if they are localized to a specific area.

15. Check for skin discolorations, e.g., ecchymosis, petechiae, purpura, erythema, and altered pigmentation. **Rationale:** These signs are indications of generalized disease states such as leukemia, vitamin deficiency, or hemophilia.

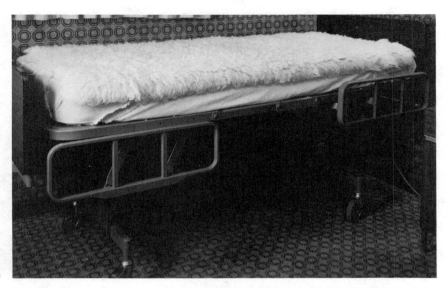

Sheepskin

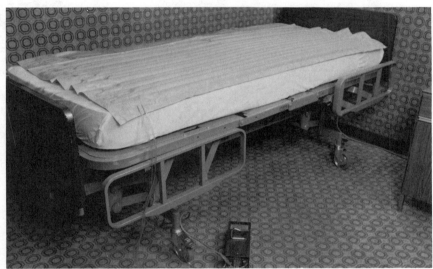

Alternating mattress

## PREVENTING SKIN BREAKDOWN

### Equipment

Skin lotion

Alcohol

### Procedure

1. Observe the patient's most vulnerable body surfaces for ischemia, hyperemia, or broken areas.
2. Change the patient's body position at least once every two hours to rotate weight-bearing areas. Observe all vulnerable areas at this time. Include right and left lateral, prone, supine, and swimming-type positioning if possible.
3. Massage patient's skin to increase circulation. Massage pressure-prone areas when patient changes position.
4. Lubricate dry, unbroken skin to prevent breakdown.
5. Keep skin clean and dry. Prevent soap, urine, feces, and excessive moisture from irritating the skin.
6. Protect healthy skin from drainage secretions.
7. Toughen skin of bedridden patients by applying alcohol to sacrum, elbows, and heels several times during the day. Use lotion once a day.
8. Keep linens clean, dry, and wrinkle-free.
9. Encourage active exercise or range-of-motion exercise.

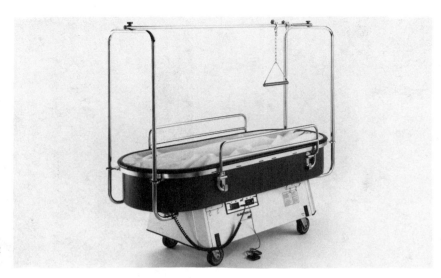

CLINITRON® II Therapy Unit from Support Systems International, Inc.

10. Encourage patient to eat a well-balanced diet with protein-rich foods and adequate fluids.

11. Teach patient and family how to prevent pressure areas and decubitus ulcer formation.

## CHARTING  *for Skin Integrity*

☐ Patient's skin condition: odor, temperature, turgor, sensation, cleanliness, integrity

☐ Patient's mobility

☐ Turning frequency and patient positioning

☐ Type of care given, e.g., massage, bathing

☐ Patient's complaints about skin and/or decubitus ulcer

☐ Time and method used to obtain wound specimen

☐ Type of lesion; location, size, shape, color

☐ Alterations in sensation in skin lesion area

☐ Skin or body odor

---

## CLINICAL PROBLEM SOLVING

**Potential Problems**

Skin is erythematous but remains intact.

**Suggested Solutions**

☐ Toughen skin with alcohol or benzoine.
☐ Obtain sheepskin, eggcrate or alternating pressure mattress.
☐ Turn patient and massage area every two hours.

Patient cannot be positioned in a manner to avoid erythematous areas entirely.

☐ Turn at least every hour.
☐ Do not turn on erythematous site.
☐ Massage area very well with each change in position.
☐ Use protocol for Stage 1 ulcer treatment on affected area.

Skin integrity is interrupted, even with skin care.

☐ Use aseptic technique in treating area to prevent spread of bacteria and promote wound healing.
☐ Use enzyme ointments or Duoderm beads.
☐ If skin is sensitive and breakdown occurs over large area, the use of a CLINITRON® Unit or water bed might be indicated.
☐ Follow treatment for specific stages of decubitus ulcer.

## UNIT SIX   EVENING CARE

### NURSING PROCESS DATA

#### ASSESSMENT   *Data Base*

Review patient's usual routines prior to sleep:
    Usual time of sleep and length of sleeping period.
    Personal hygiene routines.
    Temperature of room and number of blankets, etc.
    Anticipated elimination needs.
    Religious or meditation needs.

Evaluate patient's understanding and acceptance of safety precautions, such
    as use of side rails.

Assess patient's needs for comfort and security.
    Dressings.
    Medication.
    Linen change or adjustment.
    Positioning.
    Television, radio, light.
    Communicative needs.

Assess physical and emotional status during evening care.

Assess condition of back, especially bony prominences.

#### PLANNING   *Objectives*

To encourage a period of comfortable, uninterrupted rest.

To evaluate the patient's present health status.

To make observations about the patient's physical and emotional status.

To provide time for the patient and nurse to review the previous day's events.

To provide time for the patient to communicate needs and questions regard-
    ing health care.

To provide the patient with a clean, secure environment in which to sleep.

#### IMPLEMENTATION   *Procedures*

Providing Evening Care

Providing Back Care

#### EVALUATION   *Expected Outcomes*

Patient appears comfortable and ready for sleep in a safe, clean environment.

Patient has the time to talk about concerns or ask questions.

The nurse is able to evaluate the patient's health care status.

## PROVIDING EVENING CARE

### Equipment

Towels, washcloth

Clean linens if needed

Basin of warm water, soap

Dental items, i.e., toothbrush, dentifrice, denture cup

Emesis basin, cup

Fresh pitcher of water if allowed

Skin care lotion and powder if desired

Personal care items, e.g., deodorant, skin moisturizers

Bedpan, urinal, toilet paper

Miscellaneous supplies as needed, e.g., dressing, special equipment

### Preparation

1. Explain the needs and benefits of evening care; discuss how the patient can be involved.
2. Collect and arrange equipment.
3. Adjust the bed to a comfortable working height and assist the patient into a comfortable position.
4. Assure privacy.
5. Wash your hands.

### Procedure

1. Offer bedpan or urinal if patient is unable to use bathroom. Assist with handwashing.
2. If patient needs or requests a bath, provide assistance as needed.
3. Assist with mouth and dental care as needed.
4. Remove equipment, extra linens, and pillows if possible. Remove stockings, ace wraps, binders, etc.
5. Change dressings. Perform any required procedural techniques.
6. Wash face, hands, and back. Provide back massage.
7. Assist with combing or brushing hair if desired.
8. Replace stockings, binders, etc.
9. Replace soiled linen, or straighten and tuck remaining linen. Fluff pillow.
10. Straighten top linens. Provide additional blankets if desired.

11. Remove any additional equipment. Place call signal and water (if allowed) within patient's reach.
12. Administer sleeping medication if ordered.
13. Assist patient into a comfortable position.
14. Ensure that the patient's environment is safe and comfortable.
15. Raise side rails, place bed in LOW position, and turn lighting to low.
16. Wash your hands.

## PROVIDING BACK CARE

### Equipment

Basin of warm water

Washcloth

Towel

Soap

Skin care lotion

### Procedure

1. Explain the purpose of a back rub, and ask patient if he would like one.
2. Provide privacy.
3. Wash your hands with warm water.
4. Warm lotion by holding bottle under water.
5. Raise bed to comfortable height for you, and assist the patient into a comfortable prone or semi-prone position. Keep farthest side rail in UP position.
6. Drape bed clothes for warmth and untie the patient's gown. Wash back with warm water and soap if necessary.
7. Place lotion on your hands.
8. Once you place your hands on a patient's back to begin a backrub, your hands should remain in constant skin contact with the patient until backrub is complete. **Rationale:** To prevent "tickling" sensation.
9. Repeatedly move your hands up on either side of the patient's spine, across shoulders, and down the lateral aspects of the back using the effleurage stroke, applying firm and steady pressure.
10. Then rub your hands over the scapular area, extending over the upper shoulders, using a circular motion.

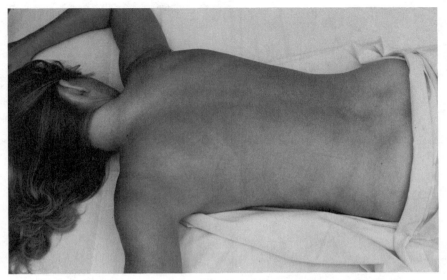

Fanfold covers to buttocks and open gown to expose back for back care.

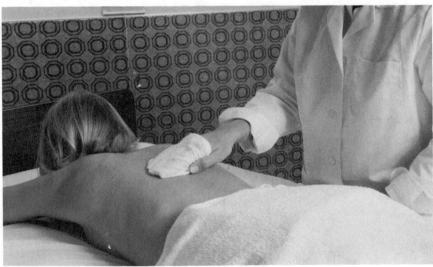

Wash back with soap and water, then dry thoroughly before beginning back rub.

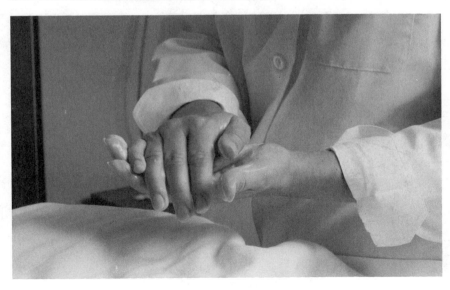

Warm lotion in hands before applying to back to avoid discomfort of cold application.

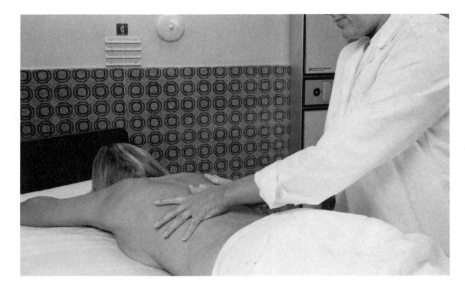

Without lifting hands from skin surface, massage in continuous motion.

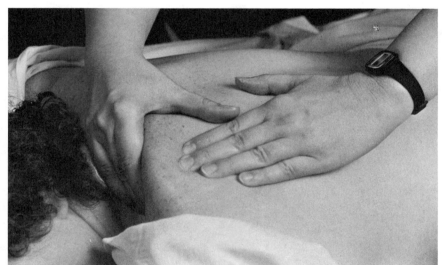

The petrissage, or kneading stroke, is used over the shoulders and along gluteal area.

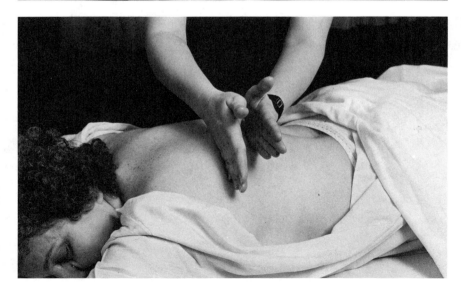

The tapotement stroke stimulates the skin as the hands move up and down the back.

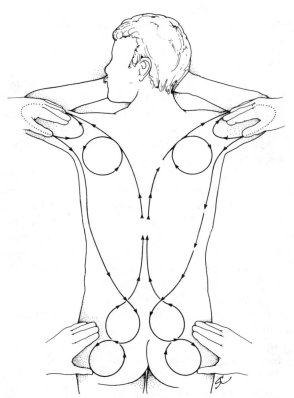

Maintain constant skin contact during back care by moving hands in figure-eight motion from shoulder to buttocks and back again.

11. Move your hands down the center of the patient's back to sacral area.

12. Massage with a figure-eight motion from the sacrum out over each buttock.

13. Finally, rub lightly up and down the back a few strokes before lifting hands from patient's back.

14. Assess skin for color, turgor, skin breakdown, or erythema while massaging.

15. Massage erythematous areas an additional amount of time to promote circulation to the area.

16. When stimulation is desired, the back and buttocks can be lightly struck with the fleshy sides of your hands, called tapotement. Using an alternating rhythm, move up and down the back several times. In addition, kneading can be accomplished by picking up the skin between the thumb and fingers as you move up the back. This movement is called petrissage.

17. Close patient's gown, pull up bedcovers, and assist patient to change position if desired. Place side rails in UP position. Place bed in LOW position.

18. Return lotion to the proper area.

19. Wash your hands.

## CHARTING  *for Evening Care*

☐  Patient's level of comfort or discomfort

☐  Type of care given, i.e., back care, evening care

☐  Any significant complaints

☐  Nature of patient teaching if done

☐  Medication required for discomfort or sleep

☐  Patient's physical and emotional status after evening care completed

---

## CLINICAL PROBLEM SOLVING

### Potential Problems

Male patient misinterprets back care from female nurse and makes sexual advances.

Patient refuses back care because he thinks you are too busy or disinterested.

Patient is unable to sleep even after evening care is given.

### Suggested Solutions

☐  Set firm limits by explaining therapeutic purpose of back care.

☐  Tell patient that if he cannot accept back care as part of the therapeutic regimen, you will stop.

☐  Make sure you offer the back care in an unhurried and meaningful manner. Do not allow the patient to misinterpret your offer for care.

☐  Return to patient and offer back care later in the evening.

☐  Encourage verbalization of fears.

☐  Check to see if sleeping medication can be given.

☐  Provide additional back care.

# TERMINOLOGY

## BEDMAKING

*Occupied bed:* The patient remains in the bed while it is being made.

*Unoccupied bed:* The patient is out of the bed while it is being made.

*Anesthesia (surgical, recovery) bed:* A bed made in a specific manner for the patient who is returning to the bed after having anesthesia or surgery.

*Open bed:* A bed being used by a patient; the linens are folded down.

*Closed bed:* A bed not being used by a patient; the linens are left to cover the bed.

### Equipment Used with Beds
Aside from the standard types of equipment used on the basic hospital bed, specialized equipment can be added to meet the patient's health care needs.

*The footboard:* Usually a solid support placed on the bed where the soles of the feet touch. It is secured to the mattress or bed frame. Footboards are used to prevent permanent plantar flexion (footdrop) and to exercise leg muscles. The footboard may also have side supports to help maintain proper alignment of feet.

*The bed cradle:* A device attached to the lower end of the bed to prevent the bed linens from resting on the patient's legs or feet. It is often used when a patient has burns, ulcers, a wet cast, or specific circulatory diseases.

*Balkan (overbed) frame:* An overhead bed bar(s) that is used to support a trapeze, or a series of pulleys and weights used for traction equipment.

### Sheets for Bedmaking

*Full sheets:* Regular full length flat sheets that can be used as the top and bottom sheet.

*Contour sheets:* Sheets that have elastic at each corner; fitted sheets.

*Drawsheets:* Sheets made of fabric, plastic, or rubber that are placed across the shoulder-to-knee area of the bed and tucked in on the sides.

*Incontinent pads:* Large, disposable pads that can be placed under the buttocks area, head, drains, or any place where excess moisture or fluid may collect on the bed.

*Pull sheets:* Sheets placed across the shoulder-to-knee area of the bed. The sides are not tucked under the mattress. The sheet is kept wrinkle-free and folded under the patient. Pull sheets are used to lift the patient in the bed.

## Levels of Personal Care

*Complete care:* The patient requires total assistance from the nurse because the patient is able to do little or nothing for him or herself. Complete bathing, skin care, oral care, nail and hair care, care of the feet, eyes, ears, and nose, and a total bed linen change are usually provided.

*Partial care:* The patient performs as much of his or her own care as possible. The nurse completes the remaining care.

*Early morning care:* This type of care may or may not be a routine in some hospitals. If early morning care is provided, it is usually given by the night shift nurses. It may include bathing the hands and face, use of the bedpan or urinal, oral care, and other preparations before breakfast.

*P.M. care (H.S. care, hour of sleep care):* P.M. care is usually provided to prepare the patient for a relaxing, uninterrupted period of sleep. Activities include oral care, partial bathing, skin care and a soothing back massage, straightening or changing the bed linen, and offering the bedpan or urinal. The patient should also be assessed for the need of food, drink, or medication before sleep.

*O.R. care:* Patients who will be undergoing surgery or diagnostic tests may be required to bathe the evening before. Partial bathing is sometimes allowed in the morning if time permits. If the patient is not allowed to have anything by mouth, care must be taken not to allow swallowing of water or dentifrice while providing oral care. The patient is usually given a clean gown. All dentures, hairpins, makeup, nail polish, contact lenses, and jewelry are removed. Valuables are locked up. The patient is encouraged to void before leaving for the operating room.

## SKIN CARE

*Acne:* Skin condition due to irritation and infection of the sebaceous glands.

*Bedsore:* A synonym for decubitus ulcer or pressure sore area of cellular necrosis due to decreased circulation.

*Blanching:* A whitish hue to an area of the skin.

*Decubitus ulcer:* A synonym for bedsore or pressure sore area of cellular necrosis due to decreased circulation.

*Ecchymosis:* Collection of blood underneath skin surface; bruise.

*Emollient:*  Soothing, softening agent applied to body surfaces.

*Epidermis:*  Superficial or top layer of skin.

*Erythema:*  Redness of skin associated with rashes, infections, and allergic responses.

*Hyperemia:*  Influx of blood into an area causing redness to the skin.

*Ischemia:*  Decreased, insufficient blood supply to body area.

*Lesion:*  An area of broken skin.

*Necrosis:*  Cellular death.

*Pediculosis:*  Infestation of lice.

*Pediculosis capitis:*  Head lice.

*Pediculosis corporis:*  Body lice.

*Pediculosis pubis:*  Crab lice.

*Petechiae:*  Pinpoint reddish spots.

*Purpura:*  Reddish-purple areas.

*Shearing force:*  Layers of skin moving upon each other.

*Turgor:*  The degree of elasticity of the skin.

## Back Care

*Effleurage:*  Long stroking motions of the hands up and down the back. Hands do not leave the skin surface. Pressure is light.

*Tapotement:*  Alternate striking of fleshy part of hands on patient's back as you move up and down the back.

*Petrissage:*  Pinching of the skin, subcutaneous tissue, and muscle as you move up and down the patient's back.

## General Terminology

**Assessment:**  critical evaluation of information; the first step in the nursing process.

**Complete bath:**  all areas of the body are bathed. This bath can be done completely by the nurse or by the patient.

**Cyanosis:**  blueness of the skin.

**Erythema:**  a redness of the skin due to congestion of the capillaries.

**Excreta:**  waste matter; materials cast out by the body.

**Fissure:**  a groove, slit, or natural division; ulcer or crack-like sore.

**Flush:**  a redness of the face and neck.

**Hypoallergenic:**  against allergy, as hypoallergenic tape.

**Incurvate:**  curved, especially inward.

**Inflammation:**  swelling, pain, heat, and redness of tissue.

**Intervention:**  the act of coming between, so as to hinder or modify.

**Jaundice:**  yellowish appearance caused by deposition of bile pigment in the skin.

**Mucosa:**  mucous membrane lining passages and cavities communicating with the air.

**Pallor:**  paleness; absence of skin coloration.

**Partial bath:**  certain parts of the body are bathed such as the face, hands, under arms, back and perineal area. Another definition of a partial bath is when the nurse bathes areas which the patient cannot reach and the patient washes all other areas.

**Pigment:**  any normal or abnormal coloring of the skin.

**Plaque:**  a patch on the skin or on a mucous surface; a blood platelet.

**Pressure point:**  area for exerting pressure to control bleeding; an area of skin that can become irritated with pressure, especially over bony prominences.

**Sensory deprivation:**  enforced absence of usual and accustomed sensory stimuli.

**Sensory overload:**  too much stimuli for the senses to adjust to at once.

**Ulcer:**  an open sore or lesion of the skin or mucous membrane of the body.

# Chapter 10

# *Personal Hygiene*

## LEARNING OBJECTIVES

Discuss oral hygiene needs of patients.

Outline the procedure for flossing teeth.

Compare and contrast oral hygiene for patients with natural teeth and dentures.

Demonstrate safety awareness when providing oral care for unconscious patients.

Identify the appropriate method of hair care according to patient's condition.

Outline the steps for shaving a male patient.

State the rationale for preventing prolonged scalp contact with solutions used to treat pediculosis.

Discuss rationale for cutting nails straight across.

Demonstrate proper draping technique for female patients.

Describe the steps in providing perineal care for male and female patients.

List the steps in administering a vaginal irrigation.

Describe nursing actions necessary to care for patients with a prosthetic eye or contact lenses.

State two suggested solutions when hearing is not improved after cleaning a hearing aid.

Demonstrate the procedure for replacing an artificial eye.

State at least two nursing diagnoses pertinent to patients requiring assistance with personal hygiene.

## HYGIENIC CARE

Unfamiliar or life threatening conditions affect the patient's adaptation to the health care system. A holistic approach on the part of the nurse provides individualized care and assists in adaptation. Basic hygiene care is an integral part of the total treatment program. Together with its role in enhancing the patient's adaptation to the hospital environment and sense of self-worth, it provides an opportunity to do a total assessment and evaluation. This time also allows for establishing a working relationship with the patient and offers an opportunity to reduce stress by discussing fears and concerns about being in the hospital or the care he is receiving.

The manner in which hygienic care is provided by the nursing staff influences the patient's perception of the staff. If the care is administered in a professional and efficient manner, the patient's confidence in the health care system is increased. The need to provide personal hygiene will depend on each patient's physical state and ability to care effectively for himself. Your first responsibility is to assess the patient's level of ability. After gathering this data, you should assist the patient as necessary, providing any assistance or teaching he may require.

**Oral Hygiene**   The condition of the oral cavity has a direct influence on an individual's overall state of health. Dental diseases require a "host" (the tooth and gum), an "agent" (plaque), and an "environment" (the presence of saliva and food, etc.). When plaque comes in contact with bacterial enzymes, carbohydrates, and acids, cavitation begins as the enamel of the tooth is decalcified. As food and plaque remain in the oral cavity, the possibility of dental decay increases. In the hospital the incidence of caries (cavities) can be decreased by using a dentifrice containing fluoride, proper brushing and flossing, and adequate nutrition.

**Hair Care**   The appearance and condition of a patient's hair can reflect his general physical and emotional status, individuality and feelings of worth, and the ability to care for himself. When complex medical care is required during illness or trauma, hair care is often neglected.

Hair care is an important aspect of regular hygiene. To prevent damage to the hair, scalp, and surrounding skin, and to promote the patient's sense of well-being, you should assess the condition of a patient's hair. Based on the assessment, provide hair and scalp care, shampooing, and shaving and intervene for special problems.

**Foot Care**   The feet are especially susceptible to discomfort, trauma, and infection due to the amount of stress they must endure as well as to their distance from main blood supplies. Many conditions can be avoided if proper foot care is taken. The more common foot problems include:

☐ Incurvated or ingrown toenails: The corners of the nail tend to press into skin, causing pain, ulceration, and infection.

☐ Cracks and fissures between toes: This problem often occurs as a result of excessively dry skin.

☐ Athlete's foot: Irritation characterized by itching, burning skin; caused by an easily transmitted fungus.

☐ Corns: High calluses caused by pressure on toes, joints, or bony prominences.

☐ Plantar warts: A virus manifested as a deep, often painful wart on the soles of the feet.

☐ Calluses: Thickened epidermis over areas of pressure.

☐ Decreased circulation to the feet: A problem that is often caused by diabetes, vascular diseases, or the constriction of major vessels to the lower extremities.

**Perineal and Genital Care**   The perineum consists of the area between the thighs and from the anterior pelvis to the anus. This area contains organs and structures related to sexual functioning, reproduction, and elimination.

Hygienic care involves cleaning the perineum and genitalia to prevent bacterial growth, which can rapidly increase in a warm, dark, moist environment. Perineal care is often provided as a routine part of bathing but may be required more frequently to prevent skin irritation, infection, discomfort, or odor.

All patients are susceptible to perineal irritation or infection. Patients who are especially vulnerable are those who are immobilized, incontinent, debilitated, postsurgical, or comatose; those who have in-dwelling catheters; those who have metabolic and fluid balance disorders; or those who require systemic medications.

Vaginal irrigations are not done as a routine hygiene measure for odor from the perineal area is rarely due to a vaginal discharge. Perineal odor is usually a reflection of inadequate perineal care. Vaginal irrigations are used prior to radiation therapy, to apply antimicrobial solutions to the area, or to apply a heat or cold treatment to the vagina.

The normal vaginal pH and flora can be altered with vaginal irrigations; therefore, the irrigation should not be given 24 hours before a culture and sensitivity of vaginal secretions or pap smear is taken. White vinegar, salt, Betadine, or tap water are solutions frequently used for vaginal irrigations.

**NURSING DIAGNOSES**    The following nursing diagnoses may be appropriate to include in a Patient Care Plan when a patient is admitted and requires basic hygienic care.

| Nursing Diagnosis (Potential) | Defining Characteristic; Etiology (Examples) |
| --- | --- |
| ☐ Oral Mucous Membrane, Alteration in, *related to* | Membrane lesions, e.g., chemotherapy, malnutrition, prolonged dehydration. |
| ☐ Self-Care Deficit, *related to* | Physical limitations, e.g., age, immobilized limb. |
| ☐ Self-Concept, Disturbance in: Self-Esteem, *related to* | Poor grooming, e.g., depression, physical disability. |
| ☐ Skin Integrity, Impairment of: Potential, *related to* | Skin breakdown, e.g., poor nursing care. |

# UNIT ONE   ORAL HYGIENE

## NURSING PROCESS DATA

### ASSESSMENT   *Data Base*

Assess whether patient wears dentures.

Evaluate patient's knowledge of oral hygiene techniques.

Assess condition of patient's oral cavity, teeth, gums, and mouth.

Assess for color, lesions, tenderness, inflammation, intactness of teeth, and degree of moisture or dryness of the oral cavity.

Observe the external and internal lips.

Assess the palate (roof and floor of mouth) and inspect under the tongue.

Assess the entire oral mucosa, noting the inside of the cheek.

Observe the tongue. Note tip, sides, back position, and underside.

Evaluate the condition of gums and teeth.

Assess the condition of throat as patient says "Ah."

If dentures or orthodontic appliances are used, observe the relationship of the appliances to the patient's oral cavity, i.e., fit, irritation, condition of dentures, etc.

### PLANNING   *Objectives*

To remove plaque and bacteria-producing agents from the oral cavity.

To allow the nurse to assess the patient's oral health status, knowledge, and routines of oral care.

To decrease the possibility of irritation or infection of the oral cavity.

To remove unpleasant tastes and odors from the oral cavity.

To provide comfort for the patient.

To provide patient teaching when appropriate.

**IMPLEMENTATION** *Procedures*

Providing Oral Hygiene

Flossing Patient's Teeth

Providing Denture Care

Providing Oral Care for Unconscious Patients

**EVALUATION** *Expected Outcomes*

The oral health status of the patient has been assessed and documented by the nurse.

Oral hygiene care is provided without complications.

Plaque and bacteria-producing agents are removed.

## PROVIDING ORAL HYGIENE

### Equipment

Toothbrush: small enough to reach back teeth; soft and rounded with non-frayed rows of nylon bristles

Dentifrice: patient's choice, preferably one containing fluoride; special paste for dentures

Cup of water

Emesis basin or sink

Dental floss: regular or fine, waxed or unwaxed, depending on patient's needs

Tissues or towel

Mouthwash if desired

### Preparation

1. Wash your hands.
2. Collect necessary equipment. Assist patient with the arrangement of equipment if necessary.
3. Assist patient to sink or provide privacy if care is to be given in bed.
4. Help patient into a comfortable semi-Fowler's position or a sitting position.
5. If dentures are present, help patient remove them if necessary. Place dentures in denture cup.
6. Inspect surface of mouth for any abnormalities. Ask patient about usual oral care routines.
7. Elicit any concerns, comments, or questions patient may have about his oral health status.
8. Determine oral hygiene needs based on findings.

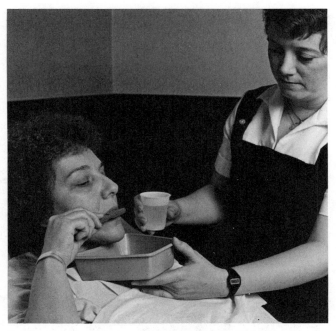

Providing oral hygiene is an essential component of patient care.

9. Assess patient's need for teaching. Consider educational level, physical, emotional and mental state, previous experiences, cultural differences, etc.
10. Assess patient's physical condition. Consider diagnoses, treatments, fluid status, drugs, diet, level of comfort, or pain.
11. Assess patient's ability to care for himself.

### Procedure

1. Wash your hands.

2. Request that patient open mouth wide and hold emesis basin under chin.

3. Direct the bristles of the toothbrush toward the gum line for all areas to be brushed. **Rationale:** Action will remove food particles from gum line and stimulate the gums.

4. Keep the brush positioned over only two or three teeth at a time. Use small rotating movements to cover the outside surfaces of all teeth.

5. Using the brushing method described above, clean the inner surfaces of all back teeth.

6. To clean the flat chewing surfaces, use a firm back-and-forth motion.

7. To clean the inner surfaces of the front teeth, use the bristles on the end of the toothbrush and rotate the brush back and forth across the teeth.

8. Lightly brush all areas of the tongue—this will improve the breath.

9. Rinse the patient's mouth thoroughly with water.

10. Inspect oral cavity and repeat brushing if necessary.

11. Floss thoroughly, using approximately 12 to 15 inches of floss loosely wrapped around one finger of each of your hands.

12. Floss between each tooth by looping floss around each edge of the tooth and sliding floss down to the gum line.

13. Rinse patient's mouth thoroughly with water.

14. Wipe off patient's mouth and chin.

15. Wash patient's brush, rinse and put it and paste away and return additional equipment.

16. Check to see that patient is comfortable.

17. Wash your hands.

## FLOSSING PATIENT'S TEETH

### Equipment

Dental floss 12–18 inches long—two pieces

Cup of water

Emesis basin

Towel

### Preparation

1. Discuss with patient when he would prefer flossing his teeth, after brushing or after morning care is completed.

2. Instruct patient in procedure if he is able to floss; otherwise, the nurse will carry out procedure.

3. Gather necessary equipment.

4. Wash your hands. **Rationale:** This is an important step, as clean hands will prevent the transmission of microorganisms to the patient's mouth.

### Procedure

1. Place patient in sitting position and move bed to HIGH position.

2. Place towel under patient's chin and emesis basin within reach.

3. Cut dental floss into two 12–18 inch lengths.

4. Wrap one length around index fingers of both hands.

5. Hold floss taut between your two hands and gently pull back and forth between each tooth.

6. Move floss up and down sides of teeth to clean plaque. Go as near gum line as possible without injury to gum. Pull floss back and forth gently, working back toward the biting surface of each tooth. Repeat other edge of each tooth, using a new section of floss. **Rationale:** Overly vigorous flossing can damage gums.

7. Floss each tooth several times until all particles of food are removed.

8. Assist patient to rinse mouth and expectorate into emesis basin.

9. Remove basin and wipe patient's mouth with towel.

10. Lower bed and return patient to comfortable position.

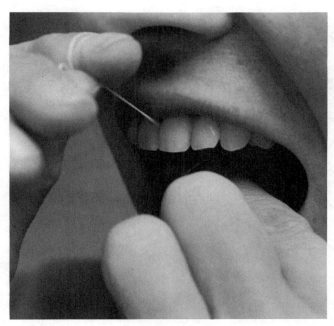

Flossing patient's teeth prevents the buildup of plaque and food particles between the teeth.

## PROVIDING DENTURE CARE

### Equipment

Denture toothbrush

Denture cup

Cleanser or effervescent tablets for dentures

### Procedure

1. Encourage patient to use his dentures. **Rationale:** Dentures improve speech, make eating easier, and improve the shape of the mouth, appearance, and self-image.

2. Wash your hands.

3. Help patient remove dentures. If patient is unable to do this, carefully place your finger on the edge of the upper denture. **Rationale:** This action breaks the seal at the roof of the mouth and allows the denture to easily slide out. Lower denture generally lifts out easily.

4. If patient is unable to clean own dentures, place them in an unbreakable container immediately and carry them to the sink. Place a paper towel or washcloth on the bottom of the sink to cushion the surface in case you accidentally drop a denture.

5. Hold one denture in your hand. With your other hand, use a toothbrush or special denture brush and a cleaning agent, such as a commercially pre-

pared paste or solution, to brush the denture. Use the same brushing motion as with natural teeth.

6. Rinse denture thoroughly in cold water.

7. If dentures are to remain out of the mouth for a period of time, as at night, store them in a clearly labeled, unbreakable container of cold water.

8. If dentures are to be worn immediately, help patient to rinse oral cavity with warm water or mouthwash.

9. You may also gently brush patient's gums and tongue.

10. Help patient replace dentures.

11. Wash your hands.

## PROVIDING ORAL CARE FOR UNCONSCIOUS PATIENTS

### Equipment

Mouthswabs (lemon/glycerin type)

Lubricant for lips

Waterpik devices and/or brush

Bulb syringe

Tongue blades

### Procedure

1. Gather equipment.

2. Wash your hands.

3. If possible, position patient on side in a semi-Fowler's position. If this is not possible, turn patient's head to the side. **Rationale:** Allows fluid to drain or be suctioned out of mouth and thus prevents aspiration.

4. Place a bulb syringe or suctioning equipment nearby to use for suctioning oral cavity as needed.

5. Brush the external surfaces of the teeth in the routine manner, using less water on the brush. You may use a tongue blade to move the cheeks and lips. Do not put your fingers in the patient's mouth. **Rationale:** Accidental biting can cause serious injuries.

6. To clean the inner surfaces of the teeth, use a padded tongue blade to separate the upper and lower sets of teeth. Brush the teeth and tongue in the usual manner.

7. Rinse the patient's mouth carefully, using very small amounts of water that can be suctioned.

8. Lubricate patient's lips with petroleum jelly.

9. Provide oral care frequently—as often as every two hours if necessary. **Rationale:** Oral care maintains adequate oral health.

10. Wash your hands.

### CHARTING *for Oral Hygiene*

☐ Findings of assessment of mouth, gums, mucous membranes, and teeth

☐ Assessment of patient's oral hygiene needs

☐ Planning steps taken to meet patient's oral hygiene needs

☐ Oral care given or observed

☐ Effectiveness of oral care on patient's teeth, gums, mucosa

☐ Patient's reaction and level of comfort

☐ Patient's participation in nurse-patient teaching

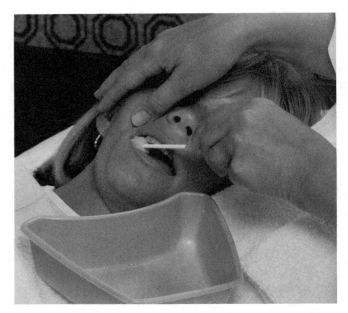

Turn the patient's head to the side to prevent aspiration when providing oral care to unconscious patients.

## CLINICAL PROBLEM SOLVING

| **Potential Problems** | **Suggested Solutions** |
|---|---|
| Even with increased oral hygiene, patient still has odorous breath. | ☐ Use antiseptic mouthwash between oral hygiene care.<br>☐ Notify the physician, as this could be a symptom of systemic disease.<br>☐ Obtain dental consultation to check for presence of dental caries or gum disease. |
| Patient complains of extreme oral mucosal irritation or sensitivity. | ☐ Request physician's order for one of the following solutions:<br>  Saline solutions: for soothing, cleansing rinses.<br>  Anesthetic solutions: to dull extreme pain in the oral cavity.<br>  Effervescent solutions, e.g., hydrogen peroxide or ginger ale: to loosen and remove debris from the mouth.<br>  Coating solutions, e.g., Maalox: to protect irritated surfaces.<br>  Antibacterial/antifungal rinses, e.g., nystatin (mycostatin): to prevent the spread of organisms that cause thrush. |
| Vigorous flossing results in bleeding and sore gums. | ☐ Give patient warm antiseptic mouthwash to relieve soreness.<br>☐ Investigate gum condition and refer for consultation. |

Patient needs care after oral surgery or oral trauma.

☐ Oral care following surgery or trauma will always be ordered by physician. No oral hygiene care should be attempted until physician has clearly defined the specific care.

☐ Suctioning equipment should always be present.

☐ Assessment of patient's head, face, neck, and general status is critical at this time.

Normal stimulation and cleaning is not sufficient to remove debris and plaque for the unconscious patient.

☐ Use toothettes, lemon/glycerin swabs.

☐ Provide mouth care with toothbrush and dentifrice at least b.i.d.

Parotid gland inflammation can occur with improper oral hygiene.

☐ Rinse mouth with mouthwash.

☐ Use lemon/glycerin swab to reach back in oral cavity along mandible to temporomandibular area.

☐ Floss teeth at least daily.

# UNIT TWO   HAIR CARE

## NURSING PROCESS DATA

### ASSESSMENT   *Data Base*

Review general physical assessment findings.

Elicit information regarding loss of hair, tenderness of scalp, or itching.

Determine patient's ability to perform own hair care.

If unable to care for own hair find out who usually assists patient.

Observe patient's hair and scalp, noting the following:
Texture.
Color.
Degree of thickness and hair distribution.
Degree of gloss or shine.
Dryness or oiliness.
Areas of irritation, rash, or scaliness on the scalp or surrounding skin.
Matting or snarls.
Pediculosis (lice).

Assess usual hair care routines, products, and appliances.

Assess method for providing hair care, e.g. in bed, on guerney, in wheelchair.

Determine patient teaching needs regarding hair care.

### PLANNING   *Objectives*

To prevent irritation to the scalp and damage to the hair.

To help maintain or improve patient's existing condition of hair and scalp.

To promote circulation to the hair follicle and growth of new hair.

To distribute oils along the hair shaft.

To promote self-esteem.

**IMPLEMENTATION** *Procedures*

Providing Hair Care
  *for Routine Hair Care*
  *for Tangled Hair*
  *for Coarse or Curly Hair*

Shampooing Hair
  *for Patient in a Chair*
  *for Patient on a Guerney*
  *for Patient on Bedrest*

Braiding Hair

Providing Hair Care for Beards and Mustaches

Shaving a Patient

**EVALUATION** *Expected Outcomes*

Hair and scalp assessment are performed without complications.

Patient's hair and scalp are clean, comfortable, and styled according to patient's preference.

Patient is comfortable and rested following shampooing.

Shaving is accomplished without discomfort.

## PROVIDING HAIR CARE

### Equipment

Blunt end comb or pick

Brush

Towel

Mirror

Hair care products and/or ornaments

### Preparation

1. Determine patient's hair care needs.
2. Wash your hands.
3. Help patient into a comfortable position to perform hair care.
4. Collect and assemble equipment.

### Procedure

*for Routine Hair Care*

1. Place all hair care items within reach.
2. Place towel over patient's shoulders.
3. Brush or comb patient's hair from scalp to hair ends, using gentle, even strokes.
4. Style hair in a manner suitable to patient.
5. Replace hair care items in appropriate place, and clean items as needed.
6. Wash your hands.

### Procedure

*for Tangled Hair*

1. Hold patient's hair above the tangle to prevent discomfort.
2. Using a wide-toothed comb, gently comb tangle. Use short, gentle strokes. Work out the tangle from the end of hair shafts toward the scalp. Work on small amount of tangle at one time. **Rationale:** Working on large tangles will result in broken ends and damaged hair shafts.
3. You may also apply small amounts of vinegar or alcohol to patient's hair to make combing the tangle easier.
4. Style the patient's hair in a manner that will prevent further tangling, e.g., a loose braid placed in an area that does not put pressure on the head.

## Procedure

*for Coarse or Curly Hair*

1. Comb hair in small sections to remove tangles.

2. Use a comb or pick to comb hair in small sections.

3. Apply a small amount of oil to dry or flaking areas of the scalp.

4. Using a wide-toothed comb or pick, gently lift hair and smooth out evenly.

5. If corn-rowing is desired, make small rows of braids close to the scalp in the patient's choice of design. (This type of braid is left in the hair for a longer period of time.)

## SHAMPOOING HAIR

### Equipment

Two bath towels

Washcloth

Shampoo

Conditioner, if desired

Hair dryer, if allowed in hospital

"Shampoo board" for patients confined to bed

### Preparation

1. Determine patient's hair care needs.

2. Wash your hands.

3. Collect and assemble equipment.

4. Help patient into a comfortable position to perform hair care.

5. Shampooing the hair can be accomplished in a variety of ways depending on the patient's usual routine and physical condition. In many institutions, a physician's order is necessary before shampooing a patient's hair.

6. If possible, the easiest way to shampoo is to assist the patient while he is in the shower. Caution should be taken to prevent the patient from becoming overly tired or weak while in the shower.

### Procedure

*for Patient in a Chair*

1. Have shampoo items readily available.

2. Drape one towel over patient's shoulders and around neck. Place another towel within reach.

3. Face patient away from sink. Lock wheels of wheelchair.

4. Pad the edge of the sink with a towel or bath blanket.

5. Ask patient to lean head and neck against sink.

6. Using a washcloth to protect patient's eyes, wet hair and gently make a lather with shampoo.

7. Rinse thoroughly and repeat if necessary.

8. Towel dry, add conditioner if desired, and rinse again.

9. Using a dry towel, pat hair dry and wrap turban style to transport back to bed.

10. Use hair dryer if available.

11. Style as desired.

12. Replace equipment.

### Procedure

*for Patient on a Guerney*

1. Have shampoo items readily available.

2. Position guerney with head end at sink.

3. Lock the brakes.

4. Put a pillow or a rolled blanket under the patient's shoulders to help elevate and extend the head.

5. Move the patient's head just beyond the edge of the guerney to allow water to run off more easily.

6. Drape one towel over patient's shoulders and around neck. Place another towel within reach.

7. Pad the edge of the sink with a towel or bath blanket.

8. Lock wheels on guerney. **Rationale:** This prevents the guerney from moving away from the sink.

9. Using a washcloth to protect patient's eyes, wet hair and gently make a lather with shampoo.

10. Rinse thoroughly and repeat if necessary.

11. Towel dry, add conditioner if desired, and rinse again.

12. Using a dry towel, pat hair dry and wrap turban style to transport back to room.

13. Use hair dryer if available.

14. Style as desired.

15. Replace equipment.

**Procedure**

*for Patient on Bedrest*

1. Place shampoo board, if available, under the patient's head. This allows water and soap to run off into a basin at the side of the bed.
2. Drape one towel over patient's shoulders and around neck. Place another towel within reach.
3. Place patient's head on shampoo board.
4. Using a washcloth to protect patient's eyes, wet hair and gently make a lather with shampoo.
5. Rinse thoroughly and repeat if necessary.
6. Towel dry, add conditioner if desired, and rinse again.
7. Using a dry towel, pat hair dry and wrap turban style.
8. Remove equipment from bed.
9. Change gown and linen if wet.
10. Use hair dryer if available. Ensure that electrical equipment is checked by maintenance department before using. **Rationale:** This will confirm that equipment is grounded and mechanically safe.
11. Style as desired.
12. Replace all equipment.
13. If a shampoo board is not available, follow these guidelines:
    a. Remove pillows so that patient is flat on the bed.
    b. Place a plastic sheet or plastic bed protector under patient.
    c. Roll a bath blanket or sheet and form a trough under patient's head. Be sure to have the trough directed over the edge of the bed.
    d. Cover entire trough with a plastic sheet.
    e. Adjust edge of trough to empty into a basin at the side of the bed.
    f. Using pitchers of water, proceed with the routine shampooing procedure.
    g. Change bed linens and clothes if they become wet.
    h. Replace all equipment.

## BRAIDING HAIR

### Equipment

Comb or brush

Barrette, ribbon, or covered elastic band

**Procedure**

1. Wash your hands.
2. Position patient in a sitting position, if possible.
3. Comb and/or brush hair. Remove tangles, especially those close to scalp, before braiding.
4. Part hair into sections equal to the number of desired braids.
5. Divide each section into three equal strands.
6. Begin braid so that base is not in a pressure area of the head. **Rationale:** If braid is directly at base of scalp, it may be uncomfortable for patient who is bedridden.
7. Weave each of the three strands, alternately placing right strand over the middle strand, then the left strand over the middle one. Move strands smoothly from one hand to the other and keep in hands at all times or the tension will be released and hair will unbraid.
8. Continue until ends of strands are reached.
9. Fasten ends with barrette or covered elastic. Put on a ribbon, if desired. **Rationale:** Avoid using rubber bands, as they damage the hair shaft.
10. Arrange braids as desired.
11. Reposition patient for comfort.
12. Wash your hands.

## PROVIDING HAIR CARE FOR BEARDS AND MUSTACHES

### Equipment

Brush or comb

Towel

Mustache scissors

### Preparation

1. Determine patient's hair care needs and procedure for mustache or beard.
2. Wash your hands.
3. Help patient to a comfortable position.
4. Collect and assemble equipment.

### Procedure

1. Observe patient's skin underneath beard or mustache.

2. If necessary, comb or brush the beard or mustache.

3. With patient's or family's direction, periodically trim patient's mustache or beard with sharp scissors.

4. Shampoo beard or mustache as needed.

## SHAVING A PATIENT

### Equipment

Razor, specific to patient's needs or wishes

Shaving cream

Aftershave lotion (optional)

Two towels

Basin of warm water

### Preparation

1. Place patient in sitting position.

2. Place towel over chest and under chin.

3. Provide mirror on overbed table.

4. Determine how the patient usually shaves, i.e., use of safety edge or electric razor; use of special products.

5. Check to see if the patient has excessive bleeding tendencies due to pathological conditions (hemophilia) or to the use of specific medications (anticoagulants or large doses of aspirin). **Rationale:** Bleeding, if accidentally cut, could lead to serious loss of blood.

---

**Clinical Alert**

According to the hospital policy, be sure to have the electric razor checked for safety aspects. Some hospitals do not allow patients to use their own electric razors.

---

### Procedure

1. If using a safety edge razor, apply a warm, moist towel to patient's skin to soften the hair.

2. Apply a thick layer of soap or shaving cream to the shaving area.

3. Holding skin taut, use firm but small strokes in the direction opposite that of hair growth.

4. Gently remove soap or lather with a warm, damp towel. Inspect for areas you may have missed.

5. Apply aftershave lotion or powder as desired.

6. Reposition patient for comfort if needed.

7. Replace equipment.

### CHARTING  *for Hair Care*

☐ Documentation of hair care assessment and needs

☐ Shampooing method, outcomes, problems encountered

☐ Patient's tolerance to hair care

☐ Shaving done

☐ Unusual bleeding from shaving

---

## CLINICAL PROBLEM SOLVING

### Potential Problems

Extreme matting, snarling, blood, or nonremovable substances appear in patient's hair.

Patient is cut during shaving procedure.

Shaving is difficult and painful for the patient.

### Suggested Solutions

☐ Never cut a patient's hair unless it is absolutely necessary. Check hospital policy regarding hair cutting.

☐ Secure permission of family or physician.

☐ Assess extent of cut and place a clean towel on the area with pressure to stop bleeding.

☐ If cut appers to be more than a nick, report to physician and fill out incident report.

☐ Place warm towels on area to be shaved for 15 minutes.

☐ Apply more shaving cream.

☐ Ensure that razor is sharp.

## UNIT THREE PEDICULOSIS

### NURSING PROCESS DATA

**ASSESSMENT** *Data Base*

Observe head (scalp), body (beard, eyebrows, arms, legs), and pubic areas for the following signs:
Small, hemorrhagic areas on the skin.
Scratches on the skin.
Habitual itching and scratching.
Insect-type bites or pustular eruptions behind the ears or hairline.
Small, white dandruff-like particles.

Assess patient's personal hygiene, living conditions, contact/exposure to others with lice, e.g., school-age children, sexual partners, siblings.

**PLANNING** *Objectives*

To remove lice from patient's hair and prevent further skin problems such as impetigo or infection.

To remove cause of itching and intense need to scratch scalp.

To control spread to others.

**IMPLEMENTATION** *Procedure*

Removing Lice

**EVALUATION** *Expected Outcomes*

Lice removed following treatment.

Patient verbalizes cause of problem and preventive measures.

## REMOVING LICE

### Equipment

Isolation bags

Treatment solution as ordered, i.e., gamma benzene hexachloride (Kwell) or nonprescription drug

Clean linen

Fine-tooth comb

Disinfectant for comb

### Procedure

1. Remove and bag patient's clothing and linens separately. Use isolation bags.

2. Notify physician and other health care providers.

3. Begin treatment as ordered by physician. Common treatment is gamma benzene hexachloride applied as a cream, lotion, or shampoo. **Rationale:** Head lice requires shampoo. Body and pubic lice requires shower with soap followed by lotion application for 24 hours.

4. Apply solution and leave in place several minutes. **Rationale:** Prolonged use of shampoo can burn scalp.

5. Rinse thoroughly.

6. Comb through hair with fine-tooth comb.

7. Repeat in 24 hours if necessary.

8. Disinfect comb and brushes with Kwell shampoo.

9. Wash clothes and linens separately from other patients' belongings.
10. Sterilize equipment as prescribed.
11. Discuss the cause, treatment, and preventive measures regarding lice infestation with patient and family.
12. Wash your hands.

**CHARTING** *for Removing Lice*

☐ Location of lice infestation
☐ Notification of physician and health care providers
☐ Action taken and the results
☐ Patient teaching activities

---

## CLINICAL PROBLEM SOLVING

**Potential Problems**

Kwell shampoo is left on too long a period of time.

Other patients or staff become infested with lice.

Lice are not eliminated with treatment.

**Suggested Solutions**

☐ Observe for irritation or burning after rinsing out the shampoo.
☐ If scalp is burned, notify physician for a medication order.
☐ Do not repeat treatment until scalp is healed.

☐ Isolate the patient's linen and personal hair grooming equipment to prevent spread of lice.
☐ Instruct patient or staff on use of Kwell shampoo.

☐ Obtain an order for shaving patient's hair.

---

# UNIT FOUR  FOOT CARE

## NURSING PROCESS DATA

### ASSESSMENT  *Data Base*

Review data from general physical assessment.

Observe the color of the patient's feet and lower extremities.

Assess temperature of each foot.

Note color, shape, condition, contour, and length of toenails.

Assess speed of color return when nailbed is depressed (capillary refill).

Inspect skin of entire foot (including corner of toes, between toes, and heels) for irritation, cracking, lesions, corns, calluses, deformities, and edema.

Assess mobility of ankle and toes. Footdrop or plantar flexion and eversion of feet can occur during prolonged bed rest.

Assess cleanliness of feet.

Inspect patient's shoes for excessive wear, proper fit, etc.

During assessment, gather data from the patient about level of comfort, pain, tenderness, etc.

**PLANNING** *Objectives*

To provide for specific foot care needs.

To encourage self-care and prevention of future problems.

To prevent infection, discomfort, deformities, circulatory problems, and odor.

**IMPLEMENTATION** *Procedures*

Providing Foot Care

Providing Nail Care

**EVALUATION** *Expected Outcomes*

Foot care provided without complications.

Patient's feet are clean and appear free of complicating conditions such as excessive moisture, calluses, corns, blisters, abrasions, or infection.

Patient and family understand the importance and techniques for proper foot care.

## PROVIDING FOOT CARE

### Equipment

Basin of warm water

Soap or emollient agent

Washcloth

Two towels

Toenail clippers

Nail file, emery board, pick, or orangewood stick

Skin care lotion or lanolin

### Preparation

1. Determine foot care needs based on patient's condition and assessment data.
2. Check physician's orders and Patient Care Plans.
3. Discuss procedure with patient.
4. Wash your hands.
5. Collect necessary equipment.
6. Help patient into a chair in a comfortable sitting position if possible.

### Procedure

1. Place towel or bath mat on floor in front of patient.

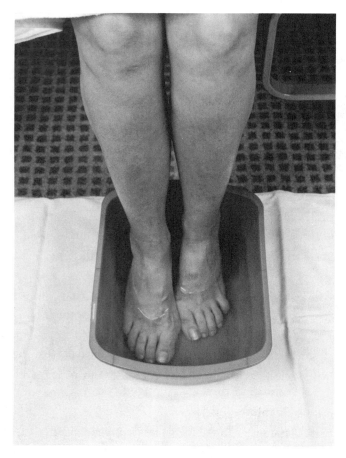

Place basin on the floor and allow patient's feet to soak.

> **Clinical Alert**
>
> Check policy of hospital regarding cutting of nails. Some health care facilities require that only a podiatrist cut nails. Do not cut diabetics' nails.

2. Place basin of warm water on towel.

3. Help patient place feet in basin.

4. Add emollient agent to water, if desired.

5. Assist patient with other personal hygiene activities while feet are soaking. Let feet soak for ten minutes.

6. Using a washcloth, gently wash patient's feet with soap and water.

7. Dry each foot thoroughly with a second towel. Dry between each toe.

8. Using nail clippers, cut straight across the nails. **Rationale:** Prevents trauma to surrounding tissue.

9. Clean underneath and on sides of nails using a file or orangewood stick.

10. If necessary, push back cuticles using an orangewood stick. Smooth rough edges with an emery board.

11. Apply lotion to entire foot focusing on callused or dry areas.

12. Assist patient in putting on clean socks and shoes or slippers.

13. Replace equipment.

14. Assist patient to bed or position for comfort in chair.

15. Wash your hands.

## PROVIDING NAIL CARE

### Equipment

Basin of warm water

Towel

Scissors or nail clippers

File or emery board

Orangewood stick

### Procedure

1. Check hospital policy on nail cutting. Some institutions do not allow nurses to cut patient's nails if the patient has diabetes mellitus, peripheral vascular disease, or a localized condition such as a fungus infection. Thick, mycotic or ingrown toenails should not be cut by the nurse. Request that a podiatrist see the patient.

2. Wash your hands.

3. Position patient for comfort.

4. Expose one extremity at a time.

5. Soak nails if softening is needed. Dry nails.

6. Cut toenails straight across with scissors or clippers. **Rationale:** Rounding off toenails may break the skin or cause ingrown toenails.

7. Smooth cut edges as necessary with file or emery board.

8. Clean under nail with orangewood stick to remove debris.

9. Reposition patient.

10. Remove and clean equipment.

11. Wash your hands.

### CHARTING  *for Foot and Nail Care*

☐  Initial assessment findings and overall status of patient's feet

☐  Foot and nail care needs and plans

☐  Foot care needs and plans

☐  Care given and results of care

☐  Any abnormalities

☐  Involvement in patient/family teaching

---

## CLINICAL PROBLEM SOLVING

**Potential Problems**

Patient has excessively dry, scaly skin, even after routine foot care.

**Suggested Solutions**

☐  Apply alkali solutions as ordered such as Epsom salts or bicarbonate of soda to soften skin and remaining scales. Repeated soakings are usually necessary.

☐ Apply lanolin.

Patient's feet are excessively moist.

☐ Give foot care twice a day.
☐ Use moisture-absorbing powder.

Patient has large calluses on feet.

☐ After soaking, obtain an order to rub a pumice stone or an abrasive material on the callused area. Calluses are never cut from the skin due to possible scarring to the epidermis.
☐ For diabetic patients, obtain services of a podiatrist.

Patient has mycotic nails.

☐ Report to physician so podiatrist can be consulted.

---

## UNIT FIVE   PERINEAL AND GENITAL CARE

### NURSING PROCESS DATA

#### ASSESSMENT   *Data Base*

Review general assessment data about patient.

Observe for signs of perineal itching, burning on urination, or skin irritation. Ask patient if he or she experiences any of these problems.

Assess patient's ability to bathe him or herself and to perform perineal care.

While providing privacy, assess the perineal/genital area for abnormal secretions, ulcerations, skin excoriations and sensitivity, drainage (amount, consistency, odor, color), swelling, enlarged lymph glands, catheter patency, and comfort.

Assess patient's learning needs related to perineal and genital care.

#### PLANNING   *Objectives*

To decrease the growth of bacteria.

To remove excessive secretions.

To promote healing after surgery and vaginal deliveries.

To prevent the spread of microorganisms for patients with indwelling catheters.

To increase patient comfort.

#### IMPLEMENTATION   *Procedures*

Draping a Female Patient

Providing Female Perineal Care

Administering a Vaginal Irrigation

Providing Male Perineal Care

**EVALUATION**  *Expected Outcomes*

Perineal care has been comfortably and effectively provided.

Perineal area is clean, odor-free, and without irritation or discharge.

## DRAPING A FEMALE PATIENT

### Equipment

Bath blanket

### Procedure

1. Bring bath blanket to bedside.
2. Identify patient and explain procedure.
3. Provide privacy.
4. Wash your hands.
5. Place bed in HIGH position and lower side rail nearest you.
6. Place bath blanket over patient's top linen so that one corner of the blanket is pointed toward the patient's head to form a diamond shape over the patient.
7. Instruct patient to hold onto bath blanket. Fanfold linen to foot of bed.
8. Request that patient flex knees and keep them apart with feet firmly on bed.
9. Wrap lateral corners of bath blanket around feet in a spiral fashion until they are completely covered.

10. The corner of the blanket between knees and extending over perineum can later be folded back over the abdomen.

## PROVIDING FEMALE PERINEAL CARE

### Equipment

Bath blanket or sheet

Two bath towels

Protective pad

Washcloth

Three or more cotton balls (optional)

Clean surgical gloves (optional)

Bedpan (optional)

Pitcher of warm water (optional)

Antifungal/antibacterial solution as ordered

### Preparation

1. Check to see if specific physician orders are to be followed.
2. Talk with patient about how she can perform care or assist with procedure.

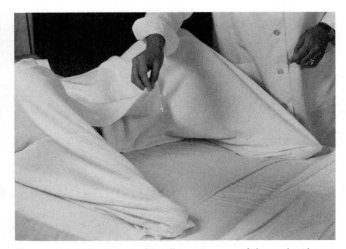

When providing perineal care, cover the patient to provide optimum privacy and warmth.

Drapes should be arranged to allow exposure of the perineal area by lifting up one edge of the drape.

3. Collect and arrange necessary equipment.

4. Provide privacy by closing door and pulling drapes.

5. Wash your hands.

6. Position patient in a comfortable position. Perineal and genital care can be provided while patient sits on a toilet or sitz bath, remains in bed in a supine position, or sits on a bedpan in a dorsal recumbent or semi-Fowler's position.

7. When care is given in bed, position patient comfortably. Drape according to procedure described above.

8. If possible, encourage the patient to bend her knees and separate her legs so that the perineal area can be cleansed.

### Procedure

1. Place a protective pad or towel and bedpan under the patient's hips.

2. The perineum is sometimes more comfortably and effectively cleansed by pouring warm water or a prescribed solution over the perineum while patient is positioned on the bedpan.

3. Tell the patient what sensations she will feel as you perform the procedure.

4. Put on gloves if desired. Separate the labia with one hand to expose the urethral and vaginal openings.

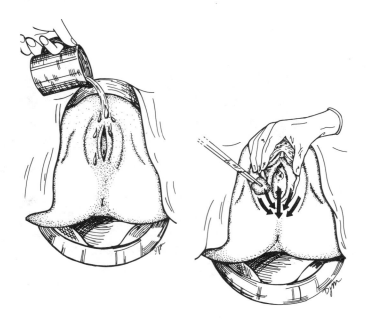

Cleansing the perineum with warm water and wiping front to back will provide effective perineal care and prevent cross-contamination.

5. With your other hand, wipe from front to back in a downward motion, using warm water or soap and water and a washcloth or cotton balls. Be sure to use a different corner of the washcloth or a different cotton ball for each downward stroke. **Rationale:** This procedure prevents cross-contamination.

6. Wash the external labia and anus.

7. Thoroughly pat dry with second towel.

8. Remove equipment and cover patient.

9. Position patient for comfort.

10. Wash your hands.

## ADMINISTERING A VAGINAL IRRIGATION

### Equipment

Irrigation set

Douche tip

Solution

Bath blanket

Waterproof pad

Bedpan

Towel or toilet tissue

IV standard

"Clean" gloves

### Preparation

1. Check physician's order and Patient Care Plan for type, amount and temperature of irrigating solution (usually 1000–2000 cc of 105°F (40.5°C).

2. Gather equipment and solution.

3. Identify patient.

4. Explain procedure to patient.

5. Provide privacy.

6. Have patient void.

7. Wash hands.

8. Hang solution container on IV standard.

9. Raise bed to HIGH position and lower head of bed.

10. Lower side rail nearest you.

11. Adjust IV standard so container base is 12–18″ above vaginal orifice.

**Procedure**

1. With patient in supine position, fanfold top bedding to foot of bed while replacing with bath blanket.

2. Place waterproof pad under patient.

3. Wash and dry perineum thoroughly if excess secretions or discharge present.

4. Position patient with knees bent and feet flat on bed.

5. Drape patient according to Draping Procedure.

6. Place on bedpan.

7. Put on "clean" gloves.

8. Encourage patient to relax and move knees apart. Cleanse external genitalia with soap and water.

9. Open clamp on tube from solution container and allow fluid to flow over perineum. **Rationale:** This procedure tests the water temperature and relaxes the patient.

10. Spread labia with gloved hand and insert douche tip 3–4″.

11. Rotate douche tip while irrigating solution flows into vagina. **Rationale:** This promotes even flow of solution to all areas of the vagina.

12. Remove douche tip from vagina when solution flow ceases.

13. Assist patient to sitting position. **Rationale:** A sitting position facilitates drainage from vagina.

14. Remove bedpan from patient. Note amount of returned solution.

15. Dry perineum with toilet tissue or towel.

16. Remove waterproof pad from under patient.

17. Remove gloves.

18. Replace top bedding and remove drape.

19. Position patient for comfort. Remove curtain.

20. Raise bed rails and place bed in LOW position.

21. Remove and clean or discard irrigation equipment. Replace equipment to appropriate area. **Rationale:** Douche tips and bags are reusable for that patient.

22. Wash your hands.

## PROVIDING MALE PERINEAL CARE

### Equipment

Bath blanket or sheet

Two bath towels

Protective pad or plastic sheet

Washcloth

Clean surgical gloves (optional)

### Preparation

1. Check to see if specific physician orders are to be followed.

2. Talk with patient about how he can perform care or assist with procedure.

3. Collect and arrange necessary equipment.

4. Provide privacy by closing door and pulling drapes.

5. Wash your hands and put on gloves if desired.

6. Cover patient with bath blanket, exposing genital area as little as possible.

### Procedure

1. If the patient has not been circumcised, retract his foreskin carefully to expose the glans penis.

2. Gently but securely hold the shaft of the penis in one hand.

3. Using a circular motion, start at the tip of the penis and wash downwards toward the shaft with soap and water. Do not repeat washing over an area without using a clean area of the washcloth. **Rationale:** This procedure prevents cross-contamination.

4. Replace the foreskin over the glans penis.

5. Wash around the scrotum.

6. Wash the anus last.

7. Rinse and dry all areas thoroughly.

8. Remove articles and cover patient.

9. Reposition patient for comfort.

10. Wash your hands.

### CHARTING  *for Perineal Care*

☐ Assessment and care needs for perineal hygiene

☐ Patient's level of understanding and teaching needs

☐ Perineal care provided and outcomes of care

☐ Time irrigation procedure performed

☐ Type, amount, and temperature of solution used for irrigation

☐ Description of returns from irrigation

☐ Response of patient to procedure

## CLINICAL PROBLEM SOLVING

**Potential Problems**

Patient has foul odor even after peri-care.

Patient develops urinary tract infection.

**Suggested Solutions**

☐ Obtain order for sitz bath.
☐ Request order for medicated solution.
☐ Request culture of discharge so the appropriate treatment can be instituted.

☐ Instruct patient on proper technique for perineal care.
☐ Instruct females to wash from anterior to posterior aspects of perineum, using different sections of cloth for each wipe.
☐ Instruct male patients to wash from urethral opening down the shaft of the penis.

## UNIT SIX   PROVIDING EYE AND EAR CARE

### NURSING PROCESS DATA

#### ASSESSMENT   *Data Base*

Assess if patient is using eyeglasses or contact lenses, has an artificial eye, or is experiencing any eye problems.

Observe patient's eyes for symmetry and clarity.

Assess the skin surrounding patient's eyes for excessive dryness, scaling, and irritation.

Observe eyelids for irritation, edema, crustation, sties, and lesions.

Observe patient's tear ducts and sclera for inflammation and excessive tearing.

Assess patient's pupils for response to light.

Observe patient's eye movements or muscle action.

Evaluate ability to hear.

#### PLANNING   *Objectives*

To ensure that the eyes and surrounding skin areas are clear, comfortable, and free of crustation.

To improve or maintain the patient's vision.

To prevent irritation and infection.

To maintain or improve the patient's appearance and self-esteem.

To increase ability to hear.

#### IMPLEMENTATION   *Procedures*

Providing Routine Eye Care

Providing Eye Care for Comatose Patient

Providing Eye Care for Patient with Glasses

Providing Eye Care for Patient with Artificial Eye

Providing Eye Care for Patient with Hard Contact Lenses

Providing Eye Care for Patient with Soft Contact Lenses

Providing Ear Care for Patient with Hearing Aid

**EVALUATION** *Expected Outcomes*

Eyes and surrounding area are clear and free of crustation.

Vision is maintained or improved.

Hearing is improved.

## PROVIDING ROUTINE EYE CARE

### Equipment

Small basin

Water or saline

Washcloth or cotton balls

### Preparation

1. Determine patient's eye care needs and obtain physician's order if needed.
2. Explain the necessity for and method of eye care to the patient. Discuss how patient can assist you.
3. Collect necessary equipment.
4. Wash your hands.

### Procedure

1. Use water or saline at room temperature.
2. Using the washcloth or cotton balls dampened in water or saline, gently wipe each eye from the inner to outer canthus. Use a separate cotton ball or corner of washcloth for each eye. **Rationale:** To prevent cross-contamination from one eye to the other.
3. If crusting is present, gently place a warm, wet compress over the eye(s) until crusting is loosened.

## PROVIDING EYE CARE FOR COMATOSE PATIENT

### Equipment

Water or normal saline

Washcloth, cotton balls, tissues

Sterile lubricant or eye preparations if ordered by the physician

Eye dropper or asepto bulb syringe

Eye pads or patches

### Procedure

1. Cleanse the eyes using a dampened washcloth or cotton balls dampened in water or saline. Gently wipe each eye from the inner to outer canthus. Use separate cotton ball or corner of wash cloth for each eye. **Rationale:** Wiping from the inner canthus to the outer prevents particles and fluid from entering the nasolacrimal duct.
2. Use a dropper to instill a sterile ophthalmic solution (liquid tears, saline, methylcellulose) every three to four hours as ordered by a physician. (See procedure for instilling eye drops.)
3. Keep patient's eyes closed if blink reflex is absent. If eye pads or patches are used, explain their purpose to patient's family. Do not tape eyes shut. **Rationale:** Corneal abrasions and drying occur when eyes lose blink reflex.

## PROVIDING EYE CARE FOR PATIENT WITH GLASSES

### Equipment

Towel

Water

Mild soap

Soft, dry cloth or lens paper

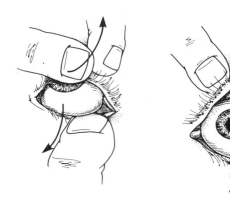

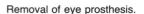

Removal of eye prosthesis.

## Procedure

1. Encourage patient to wear eyeglasses as needed.

2. Clean glasses over a protected area, i.e., a towel. Holding glasses by the frame, gently wash the glass in tepid water. Use soap if necessary. Rinse thoroughly.

3. Dry and wipe lenses with a clean, soft cloth or lens paper.

4. Label eyeglasses with patient's name.

## PROVIDING EYE CARE FOR PATIENT WITH ARTIFICIAL EYE

### Equipment

Rubber bulb or eyedropper

Water or saline

Mild soap

Washcloth

Towel

### Preparation

1. If possible, encourage patient or family member to care for patient's artificial eye.

2. If assisting with artificial eye care, assess patient's usual method for cleansing.

3. Gather equipment.

### Procedure

1. Wash your hands.

2. Remove eye prosthesis by depressing lower lid and sliding prosthesis out, or by using gentle suction with the rubber bulb of an eyedropper.

3. Flush empty socket with water or saline.

4. Clean the prosthesis with soap and water. Rinse thoroughly.

5. Lift upper eyelid and slide prosthesis into place.

## PROVIDING EYE CARE FOR PATIENT WITH HARD CONTACT LENSES

### Equipment

Towel

Commercial hard contact lens cleanser

Small container of water

Small empty basin

### Preparation

1. If possible, encourage patient or family member to care for patient's lenses.

2. If assisting with contact lens care, assess patient's usual method of cleansing.

3. Wash your hands.

### Procedure

1. Place patient in Fowler's position and place a towel under the patient's chin.

2. Place the tip of your forefinger across the lower lid below its margin.

3. Place the top of the forefinger of the other hand on the upper lid above its margin.

4. Assess for presence of lens.

5. Using a scissors motion, manipulate the two lids as the patient closes, opens, and rolls eyes.

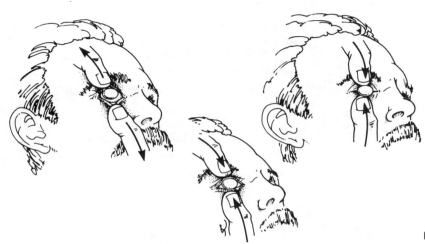

Removal of a hard contact lens.

6. Observe carefully when lens pops out to ensure you don't lose it.

7. Drop a few drops of contact lens cleaner on lens while holding lens on tip of index finger.

8. Rub contact lens between fingertip and thumb for one minute or according to directions on lens cleaner container.

9. Hold lens gently between tips of index finger and thumb over empty basin and rinse by pouring water from container over the lens.

10. Be sure lens is rinsed thoroughly before reinserting in eye.

11. If lens is not reinserted in eye, store in clean, dry contact lens storage case. Make careful note that each lens is placed in the properly marked side of container for that lens.

## PROVIDING EYE CARE FOR PATIENT WITH SOFT CONTACT LENSES

### Equipment

Towel

Contact lens container

Commercially prepared cleaning solution for soft lenses

Commercially prepared rinsing solution for soft lenses

Commercially prepared storing solution for soft lenses

### Procedure

1. Place patient in supine position and place a towel under the patient's chin.

2. Place the tip of your thumb across the lower lid below its margin.

3. Place the top of the forefinger of the same hand on the upper lid above its margin.

4. Spread eyelids apart as wide as possible.

5. Locate outer edges of soft lens which should appear as a rim around outer edge of iris.

6. Place thumb and forefinger directly on soft lens.

7. Gently remove soft lens from surface of eyeball by squeezing lens between thumbs and fingertip. (Lens bends like a piece of Saran wrap.)

8. Release eyelids.

9. Place lens in palm of hand.

10. Drop a few drops of special soft lens cleaner on lens.

11. Clean lens thoroughly by rubbing between fingertip and palm of hand for at least two minutes.

12. Clean other side of lens by repeating previous step.

13. Rinse lens thoroughly with special rinsing solution.

14. Place in lens container and fill container with soft lens storage solution.

15. Repeat entire procedure for lens in patient's other eye.

# PROVIDING EAR CARE FOR PATIENT WITH HEARING AID

## Equipment

Soap

Water

Petroleum jelly

Pipe cleaner

Cotton-tipped applicator

Hearing aid batteries

## Procedure

1. Determine ability of patient to perform all or part of cleaning procedure, and teach procedure when necessary.

2. Have patient remove hearing aid if able to do so.

3. Remove ear mold from receiver before cleaning. Do not immerse receiver in water.

4. Wash ear mold, using soap and water. A pipe cleaner may be used to clean and dry the cannula. Reconnect receiver to dry ear mold.

5. Check batteries if hearing aid has not been functioning. Insert new batteries, matching positive (+) and negative (−) signs.

6. Examine cord for breaks; replace as necessary.

7. Before inserting ear mold, cleanse outer ear gently with cotton-tipped applicator. Apply light film of petroleum jelly to external auditory canal to ease insertion of mold.

8. Turn receiver switch to "ON." Assist patient to adjust volume control to desired level. If whistling or feedback noises occur, check for tightness of fit as ear mold probably has not been inserted properly.

9. Place hearing aid in container when not in use and place in bedside stand.

## CHARTING *for Eye and Ear Care*

☐ Documentation of eye assessment and eye care needs

☐ Method and outcome of eye care provided

☐ Condition of eye and surrounding structure

☐ Condition of eye socket

☐ Response to using hearing aid

☐ Improved hearing after cleaning

☐ Patient's ability to insert, remove, and clean hearing aid

---

## CLINICAL PROBLEM SOLVING

### Potential Problems

Eyelids become crusted from exudate.

You are unable to replace the artificial eye or contact lens.

Wrong solution used on contact lens causes excessive tearing and burning sensation when lens is placed in eye.

Hearing did not improve with cleaning of hearing aid.

### Suggested Solutions

☐ Place warm, moist washcloth across eyes and leave in place for several minutes.

☐ Moisten cotton applicator stick with sterile saline and gently twist the applicator stick over crusted surface to assist in removing crust.

☐ If patient is unable to assist, ask relatives for help.

☐ Do not use force. Leave lens or eye out until someone who is able to replace it is available.

☐ Immediately remove lens from eye and place in proper storage container.

☐ Immediately rinse patient's eye with copious amounts of sterile water.

☐ Have patient checked immediately by opthalmologist for emergency care of potentially burned cornea.

☐ Check if receiver switch is "ON."

☐ Check if batteries are properly in place and that the poles match: positive (+) and negative (−).

# TERMINOLOGY

**Abrasion:** the scraping away of a portion of skin or of a mucous membrane as a result of injury.

**Adaptation:** an alteration or adjustment by which an individual can improve his relationship to the environment.

**Antibacterial:** any substance that fights against or suppresses bacteria.

**Anticoagulant:** any substance that suppresses or counteracts coagulation of blood.

**Aspiration:** to draw in or out, as by suction.

**b.i.d.:** two times daily.

**Canthus:** the angle at either end of the slit between the eyelids.

**Capillary:** minute blood vessel carrying blood and forming the capillary system.

**Cavitation:** formation of a cavity.

**Congenital:** present at birth.

**Cornea:** the clear, transparent anterior portion of the fibrous coat of the eye.

**Debilitated:** to become feeble; tired; worn-out.

**Decalcification:** the act of removing calcium, the basic component of bones and teeth.

**Decubitus:** a bedsore.

**Edema:** a local or generalized condition in which there is excess fluid in the tissues.

**Emesis:** vomiting.

**Epidermis:** the outer layer of skin.

**Eversion:** a turning outwards.

**Excoriation:** the abrasion of the epidermis or of the coating of any organ of the body.

**Expectoration:** expulsion of mucous or phlegm from the throat or lungs.

**Fissure:** a groove, slit, or natural division; ulcer or crack-like sore.

**Floss:** a waxed or unwaxed tape or thread used to clean between teeth.

**Fungus:** a vegetable cellular organism that subsists on organic matter.

**Genitals:** organs of generation; reproductive organs.

**Hemorrhage:** abnormal internal or external discharge of blood.

**Holistic:** the philosophy that an individual must be looked at as a whole rather than a sum of the parts.

**Hygiene:** the study and observance of health rules.

**Hypoallergenic:** against allergy, as hypoallergenic tape.

**Impetigo:** inflammatory skin disease marked by isolated pustules which become crusted and rupture.

**Incontinent:** inability to retain urine or feces through loss of sphincter control.

**Incurvate:** curved, especially inward.

**Intervention:** the act of coming between, so as to hinder or modify.

**Irritation:** a source of annoyance; incipient inflammation, soreness or roughness, or irritability of a body part.

**Labia:** the lips of the vulva.

**Lesion:** an injury or wound; a single infected patch in a skin disease.

**Metabolism:** the sum of all physical and chemical changes that take place within an organism; all energy and material transformations that occur within living cells.

**Microorganism:** a minute living body such as a bacterium or protozoon not perceptible to the naked eye.

**Mucosa:** mucous membrane lining passages and cavities communicating with the air.

**Nasolacrimal:** pertinent to the nose and lacrimal apparatus.

**Ophthalmic solution:** solution designed especially for the eyes.

**Oral:** concerning the mouth.

**Palate:** the roof of the mouth.

**Parotid gland:** either of the largest of the paired salivary glands, located below and in front of each ear.

**Pediculosis:** infestation with lice.

**Perineum:** the external region between the vulva and anus in a female or between the scrotum and anus in a male.

**Plaque:** a patch on the skin or on a mucous surface; a blood platelet.

**Pressure point:** area for exerting pressure to control bleeding; an area of skin that can become irritated with pressure, especially over bony prominences.

**Sclera:** the tough, white, fibrous outer envelope of tissue covering all of the eyeball except the cornea.

**Semi-Fowler's position:** semi-sitting position.

**Systemic:** pertinent to the whole body rather than to one of its parts.

**Thrush:** fungus infection of mouth or throat, especially in infants and young children.

**Ulcer:** an open sore or lesion of the skin or mucous membrane of the body.

**Urethra:** canal for the discharge of urine extending from the bladder to the outside.

**Vascular:** pertinent to or composed of blood vessels.

# Chapter *11*

# *Stress Management*

## LEARNING OBJECTIVES

Define the term stress according to Dr. Selye.

Discuss the impact of stress on the body psychologically.

Describe the body's physiological response to stress and include at least two body systems.

Explain Selye's General Adaptation Syndrome and differentiate between the three stages.

List at least three different categories of stressors.

Identify at least five danger signals of stress.

Describe the four stages of anxiety.

List two characteristics of each stage of anxiety.

Outline the factors that would be labeled causes of stress.

Discuss a specific method the patient can use to control stress.

Demonstrate three nursing actions that will assist the patient to manage anxiety.

Discuss management of the aggressive patient.

State two nursing diagnoses that relate to managing stress and anxiety.

## STRESS

Human beings experience stress as a part of their everyday existence. And, while stress is a natural component of life, it can sap energy and contribute to the presence of disease. It is a universal phenomenon and all human beings in all cultures experience some degree of stress. The concept of stress has been with man since the beginning of time, but it was not until William Osler and Walter Cannon began their investigation in the early 1900's that stress was actually linked to illness. By 1950 Dr. Hans Selye, an endocrinologist and biologist and the world expert on stress, scientifically demonstrated that stress played a major role in certain diseases such as gastric ulcers and high blood pressure. Since Dr. Selye's early research, authorities from medicine, biology, physiology, sociology, psychology, and anthropology have studied and written thousands of articles on the subject of stress. With the undeniable fact that stress affects an individual's total life, it is imperative that the nurse have a basic understanding of stress, its effect on humans, how humans cope and adapt to stress, and how she can deal with her own stress and help patients deal with theirs. The stress of life is life itself according to Dr. Barbara Brown, a nurse author who wrote about stress and biofeedback. To examine stress and its impact on human beings in this culture, we have to examine one's total life experience.

Western medicine is entering an era of transformation. The whole context of the medical profession is changing. Patients and professionals alike are examining alternatives to traditional patterns of treatment and are devising new modes of health care delivery. These changes are occurring at a time when the structure of the health care system in this country (and indeed the world) desperately needs new ways of dealing with health and illness.

And, as we change our focus from illness to health, we need new perspectives for health care.

Perhaps the greatest impetus for these changes has come about in response to new knowledge about the role of stress in our lives. Dr. Selye believed that efforts to manage and find cures for diseases are an ineffective approach to creating wellness. He and other prominent scientists think that the only viable approach is to examine man's ability to cope and adapt to stress. At the second international conference on stress held in Monte Carlo eminent physician Dr. Arnold Fox stated that stress is either the main cause or a strong contributing factor in all diseases of mankind. Most of these scientists now attribute 70 to 80 percent of all diseases to stress.

Dr. Brown, however, believes that 100 percent of diseases have stress factors at the root. The view that disease is caused by invading microorganisms or that ill people are merely victims or even that all disease can be cured by modern science is erroneous. New definitions of existing problems necessitate finding new solutions. The current emphasis on stress and stress reduction methods may be a new solution to old problems. The current emphasis on stress is relevant to our times, and we, as nurses, need to recognize and understand stress and the impact of stress on us as individuals, on our profession, and, most particularly, on our patients.

Stress is a difficult term to define precisely, for there is not one specific source or one definite response. Dr. Selye stated that stress may be viewed as the common denominator of all the body's adaptive reactions. Stress may be grief as well as joy, pleasure as well as unhappiness, cold as well as heat, fear as well as elation. In fact, stress covers the total range of mental, emotional, and physical demands on the body that will respond with predictable biochemical and general adaptation changes. Health is determined by the body's being in a state of balance in which the whole organism functions in harmony. Stress can be defined as a state of arousal or agitation which throws the body out of balance. While a certain amount of stress is necessary for survival, when it becomes prolonged and intense, our adaptive responses weary and the negative aspects begin to take their toll on our bodies and our minds.

**The Impact of Stress**    Psychologically, stress may be viewed as the experience an individual has when the demands placed on the body exceed the ability to cope, thus, the body is thrown out of balance. Physiologically, stress initiates certain bodily processes, such as the "fight or flight" mechanism, which result in a threat to homeostasis. Early in the 1900s Dr. Cannon, a Harvard physiologist, coined the term "homeostasis." As a result of his work, certain adjustment mechanisms of the body, such as blood sugar level, temperature, hydration, etc., were identified. According to Dr. Cannon, the stress response resulted in these mechanisms being activated, which in turn threw the body out of balance.

Rather than a specific response, Dr. Selye focused on a general adaptation process as a response to stress. This process is the body's attempt to adapt and maintain homeostasis. Dr. Selye further defined stress as the rate of wear and tear on the body and stated that the only freedom from stress is death.

Dr. Selye's general adaptation syndrome occurs in three stages. The first stage, *the alarm stage,* occurs when a generalized response throughout the body responds to stressors such as trauma, infection, pain, cold, heat, fear. The purpose of the alarm reaction is to mobilize the body's defenses to meet the stressor. Biochemically, during the alarm stage, the hormonal levels

**TABLE 1** SELYE'S STRESS ADAPTATION SYNDROME

| STAGE | GENERAL FUNCTION | INTERPERSONAL | BEHAVIORAL | AFFECTIVE | COGNITIVE | PHYSIOLOGICAL |
|---|---|---|---|---|---|---|
| 1 Alarm reaction | Mobilization of body defenses | Interpersonal communication effectiveness decreases | Task oriented Increased restlessness Apathy, regression Crying | Feelings of anger, suspiciousness, helplessness Anxiety level increases | Alert Thinking becomes narrow and concrete Symptoms of thought blocking, forgetfulness, and decreased productivity | Muscle tension Increase in epinephrine and cortisone Stimulation of adrenal cortex and lymph glands Increase in blood pressure, heart rate, blood glucose |
| 2 Stage of resistance | Adaptation to stresses Resistance increases | Interpersonal communication self-oriented Uses interpersonal relationships to meet own needs | Automatic behaviors Self-oriented behaviors Fight or flight behavior apparent | Increased use of defense mechanisms Emotional responses may be automatic or exaggerated | Thought processes more habitual than problem solving oriented | Hormonal levels return to pre-alarm stage All physiological responses return to normal or are channeled into psychosomatic symptoms |
| 3 Stage of exhaustion | Depletion or exhaustion of organs and resources Loss of ability to resist stress | Disintegration of personal interactions Communication skills ineffective and disorganized Self-oriented | Restless, withdrawn, agitated; may become violent or self-destructive Diminished productivity | Depressed, flat, or inappropriate Exaggerated or inappropriate use of defense mechanisms Decreased ability to cope | Thought disorganization, hallucinations, preoccupation Reduced intellectual processes | Exhaustion, with increased demands on organism Adrenal cortex hormone depletion Death, if stress is continuous and excessive |

from the adrenal cortex increase. The anti-inflammatory hormones, the adrenocorticotropin hormones, cortisone, and cortisol are produced along with pro-inflammatory hormones, aldosterone, and desoxycorticosterone. This is the shock phase when the autonomic nervous system comes into full play. The second stage, *the resistance stage,* occurs when the body's defenses are mobilized to produce hormones to cope with the alarm stage. The body chemistry either repels or adapts to the stressor. During this phase the organism is successful in adapting to the stressor, and the biochemical changes resulting from the alarm phase return to the pre-alarm stage. Any life change causes alarm and resistance and the stress accrued through life reduces the body's adaptive abilities. Continuous high degrees of stress will deplete the organism's adaptive abilities at a much greater rate than normal stress levels. *The final stage* occurs when the stress is prolonged and the body can no longer cope effectively. The result is exhaustion and the body may become ill with disease. The organism's adaptive abilities are depleted and the organism loses its ability to deal with the stress. The organism goes into shock, and if the stress is not alleviated, the result may be the death of the organism.

The general adaptation syndrome varies widely in intensity. A reaction to positive stimuli, such as getting married or learning you are going to have a baby, will activate a stress response, but it may result in less damage than a negative stressor even though it does temporarily throw the body out of balance. Furthermore, a person does not respond with the same intensity to all negative stressors. For example, you would not respond with the same degree of intensity to jumping in a cold pool as you would to turning a corner and seeing a man pointing a gun at you.

The local adaptive syndrome is the manifestation of stress in a limited part of the body. The body responds locally to the stressor, such as a burn or a cut to a finger. The local response may also trigger a general response if the ability of the body to respond to the specific area is greatly affected by the condition of the whole organism. An upper respiratory infection causes a much different response within a healthy child than in a child with cystic fibrosis. The better the organism as a whole is at adapting to stress, the more effective the local adaptive response.

**Response to Stress**  Responses to stress then, can be categorized into several different patterns: the *physiological response*, where there is loss or gain in weight over time, increase in hormone levels, increase in blood pressure, or a psychosomatic symptom; the *psychological response*, which may also result in a psychosomatic illness or psychiatric manifestations, such as depression, mania, withdrawal from reality, or anxiety; and, the *behavioral response*, where one hits out, becomes aggressive (fights), or withdraws; one may also become immobilized, or turn inward (physical or emotional flight). The *interpersonal mode* can reflect stress where communication effectiveness decreases, relationships deteriorate, trust in others diminishes and the ability to form and maintain close, intimate, loving ties with another person decreases. Finally, the *affective response* may be present where one's emotions are affected so that anxiety is high and emotions are unstable, labile, unpredictable, and inappropriate to the situation. All of the above modes of response relate to the negative elements of response patterns. Of course, these modes can be used in a positive way so that stress becomes nondetrimental. There is no way to eliminate the stressors, but individuals can learn to minimize the harmful effects and utilize response modes in a positive way.

---

**Danger Signals of Stress**
Depression
Uncontrolled hyperactive behavior
Lack of concentration
Feelings of unreality
Loss of control
Pervasive high anxiety level
Physical manifestations of:
    Irregular heartbeats
    Tremors, tics
    Gastrointestinal disturbance
    Skin disturbance
    Changes in respiratory patterns
Insomnia
Disease

---

Stressors may be chemical, physical, developmental, and emotional. Graduating from nursing school, being promoted, failing to be promoted, having arguments, and playing a tough game of racketball are all stressful events and require adaptation and change at some level. By understanding stress, we can more easily identify stress factors and their effects on patients who need and/or seek health care. Whether a patient is having a baby, undergoing open heart surgery, or seeking counseling for emotional problems, each of these individuals is experiencing stress in his or her own particular manner. How the individual adapts or fails to adapt depends on several factors: personality and emotional makeup and past experiences in dealing with stress (response repertoire).

People are able to create many different forms of disease as well as emotional and spiritual scars. And the more we use our reserves of adaptation energy, the more likely we are to age and hasten our death. In fact, Dr. Selye warned that there is no evidence that the basic reserves of energy for adaptation can be restored. These may be genetically programmed. The more reserves you use handling everyday stress, the less you have for major crises or for growing older. The latest research indicates that there is a direct relationship between the amount of stress encountered in everyday life and aging.

It is important to remember that the stress syndrome can be both positive and negative. Any change or alteration in the balance of life can create stress. The Holmes and Rahe stress scale is an excellent example of the varying conditions in life that result in stress. We are all unique individuals and we respond differently to various stressors. Thus, it does not matter whether the stress is positive or negative, light or severe. What matters is how we develop adaptive mechanisms to cope with these stressors. The ability to cope or solve a problem can be translated as the ability to withstand stress and create life experiences that do not work against you. The implications of stress theory—that by being able to withstand stress, by coping with it, diluting it when it occurs, or eliminating it you can actually affect your life—are tremendously exciting. It means that you are not doomed to inevitable illness later in life. You are not preprogrammed for premature aging. The fact is you control your own health. To quote the *Journal of the American Medical Association*, "Nature did not intend us to grow old and ill; we were designed to die young in old age but free of disease."

Along with coping with her own stress, it is the responsibility of the nurse to be aware that patients suffer from the stress phenomena and that part of the nurse's role is to assist patients to adapt and cope with stress. How can this behavioral objective be implemented?

*First, the nurse must have an understanding of the role of stress.*

- ☐ Understand and accept the theory of stress—what it is and what it does to the body.
- ☐ Be cognizant of the manifestations of stress: tiredness, apathy, frequent illness, lack of interest or aliveness, unwillingness to seek out new challenges, inability to cope with change, and many other symptoms.
- ☐ Elicit the factors that alter resistance to stress (illness, hospitalization, pain, medication, family pressures, etc.).
- ☐ Assist in making a plan and implementing it, designing specific actions to reduce stress, such as relaxation methods.
- ☐ Educate the individual about how to control his or her own stressors.

*Second, the nurse may carry out specific behaviors in the hospital setting.*

- ☐ Assist in the reduction of negative aspects of stress.

# Stress Model

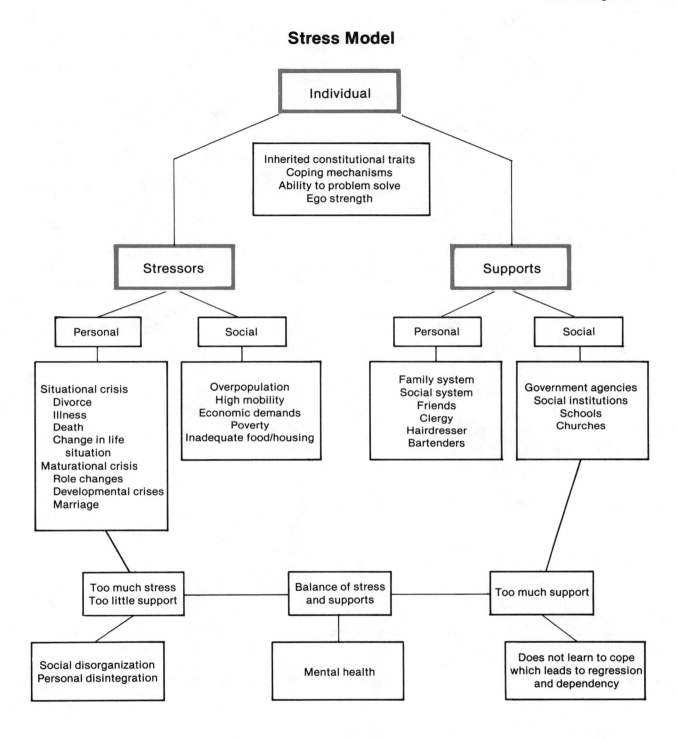

☐ Counsel the patient and family on the theory of stress; together, examine how the patient's particular stressors impact his lifestyle.

☐ Reinforce the adaptive process of the patient by meeting his needs, listening to concerns, administering care, and providing emotional support.

**ANXIETY**    Anxiety is a phenomenon that is experienced by most people during their everyday activities. The intensity may vary, but the impact is a variably potent stressor. In other words, the more intense and constant the anxiety, the more stress the individual experiences.

Anxiety is a form of energy whose presence is inferred from its effect on attention, behavior, learning, and perception.

It is a response to tensions and subjectively experienced as a painful, vague uneasiness or diffuse apprehension.

Anxiety is a result of conflicts between the personality and the environment or between different forces within the personality.

The causative conflicts and/or threats are undefined in the conscious mind of the person.

Varying degrees of anxiety are common to all human beings at one time or another.

The amount or level of anxiety is related to both the degree of threat to the self and the degree to which behavior reduces the anxiety.

Anxiety is always found in emotional disorders and is easily transmitted from one individual to another.

Constructive use of anxiety is healthy; it is often an incentive for growth.

The larger the capacity to handle anxiety, the more control an individual has over his or her environment.

---

**Danger Signals of Anxiety**
Poor concentration
Narrowed perception or tunnel vision
Hyperactivity
Poor appetite
Tension headache
Insomnia
Physical manifestations
    Tachycardia
    Gastrointestinal disturbances
    Increased urinary output
    Numbness and tingling of extremities

---

**Stages of Anxiety**    There are stages of anxiety that range from mild to severe and panic. The absence of all anxiety (ataraxia) is uncommon. It can most often be observed in persons who have taken drugs. The following stages illustrate the characteristics of each level of anxiety.

*Mild*

Patient's senses are alert.
Attentiveness is increased.
Motivation is increased.

*Moderate*

Patient's perception is narrowed and attention is selective.
The degree of pathology depends on the individual.
State may be detected in complaining, arguing, teasing behaviors.
Anxiety may be converted to physical symptoms, such as headaches, low back pain, nausea, and diarrhea.

*Severe*

> All senses are gravely affected.
> Behavior becomes automatic.
> Energy is drained.
> Defense mechanisms are used to control anxiety.
> State cannot be used constructively by person.
> Psychologically, state is extremely painful.
> Nursing action is always indicated for this state.

*Panic*

> Individual is overwhelmed.
> Personality may disintegrate.
> The patient may engage in wild, desperate, ineffective behavior.
> Patient should be watched to prevent possible bodily harm to self and others.
> Patient cannot tolerate panic state very long and soon cannot control his or her behavior; patient feels helpless; patient is momentarily psychotic.
> Condition is pathological.
> Immediate intervention is needed: physical restraint, tranquilizers, nonstimulating environment, constant presence of the nurse.

The following nursing diagnoses may be appropriate to include in a Patient Care Plan when the components are related to decreasing stress and promoting adaptation.

**NURSING DIAGNOSES**

| Nursing Diagnosis (Potential) | Defining Characteristic; Etiology (Examples) |
|---|---|
| ☐ Anxiety, *related to* | Increased stress, e.g., illness, trauma, loss. |
| ☐ Coping, Ineffective Individual, *related to* | High stress on human organism, e.g., individual inability to adapt, length and duration of stressor. |
| ☐ Health Maintenance, Alteration in, *related to* | High stress level, e.g., illness, abuse, psychological factors. |
| ☐ Social Isolation, *related to* | Maladaptive coping to stressor, e.g., long-term or high level of stress. |

# UNIT ONE   STRESS AND ADAPTATION

## NURSING PROCESS DATA

### ASSESSMENT   *Data Base*

Identify the patient who demonstrates stressed behavior.

Evaluate, with the patient, the past and present stressors that the patient has experienced.

Evaluate the stressors' effect on the patient's body and look for signs of distress in the body.

> **Clinical Alert**
>
> *Cardiovascular system:* increased pulse and blood pressure, evidence of angina, arrhythmias, migraine headaches, disturbance of heat and cold mechanisms.
>
> *Gastrointestinal system:* ulcers, ulcerative colitis, constipation or diarrhea, imbalance in sugar absorption.
>
> *Musculoskeletal system:* backache, tension headaches, arthritis, proneness to accidents.
>
> *Autoimmune system:* infections, flu, allergies, rheumatoid arthritis, cancer.

Assess patient's level of energy and degree to which it is depleted.

Evaluate patient's awareness of thoughts, attitudes, values, and beliefs that influence stress response and adaptation.

Assess present level of distress in the patient's body.

Assess possible causes of stress that are affecting the patient.

Assess the factors that influence how the patient responds to stress. Characteristics of the stressful event: magnitude, intensity, duration; Patient's biological and psychological inclinations. Sound support system.

### PLANNING *Objectives*

To identify presence of stress in patient.

To identify how stress impacts the body.

To identify the current sources that result in stressed behavior.

To determine the patient's responses to stress.

To evaluate stress interventions that will have a positive effect on stressed patient.

### IMPLEMENTATION *Procedures*

Determining Impact of Stress on Patient

Determining the Response Patterns to Stress

### EVALUATION *Expected Outcomes*

Patient is able to evaluate the general stressors and identify sources of stress in his life.

Patient is aware of response patterns to stress and is able to alter patterns appropriately.

## DETERMINING IMPACT OF STRESS ON PATIENT

### Procedure

1. Discuss the concept of stress with patient to elicit understanding of the impact on body.
   a. Stress is a physical, chemical, or emotional factor that causes bodily or mental tension and that may be a factor in disease causation.
   b. Stress is a state resulting from factors that tend to alter an existing equilibrium.

---

**Dr. Selye's definition of stress.**
- A state manifested by a specific syndrome that consists of all the nonspecifically induced changes within the biologic system.
- The body is the common denominator of all adaptive responses.
- Stress is manifested by the measurable changes in the body.
- Stress causes a multiplicity of changes in the body.

---

2. Provide a relationship where patient feels free to discuss life patterns that relate to stress.
3. Discuss the impact of stress on patient. **Rationale:** Directing the conversation to the emotional, mental, and social areas of life will assist the patient in examining the impact of stress.
4. Assist in formulating a plan with the patient to reduce or eliminate at least some sources of stress.

## DETERMINING THE RESPONSE PATTERNS TO STRESS

### Procedure

1. Discuss the patient's body response to stress. **Rationale:** The body's response to stress is a self-preserving mechanism that automatically and immediately becomes activated in times of danger.
   a. Caused by physical or psychological stress: disease, injury, anger, or frustration; or by changes in internal and/or external environment.
   b. There are a limited number of ways an organism can respond to stress (e.g., a cornered amoeba cannot fly).
2. Assist patient to understand response patterns.
3. Provide problem-solving assistance so the patient can examine new, more appropriate response patterns.
4. Refer patient to resources (therapy classes, books, relaxation tapes) that will assist in developing new responses.

### CHARTING *for Stress Response*

- Identify stressed behavior observed in patient
- Separate physical from emotional and environmental stressors
- Relate how patient is responding to stress
- Pertinent verbalization of patient related to stress

---

## CLINICAL PROBLEM SOLVING

### Potential Problems

Patient moves into the stage of exhaustion and stress becomes dangerous to health.

Patient refuses to acknowledge stress is impacting on his life.

### Suggested Solutions

- Immediately take measures to remove stressors through medication, complete rest, etc.
- Implement specific stress reducing measures such as relaxation processes, visualization, biofeedback, etc.

- Attempt to elicit feelings of patient before giving information about the role of stress and effect on one's body.
- Refer patient to resources, articles, and knowledgeable persons who can discuss the impact of stress and the importance of eliminating stressors.

# UNIT TWO  ANXIETY

## NURSING PROCESS DATA

### ASSESSMENT  *Data Base*

Assess patient's degree of anxiety by determining the patient's ability to focus on what is happening to him or her in a situation.

Mild anxiety: Patient is able to focus realistically on most of what is happening within and to self.

Moderate anxiety: Patient is able to partially focus on what is happening; focus is limited.

Severe anxiety: Patient cannot focus on what is happening to him or her; focus is scattered.

Assess patient's physiological reactions.
Increased heart rate.
Increased or decreased appetite.
Increased blood supply to skeletal muscles.
Tendency to void and defecate.
Dry mouth.
"Butterflies" in stomach, nausea, vomiting, cramps, diarrhea.
"Flight or fight" response.
Tremors.
Dyspnea.
Palpitations.
Tachycardia.
Numbness of extremities.

Evaluate patient's psychological reactions.
Lack of concentration on work.
Feelings of depression and guilt.
Harbored fear of sudden death or insanity.
Dread of being alone.
Confusion.
Tension.
Agitation and restlessness.

### PLANNING  *Objectives*

To identify behavior and/or symptoms related to anxiety.

To decrease anxiety level.

To assist patient to develop more effective coping mechanisms for handling anxiety.

To assist patient to channel anxiety-produced energy into constructive behavior.

To aid patient in gaining a degree of insight into the source of anxiety.

To give patient support in changing life-style patterns that cause anxiety.

To provide a nurse-patient relationship as a means of assisting the patient to handle anxiety.

**IMPLEMENTATION** *Procedures*

Assisting the Patient to Manage Anxiety

Managing the Aggressive or Combative Patient

**EVALUATION** *Expected Outcomes*

Anxiety level is decreased as evidenced by patient being more attentive, more alert and displaying more control of own behavior, i.e., patient is able to sit with nurse rather than pace.

Patient is able to verbalize anxious thoughts.

Patient is able to discuss anxious feelings.

Patient is able to learn new ways of coping with anxiety.

Patient is able to manage anxiety to the point where he does not become aggressive or combative.

## ASSISTING PATIENT TO MANAGE ANXIETY

### Procedure

1. Identify anxious behavior and the level of anxiety that determines degree of intervention.

2. Remain with an anxious patient. **Rationale:** Anxiety level will increase if patient is left alone.

3. Recognize anxiety in self.

4. Maintain appropriate attitudes toward patient.
   a. Acceptance.
   b. Matter-of-fact approach.
   c. Willingness to listen and help.
   d. Calmness and support.

5. Recognize if additional help is required for intervention. **Rationale:** Letting the patient and the situation get out of control will only increase the patient's anxiety.

6. Provide activities that decrease anxiety and provide an outlet for energy.

7. Establish a person-to-person relationship.
   a. Allow patient to express feelings.
   b. Proceed at patient's pace.
   c. Avoid forcing patient.
   d. Assist patient in identifying anxiety.
   e. Assist patient in learning new ways of dealing with anxiety.

8. Provide appropriate physical environment.
   a. Nonstimulating.
   b. Structured.
   c. Designed to prevent physical exhaustion or self-harm.

9. Administer medication as directed and needed. **Rationale:** Severely anxious patients will benefit by stat medication to reduce level.

## MANAGING THE AGGRESSIVE OR COMBATIVE PATIENT

### Procedure

1. Observe patient acutely for clues that the patient is getting out of control. **Rationale:** Noting rising anger—verbal and nonverbal behavior and erratic or unpredictable responses to staff or other patients will give cues to patient's control level.

2. Intervene immediately when loss of control is imminent. **Rationale:** The quicker the intervention, the less likely the patient will lose total control.

3. Use a nonthreatening approach to the patient.

4. Set firm limits on unacceptable behavior.

5. Maintain calm manner and do not show fear.

6. Avoid engaging in an argument or provoking the patient.

7. Remove the patient from the situation as soon as possible.

8. Attempt to calm the patient so that he or she may regain control.

9. Be supportive and stay with the patient.

**CHARTING** *for Managing Anxiety*

☐ Level or degree of patient's anxiety

☐ Behavior, thoughts, or feelings that patient expresses that indicate anxiety

☐ Degree of patient's understanding, insight, etc. into source of anxiety

☐ Measures that nurse takes to assist patient to lower anxiety

---

## CLINICAL PROBLEM SOLVING

**Potential Problems**

Patient becomes extremely defensive when nurse attempts to discuss coping mechanisms.

**Suggested Solutions**

☐ Avoid criticizing patient's behavior and use of adjustment mechanisms.

☐ Assist patient at own pace in learning new or alternative adjustment patterns for healthier adaptation.

Patient's anxiety level increases sharply during interaction with the nurse.

☐ Use techniques to alleviate the patient's anxiety—engage in activity; encourage the patient to describe anxious feelings; provide prn medication.

☐ Use a firm, supportive approach to explore any ineffective use of adjustment patterns.

---

## TERMINOLOGY

**Adaptive reaction:** a response by which the person attempts to improve or alter his or her condition in relation to the environment.

**Alleviate:** to make more bearable; reduce (pain, grief, or suffering).

**Anxiety:** a state of uneasiness and distress; diffuse apprehension.

**Apathy:** indifference; insensibility; without emotion; sluggish.

**Apprehension:** a fearful or uneasy anticipation of the future; dread.

**Ataraxia:** the absence of all anxiety.

**Autonomic nervous system:** the part of the nervous system that regulates the functioning of internal organs and glands; it controls such functions as digestion, respiration, and cardiovascular activity.

**Cerebral cortex:** the extensive outer layer of grey tissue of the cerebral hemispheres (brain), responsible for higher nervous functions.

**Coping mechanisms:** means by which an individual adjusts or adapts to a threat or a challenge; actions that assist in maintaining homeostasis.

**Defense mechanism:** conscious or unconscious processes used to protect oneself from threats or to alleviate anxiety.

**Delusion:** a fixed, false belief.

**Dynamics of homeostasis:** danger or its symbols, whether internal or external, resulting in the activation of the sympathetic nervous system and the adrenal medulla. The organism prepares for fight or flight.

**Emotional:** affected by strong feelings, as of joy and sorrow.

**Fight or flight:** one's immediate response to stress that is, although archaic and often inappropriate, part of our central nervous system biological heritage.

**General adaptation syndrome:** a general theory of stress response formulated by Dr. Hans Selye; describes the action of stress response in three stages—the alarm reaction, the stage of resistance, and the stage of exhaustion.

**-Genic:** suffix indicating generation or production.

**Hallucination:** false perception having no relation to reality and not accounted for by external stimuli.

**Health:** the state of physical, psychological, and sociological well-being.

**Holistic:** a way of looking at individuals and organisms as a whole rather than a sum of the parts.

**Homeostasis:** the maintenance of a constant state in the internal environment through self-regulatory techniques that preserve an organism's ability to adapt to stress.

**Hypertension:** a condition in which the patient has a higher blood pressure than judged to be normal.

**Illness:** a state characterized by the malfunction of the biopsychosocial organism.

**Impulsive:** act of driving onward with sudden force.

**Insomnia:** inability to sleep.

**Lifestyle:** the manner in which one is accustomed to living.

**Meditation:** the act of reflecting upon or pondering; contemplation.

**Musculo:** pertaining to the muscles.

**Musculoskeletal:** pertaining to the muscles and the skeleton.

**Neuro:** prefix pertaining to nerves.

**Pain:** a sensation in which a person experiences discomfort, distress, or suffering.

**Parasympathetic nervous system:** a division of the autonomic nervous system that regulates acetylcholine and conserves energy expenditure; it slows down the system.

**Perspective:** subjective evaluation of relative significance; a view.

**Pressure:** the act of bearing down; exerting force.

**Psychogenic:** of mental origin.

**Relaxation:** a lessening of tension or activity in a part.

**Stamina:** constitutional energy; strength; endurance.

**Stress:** a nonspecific response of the body to any internal or external event or change that impinges on a person's system and creates a demand.

**Stressor:** a specific demand that gives rise to a coping response.

**Sympathetic nervous system:** a division of the autonomic nervous system that controls energy expenditure and mobilizes for action when confronted with a threat.

**Tachycardia:** abnormal rapidity of heart action; above 100 beats/minute.

**Tranquilizer:** a drug which acts to reduce tension and anxiety without interfering with normal mental activity.

**Wellness:** a state of physical, psychological and sociological well-being of a whole person. Synonym for health.

Chapter **12**

# Nurse-Patient Relationship

**LEARNING OBJECTIVES**

Describe the components of a nurse-patient relationship.

Identify at least three principles underlying a helping relationship.

Discuss the phases in a nurse-patient relationship.

Define the concept of patient teaching.

Describe what is meant by the term learning theory.

Outline the process of collecting patient data.

Explain the major steps of implementing a teaching strategy.

Describe the key points of charting for patient teaching.

State two nursing diagnoses that relate to nurse-patient relationship and patient teaching.

## RELATIONSHIP THERAPY

Nurses are given the unique opportunity to share part of who they are with others who have asked directly or indirectly for assistance. It is within this interpersonal framework that the nurse-patient relationship begins to develop and take on its individual characteristics.

Both individuals bring into the relationship their thoughts, feelings, sense of self or self-worth, behavior patterns, abilities to adapt and cope, belief systems, and points-of-view about life and how they interact with it. Within all these complex variables, there is a commonly shared point at which the nurse-patient relationship begins.

This relationship may be defined as the interaction between the nurse and a patient with shared therapeutic goals and objectives. Characteristics of the relationship include acceptance, honesty, understanding, and empathy of the nurse toward the patient who is willingly or unwillingly seeking help. Generally, it is important for the nurse to view the patient as a unique individual who is responsible for his or her own feelings, actions, and behaviors and who is an active participant in a health care program. The relationship will be more effective if the patient shows a willingness to accept responsibility and actively participates in the therapeutic relationship. In psychiatry, however, this is not always possible, and the nurse must begin the relationship by accepting the level at which the patient is able to participate. This, at times, is a difficult and frustrating process. The goal of relationship therapy is to assist the patient to identify and meet his own needs. The nurse may assist the patient in reaching the goals by demonstrating acceptance so that the patient can experience the feeling of being accepted as an individual; by developing mutual trust through consistent, congruent nursing behaviors; by providing corrective emotional experiences to increase self-esteem; and finally by creating a safe, supportive environment. Some degree of emotional involvement and honest, open communication is essential throughout the relationship. The nurse must encourage the patient to express his feelings within safe limits.

**Relationship Principles**    The nurse-patient relationship is an interaction between a nurse and a patient; an interaction that has therapeutic goals, objectives, and tasks. Characteristics of the relationship include acceptance, honesty, understanding, and empathy. Generally, it is important for the nurse to view the patient as a unique being who is responsible for his own feelings, actions, and behaviors.

The relationship is more effective, however, if the patient shows a willingness to accept responsibility for himself and actively participates in the therapeutic relationship.

Principles underlying a helping relationship include:

Awareness of the total patient including physical needs.
Some degree of emotional involvement while maintaining objectivity.
The setting of appropriate limits and consistency.
Empathetic understanding focusing on the patient.
Open, honest, clear communication.
Encouragement of the expression of feelings.
Focus on "here and now."

Dangers to the relationship include overemotional involvement and judgmental attitudes on the part of the nurse and the staff.

## Phases in Nurse-Patient Relationship Therapy

*Initiation or orientation phase.*

☐  Establish boundaries of the relationship.

☐  Identify problems.

☐  Assess anxiety levels of self and patient.

☐  Identify expectations.

*Continuation or active working phase.*

☐  Promote attitude of acceptance of each other to decrease anxiety.

☐  Use specific therapeutic and problem-solving techniques to develop a working relationship.

☐  Continually assess and evaluate problems.

☐  Focus on increasing patient's independence and decreasing patient's reliance on the nurse.

☐  Maintain the goal of patient's confronting and working through identified problems.

*Termination phase.*

☐  Plan for the conclusion of therapy early in the development of the relationship.

☐  Maintain initially defined boundaries.

□ Anticipate problems of termination:

Patient may become too dependent on the nurse; encourage patient to become independent.

Termination may recall patient's previous separation experiences, causing feelings of abandonment, rejection, and depression. Discuss patient's previous experiences.

□ Discuss patient's feelings about termination.

## PATIENT TEACHING

Patient teaching as a legitimate process within the health care system had its "coming of age" during the 1970s. Factors contributing to this advancement of patient teaching included a shift from the focus on treatment of acute, infectious, and curable diseases to the treatment of chronic, degenerative, noncurable diseases with multiple causes; increased involvement of consumers in their health care, including issues such as patient rights, informed consents, and patient access to records; recognition of the cost benefits of patient education; emergence of the self-care movement with its emphasis on the individual's responsibility for his or her state of health; and development of health education and patient teaching theories through scientific research.

The goal of patient teaching is to impact and influence behavioral changes by the individual that will promote the person's health status. The dynamics of human behavior and the forces that influence behavioral changes are highly complex, and there is simply no "one right way" to go about the process of educating patients in order to achieve this goal.

**Learning Theories**   Since learning influences behavior, learning theories provide a framework for the education process. It is beyond the scope of this text to describe all learning theories, but two such theories provide a broad perspective. The cognitive theory emphasizes learning as an understanding of and insight into interrelationships involving perceptions, concepts, feelings, ideas; this type of learning also involves thinking and reasoning. Association theory, on the other hand, emphasizes learning by stimulus-response associations, and includes classical and operant conditioning, rote, and trial-and-error learning. While far apart in philosophy as to why and how learning occurs, proponents of both theories agree that behavior change is the outcome of learning and occurs as a result of practice. The nurse can choose to utilize those principles that are applicable to each teaching situation, whether it is use of behavior modification techniques (association theory) as part of a weight loss program or use of problem-solving games (cognitive theory) as part of group discussions for diabetics.

**Goals of Learning**   The goals of learning can be classified as follows: cognitive (intellectual), affective (values, attitudes, feelings), and psychomotor (motor skills). These areas provide a framework for setting objectives and evaluating expected outcomes for specific teaching situations. Of utmost importance is the recognition that the mere transmission of knowledge, such as a lecture, does not constitute learning. It is only one aspect. A change in the listener's attitude or value system must also occur before one's behavior changes, regardless of the knowledge one possesses.

The patient teaching process is an important component of nursing care, although in actual practice many barriers to its realization exist. Some of these are created by health care providers themselves. The description of the patient education process as an action or skill within the nursing process provides a framework for the integration of both the nursing process and patient education within the practice of nursing.

The following nursing diagnoses may be appropriate to include in a Patient Care Plan when the components are related to establishing and maintaining a nurse-patient relationship or patient teaching.

| Nursing Diagnosis (Potential) | Defining Characteristic; Etiology (Examples) |
|---|---|
| NURSE-PATIENT RELATIONSHIP | |
| ☐ Communication, Impaired: Verbal, *related to* | Inadequate language skills, e.g., cognitive impairment. |
| | Perceptual and/or psychological deficit, e.g., emotional disturbance. |
| | Aphasia, e.g., pathophysiological disruption. |
| ☐ Social Isolation, *related to* | Loneliness, limited interactions, e.g., hospitalization. |
| PATIENT TEACHING | |
| ☐ Health Maintenance, Alteration in, *related to* | Lack of knowledge and/or understanding, e.g., poor teaching strategies, poor learning skills. |
| ☐ Knowledge Deficit, *related to* | Inadequate understanding of condition, e.g., insufficient data gathering, poor communication skills. |
| ☐ Noncompliance, *related to* | Intellectual or psychological alterations, e.g., denial, cognitive impairment, religious beliefs. |

## UNIT ONE   NURSE-PATIENT RELATIONSHIP

### NURSING PROCESS DATA

**ASSESSMENT**   *Data Base*

Determine the purpose of establishing a nurse-patient relationship.

Consider the overall condition of patient to determine if patient will be able to benefit from a nurse-patient relationship.

A specific relationship could feed into secondary gains of anxiety.

An individual with chronic organic brain disorder would not benefit from a relationship per se.

Identify patient expectations of a therapeutic relationship to determine if you will be able to meet these needs.

Examine your own feelings and expectations to evaluate potential impact on such a relationship.

### PLANNING *Objectives*

To provide an environment where patient can feel secure enough to alter behavior patterns.

To allow a patient to experience a positive, satisfying relationship.

To enable patient to test out more adaptive ways to handle anxiety.

To provide a climate conducive to raising the patient's self-esteem.

To allocate enough time to complete planned process of interaction.

To terminate relationship successfully.

### IMPLEMENTATION *Procedures*

Initiating a Nurse-Patient Relationship

Facilitating a Nurse-Patient Relationship

Terminating a Nurse-Patient Relationship

### EVALUATION *Expected Outcomes*

Principles of therapeutic communication are utilized.

Boundaries of professional relationship are maintained.

The appropriate environment for interaction is established.

Termination of the relationship is completed successfully.

## INITIATING A NURSE-PATIENT RELATIONSHIP

### Procedure

1. Address the patient's symptoms and problems and communicate a willingness to help alleviate these discomforts. Establish mutual goals.
2. Assess the patient's need for and ability to handle trust and then approach the patient accordingly. **Rationale:** Open, honest, congruent communication and consistent behavior help lay the groundwork for trust.
3. Demonstrate to the patient that you can be trusted and that you care. Do what you say you will do and only make promises you are willing to keep. **Rationale:** The most important element of the initiating phase is the beginning of trust. Without trust the nurse-patient relationship will be ineffective.

4. Set limits on the patient's behavior to protect the patient from himself and to show that you care enough to intervene when his behavior is inappropriate.
5. Avoid approaching the patient in an overpowering manner. This will only frighten an already anxious patient.
6. Do not assume a cool, aloof manner since the patient may interpret this as meaning you do not care and are not interested.

## FACILITATING A NURSE-PATIENT RELATIONSHIP

### Procedure

1. Assume the role of facilitator in the relationship.
2. Accept patient as having value and worth as an individual. **Rationale:** Basic acceptance is a fundamental prerequisite of a relationship.

3. Maintain relationship on a professional level.

4. Provide an environment conducive to patient's experiencing corrective emotional experiences.

5. Keep interaction reality-oriented, that is, in the here and now. **Rationale:** Discussion of past or future experiences will not result in a change of behavior now.

6. Listen actively.

7. Use nonverbal communication to support and encourage patient.
   a. Recognize meaning and purpose of nonverbal communication.
   b. Keep verbal and nonverbal communication congruent.

8. Focus content and direction of conversation on patient.

9. Interact on patient's intellectual, developmental, and emotional level.

10. Focus on "how," "what," "when," "where," and "who." **Rationale:** Asking "why" will place the patient on the defensive because it requires that he justify his behavior.

11. Teach patient problem-solving to correct maladaptive patterns.

12. Help the patient to identify, express, and cope with feelings.

13. Help patient develop alternative coping mechanisms.

14. Recognize a high level of anxiety and assist patient to deal with it.

## TERMINATING A NURSE-PATIENT RELATIONSHIP

### Procedure

1. Work closely with the patient in planning the termination from the beginning of the relationship. **Rationale:** This approach promotes the patient's independence and increases the patient's sense of self-esteem.

2. Remember that expression of feelings by both the nurse and the patient is a necessary component of this phase. **Rationale:** Verbalization can, in itself, be a growth-producing experience by providing time for the nurse and patient to share their feelings of caring and acknowledging areas of growth.

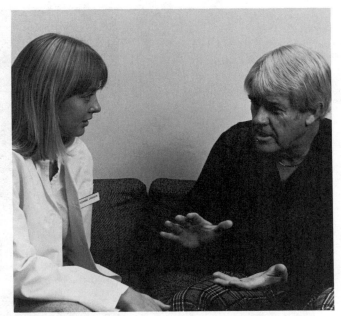

Create a safe and comfortable milieu for the nurse-patient relationship that will encourage the patient to openly express thoughts and feelings.

3. Anticipate problems of termination and plan for their resolution. **Rationale:** Saying goodbye is often uncomfortable and difficult for both the patient and the nurse.

4. Be aware that the patient's behavior may reflect overdependence, depression, and withdrawal. Allow this behavior to be expressed and help the patient to work it through.

5. Do not terminate the relationship too abruptly or allow it to persist beyond the patient's needs.

6. A satisfactory termination of the relationship will enable the patient to move on to other relationships with positive feelings.

### CHARTING  *for Nurse-Patient Relationship*

☐ Primary goals of nurse-patient relationship and identified patient needs

☐ Ongoing process of relationship therapy including patient's expressed feelings, thoughts, etc.

☐ Patient's behavior and changes in behavior, both positive and negative

☐ Cues to other team members on how best to relate to this particular patient

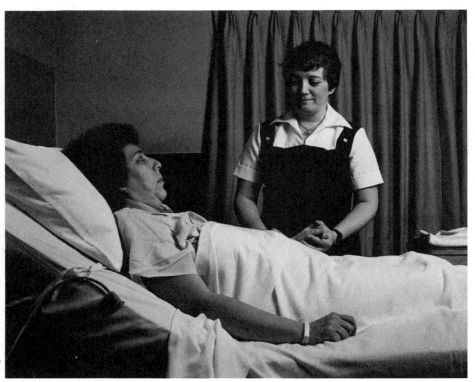

Establish a nurse-patient relationship before beginning patient care.

## CLINICAL PROBLEM SOLVING

| Potential Problems | Suggested Solutions |
|---|---|
| Patient refuses to participate in a nurse-patient relationship. | ☐ Adhere to patient's request and do not force or impose relationship therapy.<br>☐ Continue to offer relationship therapy at intervals.<br>☐ Suggest that another team member attempt to establish a relationship. |
| Nurse-patient relationship frequently degenerates into a social conversation. | ☐ Reevaluate the goals for the relationship and remind patient of terms originally established.<br>☐ Set firm limits and continually reexamine progress. |
| Termination of the nurse-patient relationship is not successful. | ☐ Reexamine the process of termination (termination should begin at the beginning of the relationship).<br>☐ Devote more interaction time to this aspect of the relationship.<br>☐ Attempt to elicit feelings about termination from the patient as well as examining your own feelings.<br>☐ Allow the patient's behavior to be expressed without making value judgments and assist the patient to discuss his feelings. |

## UNIT TWO   PATIENT EDUCATION

### NURSING PROCESS DATA

**ASSESSMENT**   *Data Base*

Determine the need for patient teaching program.

Determine appropriate setting for individual patient.

Identify patient learning needs.

Assess knowledge and skill level of patient.

Assess readiness and/or openness to learning.

Assess appropriate methodology for patient teaching sessions.

Assess appropriate adjunctive materials, such as audiovisual aids, to enhance learning process.

**PLANNING**   *Objectives*

To increase patient's knowledge that will positively affect health status.

To increase patient's self-esteem by encouraging participation in treatment program.

To acknowledge individual responsibility for health behaviors and health status.

To improve patient's ability to make informed decisions affecting health status.

To facilitate behavioral changes that are conducive to optimum health status.

**IMPLEMENTATION**   *Procedures*

Teaching a Patient

Collecting Patient Data

Determining Readiness to Learn

Implementing the Teaching Strategy

**EVALUATION**   *Expected Outcomes*

Patient's knowledge regarding his or her health status has increased.

Patient's ability to make informed and effective health-related decisions, based on accurate information and awareness of self, has improved.

Effective utilization of the health care delivery system has been promoted.

## TEACHING A PATIENT

### Equipment

Room or suitable setting where teaching is to occur

Teaching strategies

Audiovisual equipment

Charts and illustrations

Written materials such as outlines or other handouts

Equipment for demonstration and return demonstration

Form such as teaching Kardex or patient chart to document when teaching is completed

## Procedure

*for Preparing for Patient Teaching*

1. Avoid judging patient input to prevent patient telling the nurse what patient thinks the nurse wants to hear.
2. Utilize "how" questions to facilitate communication. **Rationale:** "How" is more effective than "why" in a question, as "why" tends to set up a defensive reaction to the question.
3. Utilize verbal and nonverbal behavior and congruence of both to provide important data.
4. Utilize observation skills.
5. Request demonstration of a skill previously learned or currently used to assess performance level. **Rationale:** How well patient demonstrates skill assists you in evaluating effectiveness of teaching.

## Procedure

*for Collecting Patient Data*

1. Identify personal characteristics.
   a. Age/sex.
   b. Educational level.
   c. Marital status.
   d. Family composition and living situation.
   e. Ethnic group and cultural practices pertinent to learning.
2. Identify support systems available.
3. Identify values and attitudes toward self and others having his or her particular disease or condition.
4. Assess knowledge of anatomy and physiology (normal and disease-related) by specific questioning.
5. Evaluate capacity and ability to perform specific skills, including those previously learned.
6. Check knowledge of rationale behind specific skills.
7. Evaluate patterns of coping.
   a. Past experiences of self and others in relation to the disease.
   b. Perception by patient of how ill he or she is at this time.
   c. Reactions to stress and ways of managing anxiety.

d. Current level of self management.
e. Willingness of patient to change.

## Procedure

*for Determining Readiness to Learn*

1. Determine patient's physiological readiness.
   a. Degree of physical comfort of patient, such as lack of pain, level of alertness.
   b. Acuteness of the illness and its influence on the patient's ability to learn.
   c. Environmental factors such as safety and supervision while practicing a new skill.
2. Evaluate patient's psychological readiness.
   a. Patient's feeling state and its influence on receptivity to learning. **Rationale:** An angry and hostile patient is not going to hear much information until his or her anger is acknowledged or worked through.
   b. Psychological barriers in the external environment and their impact.
   c. Intellectual capacity and level of comprehension of patient.

## Procedure

*for Implementing the Teaching Strategy*

1. Gather teaching materials appropriate for patient's learning needs and teaching strategy.
2. Sit down with patient in designated setting.
3. Set goals for individualized teaching.
4. Assess teaching situation for any modifications needed and adjust plans accordingly.
5. Verbalize (teach) content to patient(s).
6. Utilize appropriate communication skills.
7. Request feedback (evaluation interchange) during the teaching process. **Rationale:** Feedback allows you to make modifications as indicated or as appropriate.
8. Adhere to agreed-upon starting and ending times; negotiate any changes.
9. Provide closure to teaching situation by summarizing and reiterating agreements made, actions to be taken, or subsequent events to follow.
10. Provide positive reinforcement if you have not done so previously.
11. Terminate teaching session by establishing time for next patient contact.

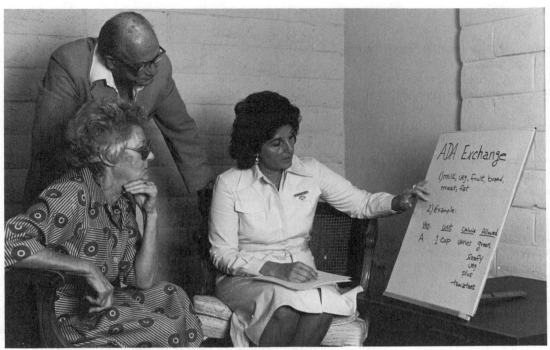

For patient teaching to be effective, provide a comfortable, quiet environment.

12. Do post-assessment of your own participation and plan for corrections and/or improvements in presentation.

## CHARTING *for Patient Teaching*

☐ Topics or subjects covered as a part of patient education process such as: medications, procedures, dietary plan, activity restrictions, or follow-up care

☐ What information or equipment was sent home with patient

☐ Degree of patient's participation in the teaching activity

☐ Progress in meeting the expected outcomes of teaching

☐ Emotional response to the learning process

---

## CLINICAL PROBLEM SOLVING

### Potential Problems

Patient's health status has not improved as a result of the teaching program.

Patient is hostile to teaching program.

### Suggested Solutions

☐ Request assistance from in-service consultant for determining which aspects of the teaching program were not successful and why.
☐ Assist in revising parts of the program and restructure for individual patient needs.

☐ Attempt to determine underlying reason for hostility.
☐ Terminate teaching program for now but tell patient you will return tomorrow or at a later time.

## TERMINOLOGY

**Adjunct:** something attached to another thing but in a dependent or subordinate position.

**Anxiety:** a troubled feeling; distress over real or imagined threat to one's mental or physical well-being.

**Body image:** the mental picture one has of one's body and, frequently, judgments of it.

**Climate:** the meteorological conditions, including temperature, precipitation and wind, that characteristically prevail in a region.

**Cognitive:** awareness with perception, reasoning, intuition, and memory.

**Cognitive thinking:** process by which one acquires knowledge, makes plans, and solves problems.

**Coping mechanism:** the means by which one adjusts or adapts to stress.

**Depression:** a mental state characterized by dejection, lack of hope, and absence of cheerfulness.

**Dynamic:** pertinent to vital force or inherent power; opposed to static.

**Empathy:** objective awareness of and insight into the feelings, emotions, and behavior of another person and their meaning and significance.

**Ethnic:** characteristic of a religious, racial, national, or cultural group.

**Facilitate:** to make an action or process easier.

**Fear:** fright, dread; the emotional reaction to a perceived threat.

**Feedback:** the return of information to the place of origin.

**Grief:** the emotional reaction that follows the loss of a love-object. Somatic symptoms include becoming easily fatigued, anorexia, insomnia, and feelings of sadness and sorrow.

**Hostility:** the state of being hostile; antagonism; enmity.

**Identity:** the collective aspect of a set of characteristics by which a thing is definitely recognizable or known; may include behavioral and personal characteristics of an individual.

**Learning theory:** theory of the way or method by which one gains wisdom, knowledge, and skill.

**Limit:** the point, edge, or line beyond which something cannot proceed; the furthest confines or bounds.

**Maladaptive:** inability to, or faulty adjustment or adaptation.

**Negotiation:** arranging or settling by conferring or discussing.

**Noncompliance:** failure or refusal to comply or go along with something.

**Operant conditioning:** conditioning or influencing behavior by rewarding an individual for certain forms of behavior.

**Overdependence:** the state of needed or relying upon someone or something too much.

**Principle:** a rule or standard; a basic truth, law or assumption.

**Reinforcement:** giving more force or effectiveness to; support, strengthen.

**Self-esteem:** the way one judges one's self, regards one's self, or considers one's self to be.

**Stimulus-response:** a change in environment that causes response or reaction; action and reaction.

**Strategy:** a plan of action.

**Termination:** the end of something; a limit or boundary; conclusion or cessation.

**Trial and error:** an empirical method of finding a satisfactory solution to a problem for which there is no conveniently applicable theory; consists of repeating experimental trials until error is sufficiently reduced or eliminated.

Chapter **13**

# *Vital Signs*

## LEARNING OBJECTIVES

State one etiology, its defining characteristics, and the related nursing diagnosis.

Identify the cardinal signs that reflect the body's physiological status.

List three mechanisms that increase heat production.

Explain how disease alters the "set point" of the temperature regulating center.

Define hypothermia and list the symptoms of this condition.

Differentiate between the oral, rectal, and axillary methods of taking a patient's temperature.

Describe two nursing actions that can be performed when temperature is not within normal range.

Describe at least three different types of pulses.

Discuss the pulse and indicate how it is an index of heart rate and rhythm.

Compare normal heart rate for adults and children.

Compare respiratory rate and rhythm to pulse and blood pressure.

Identify the characteristics of peripheral pulses.

Define the term respiration.

List the normal respiratory rate for adults and children.

Explain four types of abnormal respiratory patterns.

Identify four factors that affect blood pressure.

Demonstrate the method of palpating brachial systolic arterial blood pressure.

## VITAL SIGNS

Vital signs, also termed cardinal signs, reflect the body's physiological status and provide information critical to evaluating homeostatic balance. Vital signs include four critical assessment areas: temperature, pulse, respiration, and blood pressure. The term vital is used because the information gathered is the clearest indicator of overall patient status. These four signs form baseline evaluative data necessary for an ongoing evaluation of a patient's condition. If the nurse has established the normal range for a patient, deviations will be more easily recognized.

Routine vital signs are important to assess on every patient and should be accomplished by a staff member who is familiar with the patient's health history so results can be evaluated against previous data. Vital signs should be taken at consistent intervals. The more critical the patient's condition, the more often these signs need to be taken and evaluated. They are not only indicators of a patient's present condition but also cues to a positive or negative change in a patient's status.

Obtaining the total picture of a patient's health status is a major objective of patient care. Although vital signs yield important information in themselves, they gain even more relevance when compared to the patient's diagnosis, laboratory tests, history, and records.

Temperature represents the balance between heat gain and heat loss and is regulated in the hypothalamus of the brain. Variations in temperature indicate the health status of the body; if hyperthermia is present due to pyrogens, nervous system disease, or injury, the thermostatic function may be out of balance.

The pulse is an index of the heart's action, and by evaluating its rate, rhythm, and volume, one can gain an overall view of the heart's action.

Respiration, the act of bringing oxygen into the body and removing carbon dioxide, yields data on the entire breathing process of a patient. When the pattern of respiration is altered, on-going evaluation will yield important cues to a patient's changing condition.

Blood pressure readings provide information about the condition of the heart, the arteries and arterioles, vessel resistance, and the cardiac output. Serial readings provide the best indication of a patient's cardiac status.

## TEMPERATURE

Temperature control of the body is a homeostatic function, regulated by a complex mechanism involving the hypothalamus. The temperature of the body's interior (core temperature) is maintained within $\pm 1°F$ except in the case of febrile illness. The surface temperature of the skin and tissues immediately underlying the skin rises and falls with a change in temperature of the surrounding environment. Core temperature is maintained when heat production equals heat loss. The temperature regulating center in the hypothalamus keeps the core temperature constant. Temperature receptors, which determine if the body is too hot or too cold, feed into the hypothalamus. When the body becomes overheated, heat-sensitive neurons stimulate sweat glands to secrete fluid. This enhances heat loss through evaporation. The vasoconstrictor mechanism of the skin vessels is reduced, thereby conducting heat from the core of the body to the body surface. Heat loss occurs through radiation, evaporation, and conduction.

**Regulatory Mechanisms**    When the body core is cooled below 98.6° F (37° C), heat conservation is affected. Intense vasoconstriction of the skin vessels results. There is also piloerection and a decrease in sweating to conserve heat. Heat production is stimulated by shivering and increased cellular metabolism.

The "set point" is the critical temperature level to which the regulatory mechanisms attempt to maintain the body's core temperature. Above the set point, heat losing mechanisms are brought into play, and below that level heat conserving and producing mechanisms are set into action.

Disease can alter the set point of the temperature regulating center to cause fever, a body temperature above normal. Brain lesions, pyrogens from bacteria or viruses, or degenerating tissue (i.e., gangrenous areas or myocardial infarction) also increase the set point. Dehydration can cause fever due to lack of available fluid for perspiration and by increasing the set point, which brings more heat conserving and producing mechanisms into play. When the "thermostat" is suddenly set higher, the patient complains of feeling cold, has cool extremities, shivers, and has piloerection. Hypoxia can occur due to increased oxygen requirements with the increased metabolism of heat production. When the "thermostat" returns to normal, heat losing mechanisms again come into play. The patient feels hot and starts perspiring. Other symptoms of fever the patient may experience are: perspiration over body surface; body warm to the touch; flushed face; feeling cold alternately with feeling hot; increased pulse and respirations; malaise and fatigue; parched lips and dry skin; and convulsions, especially with children.

When body temperature falls below the normal range, the patient experiences hypothermia and complains of being cold, shivers, and has cool extremities. Hypothermia may be caused by accidental exposure, frostbite, or GI hemorrhage. Medically induced hypothermia is now used for some surgical interventions. The ability of the hypothalamus to regulate body temperature is greatly impaired when the body temperature falls below 94° F (34.4° C) and is lost below 85° F (29.4° C). Heat production by cells is also depressed by a low temperature.

**Measuring Body Temperature**    An accurate oral or rectal temperature records the core temperature. The normal range of an oral temperature is 97° to 99.5° F, or 36° to 37.5° C. Rectal temperatures are approximately 1° F higher. Temperature may vary according to age, (lower for the aged), time of day (lower in the morning and higher in the afternoon and evening), amount of exercise, or extremes in the environmental temperature.

The thermometer is the instrument used to measure body heat. Oral and rectal (also used for axillary temperature) thermometers are glass tubes containing mercury. When exposed to heat, the mercury expands, moves up the glass, and records the body temperature. The thermometer is marked in degrees and tenths of degrees and the range is 93° to 108° F (34° to 42.2° C).

Electronic thermometers, now widely used in hospitals, are more accurate than glass thermometers. In addition, they have disposable covers, which promotes infection control, and therefore should be used when available. The electronic thermometer plugs into a receptacle and has a heat sensor that records the patient's core temperature in only a few seconds.

Heat sensitive tapes are also used to record temperature. The tape is applied to the skin, and color changes indicate the temperature level. These tapes are both disposable and nonbreakable. They are most appropriate for use with normal newborns, small children, and in situations where proper cleaning of the thermometer is difficult.

**PULSE**    The pulse is an index of the heart's rate and rhythm. Pulse rate is the number of heart beats per minute. With each beat the heart's left ventricle contracts and forces blood into the aorta. This forceful ejection of blood produces a wave that is transmitted through the arteries to the periphery of the body. The pulse is a transient expansion of an artery resulting from internal pressure changes.

The pulse wave is influenced by the elasticity of the larger vessels, blood viscosity, and arteriolar and capillary resistance. Other characteristics of the pulse wave are size or amplitude, its type or contour, and its elasticity. Old age, with its arteriosclerotic changes in the blood vessels, speeds up the pulse wave velocity. The pulse wave changes in shape as it moves toward the periphery.

**Circulatory System Control**    The circulatory system is under the dual control of autoregulation and the autonomic nervous system. This dual control allows the circulatory system to vary blood flow to meet the body's requirements.

Local control of blood flow is called autoregulation. Blood flow is adjusted to the changing metabolic activity of different tissues. At constant levels of tissue metabolism, the flow is adjusted in response to changing arterial pressure. Tissues vary in their degree of autoregulation.

The autonomic nervous system regulates circulation through the vasomotor center in the medulla oblongata. Stimulation of this area causes vasoconstriction. This condition results in increased arterial blood pressure. Stimulation also increases heart rate and cardiac contractility. On the other hand, sympathetic inhibition causes vasodilation.

The baroreceptor reflex is another important circulatory control mechanism. Baroreceptors (pressoreceptors) are located in the walls of the carotid sinus and aortic arch. Increased blood pressure causes the baroreceptors to transmit signals to the medulla, which inhibits sympathetic action. The result is vasodilation and decreased blood pressure and heart rate. With a drop in blood pressure, the opposite occurs. The baroreceptors transmit signals to stimulate the vasomotor center, which causes vasoconstriction, and increased blood pressure and heart rate.

**Heart Rate and Rhythm**    The normal heart rate is from 60 to 80 beats per minute (BPM) in the resting adult, slightly faster in women than in men, and more rapid in children and infants (90 to 140 BPM). Older people usually have a slight increase in rate (70 to 80 BPM). Tachycardia is a pulse rate over 100 beats per minute. Bradycardia is a pulse rate below 60 beats per minute.

When taking the patient's pulse be aware that many pathological conditions produce a bradycardia. Among the most common causes are decreased thyroid activity, hyperkalemia, Stokes-Adams syndrome, and increased intracranial pressure.

Tachycardia is associated with stressful conditions, hypoxia, exercise, and fever. Patient conditions such as congestive heart failure, hemorrhage and shock, diarrhea and anemia produce a tachycardia as a compensatory response to poor tissue oxygenation.

Heart rhythm is the time interval between each heart beat. Rhythm varies according to the status of the patient. Normally, the heart rhythm is regular although slight irregularities do not necessarily indicate cardiac malfunction. An intermittent pulse occurs when the normal pattern of the pulse rate is broken; if recurrent, this irregular rhythm requires cardiac evaluation as it may be indicative of cardiac disease. A consistent irregular rhythm, or arrhythmia, is indicative of cardiac malfunction.

Variance in heart rate, either increased or decreased, may be attributed to many factors such as drug intake, lack of oxygen, loss of blood, exercise, and body temperature. When evaluating a pulse rate, it is important to ascertain the normal baseline for each patient and then to determine variances from the normal for that particular patient. The heart normally pumps about 5 liters of blood through the body each minute. This cardiac output is calculated by multiplying the heart rate per minute by the stroke volume, the amount of blood ejected with one contraction. Increasing the heart rate is one of the first compensatory mechanisms the body employs to maintain cardiac output.

**Evaluating Pulse Rate**    The quality of the pulse rate is determined by the amount of blood pumped through the arteries. Normally, the amount of pumped blood remains fairly constant; when it varies, it is also indicative of cardiac malfunction. A so-called bounding pulse occurs when the nurse is able to feel the pulse by exerting only a slight pressure over the artery. If, by exerting firm pressure, the nurse cannot clearly determine the flow, the pulse is called weak or thready.

Except for the body trunk, the arterial pulse can be felt over arteries that lie close to the body surface and over a bone or firm surface that can support the artery when pressure is applied. The radial artery is palpated most frequently since it is the most accessible. The femoral and carotid arteries are used in cases of cardiac arrest to determine the adequacy of perfusion. It is important to note characteristics of peripheral pulses: 0 = absent; 1+ =

weak; $2+$ = normal; and $3+$ = full and bounding. (Use the system described in your hospital procedure manual.)

When peripheral pulses cannot be palpated, a doppler is used by the nurse to confirm presence or absence of the pulse. Remember, the pulse is not always an accurate indication of the force of cardiac contractions. If cardiac contractions are weak or ventricular filling is incomplete, the pulse will be weak; however, in the case of aortic stenosis, the pulse may be weak in spite of forceful cardiac contraction.

The pulse should be taken frequently (every five to fifteen minutes to one to two hours) on an acutely ill hospitalized patient and less frequently (every four to eight hours) on more stable hospitalized patients. Once a week or even once a month is adequate for patients in long-term care facilities. Do not wait until the next routine schedule if the patient develops unexpected symptoms or has experienced a trauma.

## RESPIRATION

Respiration is the process of bringing oxygen to the body and removing carbon dioxide. The lungs play a major role in this process. Their function is to maintain arterial blood homeostasis by maintaining the pH of the blood. The lungs accomplish this by the process of breathing.

Breathing consists of two phases, inspiration and expiration. Inspiration is an active process in which the diaphragm descends, the external intercostal muscles contract, and the chest expands to allow air to move into the tracheo-bronchial tree. Expiration is a passive process in which air flows out of the respiratory tree.

The respiratory center in the medulla of the brain and the level of carbon dioxide in the blood both control the rate and depth of respiration. Peripheral receptors in the carotid body and the aortic arch also respond to the level of oxygen in the blood. To some extent, respiration can be voluntarily controlled by breath holding and hyperventilation. Talking, laughing, and crying also affect respiration.

The diaphragm and the intercostal muscles are the main muscles used for breathing. Other accessory muscles, such as the abdominal muscles, the sternocleidomastoid, the trapezius, and the scalene, can be used to assist with respiration if necessary.

**Evaluating Respiratory Rate**   The quality of breathing is important baseline information. Normal respiration is effortless, quiet, automatic, and regular. When the breathing pattern varies from normal, it needs to be evaluated thoroughly. For example, bronchial sounds heard over the large airways are fairly loud. There is normally a pause between inspiration and expiration. Softer sounds are heard over the other lung areas, and there are no pauses between inspiration and expiration. If breathing is noisy, labored, or strained, an obstruction may be affecting the breathing pattern that could lead to major alterations in homeostasis.

In addition to evaluating the breathing pattern, it is also necessary to evaluate the rate and depth of respiration. Normal respiratory rate for a resting adult is 12 to 18 breaths per minute. The respiratory rate for infants ranges from 24 to 30 breaths per minute and is often irregular. Older children average about 20 to 26. The ratio of pulse to respiration is usually 5:1 and remains fairly constant.

The depth of a person's respiration is the volume of air that moves in and out with each breath. The tidal volume is 500 cc in the healthy adult.

Alveolar air is only partially replenished by atmosphere air with each inspiratory phase. Approximately 350 cc (tidal volume minus dead space) of new air is exchanged with the functional residual capacity volume during each respiratory cycle. Accurate tidal volume can be measured by a spirometer, but a nurse can judge the approximate depth by placing the back of the hand next to the patient's nose and mouth and feeling the expired air. Another method of estimating volume capacity is to observe chest expansion and to check both sides of the thorax for symmetrical movement.

After assessing the pattern, type, and depth of respirations, it is important to observe the physical characteristics of chest expansion. The chest normally expands symmetrically without rib flaring or retractions. In addition, observation of chest deformities should also be made, as all of these signs yield information about the respiratory process and overall health status of the patient.

## BLOOD PRESSURE

The heart generates pressure during the cardiac cycle to perfuse the organs of the body with blood. Blood flows from the heart to the arteries, into the capillaries and veins, and then flows back to the heart. Blood pressure in the arterial system varies with the cardiac cycle, reaching the highest level at the peak of systole and the lowest level at the end of diastole. The difference between the systolic and diastolic blood pressure is the pulse pressure, which is normally 30 to 50 mm Hg.

There are seven major factors that affect blood pressure.

*Cardiac Output*  The force of heart contractions and the amount of blood ejected by the heart in one minute influences blood pressure, especially systolic pressure.

*Peripheral Vascular Resistance*  Resistance to the flow of blood is due to resistant vessels under the influence of the autonomic nervous system. Peripheral vascular resistance is the most important factor in diastolic pressure.

*Elasticity and Distensibility of the Arteries*  Elasticity refers to ability of the blood vessel walls to spring back after blood is ejected into them. When blood is ejected into the aorta and large arteries, the arterial vessel walls distend. Recoil during diastole propels blood through the arterial tree and maintains diastolic pressure. Distensibility decreases with age, resulting in decreased diastolic pressure and increased systolic pressure. Arteriosclerosis is an example of a condition that will increase blood pressure.

*Blood Volume*  Increased blood volume causes an increase in both systolic and diastolic blood pressure whereas decreased blood volume causes the reverse effect. Hemorrhage will decrease blood pressure while over-hydration or excessive blood transfusions cause an increase in blood pressure.

*Blood Viscosity*  Blood viscosity influences blood flow velocity through the arterial tree. For example, increased viscosity, which occurs with polycythemia, increases resistance to blood flow whereas decreased viscosity, resulting from anemia, decreases resistance.

*Hormones and Enzymes*  These substances have an important influence on blood pressure. For example, epinephrine and norepinephrine produce a profound vasoconstrictor effect on peripheral blood vessels. Other substances, such as aldosterone (released by the adrenal cortex), renin (released by the juxtaglomerular apparatus of the kidney), and histamine all produce effects that raise or lower the blood pressure.

*Chemoreceptors*   Chemoreceptors in the aortic arch and carotid sinus also exert control over the blood pressure. They are sensitive to changes in $PaO_2$, $PaCO_2$, and pH. Decreased $PaO_2$ stimulates the chemoreceptors, which stimulate the vasomotor center. Increased $PaCO_2$ and decreased pH directly stimulate the vasomotor center, causing increased peripheral vascular resistance.

**Measuring Blood Pressure**   Measuring arterial blood pressure provides important information about the overall health status of the patient. For example, the systolic pressure provides a data base about the condition of the heart, arteries, and the arterioles. The diastolic pressure indicates vessel resistance. The pulse pressure, the difference between the systolic and diastolic pressure, provides information about cardiac output. A single blood pressure reading, however, does not provide adequate data from which conclusions can be drawn about all of these factors. Rather, a series of blood pressure readings should be taken to establish a baseline for further evaluation.

**TABLE 1**   VITAL SIGN CHART FOR CHILDREN

| AGE | NORMAL PULSE RANGE | NORMAL PULSE AVERAGE | BLOOD PRESSURE AVERAGE | RESPIRATION AVERAGE |
|---|---|---|---|---|
| Newborn | 70 – 170 | 120 | 80/45 | 40 – 90 |
| 1 year | 80 – 160 | 115 | 90/60 | 20 – 40 |
| 2 years | 80 – 130 | 110 | 95/60 | 20 – 30 |
| 4 years | 80 – 120 | 100 | 99/65 | 20 – 25 |
| 6 years | 75 – 115 | 100 | 100/56 | 20 – 25 |
| 8 years | 70 – 110 | 90 | 105/56 | 15 – 20 |
| 10 years | 70 – 110 | 90 | 110/58 | 15 – 20 |

The *indirect method* of taking a blood pressure using a sphygmomanometer and a stethoscope is accurate for most patients. New electronic blood pressure devices constantly monitor systolic, diastolic and mean readings in pre-set time intervals. These devices also provide a print-out if needed for documentation. If a stethoscope is unavailable or the brachial artery amplitude is decreased, the brachial or radial artery can be palpated with the blood pressure cuff inflated, to determine the systolic blood pressure. Those who are severely hypotensive or hypertensive, have low blood volume, or are on vasoconstrictor or vasodilator drugs should have blood pressure measured by the direct method. The *direct method* is continuous and measures mean pressures. A needle or catheter is inserted into the brachial, radial, or femoral artery. An oscilloscope displays arterial pressure waveforms.

Normal blood pressure in an adult varies between 100 to 140 mm Hg systolic and 60 to 90 mm Hg diastolic. As blood moves toward smaller arteries and into arterioles, where it enters the capillaries, pressure falls to 35 mm Hg. It continues to fall as blood goes through the capillaries, where the flow is steady and not pulsatile. As blood moves into the venous system, pressure falls until it is the lowest in the venae cavae.

Blood pressure varies widely. A blood pressure of 100/60 mm Hg may be normal for one person but may be hypotensive for another. Hypotension (90 to 100 mm Hg systolic) in a healthy adult without other clinical symptoms is little reason for concern.

Blood pressure readings are recorded in association with Korotkoff sounds. The systolic or first reading occurs with the advent of the first Korotkoff sound. The diastolic or second reading is when the Korotkoff sound changes to a more muffled sound. In some patients the sound disappears totally and this is recorded as a third reading, e.g., 120/84/52.

Routinely, the blood pressure for an acutely ill patient should be taken every 15 minutes to one to two hours and the blood pressure of more stabilized patients should be taken every four to eight hours to once a day. Patients with severe hypotension or hypertension, with low blood volume, or on vasoconstrictor or vasodilator drugs require checking every 5 to 15 minutes.

## NURSING DIAGNOSES

The following nursing diagnoses are appropriate to utilize on Patient Care Plans when the components are related to vital signs.

| Nursing Diagnosis (Potential) | Defining Characteristic; Etiology (Examples) |
|---|---|
| □ Cardiac Output, Alteration in, *related to* | Low blood pressure, rapid pulse, changes in breathing patterns, e.g., hemorrhage. |
| | Cardiac arrhythmias, e.g., hypoxia, electrolyte imbalance. |
| □ Tissue Perfusion, Alteration in, *related to* | Low blood pressure, e.g., disease state, hemorrhage, drug reactions. |

## UNIT ONE    TEMPERATURE

### NURSING PROCESS DATA

**ASSESSMENT**    *Data Base*

Determine the method most appropriate for obtaining temperature.

*Oral method*

- □ Accurate method of determining body temperature.
- □ Used only for alert and cooperative patients.
- □ Not appropriate for use with patients requiring nasogastric, nasal, or oral intubation.

*Rectal method*

- □ Appropriate for uncooperative, confused, or comatose patients or for patients on seizure precautions.
- □ Used for patients receiving oxygen or with nasal or oral intubation.

□ Appropriate for patients with wired jaws, facial fractures, or other abnormalities, or for patients with nasogastric tubes.

□ Contraindicated for patients who have had abdominal perineal resection, hemorrhoidectomy, and some cardiac patients.

*Axillary method*

□ Not accurate for adults.

□ Used with infants in a controlled environment.

□ Used in recovery rooms to avoid turning patients.

*Electronic thermometer*

□ Most accurate.

□ Prevents infection between patients.

□ Use when available

Determine number of times temperature needs to be taken daily.

Assess temperature in relationship to time of day and age of patient.

Compare temperature with other vital signs to establish baseline data.

## PLANNING  *Objectives*

To determine if core temperature is within normal range.

To provide baseline data for further evaluation.

To determine alterations in disease conditions.

## IMPLEMENTATION  *Procedures*

Taking an Oral Temperature

Using a Chemical Strip Tape

Taking a Rectal Temperature

Taking an Axillary Temperature

Using an Electronic Thermometer

## EVALUATION  *Expected Outcomes*

Temperature is within normal range.

Temperature readings are compared with age, time of day, and previous readings.

Alterations in temperature are detected early and treatment begun.

Appropriate method of temperature taking is determined for each patient.

Correct length of time is used for thermometer insertion to obtain an accurate reading.

## TAKING AN ORAL TEMPERATURE

### Equipment

Oral glass mercury thermometer

Tissues

### Procedure

1. Wash your hands.
2. Rinse thermometer in cold water if kept in a chemical solution, and wipe dry with tissue. **Rationale:** Chemical taste is bitter.
3. Grasp thermometer with thumb and forefinger and shake vigorously by flicking wrist in downward motion to lower mercury level to below 95–96°.
4. Check temperature reading on thermometer.
5. Explain procedure to patient.
6. Place thermometer in patient's mouth under tongue and ask patient to hold lips closed.
7. Leave in place 3 to 5 minutes.
8. Remove thermometer and wipe it with tissue from fingers down to bulb. Discard tissue.
9. Read temperature by rotating thermometer until the mercury level is clearly visible. Shake thermometer down and replace in bedside container.
10. Wash hands.
11. Record patient's temperature according to hospital procedure.

## USING A CHEMICAL STRIP TAPE

### Equipment

Temperature tape

Soft cloth

### Preparation

1. Obtain temperature tape from central supply.
2. Use tape indoors at room temperature and out of direct sunlight.
3. Do not use temperature tape if the patient has been eating, drinking or exercising within the last thirty minutes.
4. Check orders or Patient Care Plan that this method is appropriate for patient.
5. Explain procedure to patient.

### Procedure

1. Position patient comfortably with head slightly reclined. **Rationale:** This position facilitates getting an accurate temperature reading.
2. Grasp temperature tape firmly at both ends and press flush against a dry forehead.
3. Leave in place at least 15 seconds.
4. Read temperature while it is still on patient's forehead.
5. Read temperature as follows:
   a. The black demarcations that are numbered will change color according to the patient's temperature.
   b. Green will appear over the correct temperature.
   c. If the center portion (between the black stripes) turns blue and tan, the temperature is half–way between the two numbered stripes.
6. Remove strip from patient's forehead and clean with a soft cloth.

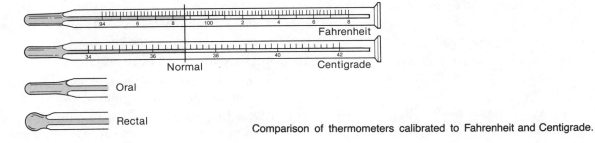

Comparison of thermometers calibrated to Fahrenheit and Centigrade.

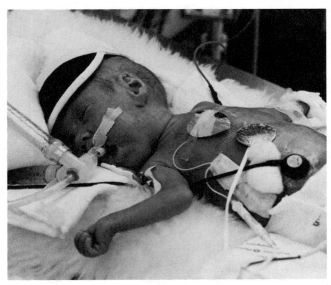

Thermister probe is another electronic device used to monitor the temperature of critically ill infants.

7. Store at patient's bedside in its protective case.

8. Reposition patient for comfort.

9. Document temperature reading in appropriate record.

## TAKING A RECTAL TEMPERATURE

### Equipment

Rectal glass mercury thermometer

Tissues

Lubricant on a paper wipe for rectal method

### Procedure

1. Wash your hands.

2. Rinse thermometer in cold water if kept in a chemical solution, and wipe dry with tissue.

3. Grasp thermometer with thumb and forefinger and shake vigorously, flicking wrist in downward motion, to lower mercury level.

4. Check temperature reading on thermometer—below 95–96°.

5. Explain procedure to patient.

6. Provide privacy; instruct and assist patient to turn on side facing away from you with knees slightly flexed.

7. Lubricate tip of thermometer with lubricant on a paper tissue.

8. Fold back bed linen to expose patient's buttocks.

9. Separate buttocks with one hand so anal sphincter opening is visible.

10. Insert thermometer into rectum approximately ½ to 1½ inches depending on the age of the patient.

11. Leave in place three to five minutes. **Rationale:** Hold in place if patient expels thermometer or is restless, for a thermometer requires at least three minutes to register temperature correctly.

12. Remove thermometer and wipe it with tissue from fingers down to bulb. Discard tissue in toilet.

13. Read temperature by rotating thermometer until the mercury level is clearly visible. Shake thermometer down.

14. Assist patient to a comfortable position.

15. Wash thermometer in warm, soapy water, rinse, and put away.

16. Wash your hands.

17. Record patient's temperature according to hospital procedure.

## TAKING AN AXILLARY TEMPERATURE

### Equipment

Glass mercury thermometer (preferably oral type)

Tissues

### Procedure

1. Wash your hands.

2. Rinse thermometer in cold water if kept in a chemical solution, and wipe dry with tissue.

3. Grasp thermometer with thumb and forefinger and shake vigorously, flicking wrist in downward motion, to lower mercury level.

4. Check temperature reading on thermometer—below 95–96°.

5. Explain procedure to patient. Provide privacy.

6. Assist patient to a comfortable position and expose axilla.

7. Place thermometer in axilla and lower patient's arm down across the chest.

8. Leave in place 8 to 10 minutes.

9. Remove thermometer and wipe it with tissue from fingers down to bulb. Discard tissue.

10. Read temperature by rotating thermometer until the mercury level is clearly visible, shake down, and replace in bedside container.

11. Assist patient to a comfortable position.

12. Wash your hands.

13. Record patient's temperature according to hospital procedure.

## USING AN ELECTRONIC THERMOMETER

### Equipment

Electronic thermometer unit with digital probe

Cover for thermometer

### Procedure

1. Remove thermometer from charger unit.

2. Place carrying strap around your neck.

3. Grasp probe at the top of the stem using your thumb and forefinger. Do not put pressure on the top because it is the ejection button.

4. Firmly insert probe into disposable probe cover.

5. Provide privacy if necessary.

*for Oral Temperature*

☐ Slide probe under front of patient's tongue and along the gum line to the sublingual pocket at the base of the tongue. **Rationale:** The larger blood vessels in the pocket are more reflective of the core temperature.

☐ Instruct patient to close lips. Lips should close at the ridge on the probe cover.

*for Rectal Temperature*

☐ Position patient on side facing away from you, separate buttocks, and insert probe 1½ in. through anal sphincter.

☐ Position probe to the side of the rectum to ensure contact with the tissue wall.

6. Remove probe when audible signal occurs. Patient's temperature is now registered on the dial.

7. Discard oral probe cover into trash by pushing ejection button. Discard rectal probe cover and tissue in bathroom.

8. Record temperature and then return probe to storage well.

9. Return thermometer unit to charging base. Ensure charging base is plugged into electrical outlet.

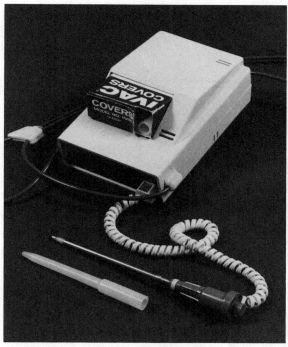

Place individual cover over temperature probe of electronic thermometer before taking patient's temperature.

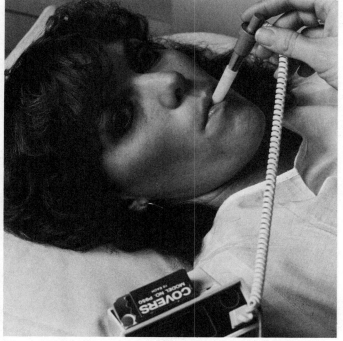

Slide probe under front of patient's tongue and along gum line to sublingual pocket.

**CHARTING** *for Temperature*

☐ Method used

☐ Temperature recorded on temp sheet and graph

☐ Nursing interventions used for alterations in temperature

☐ Condition of skin related to alterations from normothermia

☐ Signs and symptoms associated with alterations in temperature

---

## CLINICAL PROBLEM SOLVING

### Potential Problems

Fever develops.

Despite initial cooling measure, temperature remains elevated because of destruction of hypothalamus from brain disease or injury.

Temperature remains elevated because of bacterial produced pyrogens.

### Suggested Solutions

☐ Check possible sources of infection, and take preventative measures.

☐ Employ cooling methods if temperature is dangerously high, such as tepid sponge bath, ice packs, or alcohol sponge bath.

☐ Notify physician and request cooling blanket.

☐ Monitor temperature every 15 to 30 minutes.

☐ Continue to administer antipyretic drugs as ordered.

☐ Check for order to obtain culture of possible sources of infection.

☐ Give antipyretic drugs as ordered.

☐ Decrease room temperature and remove excess covers.

☐ Give tepid sponge bath.

---

## UNIT TWO   PULSE RATE

### NURSING PROCESS DATA

#### ASSESSMENT  *Data Base*

Assess appropriate site to obtain pulse.

Check pulse with health status changes.

Assess for rate, rhythm, pattern, and volume.

Take an apical pulse on patients with irregular rhythms or those on heart medications.

Obtain baseline peripheral pulses in any patient going for cardiac or vascular surgery or medical patients with diabetes, arterial occlusive diseases such as Raynaud's or Buerger's disease, atherosclerosis, or aneurysm.

Take an apical-radial pulse when deficits occur between apical and radial measurements.

Assess the need to monitor pulses with an electronic device.

**PLANNING** *Objectives*

To determine if the pulse rate is within normal range and if the rhythm is regular.

To evaluate the equality of corresponding arterial pulses.

To determine presence of peripheral pulses when palpation is ineffective.

To monitor and evaluate changes in the patient's health status.

To determine apical pulse rate before heart medications are administered.

**IMPLEMENTATION** *Procedures*

Taking a Radial Pulse

Taking an Apical Pulse

Taking an Apical-Radial Pulse

Taking a Peripheral Pulse

Monitoring Peripheral Pulses with the Doppler Ultrasound Stethoscope

**EVALUATION** *Expected Outcomes*

Pulse is palpated without difficulty.

Pulse rate is within normal range and rhythm is regular.

All peripheral pulses are equal in amplitude when compared to the corresponding pulse on the other side and when compared to the next proximal site.

Apical pulse is easily detected and counted.

## TAKING A RADIAL PULSE

### Equipment

Watch with sweep second hand

### Procedure

1. Wash your hands.
2. Place patient in comfortable position.
3. Ask about activity level within last half hour. **Rationale:** Pulse rate increases with activity.
4. Palpate arteries by using pads of the middle three fingers of your hand.
   a. Radial artery is usually used as it lies just under the skin of the inner surface of the wrist directly over the radius.
   b. Press the artery against the bone or underlying firm surface to occlude vessel and then gradually release pressure.

5. If rhythm is regular, count pulse for 30 seconds and multiply by two to obtain pulse rate.
6. If rhythm is irregular, take an apical pulse for at least one minute or longer if difficult to count. **Rationale:** It may take a minute or so to detect the irregularity and allow you to count the pulse accurately.
7. Check to see that patient is comfortable.
8. Wash your hands.
9. Record pulse rate, rhythm, pattern, and volume.

## TAKING AN APICAL PULSE

### Equipment

Watch with sweep second hand
Stethoscope

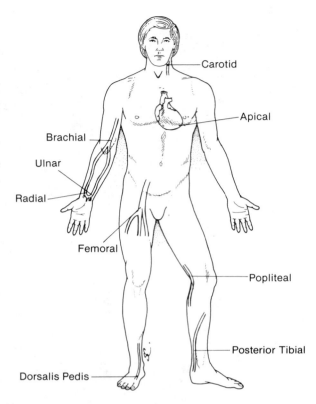

Radial artery is most commonly used site for determining pulse rate.

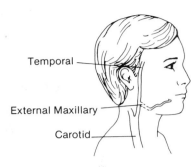

Carotid artery is used when other sites are inaccessible.

### Procedure

1. Gather equipment.
2. Wash your hands.
3. Check patient's identaband. Provide privacy.
4. Place patient in a supine or left-sided position.
5. Take patient's apical pulse.
   a. Place a stethoscope over the apex of the heart. The apex is normally located in the fifth intercostal space left of the sternum in the midclavicular line.
   b. Count the rate for one minute when taking an apical pulse.
   c. Determine if there is a pattern to the irregularity or if it is chaotically irregular. **Rationale:** The more chaotically irregular the pulse, the more dangerous the condition.
   d. Auscultate the apical pulse and palpate the radial pulse simultaneously to note a pulse deficit when the rhythm is irregular. **Rationale:** Atrial irregularities generally produce pulse deficits. Ventricular irregularities, however, usually have the same rhythm at both apical and radial areas.
   e. Assess pulse volume by feeling the pressure of the beat.
6. Check to see that patient is comfortable.
7. Wash your hands.
8. Record pulse rate, rhythm, pattern, and volume.

## TAKING AN APICAL-RADIAL PULSE

### Equipment

Watch with sweep second hand

Stethoscope

Note: If nurse is inexperienced, she should have another nurse help with procedure.

### Procedure

1. Gather equipment.
2. Wash your hands.
3. Identify patient by checking identaband.
4. Provide privacy.
5. Explain the procedure to the patient especially if two nurses are taking the pulse. **Rationale:** Patients may be apprehensive if two nurses are at the bedside at the same time, so a full explanation will help to allay fears.
6. Locate the radial pulse. The second nurse locates the apical pulse, the fifth intercostal space, the midclavicular line, and places stethoscope.
7. With your hand, signal to the other nurse when to start taking the pulse and when to stop. Both nurses simultaneously count the pulse for one full minute.

8. Position the patient for comfort.

9. Wash your hands.

10. Subtract the radial rate from the apical rate to obtain the pulse deficit.

11. Chart the apical, radial rate and pulse deficit.

## TAKING A PERIPHERAL PULSE

### Equipment

Felt tip pen

Stethoscope

### Procedure

1. Gather equipment.

2. Wash your hands.

3. Check patient's identaband.

4. Provide privacy. Explain procedure.

5. Place patient in a reclining position with the trunk of the body at a 30-degree angle.

6. Palpate peripheral pulses: radial, brachial, femoral, popliteal, dorsalis pedis, posterior tibial.
   a. For special cases, after carotid surgery, palpate temporal pulse also.
   b. With stethoscope, listen for a bruit (a whooshing sound as blood goes through a stenotic vessel).

7. Palpate pulse sites bilaterally by using pads of the middle three fingers of your hand.

8. Press the artery against the bone or underlying firm surface to occlude vessel and then gradually release pressure.

9. Assess if bilateral pulses are equal in rate, rhythm, and amplitude.
   a. If pulse is not immediately palpable, examine adjacent area. **Rationale:** This action identifies where interruption or alteration in circulation occurs in extremity.
   b. Since pulse locations differ with patients, mark pulse locations with felt tip pen, especially those that are difficult to palpate. **Rationale:** Marking allows the next nurse to find location without spending extra time.
   c. Compare presence and characteristics of peripheral pulses with previous findings. **Rationale:** This action allows early identification of alterations in circulation.

10. Palpate weak pulses gently so that you do not obliterate pulse with too much pressure.

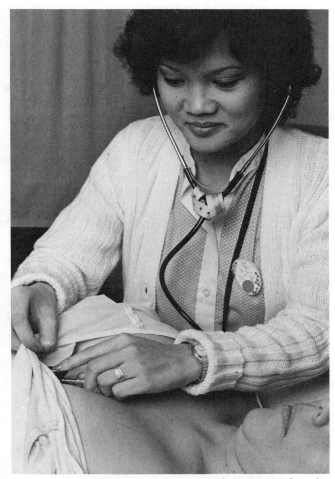

Count apical pulse for one full minute to obtain accurate pulse rate.

11. Check to see that patient is comfortable.

12. Wash your hands.

13. Record pulse rate, rhythm, pattern, and volume.

## MONITORING PERIPHERAL PULSES WITH THE DOPPLER ULTRASOUND STETHOSCOPE

### Equipment

Doppler stethoscope

Conductive jelly (not K-Y)

### Procedure

1. Gather equipment.

2. Wash your hands.

3. Explain procedure to patient.

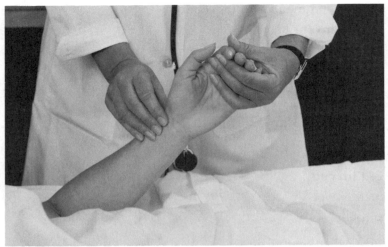

Palpate radial pulse by using tips of fingers, not thumb for accurate results.

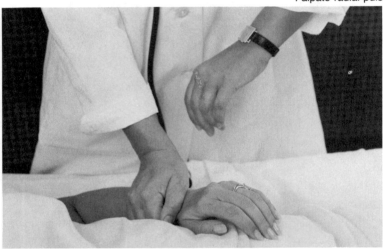

Count pulse beats for at least 30 seconds and multiply by two for rate.

4. Provide privacy.

5. Uncover extremity to be assessed.

6. Place extremity in a comfortable position.

7. Plug headset (stethoscope) into one of the two outlet jacks located next to the volume control.

8. Apply conductive gel to patient's skin. **Rationale:** The ultrasound beam travels best through gel and requires an airtight seal between the probe and the skin.

9. Hold probe (at tapered end of plastic core) against skin at a 45-degree angle to the blood vessel being examined.

10. Turn on Doppler by pressing down the "ON".

11. If pulse is not detected, move the probe over the site keeping it in direct contact with skin and adjust the volume to detect blood flow.

12. If pulse is still not detected, reapply new gel and, with light pressure, place probe over site and turn switch on. Increase volume control or check if batteries are weak.

13. Clean gel from skin and probe and replace cover over extremity.

14. Position patient for comfort.

15. Replace Doppler to appropriate place.

16. Wash your hands.

17. Document pulse findings.

**CHARTING** *for Taking a Pulse*

☐ Type of pulse taken

☐ Rate and rhythm of pulse

☐ Pulse volume

☐ Pulse deficit if any present

☐ Characteristics of all peripheral pulses—use rating scale

☐ Use of Doppler if needed

☐ Effects of nursing or medical treatments on abnormal pulse rates or rhythms

---

## CLINICAL PROBLEM SOLVING

**Potential Problems**

Apical, femoral, and carotid pulse is absent.

**Suggested Solutions**

☐ Immediately repeat procedure to validate findings and call a Code.

☐ Initiate CPR immediately and continue to assess the femoral or carotid pulse during resuscitation.

☐ For absent femoral pulse, assess for systemic circulation and presence of disorders affecting circulation to extremities.

☐ Use Doppler to assess for presence of pulse.

Irregular heart beats are present.

**Tachycardia** (pulse rate over 100 BPM in adults or 140 in children):

☐ Relieve anxiety, fear, or stress through communication and pertinent information.

☐ If patient has pain, relieve with change of position, back rub, and analgesic.

☐ Decrease heart rate by reducing an elevated temperature to normal.

☐ Take vital signs every 15 minutes to 2 hours until condition stabilizes and pulse rate is within normal limits.

☐ Obtain order and administer oxygen if patient is restless and/or agitated.

**Bradycardia** (pulse rate less than 60 in adults or less than 70 in children):

☐ Notify physician for electrocardiogram request to determine if heart block is present.

☐ If patient is on digitalis, hold the drug and notify the physician.

☐ Have atropine and temporary pacemaker available for physician if pulse is consistently slow (less than 50).

☐ Continue monitoring pulse rate every 15 minutes to 2 hours until pulse is within normal limits.

**Ectopic Beats** (premature or atrial fibrillation):

☐ Relieve pain if irregularity is due to premature beats associated with pain.

☐ Administer oxygen if patient has an order to do so.

☐ If associated with stimuli from noise, visitors, caffeinated beverages, or smoking, eliminate the cause of the stimulation.

☐ Notify physician to request a medical order for an electrocardiogram since premature beats in a patient with myocardial infarction may be potentially harmful.

□ Obtain order from physician to draw serum electrolytes, especially potassium. Low potassium levels can cause premature ventricular contractions.

□ Continue monitoring pulse rate every 15 minutes to 2 hours until irregularity is controlled.

Doppler unable to detect sounds.

□ Check that K-Y jelly is not used as salt can damage the probe.

□ Check that batteries are less than six months old. The date should be placed on all batteries.

□ Use alkaline batteries, as they last longer.

Patient is in isolation and requires vascular assessment.

□ Clean with gas sterilization after discontinuing use of Doppler.

□ Do not clean with alcohol or autoclave.

# UNIT THREE  RESPIRATIONS

## NURSING PROCESS DATA

### ASSESSMENT  *Data Base*

Assess patient's respiratory rate, depth, and position.

Evaluate any abnormalities noted during inspection and palpation or by percussion and auscultation.

Assess presence of dyspnea or cyanosis.

Assess for presence of abnormal sounds such as stertorous or sonorous breathing.

Assess if accessory muscles are used for breathing.

### PLANNING  *Objectives*

To note respiratory rate, rhythm, and depth.

To establish baseline information upon admission to the unit.

To note labored, difficult, or noisy respirations or cyanosis.

To identify alterations in respiratory pattern resulting from disease condition.

To compare if respiratory rate is within normal range with pulse and blood pressure readings.

### IMPLEMENTATION  *Procedure*

Obtaining the Respiratory Rate

### EVALUATION  *Expected Outcomes*

Regular rate of breathing and symmetrical respiratory excursion is established.

Patient exhibits quiet, effortless breathing.

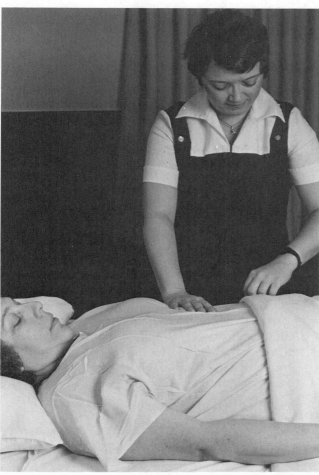

Place hand on chest when respirations are difficult to count.

BREATHING PATTERNS

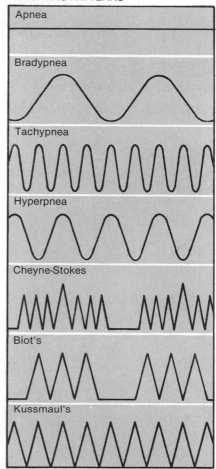

Examples of abnormal respiratory wave patterns.

## OBTAINING THE RESPIRATORY RATE

### Equipment

Watch with a second hand

### Procedure

1. Wash your hands.
2. Explain procedure to patient.
3. Check lighting to ensure it is adequate for procedure.
4. Maintain patient's privacy.
5. Place hand on chest or observe chest rise and fall and count respirations.
6. Count respirations for 30 seconds and multiply by two.
7. Observe respiratory pattern and depth of respirations.
8. Wash your hands.
9. Compare respiratory rate with previous recordings.
10. Record respiratory rate. Record if rhythm and/or depth altered from normal.

### CHARTING *for Respirations*

☐ Rate and rhythm of respirations

☐ Abnormal sounds associated with breathing

☐ Effectiveness of therapy if needed to correct respiratory problems

☐ Alterations from baseline respiratory patterns

## CLINICAL PROBLEM SOLVING

| Potential Problems | Suggested Solutions |
|---|---|

**Potential Problems**

**Suggested Solutions**

Apnea (absence of breathing) occurs.

☐ Begin artificial ventilation by mouth to mouth, mouth to nose, or other airway adjunct method at the rate of 12 per minute for an adult or 20 per minute for a child.
☐ Summon help immediately.

Tachypnea (rate faster than normal and more shallow) occurs.

☐ Relieve anxiety, fear, and stress through communication and pertinent information.
☐ Relieve fever if that is the cause.
☐ Correct respiratory insufficiency with low-flow oxygen administration, good pulmonary toilet, and deep breathing and coughing exercises.

Bradypnea (rate slower than normal) occurs.

☐ If due to respiratory depressant drugs, such as opiates, barbiturates, and tranquilizers, be prepared to assist respirations or administer mouth-to-mouth resuscitation.
☐ Administer oxygen at 6 l/min via nasal cannulae as ordered. If patient has COPD use 2 l/min.
☐ Stimulate patient to take breaths at least ten times per minute.

Hyperpnea or hyperventilation (increased rate and depth of respiration) occurs.

☐ Rest after period of exertion.
☐ Relieve fear, anxiety, or stress.
☐ Relieve fever.
☐ Encourage patient to decrease breathing rate by taking slow, deep breaths.

Hypoventilation (shallow and slow or irregular respirations) occurs.

☐ Encourage turning, coughing, and deep breathing exercises.

Cheyne-Stokes respirations (respiratory cycle in which respirations increase in rate and depth, then decrease, followed by a period of apnea) occurs.

☐ Follow physician's orders to treat underlying disease state.
☐ Monitor respirations every 15 minutes to hourly, depending on patient's status.
☐ Be prepared to administer CPR if apnea occurs.
☐ One of the indicators that death is approaching.

# UNIT FOUR   BLOOD PRESSURE

## NURSING PROCESS DATA

### ASSESSMENT   *Data Base*

Assess blood pressure initially and whenever patient's status changes.

Assess the three changes in sound during a blood pressure reading.

Assess presence of factors which can alter blood pressure readings.

Assess size of cuff needed for accurate reading.

Note any changes from prior assessments.

## PLANNING *Objectives*

To determine if arterial blood pressure reading is within normal range for the individual patient.

To assess condition of heart, arteries, blood vessel resistance, and stroke volume.

To establish a baseline for further evaluation.

To identify alterations in blood pressure resulting from a change in disease condition.

To compare blood pressure readings with pulse and respirations.

## IMPLEMENTATION *Procedures*

Taking a Blood Pressure

Palpating Brachial Systolic Arterial Blood Pressure

Taking a Flush Blood Pressure

Using a Continuous Noninvasive Monitoring Device

## EVALUATION *Expected Outcomes*

Blood pressure is within normal range (100/60 to 140/90 mm Hg).

Alterations in blood pressure are identified early and appropriate treatment initiated.

Severely altered blood pressure readings are rechecked with a different blood pressure cuff.

## TAKING A BLOOD PRESSURE

### Equipment

Sphygmomanometer with proper sized cuff (12 to 14 cm wide) for average adult arm; narrower cuffs for infants, children, and adults with thin arms; wider cuffs (18 to 20 cm) for patients with obese arms and for leg pressure readings

Stethoscope

### Procedure

1. Gather equipment. Be sure the cuff is an appropriate size for the patient. **Rationale:** If cuff is not an appropriate size for the patient, the reading will not be accurate.

2. Wash your hands.

3. Check identaband.

4. Explain procedure to patient.

5. Place patient in a relaxed reclining or sitting position with arm at heart level. Expose upper part of patient's arm. **Rationale:** If arm is above level of heart the blood pressure reading will be lower than normal.

6. Wrap cuff snugly and smoothly around the upper part of the arm (about 1 inch above antecubital space) with the center of the bladder over the brachial artery.

7. Palpate brachial artery with fingertips.

8. Place diaphragm or bell of stethoscope on the medial antecubital fossa where brachial artery is felt.

9. Place stethoscope ear pieces in ear.

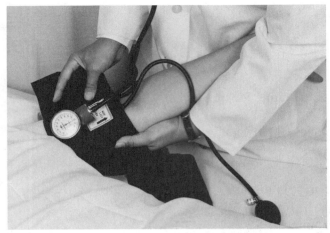

Step 1: Place patient in a reclined position with arm at heart level.

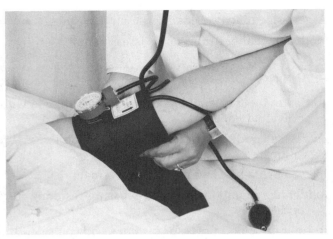

Step 2: Wrap blood pressure cuff snugly around upper arm.

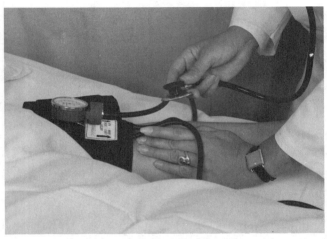

Step 3: Place bell of stethoscope where brachial artery is palpated.

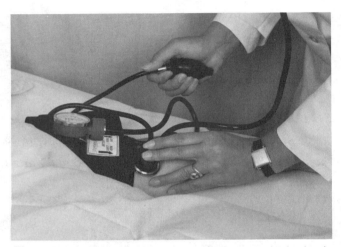

Step 4: Close valve and inflate cuff 30mm Hg above pulsation level.

10. Close valve on manometer pump.

11. Inflate cuff 30 mm Hg above level at which pulsations are no longer heard.

12. To avoid distortion, read pressure with mercury at eye level when using manometer tube filled with mercury.

13. Gradually deflate cuff by opening valve on pump (2 mm Hg per second) until the first Korotkoff's sound is heard. This is the systolic pressure.

14. Continue to deflate cuff (sounds will change in quality), continue to release pressure gradually, 2–3 mm Hg per second. Do not re-pump without letting cuff totally deflate.

15. Note when Korotkoff's sound begins to get muffled and when it disappears completely. **Ration-ale:** The first diastolic pressure occurs when the sound is muffled. The second diastolic pressure occurs when the Korotkoff's sound disappears.

16. Do not leave the cuff inflated for a prolonged period since this produces patient discomfort.

17. Completely deflate cuff before rechecking the blood pressure.

18. Remove cuff from patient's arm.

19. Check to see that patient is comfortable.

20. Compare blood pressure reading with previous recordings.

21. Wash your hands.

22. Record blood pressure and, if appropriate, blood pressure site.

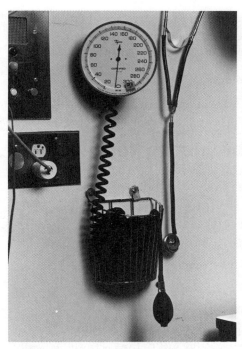

Example of wall-mounted cuneroid manometer.

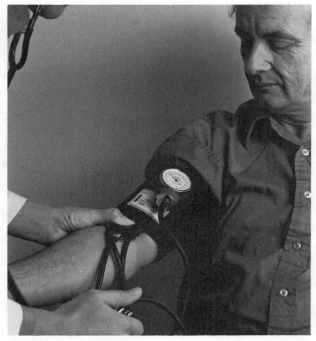

Stabilize patient's elbow with hand while taking blood pressure.

---

**Clinical Alert**

The American Heart Association recommends that all three blood pressure readings be recorded: systolic, and first and second diastolic sounds.

---

## PALPATING BRACHIAL SYSTOLIC ARTERIAL BLOOD PRESSURE

### Equipment

Sphygmomanometer with proper sized cuff

### Procedure

1. Gather equipment. Be sure the cuff is an appropriate size for the patient.
2. Wash your hands.
3. Check name and identaband.
4. Explain procedure to patient.
5. Place patient in a relaxed reclining or sitting position for 5 to 10 minutes with arm at heart level. Expose upper part of patient's arm.
6. Wrap cuff snugly and smoothly around the upper part of the arm (about 1 inch above antecu-

bital space) with the center of the bladder over the brachial artery.

7. Assess blood pressure using stethoscope. If unable to hear Korotkoff's sound, palpate for blood pressure reading.
8. Palpate brachial artery as if taking a pulse. Do not release finger pressure.
9. Inflate cuff to 30 mm Hg above last palpated pulse beat.
10. Release pressure from cuff slowly, no more than 2–3 mm Hg per second. First palpated beat is systolic pressure. Should be the same as last felt beat when inflating cuff.
11. Return equipment.
12. Wash your hands.
13. Record systolic blood pressure reading as "palpated."

## TAKING A FLUSH BLOOD PRESSURE

### Equipment

Sphygmomanometer with proper sized blood pressure cuff

Elastic bandage

## Procedure

1. Wash your hands.

2. Gather equipment.

3. Check name and patient's identaband.

4. Explain procedure to patient.

5. Place blood pressure cuff 1 to 2 inches above antecubital or popliteal space.

6. Hold extremity above level of heart.

7. Wrap elastic bandage from fingers or toes up to the blood pressure cuff. **Rationale:** Bandage application empties the capillaries and veins.

8. Keeping the extremity elevated, inflate the cuff above the last or predicted blood pressure reading on the sphygmomanometer.

9. Remove the elastic bandage and lower the extremity to the bed.

10. Release cuff pressure slowly and observe when the extremity changes from a pale to a flushed color.

11. Take the pressure reading at this point. **Rationale:** The blood pressure reading is a reading between the systolic and diastolic pressure.

12. Indicate that blood pressure was taken by the flush method when charting findings on graphic sheet or nurses' notes.

---

**Clinical Alert**

Flush pressures are taken on small infants or on adults when unable to auscultate or palpate blood pressure readings.

---

## USING A CONTINUOUS NONINVASIVE MONITORING DEVICE

### Equipment

Blood pressure cuff

Display monitor

Readout paper for monitor

### Procedure

1. Wash hands.

2. Gather equipment. Select proper size blood pressure cuff. Attach the cuff to the air hose by firmly pushing the valve from the cuff into the air hose and twisting to secure fit.

3. Squeeze the air from the cuff.

4. Wrap the cuff securely around the extremity (usually the arm).

5. Turn power switch *ON*.

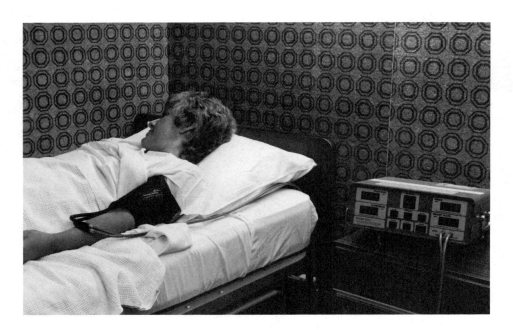

Continuous monitoring of blood presssure is done by attaching cuff to display monitor.

6. Position the extremity at the level of the heart.

7. Set arterial pressure alarm limits by pushing *Alarm* to ON and set both HIGH and LOW parameters by depressing the *Alarm* button until the parameters read out on the digital display. **Rationale:** The alarm parameters provide a safety factor by alerting the nurse when the readings exceed the parameters.

8. Test time cycles by turning wheel (found above alarm button) to 1 minute and check for cycling effects. Then, to set automatic cycle time, move the wheel to desired time increments.

9. Press *Start* button to begin timed blood pressure reading.

10. Press *Start* button for approximately 4 seconds to activate printer for readout of blood pressure. Systolic, diastolic, mean arterial pressures, and heart rates can be monitored with this system.

## CHARTING  *for Blood Pressure*

☐ Systolic blood pressure

☐ Diastolic blood pressure

☐ Level of muffled Korotkoff's sounds and their disappearance (for example: 126/80/72 mm Hg)

☐ Response to alternative nursing actions

---

## CLINICAL PROBLEM SOLVING

### Potential Problems

Blood pressure reading is abnormally high without apparent physiological cause.

### Suggested Solutions

☐ Check if cuff was too narrow.
☐ Check if cuff was not snug.
☐ Check if cuff was deflated too slowly, causing venous engorgement.
☐ Observe if mercury column, if used, was above eye level.
☐ Ask if patient was anxious or had just exercised or eaten.
☐ Check blood pressure on both arms. The normal difference from arm to arm is usually no more than 5 mm Hg.

Blood pressure reading is very low in absence of significant clinical findings.

☐ Assess if cuff is too wide.
☐ Check if mercury column was below eye level.
☐ Check if patient's arm was above heart level.
☐ Assess if Korotkoff's sounds were barely audible. Raise patient's arm and then recheck. Sounds should be louder.
☐ Identify if stethoscope was misplaced and was not on brachial artery.
☐ Take blood pressure after patient has been standing for 10 to 15 minutes if postural hypotension is suspected, if patient is taking medications that affect blood pressure, or if patient is ambulating after a period of prolonged bed rest.

Hypotension (systolic pressure is less than 90 mm Hg) develops.

☐ Take vital signs more frequently (every 15 minutes to 2 hours) until condition has stabilized.
☐ Place patient in supine position with feet and head elevated 20 degrees.
☐ Assess cause of hypotension and notify physician.

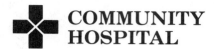

**COMMUNITY HOSPITAL**

**CLINICAL RECORD**

| DATE | | | | | | | | | | | | | | | | | | | | |
|---|---|---|---|---|---|---|---|---|---|---|---|---|---|---|---|---|---|---|---|---|
| HOSP DAY/POSTOP DAY | | | | | | | | | | | | | | | | | | | | |
| TIME | | | | 0200 | 0600 | 1000 | 1400 | 1800 | 2200 | 0200 | 0600 | 1000 | 1400 | 1800 | 2200 | 0200 | 0600 | 1000 | 1400 | 1800 | 2200 |

| KEY | PULSE | TEMP. | |
|---|---|---|---|
| | | C | F |
| | 140 | 40.6 | 105 |
| | 130 | 40.0 | 104 |
| | 120 | 39.4 | 103 |
| | 110 | 38.8 | 102 |
| | 100 | 38.3 | 101 |
| | 80 | 37.7 | 100 |
| | 80 | 37.2 | 99 |
| | 70 | 36.6 | 98 |
| | 60 | 36.1 | 97 |
| | 50 | 35.5 | 96 |

BLACK — PULSE & RESPIRATIONS
RED — TEMPERATURE

| RESPIRATIONS |
|---|
| BLOOD PRESSURE |

| HEIGHT | WEIGHT | | | WEIGHT | | | WEIGHT | | |
|---|---|---|---|---|---|---|---|---|---|
| | BREAKFAST | LUNCH | DINNER | BREAKFAST | LUNCH | DINNER | BREAKFAST | LUNCH | DINNER |
| DIET — TYPE | | | | | | | | | |
| % CONSUMED | | | | | | | | | |

| INTAKE | INTAKE & OUTPUT HOURS | 0600-1400 | 1400-2200 | 2200-0600 | 0600-1400 | 1400-2200 | 2200-0600 | 0600-1400 | 1400-2200 | 2200-0600 |
|---|---|---|---|---|---|---|---|---|---|---|
| Oral | | | | | | | | | | |
| IV | | | | | | | | | | |
| Blood - Plasma | | | | | | | | | | |
| Other | | | | | | | | | | |
| 8 Hr. Total | | | | | | | | | | |
| Output | | | | | | | | | | |
| Urine | | | | | | | | | | |
| Emesis | | | | | | | | | | |
| Stools | | | | | | | | | | |
| GI Suction | | | | | | | | | | |
| | | | | | | | | | | |
| | | | | | | | | | | |
| 8 Hr. Total | | | | | | | | | | |
| 24 Hr. Intake | | | | | | | | | | |
| 24 Hr. Output | | | | | | | | | | |
| SIGNATURE | | | | | | | | | | |

DATE:

CLINICAL RECORD

Hypertension (blood pressure consistently over 140/90 mm Hg) develops.

- ☐ Increase or administer fluids as ordered by physician.
- ☐ Observe postoperative patients for signs of bleeding.
- ☐ Administer oxygen.

- ☐ For patients with severe hypertension take vital signs more frequently (every 15 minutes to 2 hours) until condition has stabilized.
- ☐ If patient is anxious or excited, institute relaxation techniques to lower blood pressure.
- ☐ Allow patient to rest after strenuous exercise.
- ☐ Relieve pain with reassurance, change of position, and analgesia as ordered by physician.
- ☐ For patients with essential hypertension, administer antihypertensive and diuretic drugs as ordered by the physician. Evaluate response by checking blood pressure in reclining, sitting, and standing position. Instruct patient in diet therapy such as low salt, low fat, and inclusion of vitamins and garlic.
- ☐ For patients with hypoxia, relieve with oxygen administration in whichever mode is most effective.

Continuous BP monitoring system displays 00 instead of blood pressure reading. (00 indicates the unit is unable to determine parameters.)

- ☐ Check cuff placement and size to determine if appropriately placed.

---

## TERMINOLOGY

---

### Pulse Terminology

**Atrial fibrillation:** a chaotically irregular pulse rate with a pulse deficit.

**Bigeminal pulse:** pulse occurs with premature beats and is a disturbance in rhythm. The premature beat decreases the stroke volume for that beat and so is weaker than the normal beat.

**Large, bounding pulse:** pulse pressure is increased. It is felt as a slapping against the fingers because of the rapid upstroke and quick downstroke. It is seen in conditions of increased cardiac output, such as exercise, anxiety, alcoholic intake, and pregnancy. It is also noted in pathology with fever, anemia, hyperthyroidism, liver failure, complete heart block with bradycardia, and hypertension. When there is a rapid runoff of blood, such as with aortic insufficiency ("water-hammer" pulse) and patent ductus arteriosus, this type of pulse is characteristic. Increased rigidity in the aorta, which occurs with aging and arteriosclerosis, also causes this type of pulse.

**Normal pulse:** pulse pressure is about 30 to 40 mm Hg. It is smooth and rounded and is felt as a sharp upstroke and gradual downstroke.

**Premature beats:** a pacemaker outside the sinus node fires earlier than the sinus node, the normal pacemaker of the heart. Since the beat is early, the stroke volume is less because the ventricles do not have time to fill. This condition causes a pause in rhythm, which may result in a pulse deficit.

**Pulse deficit:** occurs when the heart rate counted at the apex by auscultation is greater than the heart rate counted by palpation of the radial pulse. The pulse wave is not transmitted to the periphery to produce a palpable radial pulse.

**Pulsus alternans:** rhythm is regular but the amplitude alternates from beat to beat.

**Pulsus paradoxus:** pulse diminishes in amplitude with inspiration because more blood remains in the lungs. The resulting increased negative thoracic pressure provides less return to the left ventricle and decreases stroke volume. This condition is really an exaggeration of what normally occurs during the respiratory cycle.

**Sinus arrhythmia:**   common in children and young adults. The rate accelerates with inspiration and slows with expiration.

**Small, weak pulse:**   pulse pressure is diminished. It is smooth and rounded but is felt as a gradual upstroke and prolonged downstroke. It is commonly seen in conditions resulting in decreased cardiac output, such as heart failure and shock, and with obstruction to left ventricular ejection, such as aortic stenosis.

**Tachycardia:**   abnormal rapid heart action.

## Respiratory Terminology

**Apnea:**   absence of breathing.

**Biot's:**   abrupt interruptions between a faster, deeper respiratory rate.

**Bradypnea:**   slow, regular respirations. Rate is below 10 per minute.

**Cheyne-Stokes:**   periods of apnea appear throughout cycle. Respirations become deeper and faster than normal followed by a slower rate and progressing to periods of apnea lasting up to 60 seconds.

**Hyperpnea:**   abnormal increase in depth and rate.

**Kussmaul's:**   difficult breathing that occurs in paroxysms. Called air hunger, and often precedes diabetic coma.

**Sonorous:**   loud breathing.

**Stertorous:**   loud, noisy breathing.

**Tachypnea:**   respiratory rate increased above 20 breaths per minute. Rate remains regular but shallow in pattern.

## General Terminology

**Antipyretic:**   an agent that reduces febrile temperatures.

**Apex:**   the designate of the top of a body organ.

**Arteriosclerosis:**   an arterial disease characterized by inelasticity and thickening of the vessel walls with lessened blood flow.

**Atherosclerosis:**   a form of arteriosclerosis in which there are localized accumulations of lipid-containing material within the internal surfaces of blood vessels.

**Atrial:**   pertaining to the atrium, a chamber that receives blood from the lungs and systemic circulation.

**Autoregulation:**   the intrinsic tendency of the heart to maintain constant blood flow despite changes in other factors.

**Axilla:**   armpit.

**Cardio:**   pertaining to the heart.

**Cardiogenic:**   having origin in the heart itself.

**Chemoreceptor:**   a sense organ or sensory nerve ending that is stimulated by and reacts to chemical stimuli.

**Contractility:**   having the ability to contract or shorten muscle tissue or cells.

**Diastole:**   the period in which the heart dilates and fills with blood; the period of relaxation.

**Febrile:**   feverish, increased body temperature.

**Fibrillation:**   quivering; involuntary contraction of individual muscle fibers.

**Flush blood pressures:**   obtaining a blood pressure by monitoring a change in extremity color.

**Hyperpnea:**   increased respiratory rate with deeper breathing.

**Hyperthermia:**   unusually high body temperature.

**Hypervolemia:**   abnormal increase in the volume of circulating body fluid.

**Hypothalamus:**   the part of the brain that lies below the thalamus; it maintains or regulates body temperature, certain metabolic processes, and other autonomic activities.

**Hypothermia:**   a body temperature below the average normal range.

**Hypovolemia:**   diminished blood volume.

**Infarction:**   an area of tissue in an organ or part that undergoes necrosis following cessation of blood supply.

**Ischemia:**   local and temporary anemia due to obstruction of the circulation to a part.

**Myo:**   combining form pertinent to a muscle.

**Myocardium:**   the middle muscle layer of the walls of the heart.

**Palpate:**   to examine by touch; feel.

**Peripheral:**   pertinent to the periphery, away from the central structure.

**Peripheral vascular disease:**   indicates diseases of the arteries and veins of the extremities, especially those conditions that interfere with adequate flow of blood.

**Pyrogens:**   any substance that produces fever.

**Rectum:**   lower part of the large intestine, about 12.7 cm long, between the sigmoid flexure and the anal canal.

**Sclerosis:**   hardening of a tissue part, as connective tissue.

**Shock:**   state of collapse resulting from circulatory failure, precipitated by many factors and identified by various signs and symptoms.

**Sphygmomanometer:**   instrument for indirectly determining arterial blood pressure.

**Stokes-Adams syndrome:** an altered state of consciousness caused by decreased flow of blood to the brain due to a decreased heart rate.

**Sympathetic nervous system:** a division of the autonomic nervous system; tends to be involved in the fight-flight response.

**Systole:** the period in which the heart contracts.

**Tracheobronchial:** involving the trachea (windpipe) and bronchi of the respiratory tree.

**Valsalva's maneuver:** attempt to forcibly exhale with the glottis, nose, and mouth closed, producing an increased intrathoracic pressure.

**Vaso:** part meaning a vessel, such as blood vessel.

**Vasoconstriction:** constriction of the blood vessels.

*Chapter* **14**

# *Exercise and Ambulation*

## LEARNING OBJECTIVES

Define rehabilitative nursing.

Compare and contrast preservative and restorative methods of care.

Identify the joints and the type of movement they allow.

Compare and contrast passive and active range of motion.

Demonstrate passive range-of-motion exercises using all muscle groups.

Explain the rationale of assisted ambulation for patients.

Complete a patient-teaching guide for patients requiring muscle-strengthening exercises.

Demonstrate the proper method for measuring crutches.

Name and discuss four crutch-walking gaits.

Demonstrate four crutch-walking gaits.

List the components of crutch-walking which require documentation.

Write three nursing diagnoses which are appropriate for patients requiring exercise and ambulation activities.

## REHABILITATION CONCEPTS

Rehabilitative nursing involves the prevention and correction of alterations in the musculoskeletal system. In fact, the definition of rehabilitative nursing is the process of restoring a person's ability to live and work in as normal a manner as possible. To assist patients to achieve and maintain optimal mobility, both preservative and restorative methods are used.

Preservative methods, such as exercises and assisted ambulation, include those interventions that are needed to help patients maintain their normal mobility. Because the changes that occur in the human body when a person is hospitalized are varied and subtle, preservative methods are used with every patient. Restorative methods, such as crutch walking and splinting, are used with patients who have decreased mobility caused by such factors as debilitating illness or major surgery. The purpose for applying restorative methods is to assist the patient in achieving the level of mobility the patient enjoyed before becoming ill.

The general goals for utilizing these methods are to assist the patient to strive for optimal function, to prevent further injury, and to restore normal function. In order to achieve these goals of care, it is important for the nurse to accept the philosophy underlying rehabilitative nursing: that every illness is accompanied by the intrinsic threat of disability and that this part of total patient care must begin with the initial patient contact. Finally, it is important to accept that the principles of rehabilitation are basic to the care of all patients.

When a person is hospitalized and immobile, there is a corresponding impact on his body image, his behavior, and his overall adaptation and adjustment. The greater the disability, the more these aspects of a person's life are affected. The nurse's responsibility in providing total patient care is to be aware of these responses and to take them into account when developing a Patient Care Plan.

The muscular system is a system of more than six hundred fibers that are attached to bones. The system allows for body movement under the control of the voluntary nervous system. Muscles provide for body movement or locomotion, support the body, and perform several body functions, such as the partial production of heat. The fibers of the voluntary muscles are grouped together in a sheath of connective tissue. Each bundled group of muscle fibers is surrounded by a connective tissue sheath. The sheath tissue may be continuous with fibrous tissue that extends from the muscle as a tendon.

There are several properties of muscle fibers. The first is excitability, or the capacity of a muscle to respond to stimulus without intervention of the motor nerves. Another property is contractility, the ability of a muscle to shorten, tighten, or contract. Muscles are also able to maintain steady contraction (tonicity), stretch in response to applied force (extensibility), and regain their original size and shape when applied force is removed (elasticity).

**Muscle Function**  Skeletal muscles produce body movements by pulling on the bones. Bones serve as levers, and joints serve as fulcrums of these levers. Each muscle has a point of origin and a point of insertion that are usually attached to the bone. Muscles that move a body part usually do not extend over that part. These muscles usually perform with group action; some contract, while others relax. Prime movers are muscles responsible for the primary movement of contraction. Antagonists are muscles that exert an action opposing that of the prime movers. Synergists are muscles that enhance action of the prime mover. The accessory parts to muscles are the ligaments and the tendons.

**Joints**  A joint of the body is the point at which two or more bones join together. The function of a joint is skeletal flexibility and motion. Joints are classified according to structural variations that allow for different kinds of movements. There are three main types of classification: synarthrotic, amphiarthrotic, and diarthrotic joints.

Synarthrotic joints are immovable and include those areas where tissue grows between articulating surfaces, such as the suture lines of the skull. Amphiarthrotic joints have limited movement.

Diarthrotic joints are freely movable. This type of joint is a cavity enclosed by a capsule lined with synovial membrane, which secretes a lubricant. The following types of joint movement allow for structural variations.

☐ Hinge type allows single directional movement (elbow).

☐ Ball-and-socket type allows bending (hip).

☐ Saddle type allows multidirectional shifting (thumb).

☐ Pivot type allows rotary movement.

☐ Gliding type allows limited sliding of bones against each other (wrist, ankle, invertebral joints).

☐ Ellipsoidal type.

Each of the above types of joints have specific kinds of movements which they can perform. These movements can be described in relationship to the three body planes: sagittal, transverse, and coronal. The sagittal plane divides the body into two portions with a straight vertical line between the two parts. The transverse plane divides the body into upper-lower portions with a horizontal line. The coronal plane divides the body into anterior-posterior portions at right angles to the sagittal plane. The synovial joints accomplish a variety of movements that range from flexion-extension to rotation and circumduction. For definitions of joint movements through the planes of the body refer to the following chart.

## JOINT MOVEMENTS

*Abduction:* movement of a bone away from the midline of the body or body part, as in raising the arm or spreading the fingers.

*Adduction:* movement of a bone toward the midline of the body or part.

*Eversion:* turning outward; movement of the foot at the ankle joint so that the sole faces outward.

*Inversion:* turning inward; movement of the foot at the ankle joint so that the sole faces inward.

*Flexion:* a movement that decreases the angle between two bones; the act of bending a joint.

*Extension:* a movement that increases the angle between two bones, straightening a joint.

*Hyperextension:* continuation of extension beyond the anatomical position, as in bending the head backward.

*Protraction:* movement of the clavicle (collar bone) or mandible (lower jaw) forward on a plane parallel to the ground.

*Retraction:* movement of the clavicle or mandible backward on a plane parallel to the ground.

*Pronation:* rotation of the forearm so that the palm faces backward or downward; movement of the whole body so that the face and abdomen are downward.

*Supination:* rotation of forearm so that the palm faces forward or upward; movement of the whole body so that the face and abdomen are upward.

*Circumduction:* movement of a bone in a circular direction so that the distal end scribes a circle while the proximal end remains stationary, as in "winding up" to throw a ball.

*Rotation:* movement of a bone around its own axis, as in moving the head to indicate "no" or turning the palm of the hand up and then down.

## EXERCISE

Muscles that are not used become weak and shortened. During prolonged bed rest, strength and endurance decrease rapidly. Patients can regain muscle strength and mobility by practicing specific groups of exercises daily. Promoting exercise, both passive and active, is one of the most important nursing functions. The purpose of exercises is to promote good alignment, prevent contractures, stimulate circulation, and prevent thrombophlebitis and decubiti. Exercise also prevents edema of the extremities and promotes lung expansion.

There are several types of exercises that the nurse both performs and teaches as a component of providing total patient care. Passive exercises are carried out by the therapist or nurse without assistance from the patient. These exercises enable the patient to retain as much joint range of motion as possible as well as stimulating circulation. Active exercises, while supervised by the nurse, are performed by the patient. These exercises increase muscle strength when the patient is partially immobile.

Resistive exercises, another rehabilitative measure, provide resistance in order to increase muscle power. These active exercises are performed by the individual working against resistance. Isometric or muscle-setting activities are similar to resistive exercises. These exercises maintain strength in a muscle when the joint is immobilized. They are performed by the individual without assistance.

Range-of-motion (ROM) exercises are the most common form of exercises for maintaining joint mobility and increasing maximal motion of a joint when the patient is totally or partially immobilized. These exercises are completed by the nurse or physical therapist. The therapist puts an extremity through its full range so that the joint is moved through all the appropriate planes. Before beginning these exercises, it is important that the nurse assess the general condition of the patient, establish the extent of ROM to be carried out, and ensure that the patient is comfortable. Be aware that patients might be fearful of this type of exercise and that a full explanation of what you are going to do is helpful to allay fears. Enlist the cooperation of the patient for maximum benefit. Discontinue all range-of-motion exercises if the patient complains of pain, for it is at this point that they will become counter-productive.

## AMBULATION

Ambulation is an important function that most of us accomplish automatically, that is, without thinking or conscious effort. When a person has been immobilized, confined to bed following surgery or an injury, or unable to ambulate, this seemingly simple activity can become a major hurdle to overcome. The longer a person is immobilized, the more difficult it is to regain ambulatory ability; likewise, the sooner a person begins to ambulate after being bedridden, the more easily he will regain preimmobilization status. Early ambulation decreases hospitalization time and prevents complications, such as paralytic ileus or thrombophlebitis.

The human body functions best when it is placed frequently in a vertical position. Ambulation improves physical and mental well-being. Ambulation increases muscle strength and joint mobility. It also increases respiratory exchange, gastrointestinal muscle tone, and circulation. Without stress on bones, calcium deposits occur and renal problems increase from calcium-based calculi.

Balance, coordination, and good body alignment are aspects important to walking. One must be able to move forward and maintain an upright balance; use muscles, bones, and joints correctly for coordination; and keep the head erect and vertebral column fairly straight with feet and knee caps pointed forward in order to maintain good body alignment.

The major muscle groups used for walking are the thigh and leg muscles. If these muscles have not been used or exercised because the patient has been in bed for a long time, ambulation will have to be accomplished step by step. Weak muscles cannot support a human frame for the mechanics of walking. It will be important, then, to begin the process of ambulation by administering muscle-strengthening exercises. Several different types of exercises are described above; however, the most important preambulatory preparation is quadriceps-setting and gluteal-setting exercises. Carried out several times a day, these exercises will restore muscle strength and prepare the legs for weight-bearing.

Before actually assisting the patient to walk, explain exactly what you are going to do and prepare him by doing the ambulatory procedure in stages. For example, begin with the muscle-strengthening exercises. Then, assist the patient to sit up in bed to determine if he is experiencing vertigo. Have him move to the side of the bed with his legs down, and only when he is ready and feels comfortable in doing so, assist him to stand beside the bed. Allow him to remain there with the bed as support until he feels totally secure. Finally, and with the assistance of one or two nurses (depending on the assessment of the patient's ability and readiness to ambulate), have the patient walk by taking short steps and walking only as long as he can tolerate. Do this several times a day, and it will not be long before the patient's legs are strengthened, and he can graduate to one assistant, a walker, cane, etc. Throughout this procedure, do not allow the patient to lose confidence in his ability to walk or your ability to support and assist him while regaining his independence of action.

## CRUTCHES

Crutches are an aid to walking by providing support during ambulating when the lower extremities are unable to support the body weight. Hopefully, this situation is temporary, but even if it is permanent, crutches do allow independence of movement which otherwise would not occur.

There are several safety factors that should be taken into account before assisting the patient to use crutches. The measurement from the axillary fold to the crutch bar should be 1½ to 2 inches (4 inches in front and 6 inches to the side of the toes). The handpiece should be adjusted to allow 30-degree elbow-flexion, and rubber suction tips should be placed on the bottom of the crutches. Finally, the patient should be informed that he needs well-fitting shoes with nonslip soles.

There are three types of crutches commonly prescribed for patients: axillary crutch, Lofstrand crutch, and the Canadian crutch. The type of crutch utilized by the patient will depend on the ability to ambulate, the muscle strength needed for support, and the individual needs of the patient.

## NURSING DIAGNOSES

The following nursing diagnoses may be appropriate to include in a Patient Care Plan when the components are related to exercise and ambulation needs of patients.

| Nursing Diagnosis (Potential) | Defining Characteristic; Etiology (Examples) |
|---|---|
| ☐ Activity Intolerance, *related to* | Decreased energy, stamina or desire to ambulate, e.g., depression or musculo-skeletal disease. |
| ☐ Comfort, Alteration in: Pain, *related to* | Alterations in muscle tone, e.g., muscle spasms or rigidity. |
| ☐ Home Maintenance Management, Impaired, *related to* | Poor coping measures, e.g., lack of necessary equipment or person at home. |
| ☐ Mobility, Impaired Physical, *related to* | Joint contractures, e.g., inappropriate or inadequate joint exercises by inadequately trained personnel. |
| | Limited range of motion, e.g., decreased muscle strength or restricted movement. |
| ☐ Self-Care Deficit, *related to* | Inability to ambulate, feed, bathe or dress self, e.g., traction, casts, or physical disability. |

# UNIT ONE  RANGE OF MOTION

## NURSING PROCESS DATA

### ASSESSMENT  *Data Base*

Determine patient's physical ability to perform exercises, i.e., level of consciousness, presence of casts, traction.

Ascertain patient's present level of joint movement and/or muscle strength.

Note amount of spontaneous movement shown by the patient.

### PLANNING  *Objectives*

To improve or maintain joint function.

To improve or maintain muscle tone and strength.

To counteract effects of prolonged bed rest or immobilization.

To prevent contractures.

To increase patient comfort.

To prepare the patient for ambulation.

### IMPLEMENTATION  *Procedures*

Performing Passive Range of Motion

Teaching Active Range of Motion

### EVALUATION  *Expected Outcomes*

Patient experiences improved range of motion and muscle tone.

Patient is comfortable following range-of-motion exercises.

Patient is able to ambulate without difficulty following a period of bed rest.

## PERFORMING PASSIVE RANGE OF MOTION

### Equipment

Hospital bed

### Procedure

1. Explain the rationale for the procedure to the patient.
2. Position the patient on his back with the bed as flat as possible.
3. Put all joints through range of motion.
4. When performing range-of-motion exercises the joint is protected against gravity and detrimental movement.
5. Provide support above and below the joint using a cradling or cupping support while performing the exercises.
6. All joints should be put through exercises at least twice daily and five full-range motions to each joint.
7. Encourage patient to do active exercises as soon as possible. **Rationale:** Passive exercises only help prevent contractures. They do not maintain the muscle.

**TABLE 1** RANGE OF MOTION: UPPER BODY

| | NECK | SHOULDER | ELBOW | FOREARM | WRIST | FINGERS AND THUMB |
|---|---|---|---|---|---|---|
| Flexion | Move head forward 90° with chin on chest. | Raise arm 180° from side to above head. | Bend elbow so arm moves up toward shoulder. | | Bend hand 90° toward inner arm | Make a fist so fingers are all bent inward. |
| Extension | Move head up from chest 90° —resting position. | Move arm to side of body. | Straighten elbow and return to position. | | Move hand straight pointed out. | Move fingers 90° to straight position. |
| Hyperextension | Move head backwards 90°. | Move arm to back of body 50° angle. | | | Bend hand up and back 90° toward arm. | Move fingers up toward back of hand. |
| Abduction | | Hold arm away from side 180° to above head. | | | Bend wrist out away from arm. | Spread fingers as much as possible. |
| Abduction | | Move arm from above head to side. | | | Bend wrist inward toward radius. | Move fingers and thumb together. |
| External Rotation | | Hold arm out to side with elbow bent 45°; move forward so palm faces forward. | | | | |
| Internal Rotation | | Move arm to side at shoulder level with elbow bent 45°. Lower arm so palm faces back. | | | | |
| Rotation | Move head in circular motion—90° left, then 90°right. | | | | | |
| Circumduction | | Move arm in full circle. | | | | |
| Supination | | | | Rotate forearm 90° so palm is up. | | |
| Pronation | | | | Rotate forearm 90° so palm is down. | | |

**TABLE 2** RANGE OF MOTION: LOWER BODY

| | TRUNK | HIP | KNEE | ANKLE | TOES |
|---|---|---|---|---|---|
| Flexion | Bend forward 90°. | Move leg forward and up 90°. | Bend knee 90°; foot moves back and up. | | Point down 90°. |
| Extension | Stand in straight position. | Move leg in straight alignment with trunk. | Move foot 90°, with knee straight and leg in line with body. | | Straight out from foot. |
| Hyperextension | Bend backward 30°. | Move leg backward 50°. | | | Point up 45°. |
| Lateral Flexion | Bend to both sides 45°. | | | | |
| Plantar Flexion | | | | Move foot down 45°. | |
| Internal Rotation | | Turn leg and foot inward 90°. | | | |
| External Rotation | | Turn leg and foot outward 90°. | | | |
| Circumduction | | Move leg in circle 360°. | | | |
| Abduction | | Move leg away from body 45°. | | | Spread apart 15°. |
| Abduction | | Move leg toward body 45°. | | | Bring together in normal position. |
| Rotation | Move in circle 360° from waist. | | | | |
| Dorsiflexion | | | | Raise foot up 45°. | |
| Eversion | | | | Move sole of foot lateral to outside. | |
| Inversion | | | | Move sole of foot medial to inside. | |

## TEACHING ACTIVE RANGE OF MOTION

### Equipment

Hospital bed

Sturdy nonslip shoes or slippers

### Procedure

1. Explain the rationale for the procedure to the patient.
2. Demonstrate the exercises that the patient should perform.
3. Watch as the patient does the exercises.
4. Assist with the exercises as needed.
5. Correct any problems you notice in the patient's performance.
6. Encourage patient to perform as much of the exercises as possible.
7. Instruct patient to do range-of-motion exercises every four hours, exercising all joints.

### CHARTING *for ROM Exercises*

☐ Amount of time needed to complete exercises

☐ Any changes in condition of joint or joint mobility

☐ Movements that caused unusual pain or discomfort

☐ Amount of patient participation

☐ Specific joints put through range of motion

☐ Alterations in usual procedure

---

## CLINICAL PROBLEM SOLVING

### Potential Problems

Patient continues to lose mobility and strength despite nursing intervention.

Patient experiences pain and discomfort during range-of-motion exercises.

### Suggested Solutions

☐ Discuss the need for additional measures to improve joint range with the health team.
☐ Assess the patient for the need to use splints and braces to maintain the best physiologic position between exercise periods and discuss your findings with the physician.

☐ Assess amount and type of pain and report findings to physician.
☐ Reevaluate your technique to ensure you are performing the exercises correctly.
☐ Check with physician about premedicating the patient before exercises are initiated.

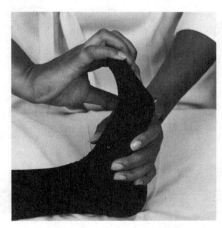

Dorsiflexion.

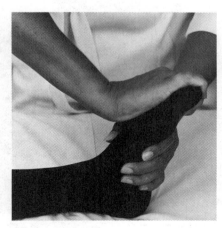

Plantar flexion.

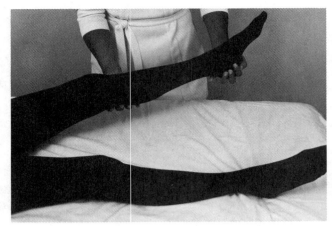

Abduction (moving away from body).

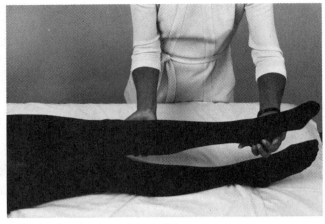

Adduction (moving toward the body).

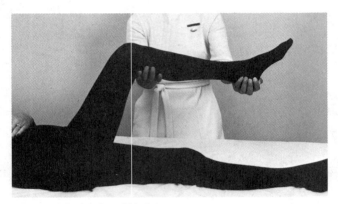

Flexion of the knee and hip joint.

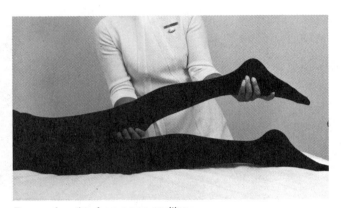

Range of motion from prone position.

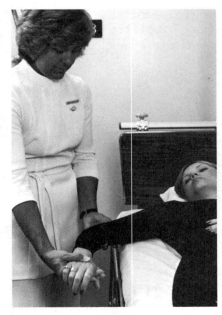

Internal rotation of shoulder.

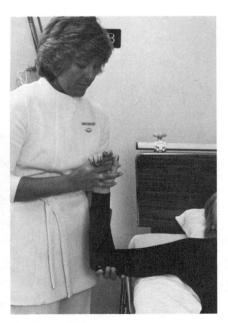

Rotation midpoint.

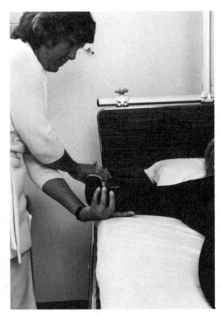

External rotation of shoulder.

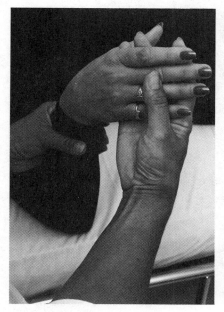

Rotation of the wrist.

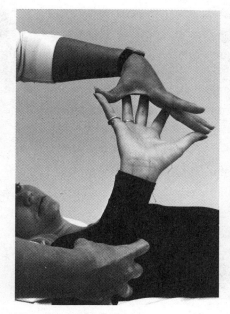

Extension of finger joints.

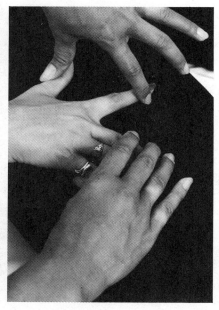

Adduction-abduction finger exercises.

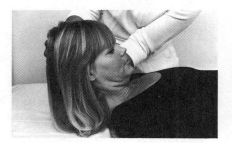

Flexion of the neck.

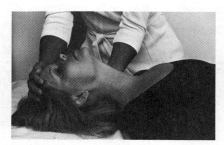

Extension of the neck.

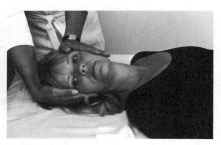

Rotation of the neck.

# UNIT TWO   AMBULATION

## NURSING PROCESS DATA

### ASSESSMENT   *Data Base*

Assess patient for dizziness when moved into an upright sitting position.

Determine if patient feels pain from operative site.

Note weakness in patient's legs.

Observe patient's balance.

### PLANNING   *Objectives*

To promote increased feelings of physical and mental well-being.

To develop increased tolerance for exercise.

To decrease hospitalization time.

To regain independence of action by regaining ability to walk.

To prevent paralytic ileus by increasing abdominal wall and gastrointestinal tract muscle tone.

To prevent thrombophlebitis by increasing circulation in the legs.

To promote healing by increasing circulation and muscle contraction.

### IMPLEMENTATION *Procedures*

Ambulating with Two Assistants

Ambulating with One Assistant

Ambulating with a Walker

Ambulating with a Cane

### EVALUATION *Expected Outcomes*

Increased feelings of physical and mental well-being.

Balance and muscle tone improved.

Patient progresses from needing assistance with ambulation to becoming independent in ambulation.

Complications of immobility are prevented with ambulation.

## AMBULATING WITH TWO ASSISTANTS

### Equipment

Robe or second hospital gown (put on backwards so that patient is not exposed)

Shoes or slippers that fit well and have nonslip soles

### Procedure

1. Explain the rationale for the procedure to the patient.

2. Help the patient sit on the side of the bed after placing bed in LOW position.

3. Assess the patient for dizziness or faintness. Keep the patient in this position until he is able to stand without becoming dizzy. **Rationale:** Orthostatic hypotension can occur with prolonged bed rest.

4. Position one nurse on each side of the patient.

5. Have each nurse grasp the patient's upper arm with the hand that is closest to the patient.

6. Have each nurse grasp the patient's hand with the other hand.

7. Encourage the patient to maintain good posture and look straight ahead, not down.

8. Ask the patient to lift each foot to take a step. The patient should not shuffle. Walk the patient only as far as he is capable of walking and returning without exhaustion.

## AMBULATING WITH ONE ASSISTANT

### Equipment

Robe or second hospital gown (put on backward so that patient is not exposed)

Shoes or slippers that fit well and have nonslip soles

### Procedure

1. Explain the rationale for the procedure to the patient.

2. Help the patient sit on the side of the bed after placing bed in LOW position.

3. Assess the patient for dizziness or faintness. Keep the patient in this position until he is able to stand without becoming dizzy.

4. Help the patient to stand.

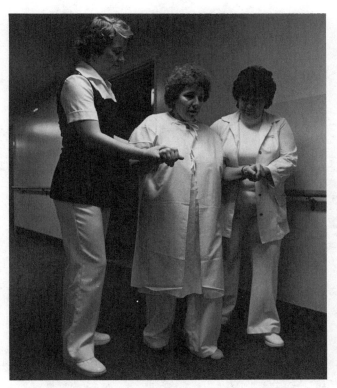

Support is provided by two nurses when patient's condition requires.

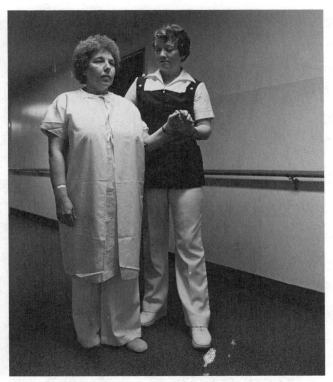

Grasp the patient's upper arm and hand when one nurse ambulates.

5. Grasp the patient's upper arm with the hand that is closest to the patient.

6. Grasp the patient's hand with the other hand. If the patient has a weaker side, stand on that side. For a patient with CVA, stand on unaffected side. **Rationale:** Flaccid muscles on affected side will not provide sufficient muscle strength for you to grasp and support patient.

7. Encourage the patient to maintain good posture and to look straight ahead, not down.

8. Ask the patient to lift each foot to take a step.

---

**Clinical Alert**

If the patient is collapsing, try to break the fall with your body and guide patient to the floor.

If the patient is unsteady or appears to be falling, support his body, especially the head and trunk, maintaining your body in good alignment with line of gravity within your base of support. This alignment will prevent injury to yourself, while giving the patient adequate support. If necessary, guide the patient all the way to the floor.

---

The patient should not shuffle. Walk the patient only as far as he is capable of walking and returning without exhaustion.

## AMBULATING WITH A WALKER

### Equipment

Robe or second hospital gown (put on backward so that patient is not exposed)

Shoes or slippers that fit well and have nonslip soles

Walker (if patient uses one)

### Procedure

1. Explain the rationale for the procedure to the patient.

2. Help the patient stand.

3. Tell patient to grasp the upper handles of the walker.

4. Have the patient move the walker forward, keeping all four feet of the walker on the floor.

5. When the walker is stable, tell the patient to walk into it.

6. Make sure the patient lifts his feet to walk.

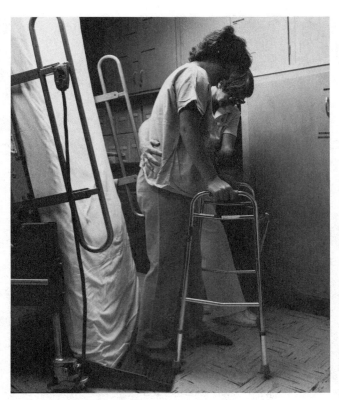

Instruct patient to lift feet while ambulating with walker.

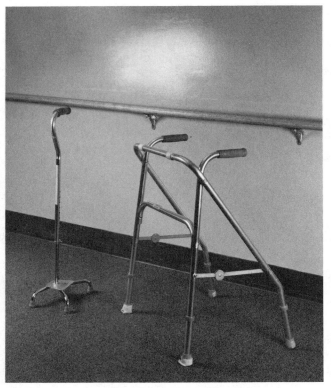

Walker and tripod cane are frequently used for stroke patients.

## AMBULATING WITH A CANE

### Equipment

Appropriate type of cane
    Straight-legged cane
    Tripod or three-pronged cane
    Quad cane
Sturdy shoes with nonskid soles

### Procedure

1. Check physician's orders and Patient Care Plan to ensure patient is ready to utilize a cane for ambulation.

2. Ascertain that cane will provide sufficient support for the patient.

3. Explain the purpose of using a cane for ambulation.

4. Demonstrate use of cane if patient is unfamiliar with its use.

5. Assist patient to put on appropriate shoes and socks for walking.

6. Assist patient to standing position with feet firmly on the floor.

7. Instruct patient to hold cane on the strongest side of the body.

8. Place cane about 12 inches in front of the foot and slightly to the side. **Rationale:** This position provides the best balance as the patient's center of gravity is within the base of support.

9. Determine that patient can maintain balance and does not feel dizzy before taking the first step.

10. Instruct patient to move unaffected (or stronger) leg forward ahead of cane and weaker leg. **Rationale:** This procedure allows the weight to be distributed first to the unaffected leg and cane, then to the affected leg and cane.

11. Assist patient to move unaffected (or stronger) leg forward ahead of cane and weaker leg. **Rationale:** This procedure allows the weight to be distributed first to the unaffected leg and cane, then to the affected leg and cane.

12. Accompany patient by walking beside him on the affected side. **Rationale:** If the patient loses his balance, supporting patient on affected side will be most effective. Simply insert your hand and arm underneath the patient's axilla and support his arm with your other hand.

13. Evaluate patient's ability to use the cane and instruct about its use as needed.

14. Reinforce the patient's achievement to assist him to gain confidence in ambulating.

15. Continue to accompany patient until the time for walking is completed.

16. Assist patient to return to the room and to bed if indicated.

17. Position patient for comfort.

18. Assess patient's response to ambulation.

19. Wash hands.

20. Chart patient's progress and evaluate plan for increased periods of ambulation in terms of patient's capability.

### CHARTING  *for Ambulation*

☐  Patient's ability to balance

☐  Time and distance of ambulation

☐  Use of correct procedure for walker or cane

☐  Patient's perceptions of ambulation

---

## CLINICAL PROBLEM SOLVING

| **Potential Problems** | **Suggested Solutions** |
|---|---|
| Patient becomes dizzy or feels faint. | ☐ If in the patient's room, help the patient return to the chair or bed.<br>☐ If in the hall, ease the patient down the wall to the floor. Do not attempt to hold the patient.<br>☐ Summon help if possible. |
| Patient is too weak to ambulate. | ☐ Provide active and passive ROM.<br>☐ Begin ambulation protocol as soon as possible. |
| Patient is heavy or has poor balance. | ☐ Ask other nurses or staff to help you ambulate the patient until he is able to walk on his own.<br>☐ If necessary, enlist the aid of a stronger assistant whose presence may give the patient additional psychological as well as physical support.<br>☐ Gradually increase ambulation as muscle tone improves and balance improves. |
| Patient feels he is unable to ambulate. | ☐ Ambulate more frequently for shorter periods and with more assistance to increase confidence.<br>☐ Medicate at least one hour before ambulation to decrease pain.<br>☐ With abdominal surgery, check with physician for an order for a binder to decrease fear of dehiscence and pain.<br>☐ Establish rapport with the patient so you can discuss fears about ambulation. |

---

# UNIT THREE  CRUTCH WALKING

## NURSING PROCESS DATA

### ASSESSMENT  *Data Base*

Assess the strength of the patient's arm, back, and leg muscles.

Observe patient's ability to balance himself.

Note any unilateral or unusual weakness.

Check patient's medical history to find out exactly why the patient needs crutches.

### PLANNING   *Objectives*

To improve patient's ability to ambulate when he has lower extremity injury.

To increase muscle strength, especially in the arms and legs.

To increase feeling of well-being when patient can ambulate.

To promote joint mobility.

### IMPLEMENTATION   *Procedures*

Teaching Muscle-Strengthening Exercises

Measuring Patient for Crutches

Teaching Crutch Walking—Four-Point Gait

Teaching Crutch Walking—Three-Point Gait

Teaching Crutch Walking—Two-Point Gait

Teaching Swing-To Gait and Swing-Through Gait

Teaching Upstairs and Downstairs Ambulation with Crutches

### EVALUATION   *Expected Outcomes*

Patient's ability to ambulate is improved.

Muscle strength of patient's arms and legs is improved.

Patient experiences a feeling of well-being.

## TEACHING MUSCLE-STRENGTHENING EXERCISES

### Equipment

Books, boards or other firm surface for each hand

### Procedure

1. Explain the rationale for the exercises to the patient.
2. Check the patient care plan for orders.
3. Demonstrate the exercises that patient will practice.
   *Quadriceps setting exercises:*
   a. Try to hyperextend the patient's leg by pushing the popliteal area (the area behind knee) into the bed and lifting heel off the bed.
   b. Instruct patient to contract muscle for a count of 5, then relax for a count of 5.
   c. Have patient repeat exercise two to three times, gradually working up to 10 to 15 times an hour.
   *Gluteal setting exercises:*
   a. Tell patient to pinch his buttocks together for a count of 5 and then to relax for a count of 5.
   b. Have patient repeat exercise 10 to 15 times an hour.
   *Push-ups in sitting position:*
   a. Tell patient to sit up in bed with arms at sides.
   b. Put books, boards, or something firm under the patient's hands and have the patient push down, raising hips off the bed. (This exercise may also be practiced while sitting in a chair.)
   c. Have patient repeat exercise until he can do 10 to 15 push-ups an hour.

*Push-ups in prone position:*

  a.  Tell patient to lie prone in bed.

  b.  Ask patient to place hands on the bed, close to the shoulders.

  c.  Tell patient to extend arms and to push the upper part of the body into an upright position.

  d.  Have patient repeat exercise until he can do 10 to 15 push-ups an hour.

4.  Monitor as the patient performs the exercises and correct any problems that may occur.

5.  Assess the patient for increasing strength as he continues to practice the exercises.

## MEASURING PATIENT FOR CRUTCHES

### Equipment

Measuring tape

Hardsoled street shoes

### Procedure

1.  Explain the rationale for the procedure to the patient.

2.  Tell patient to put on the shoes he will be wearing when using the crutches.

3.  Ask patient to lie flat in bed with arms at sides.

4.  Measure the distance from the patient's axilla (armpit) to a point six to eight inches out from heel.

5.  Adjust hand bars on the crutches so that the patient's elbows will always be slightly flexed.

6.  Tell the patient to stand with the crutches under the arms.

7.  Measure the distance between the patient's axilla and the arm pieces on the crutches. You should be able to put two of your fingers in the space between the axilla and the crutch bar. **Rationale:** Crutches that do not fit the patient correctly or crutches that are used incorrectly can damage the brachial plexus and cause paralysis of the arms.

## TEACHING CRUTCH WALKING FOUR-POINT GAIT

### Equipment

Properly fitted crutches

Regular, hardsoled street shoes

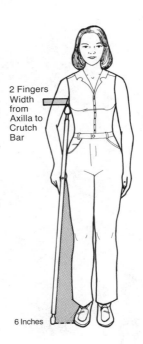

2 Fingers Width from Axilla to Crutch Bar

6 Inches

### Procedure

1.  Explain the rationale for the procedure to the patient.

  a.  The gait is rather slow but very stable.

  b.  The gait can be performed when the patient can move and bear weight on each leg.

2.  Demonstrate the crutch-foot sequence to the patient.

  a.  Move the right crutch.

  b.  Move your left foot.

  c.  Move the left crutch.

  d.  Move your right foot.

3.  Help the patient practice the gait. Be ready to help with balance if necessary.

4.  Assess patient's progress and correct mistakes as they occur.

## TEACHING CRUTCH WALKING THREE-POINT GAIT

### Equipment

Properly fitted crutches

Regular, hardsoled street shoes

### Procedure

1.  Explain the rationale for the procedure to the patient.

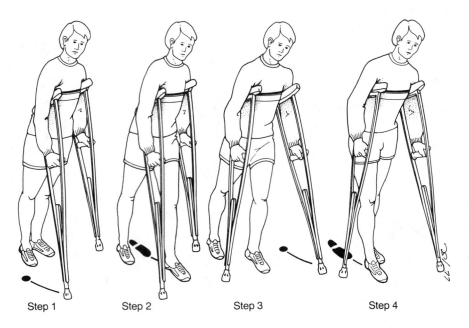

Step 1  Step 2  Step 3  Step 4

Four-point gait.

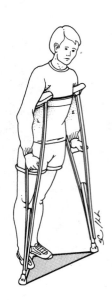

Tripod crutch stance.

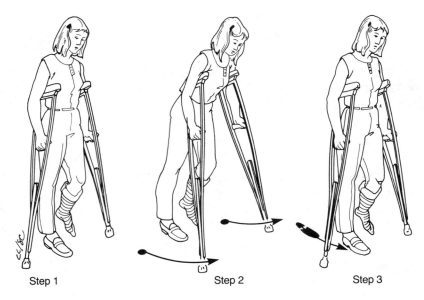

Step 1  Step 2  Step 3

Three-point gait.

   a. The gait can be performed when the patient can bear little or no weight on one leg or when the patient has only one leg.

   b. This gait is fairly rapid and requires strong upper extremities and good balance.

2. Demonstrate the crutch-foot sequence to the patient.

   a. Two crutches will support the weaker extremity.

   b. Balance your weight on the crutches.

   c. Advance forward on the foot that can bear your weight.

3. Help the patient practice the gait.

4. Assess the patient's progress and correct any mistakes as they occur.

5. Remain with patient until crutch safety is assured.

# TEACHING CRUTCH WALKING TWO-POINT GAIT

### Equipment

Properly fitted crutches

Regular, hardsoled street shoes

### Procedure

1. Explain the rationale for the procedure to the patient.
   a. This procedure is a rapid version of the four-point gait.
   b. This gait requires more balance than the four-point gait.
2. Demonstrate the crutch-foot sequence to the patient.
   a. Advance your right foot and the left crutch simultaneously.
   b. Advance your left foot and the right crutch simultaneously.
3. Help the patient practice the gait.
4. Assess the patient's progress and correct any mistakes as they occur.

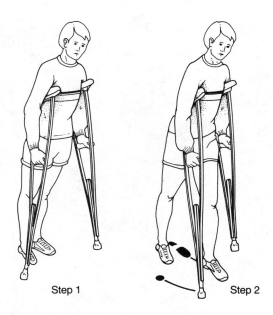

Step 1          Step 2

Two-point gait.

# TEACHING SWING-TO GAIT AND SWING-THROUGH GAIT

### Equipment

Properly fitted crutches

Regular, hardsoled street shoes

### Procedure

1. Explain the rationale for the procedure to the patient.
   a. These gaits are usually performed when the patient's lower extremities are paralyzed.
   b. The patient may use braces.
2. Demonstrate the crutch-foot sequence to the patient.
   a. Move both crutches forward.
   b. Swing-to gait: Lift and swing your body to the crutches.
   c. Swing-through gait: Lift and swing your body past the crutches.
   d. Bring crutches in front of your body and repeat.
3. Help the patient practice the gaits.

4. Assess the patient's progress and correct any mistakes as they occur.

# TEACHING UPSTAIRS AND DOWNSTAIRS AMBULATION WITH CRUTCHES

### Equipment

Properly fitted crutches

Regular, hardsoled street shoes

### Procedure

1. Explain the rationale for the procedure to the patient.
2. Demonstrate the procedure using a three-point gait.
   *Going downstairs:*
   a. Start with your weight on the uninjured leg and crutches on the same level.
   b. Put crutches on the first step.
   c. Put your weight on the crutch handles and transfer your unaffected extremity to the step where you placed the crutches.
   d. Repeat until patient understands the procedure.
   *Going upstairs:*
   a. Start with the crutches and your unaffected extremity on the same level.

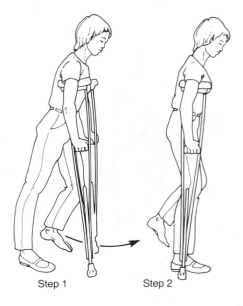

Swing-to gait.

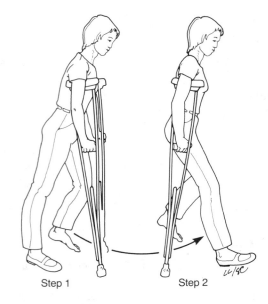

Swing-through gait.

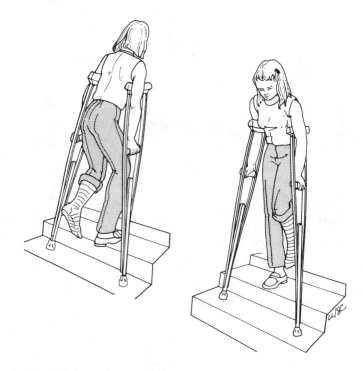

Manipulating stairs up and down.

b. Put your weight on the crutch handles and lift the unaffected extremity onto the first step of the stairs.

c. Put your weight on the unaffected extremity and lift your other extremity and the crutches to the step.

d. Repeat until patient understands the procedure.

3. Help the patient practice.

4. Make sure that the patient has adequate balance. Be ready to assist if necessary.

5. Assess the patient's progress and correct any mistakes as they occur.

### CHARTING   *for Crutch Walking*

☐   Time and distance of ambulation on crutches

☐   Balance

☐   Problems noted with technique

☐   Remedial teaching

☐   Patient's perceptions of ambulation with crutches

## CLINICAL PROBLEM SOLVING

### Potential Problems

Patient states he is frightened of the crutches.

### Suggested Solutions

☐   Observe as the patient practices the procedures to make sure that he is completing the steps correctly for each gait.

□ Explain that it will take time to become proficient.

□ Reassure the patient that he will improve with continued practice.

□ Assess the patient's ability to use the crutches and evaluate level of confidence.

□ Check with physician about obtaining an order for a walker until the patient feels more confident.

Patient fears falling while dependent on crutches.

□ Slow down crutch protocol until patient gains confidence at every level of mastery (e.g., four-point gait to two-point gait).

□ Remain with patient and give verbal reassurance and feedback for improvement.

Shoulder girdle is too weak to bear patient's weight for crutch support.

□ Increase exercise of shoulder (biceps and triceps setting) to gain strength.

□ Request that physician write order for overhead frame with trapeze for shoulder exercise sets.

Slipping occurs with crutch walking

□ Check crutch tips to ensure they cover all metal or wood.

□ Observe the patient's stance or gait to determine if it is too broad.

□ Be sure that floor surface is dry and free of scatter rugs.

Patient complains of numbness and tingling in fingers when crutch walking.

□ Remeasure distance between axilla and crutch bars to determine if two finger breadths can be inserted.

□ Observe patient's gait to determine if he is leaning on crutch inappropriately.

---

## TERMINOLOGY

**Abduction:** movement of a bone away from the midline of the body or body part, as in raising the arm or spreading the fingers.

**Adduction:** movement of a bone toward the midline of the body or part.

**Alignment:** arranged in a straight line.

**Ambulate:** walking; able to walk.

**Antagonists:** muscles that exert an action opposing that of prime mover.

**Atrophy:** a wasting of any organ or body part due to lack of nutrients or oxygen.

**Cardiovascular:** pertaining to heart and blood vessels.

**Circumduction:** movement of a bone in a circular direction so that the distal end scribes a circle while the proximal end remains stationary, as in "winding up" to throw a ball.

**Contractility:** ability of muscle to shorten, tighten, and contract.

**Dorsiflexion:** flexion of the foot at the ankle joint; the act of turning the foot and toes upward, as in standing on the heel.

**Elasticity:** ability of strained muscle to regain original size and shape when applied force is removed.

**Eversion:** turning outward; movement of the foot at the ankle joint so that the sole faces outward.

**Excitability:** capacity of muscle to respond to stimulus without intervention of motor nerves.

**Extensibility:** ability of muscle to stretch in response to applied force.

**Extension:** a movement that increases the angle between two bones, straightening a joint.

**Fibrotic:** pertinent to fibrosis, the formation of fibrous material.

**Flexion:** a movement that decreases the angle between two bones; the act of bending a joint.

**Fracture:** any break or crack in a bone.

**Hyperextension:**   continuation of extension beyond the anatomical position, as in bending the head backward.

**Inversion:**   turning inward; movement of the foot at the ankle joint so that the sole faces inward.

**Ligament:**   a band or sheet of strong fibrous connective tissue connecting the articular ends of bones serving to bind them together and to facilitate or limit motion.

**Mobility:**   state or quality of being mobile; facility of movement.

**Musculoskeletal:**   pertaining to the muscles and bones.

**Paralysis:**   temporary or permanent loss of function, especially loss of sensation or voluntary motion.

**Plantar flexion:**   extension of the foot at the ankle joint; the foot and toes are turned downward toward the sole of the foot, as in standing on tiptoe.

**Posture:**   attitude or position of body.

**Prime movers:**   muscles responsible for the primary movement of contraction.

**Pronation:**   rotation of the forearm so that the palm faces backward or downward; movement of the whole body so that the face and abdomen are downward.

**Prone:**   lying horizontal with face downward.

**Protraction:**   movement of the clavicle (collar bone) or mandible (lower jaw) forward on a plane parallel to the ground.

**Proximal:**   nearest the point of attachment or reference point.

**Retraction:**   movement of the clavicle or mandible backward on a plane parallel to the ground.

**Rotation:**   movement of a bone around its own axis, as in moving the head to indicate "no" or turning the palm of the hand up and then down.

**Sprain:**   injury caused by wrenching or twisting of a joint that results in tearing or stretching of the associated ligaments.

**Strain:**   injury caused by excessive force or stretching of muscles or tendons around the joint.

**Supination:**   rotation of forearm so that the palm faces forward or upward; movement of the whole body so that the face and abdomen are upward.

**Synergists:**   muscles that enhance action of prime mover.

**Tendons:**   fibrous connective tissue serving for the attachment of muscles to bones and other parts.

**Tonicity:**   ability of muscle to maintain steady contraction which determines its firmness.

**Ulcer:**   an open sore of the skin or mucous membrane.

# Chapter *15*

# *Medication Administration*

**LEARNING OBJECTIVES**

Explain the concepts of absorption, transportation, biotransformation, and excretion.

State the "five rights" for administering medications.

List the seven parts of a drug order.

Differentiate between unit dose and the more traditional method of medication administration.

Describe the medication cart and its purpose.

Identify three nursing actions that will prevent drug injuries.

Outline the method of calculating oral dosages of drugs.

List at least four assessment factors important for administering parenteral medications.

Outline the steps in preparing for injecting parenteral medications.

State the purpose for using the Z-tract method of injection.

List two insulin types, their action, onset, peak, and duration.

Describe the assessment factors used before applying medications to the skin and mucous membranes.

Outline the steps in applying a topical vasodilator medication.

State four alternative techniques for alleviating patient pain during injections.

Describe the information that should be included in charting injections.

Outline the steps for instilling eye drops.

Differentiate between the positions for instilling ear medications in adults and children.

List the steps for inserting a rectal suppository.

Discuss the Controlled Substance Act of 1970.

## THERAPEUTIC AGENTS

Therapeutic agents are drugs or medications which, when introduced into a living organism, modify the physiological functions of that organism. The term "therapeutic agent" usually refers to a chemical compound. If this substance has an effect on body functions, it can also be a vitamin, mineral, herb, or even a natural food. In this chapter, the term "therapeutic agents" refers to drugs and their actions.

## DRUG METABOLISM

Drug metabolism in the human body is accomplished in four basic stages: absorption, transportation, biotransformation, and excretion. In order for a drug to be completely metabolized, it must first be given in sufficient concentration to produce the desired effect on body tissues. When this "critical drug concentration" level is achieved, body tissues change.

**Absorption**  The first stage of metabolism refers to the route a drug takes from the time it enters the body until it is absorbed in the circulating fluids. Drugs are absorbed by the mucous membranes, the gastrointestinal tract, the respiratory tract, and the skin. The mucous membranes are one of the most rapid and effective routes of absorption because they are highly vascular.

Drugs that are given by mouth are absorbed in the gastrointestinal tract. Portions of these drugs dissolve and are absorbed in the stomach. The rate of absorption depends on the pH of the stomach's contents, the food content in the stomach at the time of ingestion, and the presence of disease conditions. Most of the drug concentrate dissolves in the small intestine where the large vascular surface and moderate pH level enhance the process of breaking down the drug.

Parenteral methods are the most direct, reliable, and rapid route of absorption. This method of administration includes intradermal, subcutaneous/intramuscular, intravenous, and intra-arterial injections. The actual administration site will depend on the type of drug, its action, and the patient. For example, a patient with a severe allergic reaction will receive epinephrine intravenously since this is the fastest route for drug absorption in an emergency situation.

Another route of administration that is faster than the gastrointestinal tract but not as rapid as parenteral injections is inhalation or nebulization of medications through the respiratory system. Drugs administered through the respiratory tract must be made up of small particles that can pass through to the alveoli in the lungs.

The final mode of absorption is the skin. Most drugs, when applied to the skin, produce a local rather than a systemic effect. The degree of absorption will depend on the strength of the drug as well as where it is applied on the body surface.

**Transportation**   The second stage of metabolism refers to the way in which a drug is transported from the site of introduction to the site of action. When a drug enters or is absorbed by the body, it binds to plasma protein in the blood and is transported through circulation to all parts of the body. As a drug moves from the circulatory system, it crosses cell membranes and enters the body tissues. Some of the drug is also distributed to and stored in fat and muscle, where greater masses of tissue attract the drug.

The amount of the drug that is distributed to body tissues depends on the permeability of the membranes and the blood supply to the absorption area.

**Biotransformation**   The third stage of metabolism takes place as the drug, which is a foreign substance in the body, is converted by enzymes into a less active and harmless agent that can be easily excreted. Most of this conversion occurs in the liver, although some conversion does take place in the kidney, plasma, and intestinal mucosa.

**Excretion**   The final stage in metabolism takes place when the drug is changed into an inactive form or excreted from the body. The kidneys are the most important route of excretion because they eliminate both the pure drug and the metabolites of the parent drug. During excretion, these two substances are filtered through the glomeruli, secreted by the tubules, and either reabsorbed through the tubules or directly excreted. Other routes of excretion include the lungs (which exhale gaseous drugs), feces, saliva, tears, and mother's milk.

**Factors That Affect Drug Metabolism**   There are many factors that affect drug metabolism. They include personal attributes, such as body weight, age, and sex; physiological factors, such as state of health or disease processes; acid-base and fluid and electrolyte balance; permeability; diurnal rhythm and circulatory capability. Genetic and immunologic factors play a role in drug metabolism, as do psychological, emotional, and environmental influences, drug tolerance, and cumulation of drugs. Responses to drugs vary, depending on the speed with which the drug is absorbed into the blood or tissues and the effectiveness of the body's circulatory system.

## DRUG ADMINISTRATION

The method of drug administration influences the action of that drug on the body. To obtain a systemic effect, a drug must be absorbed and transported to the cells or tissues that respond to them. How a drug is administered will depend on the chemical nature and quantity of the drug, as well as the desired speed of effect and the overall condition of the patient. Common routes of administration to obtain systemic effects include the following: oral, sublingual, rectal, inhalation, and parenteral. Parenteral injections are commonly administered in these sites: intradermal, subcutaneous, intramuscular, and intravenous.

**Source and Naming of Drugs**  The primary sources from which drugs are compounded are roots, bark, sap, leaves, flowers, and seeds of plants. Other natural sources include animal organs or organ cells and secretions and mineral sources. Synthetic drugs, such as sulfonamides, are made in a laboratory from chemical substances.

Most drugs are given chemical, generic, and trademark names. The chemical name, for example, ethyl, 1-methyl-4-phenylisonipecotate hydrochloride, refers to the chemical derivation of the drug. The generic name, i.e., meperidine hydrochloride, is shorter and simpler and reflects the chemical family to which the drug belongs. Demerol is a trademark name; and this is the most common way in which a drug is known. Once a drug is registered with a brand name (Demerol), that drug can be manufactured only by its legal owner.

**Safety Procedures**  When you administer drugs, you must follow certain safety rules, which are also known as "The Five Rights." These rules should be carried out each time you give a drug to a patient.

*The Five Rights*

☐ Right medication.
  Compare drug card, medication sheet or drug Kardex with drug container three times.
  Know action, dosage, and method of administration.
  Know side effects of the drug.

☐ Right patient—check the patient's ID band and door number.

☐ Right time.

☐ Right method of administration.

☐ Right amount.
  Check all calculations of divided doses with another nurse.
  Check heparin, insulin, and intravenous digitalis doses with another nurse.

**Documenting the Medication**  A medication administered to a patient must have a physician's order or prescription before it can be legally administered. The physician's order is a verbal or written order, which is recorded in a book or file or in the patient's chart. If an order is given verbally over the telephone, you must write a verbal order in the patient's chart for the physician to sign at a later date. Written orders are safer because they leave less room for potential misunderstanding or error.

A drug order should consist of seven parts:

☐ The name of the patient

☐ The date the drug was ordered

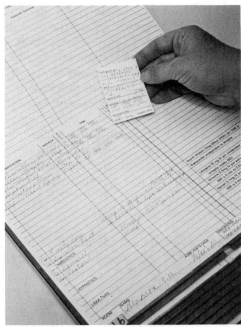

Check medication card against Kardex or order sheet before pouring meds.

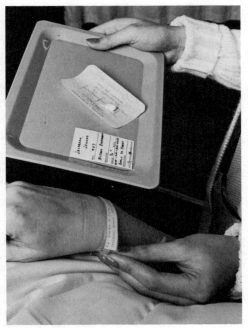

Check patient's identaband and ask name before administering medications.

☐ The name of the drug

☐ The dosage

☐ The route of administration and any special rules of administration

☐ The time and frequency the drug should be given

☐ The signature of the individual who ordered the drug

There are two basic types of drug orders: routine and one-time only drug orders. A routine medication is administered according to instructions until it is cancelled by another order. Routine medication orders can also be used for p.r.n. drugs. These drugs are administered when the patient needs the medication, not necessarily on a routine time schedule. Medication for bowel elimination is a type of p.r.n. drug that is not necessarily administered every day. When you administer medications, you should assess the continued validity of any routine order. Physicians occasionally forget to cancel an order when it is no longer appropriate for a patient's condition. One-time only orders are administered as stated, only one time. These orders may be given at a specified time or "stat," which means immediately.

If you prepare a medication, you must also give it to the patient and chart it after the patient has taken the required dosage. If a patient refuses a medication, you should chart that the medication was refused and report this information to the physician. When you chart medications, be sure to use the correct abbreviations and symbols.

If you find an error in a drug order, such as an inaccurate dose or method of administration, it is your responsibility to question the order. If you cannot understand or read the order, verify it with the physician. Do not guess at the order as this constitutes gross negligence. In many hospitals it is the pharmacist's responsibility to contact physicians when medication orders are unclear.

Always report medication errors to the physician immediately so that potential danger to the patient is minimized. While no nurse or doctor would intentionally commit an error, errors do occur. When they do, it is important that measures be taken immediately to assess and evaluate the patient's status and to institute a plan of action to reverse the effects of the medication.

Errors in medication should also be documented in a medication incident report and on the patient's record. This documentation is necessary for both legal reasons and nursing audits. Nursing audits are conducted to determine if an error in medication indicates one primary problem, a particular source of problems, or a range of problems that seem to have no connection.

Each hospital has its own policies and protocols for administering medications. Before administering any drugs, you must find out what these policies are and perform them accordingly.

## NURSING DIAGNOSES

The following nursing diagnoses may be appropriate to include in a Patient Care Plan when the components relate to a patient who requires treatment with medications.

| Nursing Diagnosis (Potential) | Defining Characteristic; Etiology (Examples) |
|---|---|
| ☐ Health Maintenance, Alteration in, *related to* | Inability to manage own disease process, e.g., age, cognitive, psychosocial or physiological limitations. |
| ☐ Knowledge Deficit, *related to* | Inadequate understanding, e.g., insufficient information, poor communication, cognitive impairment due to physiological change. |
| ☐ Noncompliance, *related to* | Inadequate knowledge base, denial, poor judgment, anxiety, e.g., cognitive, psychological, or aging factors, negative drug side effects. |

## UNIT ONE  PREPARATION FOR DRUG ADMINISTRATION

### NURSING PROCESS DATA

**ASSESSMENT**  *Data Base*

Assess route for drug administration.

Assess specific drug action for patient.

Observe for signs and symptoms of side effects or adverse reactions.

Assess need for and accuracy of drug calculations.

**PLANNING**  *Objectives*

To administer medications using correct route.

To determine appropriate drug actions.

To identify when side effects or adverse reactions occur.

To accurately calculate drug dosages.

## IMPLEMENTATION  *Procedures*

Preparing for Drug Administration

Converting Medications

Calculating Oral Dosages

Calculating Parenteral Dosages

Using a Unit Dose System

Preventing Drug Injuries

## EVALUATION  *Expected Outcomes*

Medications are administered by correct route.

Medication actions and side effects are identified.

Drug dosages are calculated accurately.

## PREPARING FOR DRUG ADMINISTRATION

### Equipment

Pharmacology textbook

Physician's Desk Reference

Hospital Formulary

Index cards

### Procedure

*Before clinical practice*

1. Check all medications your patient is receiving.

2. Determine which drugs are unfamiliar to you.

3. Research unfamiliar drugs using one of the references listed above.

4. Write out drug information on an index card. Include the following information.
   a. Generic and trade name.
   b. Drug classification.
   c. Pharmacological actions.
   d. Usual dosage, route of administration.
   e. Major uses.
   f. Side effects.
   g. Nursing implications.

5. Review procedure for medication administration, e.g., IM, Sub Q, Oral.

6. Calculate dosages if necessary.

7. Review safety procedures of "The Five Rights."

*During clinical practice*

1. Obtain all medication cards (if unit dose system is not used) for drugs to be given during your clinical practice.

2. Check each patient's medication cards against the Kardex card before beginning patient care.
   a. Start with medication listed first on the Kardex card.
   b. Find the appropriate medication card.
   c. Check that the Kardex card and medication card contain the same data: right dosage, time intervals, route of administration.
   d. Check that all medications listed on the Kardex have corresponding medication cards.
   e. If information on the Kardex and Medication cards do not correlate, check the physician's orders for the correct information.

3. If discrepancies exist between the information on your drug card and the ordered drug, check another reference source for information. If you are unable to verify information, consult with the pharmacist and/or physician. **Rationale:** Always verify when dosages or times seem inappropriate. This is for the safety of the patient.

4. Check if the patient has allergies to drugs or food by reading the History and Physical findings, Pa-

tient Care Plan and Kardex. Check the patient's identaband for allergies.

5. Separate medication cards into time frames (e.g. 9– 12– 1 –5) when drugs are to be given. Place drug cards in appropriate place for the drugs that are not to be given on your shift.

6. Take cards to medication room or medication cart and proceed to prepare for administering medications. Only set up the drugs to be administered for the specific time period. Do not set up drugs for the entire day.

## CONVERTING MEDICATIONS

### Equipment

Orders for dosage of medication

Dosage of medication on hand

### Procedure

1. To convert milligrams to grains, use the following formula:

$$\frac{1 \text{ gr}}{\text{Mg in gr}} = \frac{\text{Dose desired}}{\text{Dose on hand}}$$

$$\frac{1}{60} = \frac{x}{180}$$

$$60x = 180$$

$$x = 3 \text{ grains}$$

2. You may also make this conversion as a ratio:

1 gr:60 mg: :x gr:180 mg     $60x = 180$
$x = 3$ grains

3. Check equivalency tables in the drug supplement.

## CALCULATING ORAL DOSAGES

### Equipment

Orders for dosage of medication needed

Dosage of medication on hand

### Procedure

1. To calculate oral dosages, use the following formula. (D and H must be in same unit of measure.)

$$\frac{D}{H} = X$$

where D = dose desired
H = dose on hand
X = dose to be administered

*Example:* Give 500 mg of Ampicillin when the dose on hand is in capsules containing 250 mg.

$$\frac{500 \text{ mg}}{250 \text{ mg}} = 2 \text{ capsules}$$

2. To calculate oral dosages of liquids, use the following formula:

$$\frac{D}{H} \times Q = X$$

where Q = quantity

*Example:* Give 375 mg of Ampicillin when it is supplied as 250 mg/5 ml.

$$\frac{375 \text{ mg}}{250 \text{ mg}} \times 5$$

$$1.5 \times 5 = 7.5 \text{ ml}$$

You can also set up a direct proportion and, following the algebraic principle, cross-multiply:

$$\frac{375 \text{ mg}}{X} = \frac{250 \text{ mg}}{5 \text{ ml}}$$

$$250 X = 1875$$

$$X = 7.5 \text{ ml (of strength 250 mg/5 ml)}$$

## CALCULATING PARENTERAL DOSAGES

### Equipment

Orders for dosage of medication needed

Dosage of medication on hand

### Procedure

1. To calculate parenteral dosages, use the following formula:

D = dose desired
H = dose on hand
Q = quantity
X = amount to be administered

$$\frac{D}{H} \times Q = X$$

*Example:* Give patient 40 mg Gentamicin. On hand is a multidose vial with a strength of 80 mg/2 ml.

$$\frac{40}{80} \times 2 = 1 \text{ ml}$$

2. Check your calculations before drawing up the medications.

3. See Calculations of Solutions in Drug Supplement.

## USING A UNIT DOSE SYSTEM

### Equipment

Medication records in binder or Kardex

Medication cart

Medication keys

### Procedure

*for Oral Meds*

1. Open medication cart, take out patient's medication drawer, and open binder to patient's medication record.

2. Starting at the top of the medication record, check each medication in order against the medication packages in the drawer. Ensure that all doses for your shift are there. **Rationale:** If dose is missing, or too many doses remain, check medication record for possible error in administration.

3. Check each drug and medication record for dose, time and route of administration.

4. Check physician's orders for any discrepancy between medication record and drug package.

5. Take medication cart to the patient's room.

6. Wash your hands.

7. Start at top of medication record and find each drug to be given at that time.

8. Place the individually wrapped drugs in a medication cup. Do not take drugs out of wrapper. The package is a double check before giving med to patient.

9. Check the room number against the medication record, and lock the medication cart before entering the room.

10. Check patient's identaband and ask patient to state name.

11. Check medication name and dosage on the package before opening and placing in medication cup. **Rationale:** This is another safety check to ensure proper dosage.

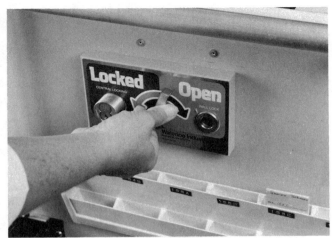

Unlock medication cart by turning knob to OPEN.

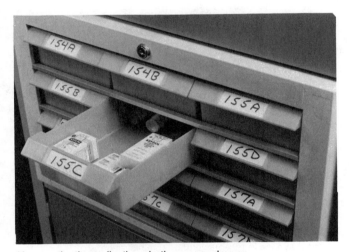

Keep patient's medications in the proper drawer.

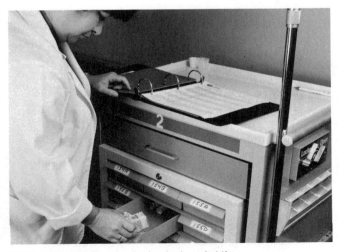

Check all medications at the beginning of shift.

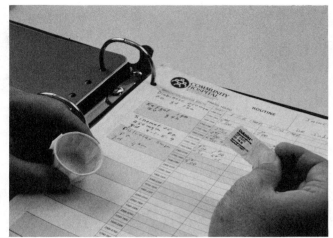

Check individually wrapped medication with record.

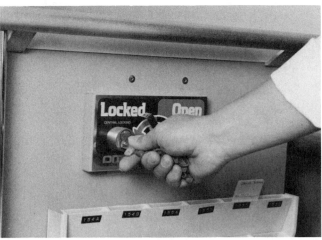

Lock medication cart before administering drug.

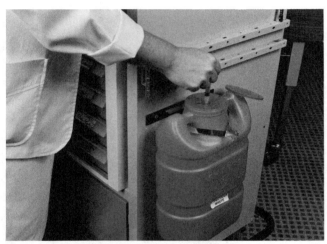

Discard syringe in receptacle after administration.

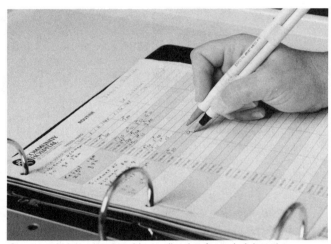

Chart medication in record immediately after administration.

12. Assist patient to sitting position. Hand medication cup and glass of water to patient. Name drug, describe its use, and answer any questions.

13. Ensure patient swallows medications.

14. Position patient for comfort.

15. Dispose of medication wrappers and cup.

16. Chart medications in medication record.

17. Take medication cart to next patient room or medication room.

*for Parenteral Meds*

1. Open medication cart, take out patient's medication drawer, and open binder to patient's medication record.

2. Starting at the top of the medication record, check each medication in order against the medication packages in the drawer. Ensure that all doses for your shift are there.

3. Check each drug and medication record for dose, time and route of administration.

4. Check physician's orders for any discrepancy between medication record and drug package.

5. Take medication cart to the patient's room.

6. Wash your hands.

7. Start at top of medication record and find each drug to be given at that time.

8. Prepare parenteral medications according to procedure.

9. Place syringe and alcohol swab on tray (if hospital policy) or carry to room in your hand.

10. Check the drug name and dosage again.

11. Check the room number against the medication record, and lock the medication cart before entering the room.

12. Check patient's identaband and ask him to state his name.

13. Provide privacy and place patient in appropriate position for type of parenteral medication to be administered.

14. Follow procedure for administering parenteral medications.

15. Position patient for comfort.

16. Discard syringe in container.

17. Wash your hands.

18. Chart medications in medication record.

19. Take medication cart to next patient's room or to medication room.

## PREVENTING DRUG INJURIES

### Equipment

Locked medication cart

Drug room or locked medication cabinet

### Use of Medication Cart

☐ Generally used with unit dose medication system.
☐ This system allows medications to be dispensed directly from cart outside patient's room.
☐ Cart remains locked at all times while nurse is dispensing medications to patient.
☐ Cart may be left unattended in hallway but it must remain locked.
☐ Pharmacy restocks carts once every 24 hours.

### Procedure

1. Keep all medicines in locked carts or cupboards.

2. Remove drugs from bedside unless there is a physician's order.

3. Keep narcotics in double-locked cabinets. Count all narcotics at the end of each shift.

4. Keep all poisonous solutions and materials in a secure area away from medicines.

5. Clearly label and separate topical medicines from parenteral or oral medicines.

6. Provide complete instructions to patients regarding medicines to be used at home. Make sure every physician involved with a patient is aware of the medications the patient is taking home.

Computerized narcotic sign-out record.

## NURSING RESPONSIBILITIES FOR NARCOTIC ADMINISTRATION

1. Check medication card or sheet for narcotic orders.
2. Check time frame since last narcotic administered.
3. Open narcotic box or cupboard and find appropriate narcotic container.
4. Count the number of pills, ampules, or injectable cartridges in container.
5. Check the narcotic sign-out sheet and check that the number of narcotics matches the number of sign-out sheets.
6. Rectify the situation before proceeding with narcotic administration if narcotics and sign-out sheets do not coincide.
7. Sign out for the narcotic on the narcotic sheet after taking narcotic out of drawer or cupboard.
8. Lock drawer on cupboard after taking out medication.
9. Sign out narcotics on medication record according to usual procedure.
10. Check narcotics every 8 hours. One off-going and one on-going nurse check the narcotics. The number of sign-out sheets must match the remaining number of narcotics. Each narcotic sheet is checked for accuracy.
11. Return the counter (if used) to the pharmacy with the completed narcotic sign-out sheet when the sheet is filled. A new narcotic supply and narcotic check sheet are signed out in the pharmacy. The nurse receiving the narcotics signs the drug record receipt.

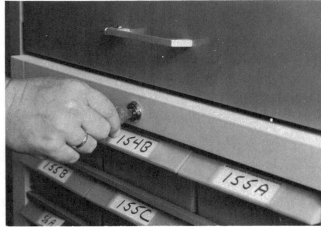

Lock narcotic drawer after removing medication.

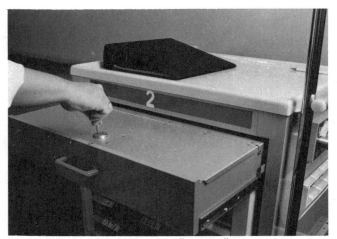

Double lock narcotics drawer according to policy.

7. Have another nurse check mathematical calculations for dosages of drugs such as insulin before administering to patients.

8. Report any errors in the administration of medicines to the charge nurse immediately. Complete a written report if required.

# UNIT TWO   ORAL MEDICATIONS

## NURSING PROCESS DATA

### ASSESSMENT   *Data Base*

Assess that oral route is the most efficient means of medication administration.

Check medication orders for completeness and accuracy.

Assess that five rights for medication administration are followed.

Determine patient's physical ability to take medication as ordered.
>   Swallow reflex present.
>   State of consciousness.
>   Signs of nausea and vomiting.
>   Uncooperative behavior.

Check to make sure you have the correct medication for the patient.

Evaluate correct dosage when calculation is needed.

Observe that patient swallowed medications after administered.

### PLANNING *Objectives*

To ensure that patient metabolizes medication without feelings of nausea or vomiting.

To offer the most common, easiest, and least expensive route of administering medications.

To provide a sustained drug action and increased absorption time.

### IMPLEMENTATION *Procedures*

Preparing Oral Medications

Administering Oral Medications to Adults

Administering Oral Medications to Children

### EVALUATION *Expected Outcomes*

Patient is able to ingest and metabolize medication without feeling nauseated or vomiting.

Patient emotionally accepts medication.

Patient experiences a sustained action of drug and a positive effect on the body.

## PREPARING ORAL MEDICATIONS

### Equipment

Medication: tablet, capsule, or liquid

Water (none if liquid preparation), juice, or milk (if not contraindicated by drug absorption) to prevent gastric irritation

Mortar and pestle for crushing pills (if needed)

Drug card, medication sheet, drug Kardex

Drug cart, if unit dose system is used

### Procedure

1. Obtain patient's medication record. Medication record may be a drug card, medication sheet, or drug Kardex, depending on the method of dispensing medications in your facility.

2. Compare the medication record with the most *recent* physician's order.

3. Check medication three times before taking to patient:
   a. When taking medication from storage area.
   b. Before placing medication into medicine cup.
   c. Before placing medicine bottle back into storage area (unless you are using the unit dose system).

4. Wash your hands.

5. Gather necessary equipment.

6. Remove the medication from the drug box or tray on medication cart.

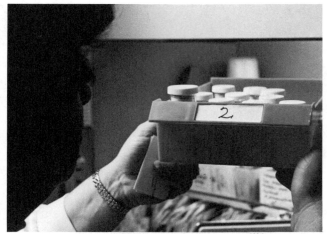

Check medication with card when taking from the storage area.

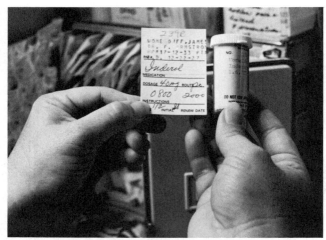

Compare medication card with printed label on drug container.

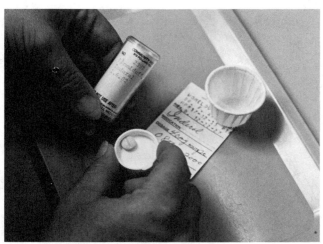

Drop tablet into lid before placing in cup and check against card.

7. Compare the label on the bottle or drug package to the medication record.

8. Correctly calculate dosage if necessary and check the dosage to be administered.

9. Pour the medication from the bottle into the lid of the container and then into the medicine cup. With unit dosage, take drug package from medication cart tray and place in medication cup. Do not remove drug from drug package.

10. When pouring a liquid, set medicine cup on a firm surface and read fluid level at the lowest point of the meniscus.

11. Check medication label again to ensure correct drug and dosages if drug is not prepackaged.

12. Place medication cup on a tray, if not using medication cart.

13. Return the multidose vial bottle to the storage area. If medication to be given is a narcotic, sign out the narcotic sheet with your name.

## ADMINISTERING ORAL MEDICATIONS TO ADULTS

### Equipment

Medication: tablet, capsule, or liquid

Water (none if liquid preparation), juice, or milk (if not contraindicated by drug absorption) to prevent gastric irritation

Mortar and pestle for crushing pills (if needed)

Drug card, medication sheet, drug Kardex

Drug cart, if unit dose system is used

### Preparation

*see Preparing Oral Medications*

### Procedure

1. Take medication tray or cart to patient's room; check room number against medication card or sheet.

2. Place patient in sitting position, if not contraindicated by his condition.

3. Check the patient's identaband and ask patient to state name so that you are sure you have correctly identified him.

4. Tell the patient what type of medication you are going to give and explain the actions this medication will produce.

5. If prepackaged medication is used, read label, take medication out of package, and put into medication cup.

6. Give the medication cup to the patient.

7. Offer a fresh glass of water, or other liquid, to aid swallowing and give assistance with taking medication.

8. Make sure the patient swallows the medication.

9. Discard used medicine cup.

10. Position patient for comfort.

11. Record the medication on the appropriate forms.

---

□ Tablets and capsules are given with water to prevent antagonism of chemical properties of the drug.

□ Cough syrups and antacids are not followed by water because they dilute the topical effect.

□ Crushed pills or liquids may be mixed with a small quantity of bland food, if not contraindicated by the patient's diet.

---

## ADMINISTERING ORAL MEDICATIONS TO CHILDREN

### Equipment

Medication: tablet, capsule, or liquid

Water (none if liquid preparation), juice, or milk (if not contraindicated by drug absorption) to prevent gastric irritation

Mortar and pestle for crushing pills (if needed)

Drug card, medication sheet, drug Kardex

Drug cart, if unit dose system is used

### Preparation

*see Preparing Oral Medications*

### Procedure

1. Follow the procedure for Preparing and Administering Oral Medications. Keep the following guidelines in mind:
   a. Play techniques may help to elicit a young child's cooperation.
   b. Remember: the smaller the quantity of diluent (food or liquid), the greater the ease in eliciting the child's cooperation.
   c. Never use a child's favorite food or drink as an enticement when administering medication because the result may be the child's refusal to eat or drink anything.
   d. Be honest and tell the child that you have medicine, not candy.

2. Assess child for drug action and possible side effects.

3. Explain medication action and side effects to parents.

### CHARTING  *for Oral Medications*

□ Appropriate medication form for facility used

□ Name of drug

□ Dosage

□ Times ordered

□ Time administered

□ Method of administration

□ Initials of nurse administering drug

□ In nurses' notes, comments made on patient tolerance, concerns, and other appropriate information

---

## CLINICAL PROBLEM SOLVING

### Potential Problems

Patient has an allergic or anaphylactic response to the medication.

### Suggested Solutions

□ Immediately stop or hold medication.

□ Notify physician at once; prepare to administer antihistamine.

□ If reaction is severe:
   Keep patient flat in bed with head elevated.
   Take vital signs every 10 to 15 minutes.
   Assess for hypotension or respiratory distress—if latter present administer oxygen via nasal prongs at 6 1/minute.

Have emergency equipment available.

Provide psychological support to patient to alleviate fears.

Record type and progression of allergic reactions.

Patient has difficulty swallowing tablets or capsules.

☐ Use mortar and pestle to crush medications and administer to patient mixed with juice or a food substance such as applesauce.

☐ If totally unable to swallow medications, ask physician to order same or comparable medication by liquid or parenteral route.

---

## UNIT THREE   SUBLINGUAL MEDICATIONS

### NURSING PROCESS DATA

#### ASSESSMENT   *Data Base*

Assess that the drug can be administered sublingually.

Assess patient's ability to understand and follow verbal directions.

Check to see if the area underneath patient's tongue is excoriated and/or painful. If so, do not give medication.

#### PLANNING   *Objectives*

To provide the most appropriate route for fast absorption of drugs such as nitroglycerin and glucose.

To provide the most efficient method of absorption.

To enable patient to experience therapeutic effect.

#### IMPLEMENTATION   *Procedure*

Administering Sublingual Medications

#### EVALUATION   *Expected Outcomes*

Therapeutic effect is achieved as chest pain is relieved following administration of nitroglycerin given sublingually.

Therapeutic effect is experienced within minutes of administration of quick-acting glucose.

---

## ADMINISTERING SUBLINGUAL MEDICATIONS

### Equipment

Medication (kept in dark bottle as nitroglycerin is light-sensitive and loses its potency when exposed to light)

Medication card or appropriate method for correctly identifying patient and medication

### Procedure

1. Follow the procedures for preparing and administering oral medications, with these exceptions:
   a. Explain that patient must not swallow drug or

Sublingual medications, such as nitroglycerin or fast-acting glucose, can be administered to nonresponsive patients because they dissolve rapidly and quickly with no chance of aspiration.

drink any liquid until the drug is completely absorbed.

b. Ask patient to place drug under his tongue or to hold tongue up so that you can place medication under the tongue. **Rationale:** Absorption is enhanced by the thin layer of epithelium underneath the tongue, as well as by the vast network of capillaries in that area.

2. Evaluate patient for drug action and possible side effects.
3. Document actions of drug or patient's response in nurses' notes to monitor effects closely.

## CHARTING   *for Sublingual Medications*

☐ Appropriate medication form for facility used

☐ Name of drug

☐ Dosage

☐ Method of administration

☐ Time administered

☐ Initials of nurse administering drug

## CLINICAL PROBLEM SOLVING

**Potential Problems**

Patient's condition is unchanged with administration of nitroglycerin.

Comatose condition is unaltered with administration of glucagon sublingually.

**Suggested Solutions**

☐ Check bottle for expiration date, as potency decreases after six months.

☐ Administer second tablet in five minutes. (You may give patient three tablets in a 15-minute period.)

☐ Give glucagon sublingually or intravenously if ordered to determine if glucose dose increases blood glucose level and reverses insulin reaction.

☐ Assess for conditions other than hypoglycemia or insulin reaction that may be eliciting comatose response.

# UNIT FOUR   PARENTERAL MEDICATIONS

## NURSING PROCESS DATA

### ASSESSMENT   *Data Base*

Check that appropriate method for administration of drug was ordered.

Assess condition of administration site for presence of lesions, rash, inflammation, lipid dystrophy, ecchymosis, etc.

Assess for tissue damage from previous injections.

Assess patient's level of awareness.

Check patient's written and verbal history for past allergic reactions. Do *not* rely solely on patient's chart.

Review patient's chart noting previous injection sites, especially insulin and heparin administration sites.

**PLANNING** *Objectives*

To perform the injection as painlessly as possible.

To ensure proper drug administration.

To observe and report side effects of the drugs administered.

To alternate injection sites according to protocol.

**IMPLEMENTATION** *Procedures*

Preparing Injections

Administering Intradermal Injections

Administering Subcutaneous (Sub Q) Injections

Administering Insulin Injections

   *for One Insulin Solution*

   *for Two Insulin Solutions*

Administering Intramuscular (IM) Injections

Using Z-Track Method

**EVALUATION** *Expected Outcomes*

Injection is completed without technical complications.

Injection is as painless as possible.

Injection sites are rotated.

## PREPARING INJECTIONS

### Equipment

Medication tray

Alcohol wipes

Vials or ampules of medications

Bottle of diluent (when necessary)

Syringe with appropriate needles:

*Intradermal injections:* short bevel, 26-gauge, ½ to ⅜" needle

*Subcutaneous injections:* 25–gauge, ⅜" to ⅝" needle

*Intramuscular injections:* deltoid muscle requires 23- to 25-gauge, ⅝" needle; needle size for thigh and buttock area varies 1" to 1½"; oil base requires 20-gauge needle; water requires 22-gauge needle; 18- to 23-gauge needles can be used in varying lengths from 1" to 1½". 18-gauge needles are rarely used.

Dry 2 × 2 gauze pad

Bandaid (optional)

### Procedure

1. Obtain patient's medication record. Medication record may be a drug card, medication sheet, or drug Kardex, depending on the method of dispensing medications in your facility.

2. Compare the medication record with the most recent physician's order.

3. Wash your hands.

4. Obtain equipment for injections. **Rationale:** The larger the gauge needle, the smaller the diameter of the cannula.

5. Assemble the needle and syringe maintaining sterility. Select the appropriate size needle. **Rationale:** Consider the size of the patient's muscle mass and the viscosity of the medication in choosing needle size.

6. Open the alcohol wipe and cleanse the top of the vial or break top of ampule.

7. Remove the needle guard and place on alcohol wipe or medication tray.

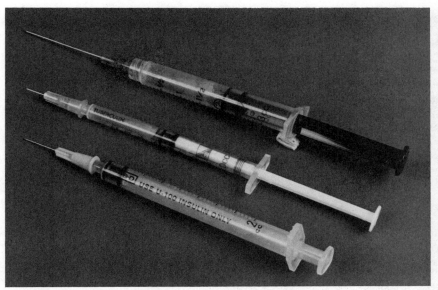

Photo depicts 3cc syringe on the top, tuberculin syringe in the middle, and insulin syringe on the bottom.

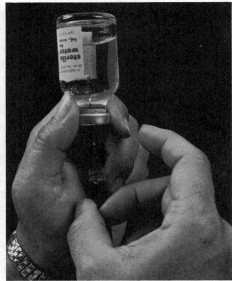

Inject an amount of air equal to the amount of liquid to be withdrawn.

## Types of Injections

*Intradermal or Intracutaneous Injections*

□ Injection sites: inner aspect of forearm or scapular area of back
□ Purpose: for antigens for skin or for tuberculin tests
□ Amount injected: ranges from 0.01 to 0.1 cc
□ Absorption rate: slow

*Subcutaneous Injections*

□ Injection sites: abdomen, lateral aspects of upper arm or thigh
□ Purpose: for medications that are absorbed slowly, to produce a sustained effect
□ Amount injected: variable—small amount of fluid, no more than 1 cc. If repeated doses are necessary, as with insulin for a diabetic, rotate injection sites

*Intramuscular Injections*

□ Injection sites: lateral aspect of thigh (vastus lateralis), buttocks (gluteus maximus), ventral gluteal area, upper arm (deltoid)
□ Purpose: to promote rapid absorption of the drug; to provide an alternate route when drug is irritating to subcutaneous tissues; to provide a less painful route for parenteral medications
□ Amount injected: variable—may be large amount of fluid. If more than 5 cc, use two syringes
□ Absorption rate: depends on circulatory state of patient

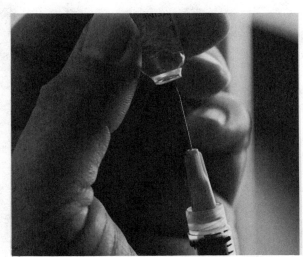

Insert needle into vial without injecting air while withdrawing the medication.

8. Pull back on barrel of syringe to quantity desired if using a vial.

9. Pick up vial, check for correct medication, insert needle into vial, and inject air in an amount equal to the solution to be withdrawn by pushing barrel of syringe down. If using an ampule, break off top at colored line, insert syringe, and withdraw medication. **Rationale:** Do not inject air into ampule as injecting air causes a displacement and possible loss of medication through leakage.

10. Extract the desired amount of fluid. Remove needle from container and cover needle with guard.

11. Double-check drug and dosage against drug card or medication sheet and vial or ampule.

12. Place syringe on tray if tray available.

13. Check label and drug card or medication sheet for correct drug and dose.

14. Return multidose vial to correct storage area or discard used vial or ampule.

## ADMINISTERING INTRADERMAL INJECTIONS

### Equipment

Tuberculin syringe, 26-gauge ½" needle

Medication vial

Alcohol swab

2 × 2 pad

### Preparation

*see Preparing Injections*

### Procedure

1. Take medication to patient's room. Check room number against medication card or sheet.

2. Check patient's identaband and ask patient to state name.

3. Explain the medication's action and the procedure for administration to patient.

4. Wash your hands.

5. Select the site of injection.

6. Cleanse the area with an alcohol wipe, wiping in circular area from inside to outside. **Rationale:** To cleanse from most clean to least clean area.

7. Take off needle guard and place on tray.

8. Grasp patient's forearm from underneath and gently pull the skin taut.

9. Insert the needle at a 10- to 15-degree angle with the bevel of needle facing up.

10. Inject the medication slowly. Observe for wheals and blanching (normal finding) at the site. **Rationale:** Indicates the drug is injected under the epidermis.

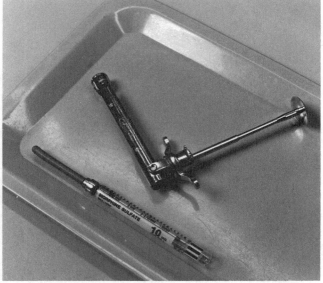

Tubex syringes are always used with prefilled medication carpujects.

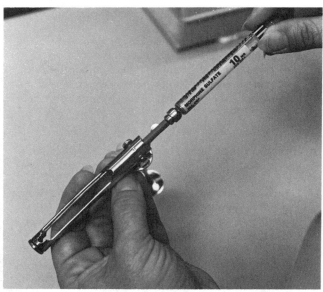

Insert carpuject firmly into tubex syringe and twist until secure.

11. Withdraw the needle, wiping the area gently with a dry 2 × 2 pad. **Rationale:** To prevent dispersing medication into the subcutaneous tissue by applying pressure to the site.

12. Return the patient to a comfortable position.

13. Discard supplies in appropriate area.

14. Chart the medication and site used.

---

### Techniques for Alleviating Pain During Injections

☐ Encourage patient to relax area to be injected: place patient on side with flexed knee or out flat on abdomen, if giving injection in buttock.

☐ Reduce puncture pain by "darting" needle.

☐ Prevent antiseptic from clinging to needle during insertion by waiting until skin antiseptic is dry.

☐ If you must draw needle through rubber stopper, use a new needle for injection of medication.

☐ Avoid injecting sensitive or hardened body areas.

☐ After needle is under skin, aspirate to be certain that needle is not in a blood vessel.

☐ Inject medication slowly.

☐ Maintain grasp on syringe; do not move needle, once inserted.

☐ Withdraw needle quickly after injection.

☐ Massage relaxed muscle gently to increase circulation and to distribute medication.

---

## ADMINISTERING SUBCUTANEOUS (SUB Q) INJECTIONS

### Equipment

3 cc syringe with ⅝″ needle

Medication vial or ampule

2 alcohol swabs

### Preparation

*see Preparing Injections*

### Procedure

1. Take medication to patient's room.

2. Set tray on a clean surface, not the bed.

3. Check patient's identaband and ask patient to state name.

4. Explain action of medication and procedure of administration.

5. Provide privacy when injection site is other than on the arm.

6. Wash your hands.

7. Select site for injection by identifying anatomical landmarks. Remember to alternate sites each time injections are given.

8. Cleanse area with alcohol wipe. Using a circular motion, cleanse from inside outward.

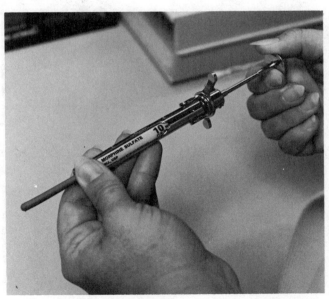

Twist tubex plunger until it fits firmly and tightly into rubber stopper.

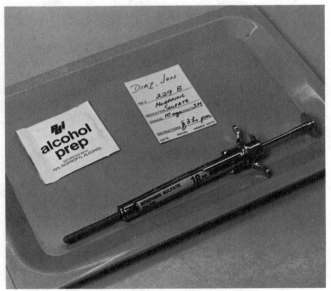

Administer injection using the same technique as with any syringe.

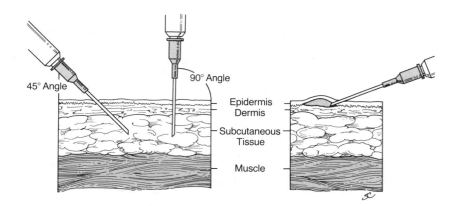

45° Angle

90° Angle

Epidermis
Dermis

Subcutaneous
Tissue

Muscle

Insert needle at 45- or 90-degree angle into tissue for subcutaneous injection.

Insert needle at 15-degree angle just under the epidermis for intradermal injection.

9. Take off needle guard.

10. Express any air bubbles from syringe.

11. Insert the needle at a 45-degree angle while forming a cushion of subcutaneous tissue by gently pinching the tissue. **Rationale:** The angle allows medication to reach the sub q layer but not the muscle.

12. Pull back on the plunger to check if needle is in a blood vessel.

13. Inject the medication slowly.

14. Withdraw needle quickly, and massage area with alcohol wipe to aid absorption. Put on bandaid if needed.

15. Return patient to a position of comfort.

16. Discard used supplies in proper areas. Remember to break needle from syringe and discard needle in safety container.

17. Chart the medication and site used.

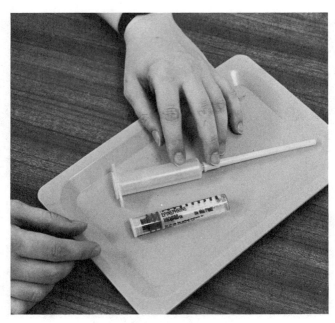

Emergency drugs are found in unit dose syringes.

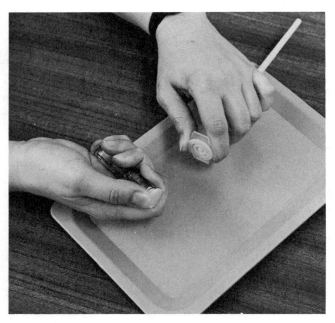

Remove caps from vial and injector.

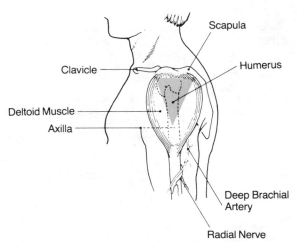

Administer IM or subcutaneous injection in deltoid area. Use shaded area as a guide for injection site.

## ADMINISTERING INSULIN INJECTIONS

### Equipment

Insulin(s)

Insulin syringe with needle

Medication sheet or card

2 alcohol wipes

### Preparation

*see Preparing Injections*

### Procedure

*for One Insulin Solution*

1. Check medication orders, injection site, and rotation chart. Insulin does not need to be refrigerated.

2. Wash your hands.

3. Gather equipment: obtain specific insulin syringe for strength of insulin being administered (U40, U100).

4. Rotate insulin bottle between hands. **Rationale:** This brings solution into suspension for insulins other than regular.

5. Wipe top of insulin bottle with alcohol.

6. Take off needle guard and place on tray.

7. Pull plunger of syringe down to desired amount of medication and inject that amount of air into the insulin bottle.

8. Do not inject air directly into insulin solution. **Rationale:** This causes bubbles in the solution. Bubbles can alter the actual dosage being administered.

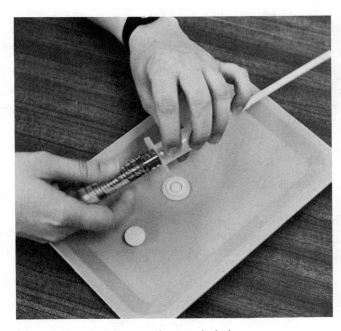

Insert vial into the injector and rotate clockwise.

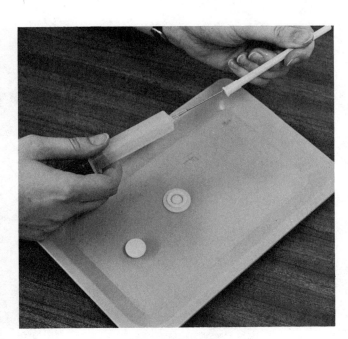

Twist and pull to remove cover from needle.

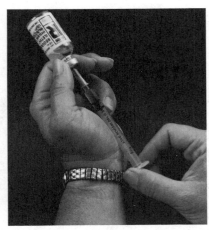

Use specific insulin syringe for strength of
insulin being administered.

**TABLE 1** INSULIN TYPES AND ACTION

| TYPES | ONSET | PEAK | DURATION |
|---|---|---|---|
| Rapid Acting | | | |
| Regular | ½ to 1 | 2 to 4 | 6 to 8 |
| Semilente | ½ to 1 | 2 to 8 | 10 to 16 |
| Intermediate Acting | | | |
| NPH | 1 to 1½ | 8 to 12 | 24 |
| Lente | 1 to 1½ | 8 to 12 | 24 |
| Long Acting | | | |
| Protamine zinc (PZI) | 4 to 8 | 14 to 20 | 24 to 36 |
| Ultralente | 4 to 8 | 16 to 24 | 36 |

9. Draw up ordered amount of insulin into syringe and remove needle from vial.

10. Expel air from syringe.

11. Replace needle guard.

12. Check medication card, bottle, and syringe with an RN for accuracy.

13. Take medication to patient's room.

14. Double-check site of last injection with patient.

15. Provide privacy.

16. Wash your hands.

17. Follow protocol for administration of medications by subcutaneous injections.

*for Two Insulin Solutions*

1. Check medication orders, injection site, and rotation chart. Insulin does not need to be refrigerated.

2. Wash your hands.

3. Gather equipment: obtain specific insulin syringe for strength of insulin being administered (U40, U100).

4. Rotate insulin bottle between hands. This brings solution into suspension for insulins other than regular.

5. Wipe top of insulin bottles with alcohol.

6. Take needle guard off and place on tray.

7. Pull plunger of syringe down to desired units of insulin.

8. Insert needle and inject prescribed amount of air into intermediate acting (NPH, lente) or long acting (PZI, ultralente) bottle.

9. Pull needle out of insulin bottle and withdraw plunger to prescribed regular insulin dosage.

10. Inject air into regular bottle and withdraw medication. Check dose with another nurse.

11. Expel all air bubbles.

12. Insert needle into second insulin bottle taking care not to push any regular insulin into bottle. This can be avoided by putting gentle "pull back" pressure on plunger with your small finger when inserting needle into bottle. **Rationale:** This prevents insulin from being injected into second bottle and thus having incorrect amount of regular insulin.

13. Invert bottle and pull back on plunger to obtain prescribed amount of insulin. Remember the total insulin dose will include the amount of regular insulin already drawn up into syringe.

14. Expel air from syringe.

15. Replace needle guard.

16. Check medication card, bottle, and syringe with another nurse for accuracy.

17. Take medications to patient's room.

18. Double-check site of last injection with patient.

19. Provide privacy.

20. Wash your hands.

21. Follow protocol for administration of medications by subcutaneous injections.

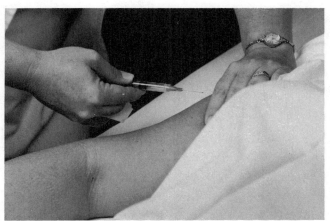

Insert needle at 45° or 90° angle to inject into subcutaneous tissue.

**TABLE 2** PURIFIED PORK INSULIN PREPARATIONS

*Actrapid*
Short acting
Rapid effect
Duration: 6 to 8 hours
Method: IV and sub q

*Semitard*
Prompt purified pork insulin
Short acting
Duration 12 to 16 hours
Zinc suspension
Method: sub q

*Monotard*
Purified pork insulin
Intermediate acting
Duration: 24 hours
Zinc suspension
Method: sub q

*Lentard*
Purified pork and beef insulin
Intermediate acting
Duration: 24 hours
Zinc suspension
Method: sub q administration only

*Ultratard*
Extended purified beef insulin
Long acting
Duration: 36 hours
Zinc suspension
Method: sub q

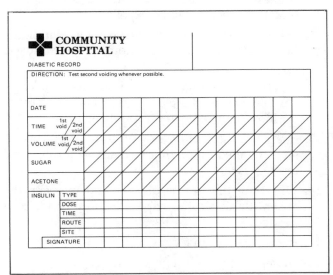

Document pertinent diabetic information on record.

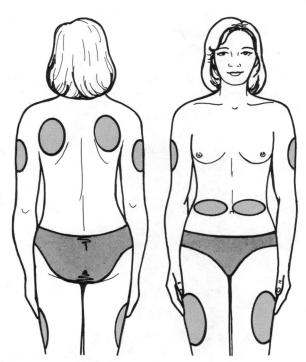

Rotate sites for subcutaneous injections given routinely.

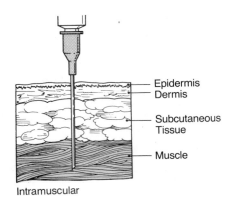

Insert needle at 90-degree angle for intra-muscular injections.

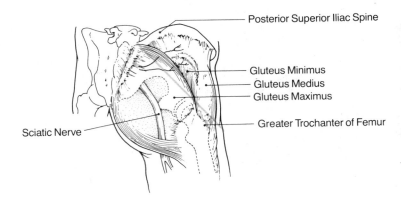

Place injection in gluteus medius above and outside the diagonal line for intramuscular injections.

# ADMINISTERING INTRAMUSCULAR (IM) INJECTIONS

## Equipment

Medication vial or ampule

3cc syringe with 1″ to 1½″ needle

2 alcohol swabs

## Preparation

*see Preparing Injections*

## Procedure

1. Take medication to patient's room. Check room number against medication card or sheet.

2. Set tray on a clean surface, not the bed.

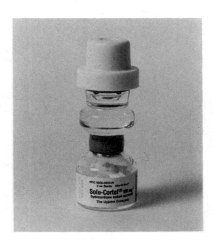

Mix-O-Vial contains solute and solvent.

3. Check patient's identaband and have patient state name.

4. Explain the procedure to patient.

5. Provide privacy for patient.

6. Wash your hands.

7. Select the site of injection by identifying anatomical landmarks. Remember to alternate sites each time injections are given.

8. Cleanse the area with alcohol wipe. Using a circular motion cleanse from inside outward.

9. Hold the syringe; take off needle cover.

10. Express air bubbles from syringe. Some clinicians suggest leaving a small air bubble at the top so that all medicine will be expelled.

11. Insert the needle at a 90-degree angle. **Rationale:** The angle permits medication to reach muscle layer.

12. Pull back on plunger. If blood returns, you know you have entered a blood vessel and need to reposition the needle and aspirate again.

13. Inject the medication slowly. **Rationale:** This allows the medication time to disperse through the tissue.

14. Withdraw the needle quickly and massage the area with an alcohol wipe. Put on a bandaid, if needed.

15. Return patient to a comfortable position.

16. Discard supplies in appropriate area.

17. Chart the medication and site used.

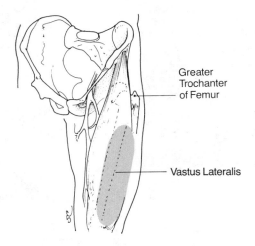

Greater Trochanter of Femur

Vastus Lateralis

Use one hand-breadth above knee and one hand-breadth below greater trochanter.

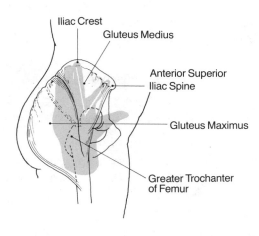

Iliac Crest

Gluteus Medius

Anterior Superior Iliac Spine

Gluteus Maximus

Greater Trochanter of Femur

Insert needle in "V" area after placing heel of hand over greater trochanter of femur.

## USING Z-TRACK METHOD

### Equipment

Syringe

2 needles (one 2″ to 3″ needle)

Alcohol swabs

Medication

### Preparation

*see Preparing Injections*

### Procedure

1. Check the medication record with physician's order.

2. Gather equipment.

3. Wash your hands.

4. Draw up prescribed medication into syringe.

5. Draw up 0.3 to 0.5 cc of air into syringe.

6. Replace needle with 3-inch needle to penetrate deep into muscle. This method is used for iron injections.

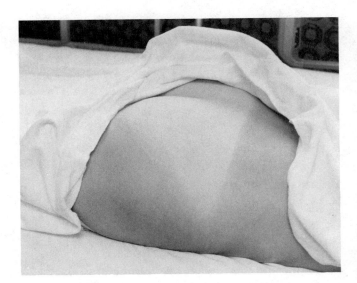

Use gluteus maximus muscle for deep intramuscular injections.

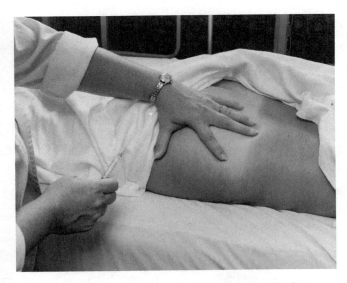

Position hand for proper placement of intramuscular injections.

7. Take medication to patient's room; check room number against medication card or sheet.

8. Check identaband and ask patient to state his name.

9. Explain reason for injection.

10. Provide patient privacy.

11. Wash your hands.

12. Place in prone position, if possible.

13. Pull skin laterally away from injection site. **Rationale:** Keeps medication from seeping into subcutaneous tissue.

14. Cleanse site with alcohol.

15. Insert needle. Pull back on plunger to check if needle is in blood vessel.

16. Inject medication slowly—and wait ten seconds keeping skin taut.

17. Withdraw needle and then release skin. Do not massage. **Rationale:** Massage of skin causes tissue damage.

18. Discard supplies in appropriate area.

19. Chart medication and site used.

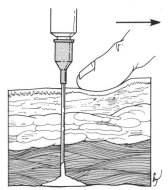

Z-Track Injection

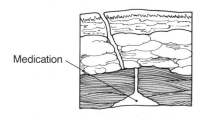

Medication

Z-track is used to prevent tracking of medications on the skin.

### CHARTING *for Parenteral Medications*

☐ Use appropriate medication form for facility

☐ Name of drug

☐ Dosage

☐ Method of administration

☐ Times ordered

☐ Time administered

☐ Initials of nurse administering drug

☐ In nurses' notes, make appropriate comments concerning patient's condition, concerns, feelings, etc.

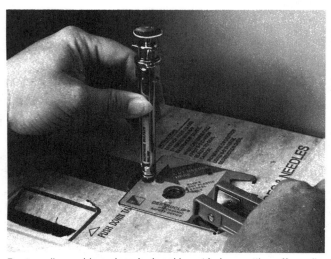

Destroy disposable syringe by breaking at hub or cutting off needle.

## CLINICAL PROBLEM SOLVING

**Potential Problems**

Pain is experienced during parenteral injections.

**Suggested Solutions**

☐ Encourage patient to relax area to be injected; place patient on side with flexed knee or out flat on abdomen with toes pointed inward if giving injection in buttock.

☐ Reduce puncture pain by "darting" needle.

☐ Prevent antiseptic from clinging to needle during insertion by waiting until skin antiseptic is dry.

<table>
<tr><td></td><td>

☐ If you must draw needle through rubber stopper, use a new needle for injection of medication. Prevents dulling of the needle.

☐ Avoid injecting sensitive or hardened body areas.

☐ Inject medication slowly.

☐ Maintain grasp on syringe.

☐ Withdraw needle quickly after injection.

☐ Massage relaxed muscle gently to increase circulation and to distribute medication unless contraindicated.

</td></tr>
</table>

**Sciatic nerve is touched with needle when administering IM injection.**

☐ Notify physician.

☐ Fill out incident report.

☐ Take greater care to identify anatomical landmarks.

☐ Locate a line from posterosuperior iliac spine to the greater trochanter of the femur; injection lateral and slightly superior to midpoint of line.

☐ Obtain order for warm, moist packs.

☐ Reassure patient that permanent damage is unlikely and pain will dissipate.

☐ Assess need for pain medication.

**Medication is administered using wrong parenteral route.**

☐ Notify physician and initiate incident report.

☐ Medications may need to be administered to reverse the action of the medication.

☐ Insulin or heparin administered IM rather than sub q. leads to slower absorption rates; therefore an assessment needs to be done to determine effectiveness of medication. (S/A to determine effectiveness of insulin and PTT level for heparin injection.)

**Ecchymosis occurs following heparin injection.**

☐ Rotate injection site. Do not inject medication into ecchymotic area.

☐ Do not massage injection site following needle withdrawal.

☐ When forming fat pad in preparation for injection site, do not pinch tightly as ecchymosis can occur.

☐ Warm, dry treatments may be administered to hasten ecchymosis reabsorption.

☐ Administer medication at room temperature to prevent tissue trauma with injections.

**Patient has an anaphylactic allergic response.**

☐ Maintain patent airway.

☐ Position patient for optimal cerebral perfusion—flat or 30-degree elevation if dyspneic.

☐ Notify physician immediately.

☐ Be prepared to carry out the following actions following physician's orders.

☐ Administer oxygen 6 l/min via nasal prongs as ordered after epinephrine for bronchodilation.

☐ Notify charge nurse to insert IV line for administering $D_5W$ solution.

□ Monitor patient for alterations in signs and symptoms to determine patient status.

□ Monitor vital signs frequently until the patient's status is stabilized.

---

# UNIT FIVE   TOPICAL MEDICATIONS

## NURSING PROCESS DATA

### ASSESSMENT   *Data Base*

Observe for open lesions, rashes, or areas of erythema and skin breakdown.

Assess for known allergies as related by the patient and/or as noted in the chart.

Observe local changes in the skin occurring from the use of the drug.

Assess for proper medication administration.

### PLANNING   *Objectives*

To promote absorption of medication more rapidly through use of certain topical medications.

To treat skin disorders or lesions caused by burns or abnormal growths.

To dilute effects of a drug (local action may be less than systemic).

To apply an agent that stops, slows, or prevents the growth of microorganisms.

To provide a local anesthetic to specified parts of the body.

### IMPLEMENTATION   *Procedures*

Applying Ointments and Salves

Applying Ointment to Burns

Applying Topical Vasodilators

### EVALUATION   *Expected Outcomes*

Skin returned to normal state.

Alleviation of symptoms for which medication was administered.

Decreased pain.

Control of microorganisms.

---

## APPLYING OINTMENTS AND SALVES

### Equipment

Medication container

Application tube (if needed)

2 × 2 pads for cleansing

Tongue blade

Gloves

Sterile gauze

Commercially prepared burn dressings

**Preparation**

1. Obtain patient's medication record. Medication record may be a drug card, medication sheet, or drug Kardex, depending on the method of dispensing medications in your facility.

2. Compare the medication record with the most *recent* physician's order.

3. Wash your hands.

4. Gather necessary equipment including gloves or tongue blade as needed.

5. Remove the medication from the drug box or tray on medication cart.

6. Compare the label on the medication tube or jar to the medication record.

7. Place medication tube or jar (include a tongue blade with jar) on a tray if not using medication cart.

**Procedure**

1. Take medication to patient's room; check room number against medication card or sheet.

2. Check patient's identaband and ask patient to state name.

3. Provide patient privacy.

4. Wash your hands.

5. Cleanse skin surface with soap and water unless contraindicated by patient's condition. Dry thoroughly.

6. Squeeze medication from a tube or, using a tongue blade, take ointment out of jar.

7. Spread a small, smooth, thin quantity of medication evenly over patient's skin surface using your fingers or a tongue blade.

8. Protect skin surface with a dressing, if needed, so that medication cannot rub off.

9. Check to see that patient is comfortable before leaving room.

10. Return medication to appropriate storage area.

11. Wash your hands.

## APPLYING OINTMENT TO BURNS

**Equipment**

Medication container

Application tube (if needed)

2 × 2 pads for cleansing

Tongue blade

Sterile gloves

Sterile gauze (for burn dressing)

Commercially prepared burn dressings

**Preparation**

*see Applying Ointments and Salves*

**Procedure**

1. Take medication to patient's room; check room number against medication card or sheet.

2. Check patient's identaband and call patient by name.

3. Provide patient privacy.

4. Wash your hands.

5. Squeeze medication from a tube or, using a tongue blade, take ointment out of jar.

6. If *no dressing is ordered,* apply drug directly to burn area; using sterile gloves and tongue blade, cover entire burn area with medication. **Rationale:** To provide an occlusive effect.

7. If *dressing is ordered,* use sterile gloves to rub drug directly into sterile gauze. Then apply medicated gauze to burn area. (Commercially prepared premedicated gauze dressings can be applied directly to burn area, using sterile technique.) Cover medicated dressings with sterile Kerlix.

8. Check to see that patient is comfortable before leaving room.

9. Return drug and/or equipment to appropriate storage area.

10. Wash your hands.

## APPLYING TOPICAL VASODILATORS

**Equipment**

Medication container

Gloves

Premeasured paper

**Preparation**

*see Applying Ointments and Salves*

**Procedure**

1. Take medication to patient's room, check room number against medication card or sheet.

2. Check patient's identaband and call patient by name.

3. Provide patient privacy.

4. Wash your hands.

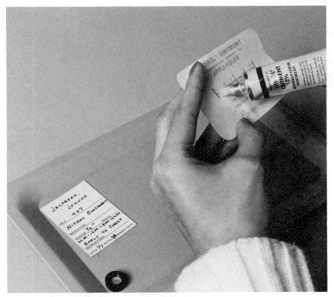

Use premeasured paper for vasodilator medication.

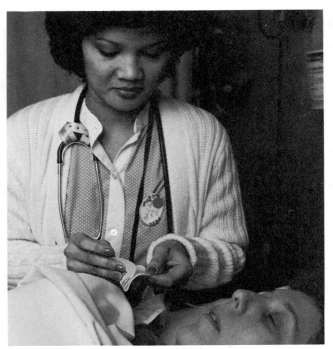

Spread paste on the paper in prescribed amount.

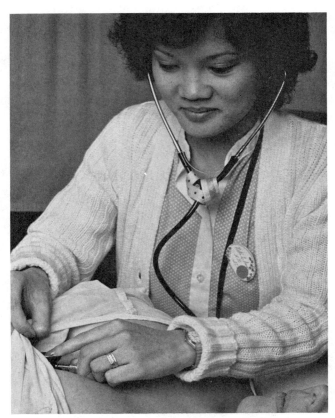

Check patient's apical pulse before applying medication.

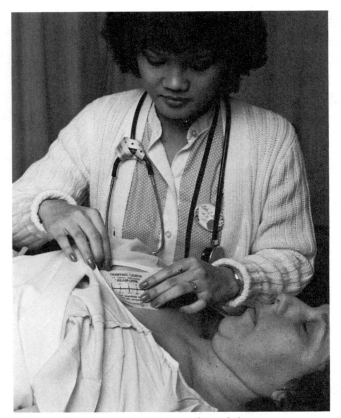

Apply medicated paper to anterior surface of chest.

5. Put on gloves. **Rationale:** To prevent absorbing any medication yourself.

6. Obtain premeasured paper, which accompanies medication tube.

7. Place prescribed medication directly on paper (usually one-half to one-inch strip).

8. Apply medicated paper to anterior surface of chest. You may apply medicated paper to any area of the body. **Rationale:** Most patients feel the medication works better if applied to the chest surface; therefore, it is most frequently used area.

9. Alternate areas of the chest with each dose of medication.

10. Check to see that patient is comfortable before leaving room.

11. Return medication to appropriate storage area.

12. Wash your hands.

### CHARTING  *for Topical Medications*

☐ Appropriate medication form for facility

☐ Name of drug

☐ Dosage

☐ Times ordered

☐ Time administered

☐ Method of administration

☐ Initials of nurse administering drug

☐ In nurses notes, make comments on skin condition, any areas of irritation, erythema, etc.

---

## CLINICAL PROBLEM SOLVING

**Potential Problems**

Skin irritation due to medication.

Patient has allergic response (hives, rash, or itching).

Headache occurs after nitroglycerine ointment applied to skin.

**Suggested Solutions**

☐ Notify the physician so that medication may be discontinued.

☐ Hold medication; notify physician.
☐ Obtain order for antihistamine if necessary.

☐ Notify physician. Usually decrease in dosage is ordered.
☐ Administer analgesic if ordered.

## UNIT SIX  EYE MEDICATIONS

### NURSING PROCESS DATA

#### ASSESSMENT  *Data Base*

Assess patient's ability to cooperate during administration, since medications are instilled into the lower conjunctival sac.

Check medication expiration date.

Assess condition of eye and surrounding areas.

#### PLANNING  *Objectives*

To provide direct route for local effect.

To decrease intraocular pressure.

To provide means for eye evaluation.

To obtain desired therapeutic effect.

> **IMPLEMENTATION** *Procedures*
>
> Instilling Eye Drops
> Medicating Upper Lid
> Medicating Lower Lid
>
> **EVALUATION** *Expected Outcomes*
>
> Patient cooperates with instillation of eye medication.
> Desired therapeutic effect is obtained.
> Eye surgery or evaluation is accomplished.
> Intraocular pressure is reduced.

## INSTILLING EYE DROPS

### Equipment

Eye drops
Cotton ball or tissue

### Preparation

1. Obtain patient's medication record. Medication record may be a drug card, medication sheet, or drug Kardex, depending on the method of dispensing medications in your facility.
2. Compare the medication record with the most *recent* physician's order.
3. Wash your hands.
4. Gather necessary equipment.
5. Remove the medication from the drug box or tray on medication cart.
6. Compare the label on the medication bottle to the medication record.
7. Check that medication is to be administered via *right method*, at *right time*, in *right amount*.

### Procedure

1. Place medication on a tray if not using medication cart.
2. Take medication to patient's room, and check room number against medication card or sheet.
3. Check patient's identaband and ask patient to state name.
4. Wash your hands.
5. Explain procedure to patient.
6. Tilt patient's head slightly backward and ask him to look up. **Rationale:** The cornea is protected as it goes up under the eyelid.
7. Squeeze the prescribed amount of medication into eye dropper. Hold dropper with bulb in uppermost position.
8. Give tissue to patient for wiping off excess medication.
9. Expose lower conjunctival sac by pulling down on cheek.
10. Drop prescribed medication into center of sac. **Rationale:** Do *not* place medication directly on cornea, since medication can cause injury to cornea.
11. Ask patient to close eyelids and move eyes. **Rationale:** This distributes solution over conjunctival surface and anterior eyeball.
12. Remove excess medication from surrounding tissue.
13. Wash your hands.
14. Replace medication in appropriate place.

## MEDICATING UPPER LID

### Equipment

Eye ointment
Cotton ball or tissue
Applicator stick

### Preparation

1. Obtain patient's medication record. Medication record may be a drug card, medication sheet, or

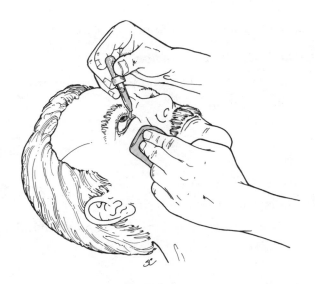

Drop eye medication in the center of lower conjunctival sac.

drug Kardex, depending on the method of dispensing medications in your facility.

2. Compare the medication record with the most *recent* physician's order.

3. Wash your hands.

4. Gather necessary equipment.

5. Remove the medication from the drug box or tray on medication cart.

6. Compare the label on the medication tube to the medication record.

7. Check that medication is to be administered via *right method*, at *right time*, in *right amount*.

## Procedure

1. Place medication on a tray if not using medication cart.

2. Take medication to patient's room, and check room number against medication card or sheet.

3. Check patient's identaband and ask patient to state name.

4. Wash your hands.

5. Explain procedure to patient.

6. Instruct patient to look down.

7. Grasp patient's lashes near center of upper lid with your thumb and index finger. Draw lid down and away from eyeball.

8. With your opposite hand, place applicator horizontally along upper part of eyelid.

9. While pressing down on applicator, quickly turn eyelid up over the applicator.

10. Squeeze ointment over entire lid starting at the inner canthus.

11. Instruct patient to close lid and move eye to assist in spreading medication, if not contraindicated.

12. Remove excess medication from surrounding tissue.

13. Wash your hands.

14. Replace medication in appropriate place.

## MEDICATING LOWER LID

### Equipment

Ointment

Cotton ball or tissue

### Preparation

1. Obtain patient's medication record. Medication record may be a drug card, medication sheet, or drug Kardex, depending on the method of dispensing medications in your facility.

2. Compare the medication record with the most *recent* physician's order.

3. Wash your hands.

4. Gather necessary equipment.

5. Remove the medication from the drug box or tray on medication cart.

6. Compare the label on the medication tube to the medication record.

7. Check that medication is to be administered via *right method*, at *right time*, in *right amount*.

### Procedure

1. Place medication on a tray if not using medication cart.

2. Take medication to patient's room, and check room number against medication card or sheet.

3. Check patient's identaband and ask patient to state name.

4. Wash your hands.

5. Explain procedure to patient.

6. Take protective guard off medication tip.

7. Gently separate patient's eyelids with your thumb or two fingers, and grasp lower lid near the margin of the lower lid immediately below

the lashes. Exert pressure downward over the bony prominence of the cheek.

8. Instruct the patient to look upward. **Rationale:** To keep cornea out of way of medication.

9. Place eye medication on the entire lower lid. Squeeze 2 cm of ointment from the tube starting at the inner canthus.

10. Ask patient to close eyelids and move eyes to assist in spreading ointment under the lids and over the surface of the eyeball.

11. With a cotton ball or soft tissue, remove the excess medication from patient's eye and cheek.

12. Wash your hands.

13. Replace medication to proper place.

### CHARTING  *for Eye Medications*

☐ Appropriate medication form for facility used

☐ Name of drug

☐ Dosage

☐ Method of administration

☐ Times ordered

☐ Time administered

☐ Initials of nurse administering drug

☐ Nurses' notes: condition of eye and surrounding tissue

---

## CLINICAL PROBLEM SOLVING

**Potential Problems**

Infection is introduced because of break in aseptic technique.

Irritation of eye occurs.

**Suggested Solutions**

☐ Medication dropper contaminated. Discard dropper and obtain new one.

☐ Review the recommended procedures for administering the medication and have another nurse observe until you perfect the skill of administering eye medications.

☐ Notify physician for new orders.

☐ Obtain orders for sterile soaks to ease pain and discomfort.

---

## UNIT SEVEN   EAR MEDICATIONS

### NURSING PROCESS DATA

#### ASSESSMENT  *Data Base*

Assess patient's ability to cooperate with instillation.

Assess patient's ability to be positioned on side.

#### PLANNING  *Objectives*

To soften ear wax.

To relieve pain and obtain desired therapeutic effect.

To apply anesthetic agent.

To provide route for antibacterial medications.

#### IMPLEMENTATION  *Procedure*

Administering Ear Medications

## ADMINISTERING EAR MEDICATIONS

### Equipment

Medication

Dropper for instilling medication

Cotton wick

### Preparation

1. Obtain patient's medication record. Medication record may be a drug card, medication sheet, or drug Kardex, depending on the method of dispensing medications in your facility.
2. Compare the medication record with the most *recent* physician's order.
3. Wash your hands.
4. Gather necessary equipment.
5. Remove the medication from the drug box or tray on medication cart.
6. Compare the label on the medication bottle to the medication record.
7. Check that medication is to be administered via *right method*, at *right time*, in *right amount*.

8. Before preparing medication for administration, warm medication bottle to body temperature.

### Procedure

1. Place medication on a tray if not using medication cart.
2. Take medication to patient's room, and check room number against medication card or sheet.
3. Check patient's identaband and ask patient to state name.
4. Explain procedure to patient.
5. Wash your hands.
6. Position patient on side, with ear to be treated in the uppermost position. **Rationale:** To allow medication to enter external ear canal.
7. Fill medication dropper with prescribed amount of medication.
8. Prepare patient for instillation of ear medication as follows:
   a. *Infant.* Draw the auricle gently downward and backward to separate the drum membrane from the floor of the cartilaginous canal.

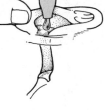

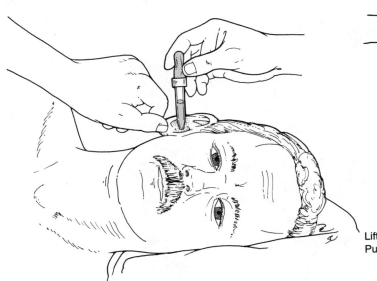

Lift auricle upward and backward for instilling medications for adults.
Pull auricle downward and backward for children.

b. *Adult.* Lift the pinna upward and backward. **Rationale:** These positions straighten out the ear canal.

9. Instill medication and insert a loose cotton wick into the canal to maintain a continuous application of the solution (optional).

10. Instruct patient to remain on his side for 15 minutes following instillation. **Rationale:** To prevent medication from escaping.

**CHARTING** *for Ear Medications*

□ Appropriate medication form for facility used
□ Name of drug
□ Dosage
□ Method of administration
□ Times ordered
□ Time administered
□ Initials of nurse adminstering drug

## CLINICAL PROBLEM SOLVING

**Potential Problems**

Patient moves unexpectedly, causing medication to run down patient's neck.

Patient complains medication is too warm.

**Suggested Solutions**

□ Repeat explanation of procedure to patient.
□ Readminister medication while holding patient in the correct position. Keep patient positioned on side for 15 minutes after instillation.

□ Check to ensure medication is heated only to 98.6° F.
□ Observe patient for any untoward effects.

# UNIT EIGHT   MUCOUS MEMBRANE DRUGS

## NURSING PROCESS DATA

### ASSESSMENT   *Data Base*

Observe for open lesions, rashes, or areas of erythema and breakdown.

Assess for known allergies as related by the patient and/or as noted in the chart.

Observe local changes in the mucous membranes.

Assess for proper medication administration.

### PLANNING   *Objectives*

To dilute effects of a drug or to dilate or contract pupil.

To apply an agent that stops, slows, or prevents infection or inflammation.

To provide local anesthesia to specified parts of the body to relieve pain or discomfort.

To provide relief of nasal congestion.

To provide more appropriate surface for absorption.

### IMPLEMENTATION   *Procedures*

Applying Medications to Mucous Membranes

Instilling Nose Drops

**EVALUATION**  *Expected Outcomes*

Mucous membrane returned to normal state.

Alleviation of symptoms for which medication was administered.

Increased comfort and relief.

Infection or inflammation controlled.

## APPLYING MEDICATIONS TO MUCOUS MEMBRANES

### Equipment

Medication container

Application tube (if needed)

Medication dropper for nasal drops

2 × 2 pads for cleansing

Tongue blade

Gloves

### Preparation

1. Obtain patient's medication record. Medication record may be a drug card, medication sheet, or drug Kardex, depending on the method of dispensing medications in your facility.
2. Compare the medication record with the most recent physician's order.
3. Wash your hands.
4. Gather necessary equipment.
5. Remove the medication from the drug box or tray on medication cart.
6. Compare the label on the medication bottle, tube, or jar to the medication record.
7. Place medication bottle, tube, or jar (include a tongue blade with jar) on a tray if not using medication cart.
8. Check drug information to determine if appropriate for application to mucous membranes.

### Procedure

1. Verify which method is most appropriate for applying medication to mouth or vagina: instilling, swabbing, spraying, irrigating, or douching.
2. Take medication to patient's room; check room number against medication card or sheet.
3. Wash your hands.
4. Provide patient privacy.

5. Complete application according to specific method of application.
6. For specific information on application methods, review drug information pamphlets that accompany medications.

## INSTILLING NOSE DROPS

### Equipment

Medication

Dropper

### Preparation

*see Applying Medications to Mucous Membranes*

### Procedure

1. Take medication to patient's room; check room number against medication card or sheet.
2. Wash your hands.
3. Place patient in sitting position with head tilted back, or in supine position with head tilted back over pillow.
4. Fill dropper with prescribed amount of medication.
5. Place dropper just inside the nares and instill correct number of drops. Repeat procedure in other nares.
6. Instruct patient not to sneeze and to keep head tilted back for five minutes to prevent medication from escaping.
7. Return medication to appropriate storage area.
8. Check to see that patient is comfortable before leaving room.

### CHARTING  *for Mucous Membranes*

☐  Appropriate medication form for facility used

☐  Name of drug

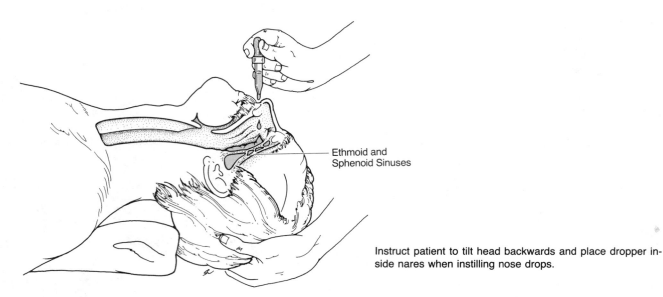

Ethmoid and
Sphenoid Sinuses

Instruct patient to tilt head backwards and place dropper inside nares when instilling nose drops.

□ Dosage
□ Method of administration
□ Times ordered
□ Time administered

□ Initials of nurse administering drug
□ In nurses' notes, discussion of status of mucous membrane, patient tolerance of medication, and observed effects of medication

## CLINICAL PROBLEM SOLVING

**Potential Problem**

Skin irritation occurs.

**Suggested Solution**

□ Hold medication and notify physician.

## UNIT NINE    SUPPOSITORY MEDICATIONS

### NURSING PROCESS DATA

#### ASSESSMENT    *Data Base*

Observe for signs of rectal irritation and/or bleeding.

Observe for hemorrhoids.

Check sphincter control.

Observe for presence of vaginal irritation or secretions.

#### PLANNING    *Objectives*

To provide alternate route when upper GI tract is malfunctioning, i.e., vomiting.

To offer alternate route when drug has offensive taste or odor.

To maintain chemical integrity of drug when digestive enzymes change the chemical properties of the drug.

To obtain high blood concentration of the drug.

To assist in bowel elimination.

### IMPLEMENTATION  *Procedures*

Inserting Rectal Suppositories

Inserting Vaginal Suppositories

### EVALUATION  *Expected Outcomes*

Medication is inserted without technical complications.

Medication enters the bloodstream and is effectively utilized.

Medications are maintained without expulsion.

Bowel elimination is achieved.

## INSERTING RECTAL SUPPOSITORIES

### Equipment

Suppository as ordered

Disposable glove or fingercot

K-Y jelly

### Preparation

1. Obtain patient's medication record. Medication record may be a drug card, medication sheet, or drug Kardex, depending on the method of dispensing medications in your facility.
2. Compare the medication record with the most recent physician's order.
3. Wash your hands.
4. Gather necessary equipment.
5. Remove the medication from the drug box or tray on medication cart.
6. Compare the label on the medication bottle.
7. Place medication and K-Y jelly on a tray if not using medication cart.
8. Check drug information to determine if appropriate for application to mucous membranes.

### Procedure

1. Take medication to room.
2. Check room number against medication card or sheet.
3. Identify patient by name; check identaband.
4. Explain procedure to patient.
5. Provide privacy.
6. Wash your hands.
7. Place patient in the Sim's (left lateral) position.
8. Remove the foil wrapper from the suppository.
9. Put K-Y jelly on tip of suppository to facilitate its insertion.
10. Using a fingercot or disposable glove, insert the suppository into the rectal canal beyond the anal sphincter. **Rationale:** Prevents suppository from slipping out.

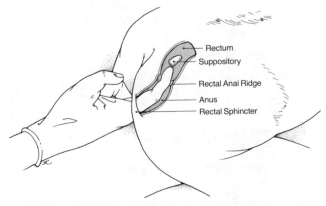

After donning a clean glove, insert rectal suppository beyond the anal-rectal ridge to ensure it is retained.

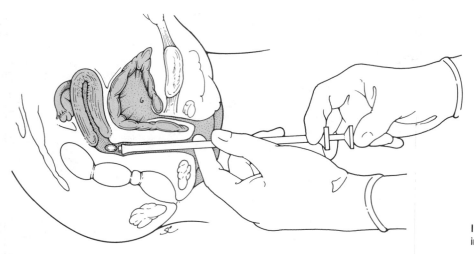

Insert vaginal suppositories at least two inches using glove or applicator as shown.

11. Instruct the patient to lie quietly for fifteen minutes until the medicine is absorbed.

12. Dispose of equipment and wash your hands.

13. Return after fifteen minutes to check on patient and make him comfortable.

14. Chart medication and results obtained.

## INSERTING VAGINAL SUPPOSITORIES

### Equipment

Suppository

Applicator if needed

Disposable glove

### Preparation

1. Obtain patient's medication record. Medication record may be a drug card, medication sheet, or drug Kardex, depending on the method of dispensing medications in your facility.

2. Compare the medication record with the most recent physician's order.

3. Wash your hands.

4. Gather necessary equipment.

5. Remove the medication from the drug box or tray on medication cart.

6. Compare the label on the medication to the medication record.

7. Place medication jar (include an applicator) on a tray if not using medication cart.

8. Check drug information to determine if appropriate for application to mucous membranes.

### Procedure

1. Take medication to patient's room and check room number against medication card or sheet.

2. Check patient's identaband and ask patient to state name.

3. Check medication route and dosage.

4. Provide privacy.

5. Wash your hands.

6. Place patient in the dorsal recumbent or Sim's position.

7. Remove the foil wrapper from the suppository. Insert into applicator.

8. Using a disposable glove, insert the suppository into the vaginal canal at least 2 inches. **Rationale:** Prevents suppository from slipping out.

9. Instruct the patient to lie quietly for fifteen minutes until the suppository is absorbed.

10. Discard equipment, wash applicator and return to appropriate place.

11. Wash your hands.

12. Return to patient after fifteen minutes to check on patient.

13. Chart medication and any evidence of discharge or odor from vagina.

### CHARTING  *for Suppository Medications*

☐ Appropriate medication form for facility used

☐ Name of drug

☐ Dosage

☐ Times ordered

☐ Time administered

☐ Method of administration

☐ Initials of nurses administering drug

☐ In nurses' notes, comments made on perineal skin condition or anal area

☐ Results from rectal suppository

## CLINICAL PROBLEM SOLVING

| Potential Problems | Suggested Solutions |
|---|---|
| Patient unable to retain suppositories. | ☐ Observe if sphincter is competent.<br>☐ Instruct patient to maintain position for at least 15 minutes in order to allow any absorption.<br>☐ Position on abdomen and hold buttocks closed.<br>☐ Notify physician so that an alternate route or a different medication can be tried. |
| Suppository fails to dissolve. | ☐ Check expiration date on package and, if necessary, obtain new supply.<br>☐ Instruct patient to maintain appropriate position so that drug is absorbed.<br>☐ Ensure that suppository has been placed in appropriate area. |

# UNIT TEN   IRRIGATIONS

## NURSING PROCESS DATA

### ASSESSMENT   *Data Base*

Identify purpose of irrigation.

Assess the area surrounding part being irrigated for signs of irritation, sloughing of tissue and edema.

Assess area being irrigated for itching, burning and pain.

Assess patient's response to irrigating solution and irrigation.

### PLANNING   *Objectives*

To administer an irrigation using appropriate technique.

To cleanse an area of excess drainage, debris or irritating substances.

To administer an antiseptic solution.

To apply heat or cold.

To remove foreign objects.

### IMPLEMENTATION   *Procedures*

Irrigating the Eye

Irrigating the Ear

Irrigating the Throat

## IRRIGATING THE EYE

### Equipment

2 sterile containers—1 round bowl, 1 curved basin

Irrigating solution, 60cc to 200cc

Sterile 10cc syringe or eye irrigating syringe

Sterile 4 × 4" gauze pad

Absorbent pad

### Preparation

1. Check physician's orders or Patient Care Plan.
2. Wash hands.
3. Gather equipment.
4. Warm irrigating solution to about 100° F.
5. Explain procedure to patient.
6. Provide privacy if appropriate.
7. Place in Fowler's position, turned slightly to affected eye side.
8. Place absorbent pad over chest. **Rationale:** This action protects clothing from becoming wet.

### Procedure

1. Open two sterile containers as with any sterile package. Place on table close to bed.
2. Pour 60cc to 200cc of irrigating solution into round bowl.
3. Draw up irrigating solution into syringe.
4. Have patient hold curved basin on cheek under eye. **Rationale:** Basin is used to catch solution.
5. Clean eyelids and eyelashes with moistened 4 × 4 gauze pad. Wipe from inner to outer canthus. **Rationale:** This method prevents contamination of opposite eye.
6. Using your thumb and forefinger, open the eye and expose lower conjunctival sac by pulling the sac down toward cheek.
7. Place the syringe over area of inner canthus pointing toward the outer canthus. Push the bar-

rel of the syringe slowly, allowing irrigating solution to flow into the conjunctival sac.

8. Continue irrigating until eye is cleansed completely or ordered amount of solution is used. Patient will need to close eyes between irrigating when large amounts of solution are used.
9. Wipe eyelid with 4 × 4 gauze from inner to outer canthus.
10. Place patient in position of comfort.
11. Dispose of equipment in appropriate area.
12. Wash your hands.

## IRRIGATING THE EAR

### Equipment

Ear syringe or asepto syringe

2 sterile containers—1 round basin, 1 curved basin

Sterile solution

Absorbent pad

Sterile cotton-tipped swabs

Sterile 4 × 4 gauze pad

### Preparation

1. Check physician's order or Patient Care Plan.
2. Wash your hands.
3. Gather equipment.
4. Explain procedure to patient.
5. Warm irrigating solution to body temperature.
6. Provide privacy if appropriate.
7. Place patient in Fowler's position.
8. Place absorbent pad over shoulder. **Rationale:** This procedure protects clothing and bed linen from becoming wet.
9. Pour irrigating solution into round basin.

### Procedure

1. Place curved basin under ear to catch irrigating solution.

2. Moisten cotton-tipped applicator swab with irrigating solution.

3. Clean the external structures of the ear and meatus with the moistened cotton-tipped applicator swab.

4. Fill the syringe with irrigating solution.

5. Open and straighten the canal by pulling the penna up and backward in adults or down for infants. **Rationale:** This action allows the solution to flow into the canal.

6. Insert the irrigating syringe tip into the meatus, and as you push the plunger, direct the flow of solution toward the top of the canal. **Rationale:** This action allows the flow to reach the entire length of the canal.

7. After the solution has ceased to flow, dry the outside of the ear with a 4 × 4 gauze pad.

8. Position the patient for comfort or on the affected side. **Rationale:** Positioning on the affected side increases the drainage of residual irrigation solution.

9. Discard equipment in appropriate area.

10. Wash your hands.

## IRRIGATING THE THROAT

### Equipment

Irrigation bag, tubing, catheter

Irrigation solution

Absorbent pad

Curved basin

### Preparation

1. Check physician's orders or Patient Care Plan.

2. Wash your hands.

3. Gather equipment.

4. Warm irrigating solution to 100° F.

5. Explain procedure to patient.

6. Provide privacy if appropriate.

7. Place in Fowler's position or position in front of the sink.

8. Place absorbent pad over chest.

### Procedure

1. Establish communication system for halting the irrigation. The patient can be instructed to bend the tubing to stop the flow of solution or tap you on the hand. If he can perform the irrigation himself, it is advisable.

2. Unclamp the tubing.

3. Direct the irrigating tip toward the throat. Move the tip slowly back and forth in the mouth to reach all areas of the throat.

4. Continue to irrigate, with interruptions as directed by the patient.

5. Clamp tubing and remove the irrigation catheter.

6. Remove equipment and place patient in bed or in position of comfort.

7. Clean equipment if to be reused or dispose of equipment in appropriate place.

8. Wash your hands.

### CHARTING  *for Irrigations*

☐  Irrigating solution

☐  Amount of solution utilized

☐  Presence of exudate, color, odor

☐  Presence of edema, erythema of surrounding area

☐  Patient's reaction to procedure

## CLINICAL PROBLEM SOLVING

### Potential Problems

Irrigating solution runs out of ear without first reaching the canal.

Difficulty is experienced in keeping eye open during irrigation.

### Suggested Solutions

☐  Reposition the ear to ensure the canal is open.
☐  Point the syringe toward the top of the canal when irrigating.
☐  Slow down the speed of the irrigation to prevent the solution from running in too quickly.

☐  Obtain assistance from another nurse as two hands may be needed to keep eye open.

Patient cannot tolerate throat irrigations.

☐ Allow patient to do own irrigations if you have been performing them. He may be less apt to gag when he can control the flow.

# ━━━ DRUG SUPPLEMENT ━━━

This section is a supplement to the conceptual base of therapeutic agents. It contains information on systems of measurements, mathematic conversion tables, calculation of solutions, drug classification by action and by body system, and basic laws governing drug dispensation.

## APOTHECARY SYSTEM

1. Older system, based on unrelated, arbitrary units of measure; gradually being replaced by metric system.
   a. Portions of a unit of measurement are designated by common fractions, e.g., one-fourth grain, written as gr ¼.
   b. Symbols for ounces and drams are similar in form and must be written clearly (e.g., ℨ is dram; ℥ is ounce).
   c. Symbols and abbreviations are placed before Roman numerals (5 grains written as gr v).

2. Common apothecary measures and symbols:

   | | |
   |---|---|
   | drop | gtt |
   | minim | m |
   | dram | ℨ |
   | ounce | ℥ |
   | grain | gr |

3. Equivalents:

   | | | |
   |---|---|---|
   | 1 drop | = | 1 minim |
   | 15 drops | = | 1 grain |
   | 60 minims | = | 1 fluid dram |
   | 8 fluid drams | = | 1 fluid ounce |
   | 16 fluid ounces | = | 1 pint |

## METRIC SYSTEM

1. French-invented system, based on rationally and related derived units; developed in the eighteenth century.
   a. Basic units of measure used in drug administration are the gram and liter.
   b. Other units are decimals, fractions, and Arabic numerals.
   c. Numbers and fractions are placed before symbols.

2. Common metric measures and symbols:

   | | |
   |---|---|
   | gram | gm |
   | kilogram | kg |
   | milligram | mg |
   | milliliter | ml |
   | liter | l |

3. Weight and volume equivalents with corresponding symbols:

   | | |
   |---|---|
   | 1 gram = 1,000 milligrams | 1 gm = 1,000 mg |
   | 1 liter = 1,000 milliliters | 1 l = 1,000 ml |

## HOUSEHOLD SYSTEM

1. System based on familiar measures used in the home.
   a. Most measures are not sufficiently accurate for measure of medicines.
   b. Pints and quarts are also used in the apothecary system.

2. Common household measures and their abbreviations:

   | | |
   |---|---|
   | pint | pt |
   | teaspoon | t |
   | tablespoon | T |
   | quart | qt |

## MATHEMATIC CONVERSION

### Approximate Equivalents

1. The metric system is the universal system of weights and measures.

2. Apothecary and metric systems do not use same size units; denominations of one system are not compatible with the other.

3. Equivalency tables are established to list measurement denominations of one system in terms of another. (See Appendix 2, Tables A, B, and C.)
   a. Conversion from one system to another can be computed, but measurements are not equivalent in absolute terms.
   b. If there is occasion to compute, have computations checked by another nurse.

## Computation

1. Drugs are not always labeled clearly as to number of tablets to administer, so computation may be necessary. Always have your computation checked by another nurse.

2. Method:
   a. Both desired (ordered) dose and dose on hand must be in same unit of measurement, e.g., grains, grams, milligrams.
   b. If not, convert so that unit of measure is the same.
      • Refer to conversion tables in Appendix 2.
      • To convert one measure unit to another, basic equivalencies must be memorized.
   c. After converting, divide desired dose by dose on hand to find amount to administer.

## CALCULATION OF SOLUTIONS

### Types of Solutions

1. Volume to volume (v/v): a given volume of solute is added to a given volume of solvent.

2. Weight to weight (w/w): a stated weight of solute is dissolved in a stated weight of solvent.

3. Weight to volume (w/v): a given weight of solute is dissolved in a given volume of solvent which results in the proper amount of solution.

### Preparing Solutions

■ Liquid to Drug Solutions

Determine the strength of the solution, the strength of the drug on hand, and the quantity of solution required.

Use this formula for preparing solutions:

$$\frac{D}{H} \times Q = X$$

where  D = desired strength
       H = strength on hand
       Q = quantity of solution desired
       X = amount of solute

*Example:* You have a 100% solution of hydrogen peroxide on hand. You need a liter of 50% solution.

$$\frac{50}{100} \times 1000 \text{ ml} = 500 \text{ ml}$$

If the strength desired and strength on hand are not in like terms, you need to change one of the terms.

*Example:* You have 1 liter of 50% solution on hand. You need a liter of 1:10 solution. 1:10 solution is the same as 10%.

$$\frac{10\%}{50\%} \times 1000 \text{ ml} = 200 \text{ ml}$$

Add 200 ml of the drug to 800 ml of the solvent to make a liter of 10% solution.

■ Volume to Volume Solutions

Use the formula:

$$\frac{D}{H} \times Q = X$$

where X = amount of stock solution used.

*Example:* Prepare a liter of 5% solution from a stock solution of 50%.

$$\frac{5\%}{50\%} \times 1000 \text{ ml} = 100 \text{ ml}$$

Add 100 ml to 900 ml of diluent to make 1 liter of 5% solution.

■ Solutions from Tablets

Use the formula:

$$\frac{D}{H} \times Q = X$$

where X = amount/number of tablets used.

*Example:* Prepare 1 liter of a 1:1000 solution, using 10 grain tablets.

$$\frac{1/1000}{10 \text{ gr}} \times 1000 \text{ ml} = X$$

First convert 10 grains to grams so the numerator and denominator are in the same unit of measure. 1 gm = 15 gr; therefore 10 gr = 2/3 gm. Now substitute the new numbers in the formula and solve for X.

$$\frac{1/1000}{2/3} \times \frac{1000}{1} \text{ ml} = X$$

$$\frac{3}{2000} \times \frac{1000}{1} = X$$

$$X = 3/2, \text{ or } 1\frac{1}{2} \text{ tablets}$$

Place 1½ tablets into the liter of solution and dissolve.

# DRUG CLASSIFICATION

## Classification by Action

*Anti-infectives*

1. Antiseptics.
   a. Inhibit growth of microorganisms (bacteriostatic).
   b. Cleanse wounds and skin infections, sterilize equipment, promote hygiene.

2. Disinfectants.
   a. Destroy microorganisms (bactericidal).
   b. Destroy bacteria on inanimate objects (not appropriate for living tissue).

*Antimicrobials*

1. Sulfonamides.
   a. Inhibit the growth of microorganisms.
   b. Reduce or prevent infectious process, especially urinary tract infections.

2. Antibiotics (e.g., penicillin).
   a. Interfere with microorganism metabolism.
   b. Reduce or prevent infectious process.
   c. Specific drug and dosage: based on culture and sensitivity of organism.

*Metabolic Drugs*

1. Hormones obtained from animal sources; found naturally in foods and plants.

2. Synthetic hormones.

*Diagnostic Materials*

1. Dyes and opaque materials: ingested or injected to allow visualization of internal organs.

2. Analyze organ status and function.

*Vitamins and Minerals*

1. Necessary to obtain healthy body function.

2. Found naturally in food or through synthetic food supplements.

*Vaccines and Serums*

1. Prevent disease and detect presence of disease.

2. Types.
   a. Antigenics: for active immunity.
      • Vaccines: attenuated suspensions of microorganisms.
      • Toxoids: products of microorganisms.
   b. Antibodies: stimulated by microorganisms or their products.
      • Antitoxins.
      • Immune serum globulin.

   c. Allergens: agents for skin immunity tests.
      • Extracts of materials known to be allergenic.
      • Used to relieve allergies.
   d. Antivenins: substances that neutralize venom of certain snakes and spiders.

*Antifungals*

Check growth of fungi.

*Antihistaminics*

1. Prevent histamine action.

2. Relieve symptoms of allergic reaction.

*Antineoplastics*

Prevent growth and spread of malignant cells.

## Classification by Body Systems

*Central Nervous System* Drugs affect CNS by either inhibiting or promoting the actions of neural pathways and centers.

1. Action-promoting drug groups (stimulants).
   a. Antidepressants: psychic energizers used to treat depression.
   b. Caffeine: increases mental activity and lessens drowsiness.
   c. Ammonia: used as a stimulant to counteract fainting.

2. Action-inhibiting drug groups (depressants).
   a. Analgesics: reduce pain by interfering with conduction of nerve impulses.
      (1) Narcotic analgesics: opium derivatives (morphine); may depress respiratory centers; must be used with caution and respiratory rate above 12.
         • A narcotic antagonist drug counteracts depressant drugs.
         • Such antagonist drugs are Lorfan, Narcan, and Nalline.
      (2) Nonnarcotic antipyretics: reduce fever and relieve pain (ASA and Tylenol).
      (3) Antirheumatics: analgesics given to relieve arthritis pain; may reduce joint inflammation.
   b. Alcohol: stimulates appetite when given in small doses; classified as a depressant.
   c. Hypnotics: sedatives that induce sleep; barbiturates (phenobarbital) and nonbarbiturates (chloral hydrate).
   d. Antispasmodics: relieve skeletal muscle spasms; anticonvulsants prevent muscle spasms or convulsions.

e. Sedatives: produce relaxed, calming effect.
f. Tranquilizers:
  (1) Relieve tension and anxiety, preoperative and postoperative apprehension, headaches, menstrual tension, chronic alcoholism, skeletal muscle spasticity, and other neuromuscular disorders.
  (2) Tranquilizers and analgesics frequently given together (in reduced dosage); one drug enhances action of the other (synergy).
g. Anesthetics: produce state of unconsciousness (general), blocks pain (local).

3. Precautions to be taken with CNS drugs:
  a. Drugs that act on CNS may potentiate other CNS drugs.
  b. Patient may be receiving other medications; find out drug name and dosage.
  c. Dependence on CNS drugs may occur.

*Autonomic Nervous System*  This system governs several body functions. Drugs that affect the ANS will also affect other system functions.

1. The ANS is made up of two nerve systems: the sympathetic and parasympathetic.
  a. Sympathetic: the protective emergency system.
  b. Parasympathetic: the stabilizing system.

2. Basic drug groups:
  a. Adrenergics: mimic the actions of sympathetic system.
    (1) Vasoconstrictors: stimulants such as Adrenalin.
      • Constrict peripheral blood vessels, increase blood pressure.
      • Dilate bronchial passages.
      • Relax gastrointestinal tract.
    (2) Vasodilators: depressants such as nicotinic acid.
      • Antagonists of epinephrine and similar drugs.
      • Vasodilate blood vessels.
      • Increase tone of GI tract.
      • Reduce blood pressure.
      • Relax smooth muscles.
      *Caution:* If drug is to be stopped, reduce the dosage gradually over a period of a week; do not stop dosage suddenly.
  b. Cholinergics: mimic actions of parasympathetic system.
    (1) Cholinergic stimulants (e.g., Prostigmin or Neostigmine).
      • Decrease heart rate.
      • Contract smooth muscle.
      • Contract pupil in eye.
      • Increase peristalsis.
      • Increase gland secretions.
    (2) Cholinergic inhibitors (anticholinergics).
      • Decrease gland secretion.
      • Relax smooth muscle.
      • Dilate pupil in eye.
      • Increase heart action.

*Gastrointestinal System*  Drugs affecting GI system act upon muscular and glandular tissues.

1. Antacids: counteract excess stomach acidity (Maalox).
  a. Have alkaline base.
  b. Used in treatment of ulcers.
  c. Neutralize hydrochloric acid in the stomach.
  d. Given frequently (two-hour intervals or more often).
  e. May not be given with water.
  f. May cause constipation, depending on type of medication.
  g. Baking soda is a systemic antacid, which disturbs the pH balance in the body. Most other antacids coat the mucous membrane and neutralize HCl.

2. Emetics; produce vomiting (emesis).

3. Antiemetics: prevent vomiting or nausea; cause drowsiness (Emetrol).

4. Digestants: relieve enzyme deficiency by replacing secretions in digestive tract.

5. Antidiarrheics: prevent diarrhea.

6. Cathartics: affect intestine and produce defecation.
  a. Provide temporary relief for constipation.
  b. Rid bowel of contents before surgery; prepare viscera for diagnostic studies.
  c. Counteract edema.
  d. Treat diseases of GI tract.
  e. Classifications:
    (1) By degree of action:
      • Laxative: mild action.
      • Cathartic: moderate action.
      • Purgative: severe action.
    (2) By method of action:
      • Increase bulk.
      • Lubricate mechanically.
      • Irritate chemically.
      • Increase or decrease water content with saline.

- Disperse detergent or wetting agent.
- Cathartics are contraindicated when abdominal pain is present.

*Respiratory System*   Drugs act on respiratory tract, tissues, and cough center; suppress, relax, liquefy, and stimulate.

1. Respiratory stimulants: stimulate depth and rate of respiration.
2. Bronchodilators: relax smooth muscle of trachea and bronchial tree.
3. Drug groups that provide cough relief:
   a. Antitussive agents (narcotic, nonnarcotic).
      (1) Sedatives: prevent cough.
      (2) Not to be accompanied by water.
   b. Demulcents: soothe respiratory tract.
   c. Expectorants: liquefy bronchial secretions; increase amount of excretions in respiratory tract.

*Urinary System*   Drugs act on kidneys and urinary tract; increase urine flow, destroy bacteria, perform other important body functions.

1. Diuretics:
   a. Rid body of excess fluid and relieve edema.
   b. Some drugs that act on the GI tract and circulatory system are also diuretic in action.
2. Urinary antiseptics.
3. Acidifiers and alkalinizers: certain foods increase body acids or alkalies.

*Circulatory System*   Drugs act on heart, blood, and blood vessels; change heart rhythm, rate, and force and dilate or constrict vessels.

1. Cardiotonics: used for heart-strengthening.
   a. Direct heart stimulants: speed heart rate, e.g., caffeine, Adrenalin.
   b. Indirect heart stimulants: e.g., digitalis.
      (1) Stimulate vagus nerve.
      (2) Slow heart rate and strengthen it.
      (3) Improve heart action, thereby improving circulation.
      (4) Do not administer if apical pulse is below 60.
2. Antiarrhythmic drugs: used clinically to convert irregularities to a normal sinus rhythm; monitor constantly with ECG when administering these drugs.
   a. Quinidine: used for its vasodepressor action.
   b. Slows heart rate.
   c. Side effects: ringing in ears.

3. Drugs that alter blood flow:
   a. Anticoagulants: inhibit the blood-clotting action (heparin).
   b. Vasodilators: maintain blood flow.
4. Blood replacement.

**Miscellaneous Drug Classifications**

1. Anticonvulsant or antiepileptic drugs: drugs that control seizures, i.e., Dilantin (Hyperplasia of the gingiva, which is a side effect, requires frequent teeth brushing and dental checks.)
2. Anti-inflammatories: drugs that reduce tissue inflammation, i.e., prednisolone. (Observe patient for gastric ulcers, Cushing's syndrome, and mood swings.)
3. Antineoplastics: drugs that stop cell division, i.e., vincristine.
4. Antiparasitics: drugs used to rid the body of parasitic worms, amoebas, and protozoans, i.e., Antepar. (Treat entire family.)
5. Antiparkinsonism agents: drugs used to control symptoms of Parkinsonism, i.e., L-dopa.
6. Antituberculosis agents: drugs used to destroy tuberculosis bacteria, i.e., PAS, INH.
7. Hallucinogenics: drugs that induce hallucinations, i.e., LSD.
8. Hormones: substances secreted by the pituitary gland and the adrenal cortex.
9. Insulin and oral hypoglycemics: animal insulin or drugs that stimulate insulin production necessary for carbohydrate utilization. (Site rotation prevents lipid dystrophy and hypertrophy.)
10. Narcotic antagonists: drugs that abolish the effect of opiates and opiate-like narcotics, i.e., Narcan.
11. Thyroid and antithyroid agents: drugs used either to stimulate or to suppress thyroid gland functions, i.e., hypothyroid (euthroid), hyperthyroid (iodine).

## GOVERNING LAWS

### Federal Food, Drug, and Cosmetic Act of 1938

1. The Act is an update of the Food and Drug Act, first passed in 1906.
2. It designates *United States Pharmacopeia* and *National Formulary* as official standards; gives the federal government the power to enforce standards.

3. Provisions of the Act:
   a. Drug manufacturer must provide adequate evidence of drug's safety.
   b. Drug manufacturer is responsible for the correct labeling and packaging of drugs.

4. The Act was amended in 1952 to include control of barbiturates by restricting prescription refills.

5. The Act was amended in 1962 to require substantial investigation of drugs and evidence that drugs are effective in terms of labeling claims.

## Harrison Narcotic Act of 1914

1. Provisions of the Act.
   a. Regulates manufacture, importation, and sale of opium, cocaine, and their derivatives.
   b. Amendments have added addictive synthetic drugs to the regulated drug listing.

2. Applications of the Act.
   a. Individuals who produce, sell, dispense (pharmacists), and prescribe (dentist, physicians) these drugs must be licensed and registered; prescriptions must be in triplicate.
   b. Hospitals order drugs on special blanks that bear hospital registry number. The following information is recorded for each dose:
      (1) Name of drug.
      (2) Amount of drug.
      (3) Date and time drug obtained.
      (4) Name of physician prescribing drug.
      (5) Name of patient receiving drug.

## The Controlled Substance Act of 1970

1. Provisions of the Act.
   a. Regulates potentially addictive drugs as to prescription, use, and possession.
      (1) Regulations refer to use in hopsital, office, research, and emergency situations.
      (2) Regulations cover narcotics, cocaine, amphetamines, hallucinogens, barbiturates, and other sedatives.
   b. Controlled drugs are placed in five different schedules or categorical listings, each governed by different regulations.
      (1) The regulations govern the manufacture, transport, and storage of the controlled drugs.
      (2) The use of the drugs is controlled as to prescription, authorization, the mode of dispensation, and administration.

2. Application of the Act for use of controlled drugs in hospital.
   a. The nurse is to keep the stock supply of controlled drugs under lock and key.
      (1) Nurse must sign for each dose (tablet, cc) of drug.
      (2) Key is held by the nurse responsible for administration of medication.
      (3) At the end of each shift, nurse must account for all controlled drugs in the stock supply.
   b. Violations of the Controlled Substance Act
      (1) Violations punishable by fine, imprisonment, or both.
      (2) Nurses, upon conviction of violation, are subject to losing their license to practice nursing.

## APPENDIX 1

### ABBREVIATIONS AND SYMBOLS FOR ORDERS, PRESCRIPTIONS AND LABELS

| | |
|---|---|
| aa | of each |
| a.c. | before meals |
| ad lib. | freely, as desired |
| b.i.d. | twice each day |
| c̄ | with |
| C | carbon |
| Ca | calcium |
| Cl | chlorine |
| dr *or* 3 | dram |
| et | and |
| GI | gastrointestinal |
| gt *or* gtt | drop(s) |
| $H_2O$ | water |
| $H_2O_2$ | hydrogen peroxide |
| IM | intramuscular |
| in. | inch |
| K | potassium |
| lb *or* # | pound |
| m | minimum (a minimum) |
| Mg | magnesium |
| N | nitrogen, normal |
| Na | sodium |
| n.p.o. | nothing by mouth |
| oob | out of bed |
| os | mouth |
| oz *or* 3 | ounce |
| p.c. | after meals |
| per | by, through |
| p.r.n. | whenever necessary |
| q.d. | every day |
| q.h. | every hour |
| q.i.d. | four times each day |
| q.s. | as much as required, quantity sufficient |
| q2h | every two hours |
| q3h | every three hours |
| q4h | every four hours |
| $R_x$ | treatment, "take thou" |
| s̄ | without |
| s̄s̄ | one-half |
| stat | immediately |
| t.i.d. | three times each day |
| tsp | teaspoon |
| WBC | white blood cell |
| ° | degree |
| − | minus, negative, alkaline reaction |
| + | plus, positive, acid reaction |
| % | percent |
| v | Roman numeral five |
| vii | Roman numeral seven |
| ix | Roman numeral nine |
| xiii | Roman numeral thirteen |

## APPENDIX 2

### CONVERSION TABLES

**TABLE A**   HOUSEHOLD EQUIVALENTS (VOLUME)

| METRIC | APOTHECARY | HOUSEHOLD |
|---|---|---|
| 0.06 ml | 1 minim | 1 drop |
| 5 (4) ml | 1 fluid dram | 1 teaspoonful |
| 15 ml | 4 fluid drams | 1 tablespoonful |
| 30 ml | 1 fluid ounce | 2 tablespoonfuls |
| 180 ml | 6 fluid ounces | 1 teacupful |
| 240 ml | 8 fluid ounces | 1 glassful |

**TABLE B**   APOTHECARY EQUIVALENTS (VOLUME)

| METRIC | | APOTHECARY |
|---|---|---|
| 1 ml | = | 15 minims |
| 1 cc | = | 15 minims |
| 0.06 ml | = | 1 minim |
| 4 ml | = | 1 fluid dram |
| 30 ml | = | 1 fluid ounce |
| 500 ml | = | 1 pint |
| 1000 ml (1 l) | = | 1 quart |

**TABLE C**   APOTHECARY EQUIVALENTS (WEIGHT)

| METRIC | | | | | APOTHECARY |
|---|---|---|---|---|---|
| 1.0 | gm | *or* | 1000 mg | = | gr xv |
| 0.6 | gm | *or* | 600 mg | = | gr x |
| 0.5 | gm | *or* | 500 mg | = | gr viiss |
| 0.3 | gm | *or* | 300 mg | = | gr v |
| 0.2 | gm | *or* | 200 mg | = | gr iii |
| 0.1 | gm | *or* | 100 mg | = | gr 1½ |
| 0.06 | gm | *or* | 60 mg | = | gr 1 |
| 0.05 | gm | *or* | 50 mg | = | gr ¾ |
| 0.03 | gm | *or* | 30 mg | = | gr ½ |
| 0.015 | gm | *or* | 15 mg | = | gr ¼ |
| 0.010 | gm | *or* | 10 mg | = | gr ⅙ |
| 0.008 | gm | *or* | 8 mg | = | gr ⅛ |
| 4 g | | | | = | 1 dr |
| 30 g | | | | = | 1 oz |
| 1 kg | | | | = | 2.2 lbs |

## TERMINOLOGY

**Absorption:** the passage of a substance through some surface of the body into body fluids and tissues.

**Addictive:** alcohol or drug that causes enslavement to some habit.

**Allergy:** an antigen-antibody reaction or sensitivity to a substance.

**Anaphylaxis:** a hypersensitive shock state due to a foreign substance, protein, or drug.

**Anesthesia:** partial or complete loss of sensation with or without loss of consciousness as a result of injury, disease, or administration of a drug or gas.

**Aseptic:** sterile; condition free from germs and infection.

**Aspirate:** to remove by suction.

**Biotransformation:** the biological process of changing a substance so that it may be metabolized or excreted.

**Bronchodilatation:** dilatation of a bronchus.

**Cardiotonic:** increasing tonicity of the heart.

**Cathartic:** an active purgative for the bowels.

**Circulation:** having to do with the movement of blood in a circular course, exiting from the aorta and coming back into the heart via the vena cava.

**Compatible:** able to mix with another substance without destructive changes.

**Congestion:** the presence of an excessive amount of blood or tissue fluid in an organ or in tissue.

**Contaminate:** to soil, stain, or pollute; to render impure.

**Contraindication:** any symptom or circumstance indicating the inappropriateness of a form of treatment otherwise advisable.

**Dosage:** the amount of medicine to be administered to a patient at one time.

**Drug:** any substance that when taken into the living organism may modify one or more of its functions.

**Dyspnea:** labored or difficult breathing.

**Ecchymosis:** a form of macula appearing in large irregularly-formed hemorrhagic areas of the skin.

**Emetic:** medicine that produces vomiting.

**Generic:** general; pertinent to a genus; distinctive.

**Hydration:** the chemical combination of a substance with water.

**Hypnotic:** an agent that induces sleep or which dulls the senses.

**Infection:** condition in which the body or body part is invaded by a pathogenic agent (microorganism or virus) which may multiply and produce effects that are injurious.

**Instillation:** slowly pouring or dropping a liquid into a cavity or onto a surface.

**Intradermal:** within the dermal layer of the skin.

**Intravenous:** within or into a vein.

**Medicine:** a drug or remedy.

**Metabolism:** all energy and material transformations which occur within living cells.

**Narcotic:** a drug that, in moderate doses, depresses the central nervous system, thus relieving pain and producing sleep; most narcotics are addictive and in excess may produce coma or death.

**Ointment:** a medicated, fatty, soft substance having antiseptic, cosmetic, or healing properties.

**Parenteral:** injection of substances into the body through any route other than alimentary; outside the intestines.

**Peristalsis:** a progressive, wavelike movement which occurs involuntarily in the intestines of the body.

**Salve:** an ointment applied to a wound; any ointment made with a base of fat, oil, petrolatum, resin, etc.

**Subcutaneous:** third tissue layer; introduced beneath the skin.

**Sublingual:** beneath the tongue.

**Synthetic:** artificially prepared.

**Systemic:** pertinent to a whole body rather than one specific area.

**Therapeutic:** having medicinal or healing properties.

**Tonicity:** state of normal tension, especially muscular, as with muscular tone.

**Vasodilator:** an agent that causes blood vessels to dilate.

*Chapter* **16**

# Nutritional Management

## LEARNING OBJECTIVES

List the six essential nutrients necessary to sustain life.

Outline the primary differences between vitamins and minerals.

Describe the primary functions of the gastrointestinal system and accessory organs.

Identify the assessment categories important for a total nutritional assessment.

Define the term therapeutic diet.

Describe a sodium-restricted diet and list at least three foods high in sodium.

Name and discuss the purpose of at least four therapeutic diets.

List what foods should be included in a postoperative surgical diet.

Explain what is meant by a postoperative diet protocol.

List the foods in at least three diabetic food exchanges that you would teach to a patient.

Outline the steps for inserting a nasogastric tube.

Identify the primary steps of administering a tube feeding.

Discuss at least two potential problems that may occur with a tube feeding and the suggested solutions.

Describe two nursing actions that are necessary to promote safe care while administering hyperalimentation solution.

## ESSENTIAL NUTRIENTS

Nutrition is comprised of essential nutrients, all of which are necessary for growth and development through the life cycle. The essential nutrients are carbohydrates, fats, proteins, vitamins, minerals, and water. When these are supplied to the body in proper balance, the body utilizes them for energy, growth and development, tissue repair, and regulation and maintenance of body processes.

**Carbohydrates** Carbohydrates are the chief source of energy and contain carbon, hydrogen, and oxygen. Carbohydrates include sugars, starches, and cellulose. Simple sugars, such as fruit sugar, are easily digested. Starches, which are more complex, require more sophisticated enzyme processes to be reduced to glucose, the end product of carbohydrate metabolism. Glucose, which is converted sugars and starches, appears in the body as blood sugar and is "burned" as fuel by the tissues. Some glucose is processed by the liver, converted to glycogen, and stored by the liver for later use.

Ingesting too many carbohydrates crowds out other important foods and prevents the body from receiving the necessary nutrients for healthy maintenance. Too few carbohydrates may lead to loss of energy, depression, ketosis, and a breakdown of body protein. Differences in individual body structure, energy expenditure, basal metabolism, and general health status will determine the amount and kind of carbohydrates that should be consumed for optimal health.

**Fats** Fats or lipids are the second important group of nutrients. Fats also provide energy. In fact, when oxidized, they are the most concentrated sources of energy and, as such, furnish the calories necessary for survival.

**TABLE 1** ESSENTIAL BODY NUTRIENTS

| | |
|---|---|
| Carbohydrates | Monosaccharides<br>    Glucose, fructose, galactose<br>Disaccharides<br>    Sucrose, lactose, maltose<br>Polysaccharides<br>    Starch, dextrin, glycogen, cellulose, hemicellulose |
| Fats | Linoleic acid, linolenic acid, arachidonic acid |
| Proteins | Amino acids<br>    Phenylalanine, lysine, isoleucine, leucine, methionine,<br>    valine, tryptophan, threonine |
| Vitamins | Fat-soluble<br>    Vitamins A, D, E, and K<br>Water-soluble<br>    Vitamins $B_1$, $B_2$, $B_6$, $B_{12}$, niacin, pantothenic acid, folacin,<br>    biotin, choline, meso-inositol, para-aminobenzoic acid, and<br>    vitamin C |
| Minerals | Major elements<br>    Calcium, chloride, iron, magnesium, phosphorous, potas-<br>    sium, sodium, sulfur<br>Trace elements |
| Water | |

Fats also act as carriers for the fat-soluble vitamins, A, D, E, and K. Consuming too much fat can lead to weight problems and poor metabolism of food products because the digestive and absorption processes are affected.

Fatty acids are the basic components of fat and comprise two main groups. Saturated fatty acids usually come from animal sources. Unsaturated fatty acids primarily come from vegetables, nuts, or seed sources. In the unsaturated group are three essential fatty acids. These acids are called "essential" because they are necessary to prevent a specific deficiency disease. Also, the body cannot manufacture them, and they are obtained only from the diet. These three acids are linoleic acid, arachidonic acid, and linolenic acid. They are necessary for healthy blood, arteries, nerves, and skin. A deficiency in this group would lead to skin problems and illness.

**Proteins** Proteins, the third essential group of nutrients, are complex organic compounds that contain amino acids. Protein is critical to all aspects of growth and development of body tissues. This substance is necessary for the building of muscles, blood, skin, internal organs, hormones, and enzymes. Protein is also a source of energy when there is insufficient carbohydrate or fat in the diet. When protein is spared, it is either used for tissue repair and maintenance or converted by the liver and stored as fat.

When proteins are digested and broken down, they form 22 amino acids. These amino acids are then absorbed from the intestine into the bloodstream and carried to the liver for synthesis into the tissues and organs of the body. They are the chemical basis for life, and if just one is missing, protein synthesis will decrease or even stop. All but eight of the amino acids can be produced by the body. These eight must be obtained from the diet. If all eight are present in a particular food, the food is a "complete protein." Foods that lack one or more of these essential amino acids are called "incomplete proteins." Most meat and dairy products are complete proteins, and most vegetables and fruits are incomplete. When several incomplete proteins are ingested, they should be combined carefully so that the result will be a balance yielding complete protein. For example, the combination of beans and rice is perfectly balanced to give a complete protein food.

It is difficult to determine the exact amount of protein needed to supply all of the essential amino acids because there are many variables. Height and weight, level of activity, and nutritional and health status all influence the amount of protein necessary for a healthy body. The National Research Council recommends that 0.42 grams of protein be consumed per day per pound of body weight. It is suggested that a person weighing 150 pounds should consume 75 grams of protein; however, recent research shows that this amount can be decreased by about one-third without negative results. It appears that as long as the essential amino acids are included in the diet, the total grams of protein can be reduced.

Protein deficiency can affect the entire body—organs, tissues, skin, and muscles, as well as certain body processes. If a child is deficient in protein, he or she may get kwashiorkor, a disease resulting in physical and mental impairment and, if severe enough, death. If an adult is deficient in protein, his stamina, mental state, and ability to withstand stress and infection is affected. Protein deficiency also interferes with recovery from diseases or surgery.

Protein is very plentiful in the body. It is an integral part of all cells and essential for growth and development. Just like fats and carbohydrates, adequate protein must be consumed in balance with other nutrients for human survival.

**Water**   While not specifically a nutrient, water is essential for survival. Water is involved in every body process from digestion and absorption to excretion. It is a major portion of circulation and is the transporter of nutrients throughout the body.

Body water performs three major functions: it gives form to the body, comprising from 50–75 percent of the body mass; it provides the necessary environment for cell metabolism; and it maintains a stable body temperature.

Almost all foods contain water that is absorbed by the body. The average adult body contains 56 quarts of water and loses about 3 quarts a day. If a person suffers severe water depletion, dehydration and salt depletion can result and can eventually lead to death. A person can survive longer without food than without water.

**Vitamins**   Vitamins are organic food substances and are essential in small amounts for growth, maintenance, and the functioning of body processes. Vitamins are found only in living things—plants and animals—and usually cannot be synthesized by the human body.

Vitamins can be grouped according to the substance in which they are soluble. The fat-soluble group includes vitamins A, D, E, and K. These vitamins are measured in international units. Each unit generally refers to the amount of the vitamin needed to produce a change in the nutritional health of a laboratory animal. The water-soluble vitamins include the B-complex vitamins, vitamin C, and the bioflavonoids. These are usually measured in milligrams.

Vitamins have no caloric value, but they are as necessary to the body as any other basic nutrient. Currently, there are about 20 substances identified as vitamins, but recent research is concerned with identifying even more of these substances since they are so essential to survival.

For many years research groups have attempted to determine basic vitamin requirements for various age groups. The most commonly used are the listings of the Recommended Dietary Allowances (RDA), based on standards established by the National Academy of Sciences.

**Minerals**     Minerals are inorganic substances, widely prevalent in nature, and essential for metabolic processes. Minerals are grouped according to the amount found in the body. Major minerals include calcium, magnesium, sodium, potassium, phosphorus, sulfur, and chlorine, all of which have a known function in the body. Major minerals are measured in milligrams. A second group, trace minerals, are iron, copper, iodine, manganese, cobalt, zinc, and molybdenum. These minerals are measured in micrograms, and their function in the body remains unclear. There remains another group of trace minerals found in scanty amounts in the body and whose function is also unclear. Minerals form 60–90 percent of all inorganic material in the body, and are found in bones, teeth, soft tissue, muscle, blood, and nerve cells.

Minerals act on organs and in metabolic processes. They act as catalysts for many reactions such as controlling muscle responses, maintaining the nervous system and acid-base balance, transmitting messages, maintaining cardiac stability, and regulating the metabolism and absorption of other nutrients. Even though they are considered separately, all minerals work synergistically with other minerals, and their actions are interrelated. A deficiency in one mineral, therefore, will affect the action of others in the body. It is essential that adequate minerals be ingested because a mineral deficiency can result in severe illness. Likewise, excessive amounts of minerals can throw the body out of balance.

Sufficient minerals can be supplied by adequate diet. Even though RDAs have not been established on all minerals, a diet that contains all the other nutrients can supply the necessary amount of minerals for the body. Many nutritionists and biochemists, however, recommend a daily basic vitamin-mineral supplement to ensure adequate levels.

# ASSIMILATION OF NUTRIENTS

Following the discussion of the essential body nutrients, it is now important to identify how these elements are broken down, absorbed, and utilized in the body. Nutrients, in most cases, are ingested through the mouth, and the body must break down these substances. This process is called digestion. It takes place in the mouth, pharynx, esophagus, stomach, and the small and large intestines.

The total daily energy requirement of an individual is the number of calories needed to replace the energy loss from the metabolic rate, plus loss from a person's exercise output, and emotional and mental state. The number of calories ingested should be directly related to maintaining an adequate energy level and supporting the body's metabolic processes.

**Gastrointestinal Tract**     The main functions of the gastrointestinal system are the secretion of enzymes and electrolytes to break down raw materials that are ingested; the movement of the ingested products through the system; the complete digestion of nutrients; and the absorption into the blood, the storage, and the excretion of the end products of digestion.

Chewing food is the first stage of digestion. When nutrients reach the stomach, both mechanical and chemical digestive processes occur. Nutrients are churned, and peristaltic waves move the material through the stomach and, at intervals with relaxation of the pyloric sphincter, into the duodenum. This chemical action creates hydrochloric acid, which provides the proper medium for pepsin to split protein into proteoses and peptones. Other chemical actions produce lipase, a fat-splitting enzyme, rennin, which coagulates the protein of milk, and the intrinsic factor, which acts on certain food components to form the antianemic factor.

As nutrients move into the duodenum and the jejunum, intestinal juices provide a large number of enzymes that break down protein into amino acids, form and convert maltase to glucose, and split nucleic acids into nucleotides. The small intestine provides for the absorption of nutrients and the large intestine for the elimination of waste products. It is here that the formation of vitamins K and $B_{12}$, riboflavin, and thiamin occurs. Also, there is absorption of water from the fecal mass.

**The Accessory Organs** The accessory organs of the gastrointestinal tract also play an important role in the utilization of nutrients. These organs include the tongue, salivary glands, teeth, liver, gallbladder, and pancreas.

The liver is especially important because it has a major role in the metabolism of carbohydrates, fats, and proteins. In the metabolism of carbohydrates, the liver converts glucose to glycogen and stores it. The liver then can reconvert glycogen to glucose when the body requires higher blood sugar. The process of releasing carbohydrates (end products) into the bloodstream is called glycogenolysis.

The liver metabolizes fats through the process of oxidation of fatty acids and the formation of acetoacetic acid. Also, the liver forms lipoproteins, cholesterol, and phospholipids and converts carbohydrates and protein to fats.

Proteins are metabolized in the liver, and deamination of amino acids takes place. Also in this process, the formation of urea and plasma proteins is completed. Finally, the interconversions of amino acids and other compounds occurs in the liver.

The gallbladder's primary function is to act as a reservoir for bile. When there are fatty materials in the duodenum, liberation of cholecystokinin is stimulated and the gallbladder contracts causing the relaxation of the sphincter of Oddi. Bile emulsifies fats through constant secretion (500–1000 ml in 24 hours).

The pancreas secretes pancreatic juices that contain enzymes for the digestion of carbohydrates, fats, and proteins. Enzymes are secreted as inactive precursors that do not become active until secreted into the small intestine. In the intestine, the enzyme trypsin acts on proteins to produce peptones, peptides, and amino acids; pancreatic amylase acts on carbohydrates to produce disaccharides; and pancreatic lipase acts on fats to produce glycerol and fatty acids.

In summary, the alimentary tract's primary function is to provide the body with a continuous supply of nutrients through utilization of a tract for ingestion and movement of food and fluids, secretion of digestive juices for breaking down the nutrients, and an absorption mechanism for utilizing foods, water, and electrolytes. Nutrients are essential for life, but their simple ingestion into the body is not sufficient for survival. They must be broken down, absorbed, and utilized efficiently if the body is to remain in proper balance or homeostasis.

Normal nutrition is based on recommended daily dietary allowances. These standards are scientifically designed for the maintenance of nearly all healthy people in the United States.

Therapeutic nutrition is a modification of nutritional needs based on the disease condition and/or the excess or deficit of a nutrition state. Combination diets, which include alterations in minerals, vitamins, proteins, carbohydrates, fats, as well as fluid and texture, are prescribed in therapeutic nutrition.

Whether a normal or a therapeutic diet is being considered, a person's cultural, socioeconomic, and psychological influences, as well as the physiological requirements, must be taken into account for effective nutrition; thus, in any given situation, the nutritional requirements must be considered within the context of the total needs of an individual.

**NORMAL AND THERAPEUTIC NUTRITION**

**Nutritional Problems in the Hospital**   In a hospital, nutrition is frequently neglected as a viable component of patient management. Studies conducted at various medical centers support the claim that patients become more malnourished the longer they remain in a hospital.

For patients who seem to be stable on admission and give no history of nutritionally related food problems, the usual hospital diet is adequate; however, these patients must be reassessed periodically to prevent nutritional problems from developing. A periodical assessment is especially important for patients hospitalized for a long period of time. In many long term care facilities, patients are weighed monthly.

For patients identified as having a nutritional problem, a nursing care plan must be developed. To manage these patients correctly, the cause of depletion must first be determined. Research indicates that poor food intake is the leading cause of malnutrition. Reasons for poor food intake include fear, anxiety, or depression prior to or during hospitalization. Some patients may not be capable of feeding themselves or may have poor fitting dentures. Treatment and therapy may limit the capability of a patient to eat or interfere with a patient's appetite. Also, some patients may have the desire to eat and a good appetite, but shortly after eating a certain food, they have cramps, pain, gas, or diarrhea or feel nauseous and/or vomit. This eventually leads to less food intake. Whatever the source, the cause of depletion must be determined to prevent further malnutrition. As patients become more and more malnourished, they lose the ability to handle foodstuffs metabolically. As their intake decreases below their nutritional requirements, their body cannot generate the epithelium of the gastrointestinal tract from the crypt cells. The villi and microvilli, needed to metabolize and absorb food, flatten and become ineffective. This leads to malabsorption, with resulting malnutrition.

**Therapeutic Management**   After determining the cause and the extent of depletion, the next step is to institute therapeutic procedures that meet the needs of the patient. In selecting nutrients, the clinician needs to evaluate the status of the patient's gastrointestinal tract to determine if modifications in nutrients are necessary. For example, can the patient split intact protein into

**TABLE 2** BASIC NUTRITIONAL ASSESSMENT

| Assessment | Normal | Abnormal |
|---|---|---|
| Appetite | Remains unchanged | Increased or decreased recently<br>Particular cravings |
| Weight | Previous weight maintained<br>Normal for patient<br>Appropriate for age and body build | Changed — increased or decreased recently<br>Rapid or slow changes in weight |
| Nutritional intake | Adequate foods and fluids to supply body nutrients<br>Nonallergic response to major food groups<br>No pattern of fad diets<br>Absence of drugs, chemicals, or other substances that influence appetite or metabolism | Elimination of certain food categories that results in limited nutrients<br>Emphasis on some food groups (sugar) to the exclusion of others (vegetables)<br>Allergic response to certain foods<br>Constant use of fad diets to lose weight<br>Use of drugs or chemicals that interfere with appetite or nutrient assimilation<br>Presence of emotional disorder (depression, anorexia, manic response) that interferes with food ingestion |
| Meal patterns | 3–6 home-prepared meals/day<br>Adequate time and calm atmosphere for meals | Fast-food or packaged foods<br>Missed meals, constant snacking, or overeating<br>Eating "on the run" or hurried |
| Physical factors | Adequate chewing and swallowing capability<br>Mouth and gums healthy so food can be ingested<br>Physical exercise adequate for calorie intake | Teeth and/or gums in poor condition or ill-fitting dentures<br>Swallowing impairs ingestion<br>Inadequate physical exercise to burn calories |
| Presence of disease | No disease process that interferes with nutrient assimilation<br>No congenital condition or postsurgery condition that interferes with nutrient assimilation | Disease present that interferes with ingestion, digestion, assimilation, or excretion<br>Congenital condition, rehabilitation phase, or postsurgery that interferes with food assimilation |
| Sociocultural-religious factors | Ability to afford adequate foods in all food categories<br>Cultural beliefs that do not eliminate whole food groups<br>Religious beliefs that do not eliminate whole food groups<br>Food does not lose all nutrient value in preparation | Economic position that precludes purchase of adequate foods<br>Religious or cultural beliefs that interfere with receiving balanced diet (macrobiotic diets)<br>Inadequate knowledge, experience, or intelligence to prepare healthy meals |
| Elimination schedule | Regular, adequate elimination of foods<br>Absence of constant flatus, discharge, or mucus | Irregular and/or painful elimination<br>Presence of constant flatus<br>Presence of discharge, blood, or mucus |

the peptides and amino acids needed for absorption? Can the patient tolerate the osmotic load of monosaccharides or disaccharides? Is the patient fat-intolerant, or does the patient need special fat? Is the patient lactose-intolerant? Can the patient eat normally?

Most of us consider that eating and meal time is a social time. Frequently, however, we place patients in uncomfortable and even unsocial positions so that eating is not a pleasure. In preparing the patient's environment for eating, try to make the patient as comfortable as possible. For example, it is important to plan painful or uncomfortable procedures so that they are not immediately before or after meals. Position the patient as near to normal as possible; that is, sitting in a chair, dangling on the side of the bed, or with the bed elevated 90 degrees. Provide a bright, non-odorous environment. If possible, position roommates so they can converse while eating if they so desire. Check the Patient Care Plan for patient preferences: cultural or religious limitations as well as allergies and personal likes or dislikes. Food trays should be checked for compliance with orders and patient preferences. If the patient is npo, be sure that a sign is posted on the unit door and that the patient does *not* receive a tray.

When you are preparing to assist the patient to eat, lower the side rail and place the tray table over the patient's lap low enough so that he can see what is on it. If the tray is not neatly arranged, rearrange it. Food appearance and presentation influence appetite. Assist the patient with whatever is needed, such as cutting meat. If the patient is unable to drink from a glass, use a straw or special cup.

Be sensitive to the patient's response to food and continually attempt to orient feeding to meet the patient's needs. If the patient has diminished sight or is blind but able to feed self, tell him what is on the tray and the position of each item. Often, it is clearer to describe position of foods by a clock; for example, chicken at 12, green beans at 3 o'clock, etc.

After therapeutic diets have been ordered, it is critical that the nurse be aware of compliance by the patient. The nurse is most closely involved with the patient and is the one who can best determine the patient's actual intake. The nurse should ensure that the patient is not receiving inappropriate foods from other sources and that the patient is actually eating the foods prescribed. If the prescribed diet is not meeting the patient's needs, an alternative method of feeding might be considered. For example, if oral feedings prove inadequate, then alternate methods such as feeding by nasogastric, nasoduodenal, or nasojejunal tube should be considered. There are a variety of delivery systems and methods of enteral feeding that are now available for adequate care of the patient. The particular choice should be based on the individual patient's needs and requirements.

When other methods have failed, parenteral nutrition may be the management of choice. This can be either administered peripherally, using isotonic concentrations of glucose, crystalline amino acids, and fats. It can also be administered through a central, high-flow vein in which hypertonic glucose, along with crystalline amino acids, fats, electrolytes, vitamins, and trace elements, may be given. This technique requires special handling and management of the patient and is the most expensive method of feeding. It should be used only if the intestines do not work adequately, if the patient is obstructed or has a fistula, if a bowel rest is required, or if the patient is so debilitated that the gastrointestinal tract is nonfunctional.

In this era of sophisticated medical and nursing management, no patient should become or remain malnourished or develop any kind of nutritional problem. As a nurse, you are responsible for meeting the patient's needs. Among these needs are adequate nutritional requirements to maintain status and to be able to successfully deal with or overcome the medical problems for which the patient is being treated.

**NURSING DIAGNOSES**

The following nursing diagnoses may be appropriate to include in a Patient Care Plan when the components of the plan are related to nutritional problems or nutritional health maintenance.

| Nursing Diagnosis (Potential) | Defining Characteristic; Etiology (Examples) |
|---|---|
| ☐ Noncompliance, *related to* | Improper nutritional intake or balance of nutrients, e.g., inadequate knowledge base, denial of disease process. |
| ☐ Nutrition, Alteration in: Less than Body Requirements, *related to* | Imbalance between caloric intake and activity level, e.g., situational alterations (mouth, teeth), physiological (gastrointestinal system alteration), psychological (manic episodes, anorexia nervosa), sociocultural (poverty, religious beliefs). |
| ☐ Nutrition, Alteration in: More than Body Requirements, *related to* | Imbalance between caloric intake and activity level, e.g., physiological (metabolic or chemical imbalance), psychological (compulsive overeating), physical (immobilized patient). |
| ☐ Self-Care Deficit: Feeding, *related to* | Inability to feed self, e.g., paralysis, casted extremity, neuromuscular disorder. |

## UNIT ONE   NUTRITION MAINTENANCE

### NURSING PROCESS DATA

#### ASSESSMENT   *Data Base*

Check appropriate dietary order.

Assess nutritional needs of patient.

Determine sociocultural orientation of patient.

Obtain diet history and determine eating habits and food preferences of patient.

Assess ability of patient to comply with diet regime.

Assess patient's fluid intake needs.

Check recommended daily dietary allowances and essential body nutrients.

Evaluate results of the following data:

Analysis of appropriate diagnostic tests.

Alterations in health status that indicate need for therapeutic vs. regular diet.

Status of GI tract, including digestion and/or absorption.

Ability of the patient to split intact protein into peptides and amino acids needed for absorption.

Ability of the patient to tolerate osmotic load of monosaccharides or disaccharides.

Ability of the patient to tolerate lactose.

## PLANNING   *Objectives*

To provide a nutritional diet based on individual needs.

To identify the patient who exhibits nutritional deficits and to determine an appropriate diet.

To provide nutritional requirements for patients unable to consume oral feedings.

To provide a diet that is tolerated physiologically and emotionally by the patient.

## IMPLEMENTATION   *Procedures*

Serving a Food Tray

Feeding a Patient

## EVALUATION   *Expected Outcomes*

Patient will receive adequate diet, fluids, electrolytes, vitamins, minerals, and trace elements.

Reasonable compliance to diet is maintained.

Diet is tolerated physiologically and emotionally by patient.

## SERVING A FOOD TRAY

### Equipment

Diet slip completed

Diet tray

Over-bed table

Utensils

Protective covering

### Preparation

1. Assist physician in determining a diet appropriate for the patient's needs.

2. Elicit food preferences of the patient.

3. Send request to the diet kitchen for the specific diet and keep diet sheets or diet rands up-to-date.

4. Check Patient Care Plan for changes in diet.

5. Medicate patient for pain twenty minutes before eating.

6. Check all diet trays before serving to ensure the diet provided is the one ordered.

7. Ensure that hot food is hot and cold food is cold.

8. Keep food trays attractive. Avoid spilling liquids on tray.

9. Assist patient to empty bladder if needed and wash hands.

10. Remove unpleasant objects from area, such as a bedpan.

### Procedure

1. Wash your hands.

2. Raise bed to HIGH position and lower side rail.

3. Assist patient to sitting position if possible.

4. Place protective covering over gown if desired.

5. Place tray on tray table. Position table so patient can see food.

6. Assist patient as needed, e.g. cut meat, open milk carton, etc.

7. Check on patient during meal to determine if assistance is necessary.

8. Reposition tray table at bedside when completed.

9. Provide hand cleaning and oral care if desired.

10. Offer bedpan or assistance to commode or bathroom.

11. Raise side rail.

12. Position bed for comfort.

13. Note amount of food eaten.

14. Remove food tray from room.

15. Wash your hands.

16. Chart amount eaten. If necessary, record I & O.

## FEEDING A PATIENT

### Procedure

1. Check Patient Care Plan for current changes in diet.

2. Wash your hands.

3. Raise bed to HIGH and lower side rail.

4. Assist patient to wash hands and face, if desired.

5. Place patient in sitting position if possible.

6. Place protective covering over gown if desired.

7. Place tray on tray table. Position table so patient can see food.

8. Stand or sit facing the patient. Bed would be in low position if you are sitting.

9. Ask patient the order in which he would like to be fed. If patient can't see, tell him what is available.

10. Encourage the patient to hold his glass, bread, finger foods.

11. Allow him time to chew and swallow.

12. Provide fluids throughout meal.

13. Alternate foods; don't feed all meat then all vegetable.

14. Allow patient to rest at intervals during the feeding.

15. Talk with patient during meal. **Rationale:** Talking with the patient makes mealtime a more pleasant time and encourages him not to hurry.

16. Reposition tray table at bedside when completed.

17. Provide hand cleaning and oral care if desired.

18. Raise side rail.

19. Position bed for comfort. Lower bed if it is raised.

20. Note amount of food eaten.

21. Remove food tray from room.

22. Wash your hands.

23. Chart amount eaten. If necessary, record I & O.

### CHARTING  *for Nutrition Maintenance*

☐  Appetite

☐  Food intake

☐  Tolerance to diet

☐  Weight

☐  I & O fluid status

## CLINICAL PROBLEM SOLVING

**Potential Problems**

Patient is unable to assimilate foods metabolically.

Patient vomits or has diarrhea.

**Suggested Solutions**

☐  Document on Patient Care Plan and make staff report of abnormal results of diagnostic tests which identify assimilation problems. Assist the physician in altering the method of feeding (enteral or parenteral).

☐  Evaluate allergic responses to food. Review history and physical to determine food allergies which may exist.

    ☐  Obtain order for clear liquid diet, gradually progressing back to regular diet.

    ☐  Assess overall health status (e.g., temperature, obstruction, etc.).

Psychosocial behavior interferes with eating.

    ☐  Modify diet to conform to patient's desires.

    ☐  Request consulation with dietician.

---

# UNIT TWO    THERAPEUTIC DIETS

## NURSING PROCESS DATA

### ASSESSMENT    *Data Base*

Assess total condition of patient—physical, emotional, and mental status.

Determine appropriateness of prescribed therapeutic diet as related to altered state of health.

Evaluate ability of patient to tolerate diet.

Assess mental state of patient in regard to compliance with diet regimen.

Refer to general assessment steps in maintaining normal nutritional status.

### PLANNING    *Objectives*

To maintain balanced nutritional status.

To meet nutritional needs based on alterations in patient's health status.

To tolerate foods and nutrients more efficiently.

To design a therapeutic diet with which patient will comply.

### IMPLEMENTATION    *Procedures*

Providing Therapeutic Diets For

| | |
|---|---|
| *Carbohydrate Control* | *Fiber Control* |
| *Protein Control* | *Bland Food Diets* |
| *Fat Control* | *Calorie Control* |
| *Renal Disease* | *Pre- and Postoperative Diets* |
| *Vitamin Control* | *Mechanical Soft Diet* |
| *Mineral Control* | *Puree Diet* |

### EVALUATION    *Expected Outcomes*

Patient complies with prescribed therapeutic diet.

Patient tolerates diet well.

Disease symptoms diminish.

Patient verbalizes knowledge of therapeutic diet.

Therapeutic diet conforms to ethnic preferences.

Therapeutic diet can be implemented in home setting.

**TABLE 3** DIABETIC EXCHANGE DIETS

| Food Group | Unit of Exchange | Calories | Food Allowed |
|---|---|---|---|
| Milk | | | |
| Whole | 1 cup | 170 | 1 cup whole milk = 1 cup skim |
| Skim | 1 cup | 80 | milk and 2 fat exchanges |
| Fruit | Varies according to allotted calories | 40 | Fresh or canned without sugar or syrup |
| Vegetables | | | |
| A | 1 cup | Vary | Green, leafy vegetables; tomatoes |
| B | 1/2 cup | 35 | Vegetables other than above |
| Bread | 1 slice | 70 | Can exchange cereals, starch items, some vegetables |
| Meat | 1 ounce | 75 | Lean meats, egg, cheese, seafood |
| Fat | 1 teaspoon | 45 | 1 teaspoon butter or mayonnaise = bacon, oil, olives, avocado |
| Unlimited foods | | | Coffee, tea, bouillon, spices, flavorings |

# PROVIDING THERAPEUTIC DIETS

## Procedures

### Carbohydrate Control

1. A hypoglycemic diet is utilized to reduce stimulation of excessive insulin by avoiding highly concentrated carbohydrate foods.
   a. Foods prescribed are high-protein, high-fat, and low-carbohydrate.
   b. Foods not allowed are high-carbohydrate; for example, sugar, syrup, candy.
2. A diabetic diet modifies the insulin disorder and controls sugar intake.
   a. Foods included on the diet are usually found on the food exchange list.
   b. Foods not allowed are refined sugars.

### Protein Control

1. A low-protein diet is utilized for renal impairment (uremia), hepatic coma, and cirrhosis (according to individual requirements).
   a. Control end products of protein metabolism by limiting protein intake.
   b. Evaluate the number of grams of protein allowed.
   c. Eliminate high-protein foods such as eggs, meat, milk, and milk products.

2. A high-protein diet is necessary for tissue building, correction of protein deficiencies, burns, liver diseases, malabsorption syndromes, undernutrition, and maternity.
   a. Correct protein loss and/or maintain and rebuild tissues by increasing intake of high-quality protein food sources.
   b. Encourage the eating of high-protein foods, such as fish, fowl, organ and meat sources, and dairy products.
   c. Suggest protein supplements (usually ordered by physician), such as Sustagen, Meritene, and Proteinum.

3. An amino acid metabolism abnormality diet is utilized for phenylketonuria (PKU), galactosemia, and lactose intolerance.
   a. Reduce and/or eliminate the offending enzyme in the food intake of protein and utilize substitute nutrient foods.
   b. Avoid milk and milk products as they constitute the main source of enzymes for the three diseases.
   c. Employ substitutes to meet daily allowances.

### Fat Control

1. A restricted cholesterol diet is utilized for cardiovascular diseases, diabetes mellitus, and high-serum cholesterol levels.
   a. Control the blood cholesterol level and/or

maintain blood cholesterol at a normal level by restricting foods high in cholesterol.

b. Limit high-cholesterol foods, such as egg yolk, shellfish, organ meats, bacon, pork, avocado, and olives.

c. Encourage low-cholesterol foods, such as vegetable oils, raw or cooked vegetables, fruits, lean meats, and fowl.

2. A modified fat diet is utilized according to individual tolerance in malabsorption syndromes, cystic fibrosis, gallbladder disease, obstructive jaundice, and liver disease.

a. Attempt to lower fat content in diet to reduce irritation of diseased organs and to reduce fat content where there is inadequate absorption of fat.

b. Low-fat diet: Avoid such foods as gravies, fatty meat and fish, cream, fried foods, rich pastries, whole milk products, cream soups, salad and cooking oils, nuts, and chocolate. Allow eggs (2 to 3 per week), lean meat, and small amount of butter or margarine.

c. Fat-free diet: Allow vegetables, fruits, lean meats, fowl, fish, bread, and cereal and restrict all fatty meats and fat.

3. A high-polyunsaturated fat diet is utilized for cardiovascular diseases.

a. Reduce intake of saturated fats and increase intake of foods rich in polyunsaturated fats. (Physician usually prescribes caloric level as well as restrictions.)

b. Avoid foods originating from animal sources, selected peanuts, olives, avocado, coconuts, chocolate, and cashew nuts.

c. Allow foods originating from vegetable sources (except for those named above), margarine, corn/soybean/safflower oil, fresh ground peanut butter, and nuts (except cashews).

### Renal Disease

1. A low-protein diet and essential amino acid diet (modified Giovannetti diet) is comprised of 20 gm of protein and 1500 mg of potassium.

a. Prevent electrolytes and byproducts of metabolism from accumulating to a fatal level between artificial kidney treatments.

b. Allow foods such as one egg daily, 6 ounces of milk, low-protein bread, fruit, vegetables, butter, oil, jelly, candy, tea, and coffee.

c. Restrict foods such as meat, chicken, fish, peanuts, and high-protein bread.

2. A low-calcium diet is utilized to prevent formation of renal calculi.

a. Decrease the total daily intake of calcium to prevent further stone formation. Total calcium intake is 400 mg per day instead of 800 mg (normal).

b. Allow foods such as milk (one cup daily), juices, tea, coffee, eggs, and fresh fruits and vegetables.

c. Restrict foods such as rye and whole grain breads and cereals, dried fruits and vegetables, fish, shellfish, cheese, chocolate, and nuts.

3. An acid ash diet is utilized to prevent precipitation of stone elements.

a. Establish a well-balanced diet in which the total acid ash is greater than the total alkaline ash daily.

b. Allow foods such as breads and cereals of any type, fats, fruits (one serving), vegetables, meat, eggs, cheese, fish, fowl (two servings), and spices.

c. Restrict foods such as carbonated beverages, dried fruits, bananas, figs, raisins, dried beans, carrots, chocolate, nuts, olives, and pickles.

4. A low-purine diet is utilized to prevent uric acid stones; also utilized for gout patients.

a. Restrict purine, which is the precursor of uric acid; 4 percent of urinary stones are composed of uric acid.

b. Allow foods such as milk, tea, fruit juices, carbonated beverages, breads, cereals, cheese, eggs, fat, and most vegetables.

c. Restrict foods such as glandular meats, gravies, fowl, fish, and high meat quantities.

### Vitamin Control

1. An increased vitamin diet is necessary for treatment of specific vitamin deficiencies.

a. Provide high-vitamin diet for patients with burns, healing wounds, raised temperatures, and infections. Also used for pregnant patients.

b. Evaluate diseases, such as cystic fibrosis and liver disease, that require water-soluble vitamins.

2. Total low-vitamin diets are not generally prescribed—although specific vitamins might be decreased for periods of illness.

| Foods Rich in Fat-Soluble Vitamins | Foods Rich in Water-Soluble Vitamins | **TABLE 4**<br>FOODS RICH IN VITAMINS |
|---|---|---|
| Vitamin A—liver, egg yolk, whole milk, butter, fortified margarine, green and yellow vegetables, fruits<br><br>Vitamin D—fortified milk and margarines, sunshine, fish oils<br><br>Vitamin E—vegetable oils and green vegetables<br><br>Vitamin K—egg yolk, leafy green vegetables, liver, cheese | Vitamin C—citrus fruits, tomatoes, broccoli, cabbage<br><br>Thiamine ($B_1$)—lean meat such as beef, pork, liver; whole grain cereals and legumes<br><br>Riboflavin ($B_2$)—milk, organ meats, enriched grains<br><br>Niacin—meat, beans, peas, peanuts, enriched grains<br><br>Pyridoxine ($B_6$)—yeast, wheat, corn, meats, liver, and kidney<br><br>Cobalamin ($B_{12}$)—lean meat, liver, kidney<br><br>Folic acid—leafy green vegetables, eggs, liver | |

**TABLE 5**  FOODS HIGH IN SODIUM AND POTASSIUM

**Foods High in Sodium**

Table salt and all prepared salts, such as celery salt

Smoked meats and salted meats

Most frozen vegetables or canned vegetables with added salt

Butter, margarines, and cheese

Quick-cooking cereals

Shellfish, and frozen or salted fish

Seasonings and sauces

Canned soups

Chocolates and cocoa

Beets, celery, and selected greens (spinach)

Anything with salt added, such as potato chips, popcorn

**Foods High in Potassium**

Fruit juices such as orange, grapefruit, banana, raw apple

Instant, dry coffee powder

Egg, legumes, whole grains

Fish, fresh halibut, codfish

Pork, beef, lamb, veal, chicken

Milk, skim and whole

Dried dates, prunes

Bouillon and meat broths

*Mineral Control*

1. A restricted sodium diet is utilized for hypertension, hepatitis, congestive heart failure, renal deficiencies, cirrhosis of liver, and adrenal corticoid treatment.

   a. Correct and/or control the retention of sodium and water in the body by limiting sodium intake. May be done by restriction of salt in the diet or in combination with medications.

   b. Restrict salt in cooking or at the table. In patients requiring dietary modification in salt intake any product containing sodium, such as soda bicarbonate, may be prohibited.

   c. Explain sodium restrictions in diet.
      Mild: 2 to 3 G sodium
      Moderate: 1000 mg sodium
      Strict: 500 mg sodium
      Severe: 250 mg sodium

2. An increased potassium diet is utilized for diabetic acidosis, extended use of certain diuretic drugs, burns (after first 48 hours), vomiting, and fevers.

   a. Replace potassium loss from the body with specific foods high in potassium or a potassium supplement. (Severe loss is managed with intravenous therapy.)

   b. Avoid no specific foods unless there is a sodium restriction because some foods high in potassium are also high in sodium.

3. A high-iron diet is utilized for anemias (hemorrhage, nutritional, pernicious), postgastrectomy syndrome, and malabsorption syndrome.
    a. Replace a deficit of iron caused by inadequate intake or chronic blood loss.
    b. Include foods high in iron content, such as organ meats (especially liver), meat, egg yolks, whole wheat products, seafood, leafy vegetables, nuts, dried fruit, and legumes.

### Fiber Control

1. A high-residue (roughage) diet is prescribed for constipation and diverticulosis.
    a. Suggest foods high in residue, such as any meat or fish, cheese, fat, milk, whole wheat breads, cereals, and especially unrefined bran.
    b. Instruct patient that foods low in carbohydrates are usually high in residue.

2. A low-residue diet is utilized for ulcerative colitis, postoperative colon and rectal surgery, diverticulitis (when inflammation decreases, diet may revert to high residue), rheumatic fever, diarrhea, and enteritis.
    a. Inform patient that low-residue foods are ground meat, fish, broiled chicken without skin, creamed cheeses, limited fat, warm drinks, refined strained cereals, and white bread.
    b. Instruct patient that foods high in carbohydrates are usually low in residue.

### Bland Food Diets

1. A bland diet is utilized to promote the healing of the gastric mucosa by eliminating food sources that are chemically and mechanically irritating. Bland diets are used for duodenal ulcers, gastric ulcers, and postoperative stomach surgery.
    a. Instruct patient that bland diets are presented in stages with the gradual addition of certain foods.
    b. Provide frequent, small feedings during active stress periods.

2. Establish regular meals and food patterns when condition permits.

**TABLE 6** BLAND DIET ALLOWANCES

1. Foods allowed
    Milk, butter, eggs (not fried), custard, vanilla ice cream, cottage cheese
    Cooked refined or strained cereal, enriched white bread
    Jello; homemade creamed, pureed soups
    Baked or broiled potatoes
2. Examples of foods that are eliminated
    Spicy and highly seasoned foods
    Raw foods
    Very hot and very cold foods
    Gas-forming foods (varies with individuals)
    Coffee, alcoholic beverages, carbonated drinks
    High-fat contents (some butter and margarine allowed)

### Calorie Control

1. A restricted calorie diet reduces the caloric intake of food below the energy demands of the body so weight loss will occur.
    a. Provide psychological support and exercise.
    b. Restrict such foods as carbohydrates and fats.

2. An increased calorie diet is utilized to meet the increased metabolic needs of the body. There is usually an increase in protein and vitamins when increased calories are ordered.

### Pre- And Postoperative Diets

1. A high-protein preoperative diet is essential for the maintenance of normal serum protein levels during and following surgery. This diet also restores nitrogen balance if protein-depleted for burn victims, the elderly, and severely debilitated patients.
    a. Provide adequate carbohydrates to maintain liver glycogen and adequate amino acids to promote wound healing.
    b. Provide a 2500-calorie diet that is high in carbohydrates, moderate in protein with high-protein supplements.
    c. Instruct patient that an elemental diet is low in residue and contains a synthetic mixture of CHO, amino acids, and essential fatty acids with added minerals and vitamins. It is bulk free and easily assimilated and absorbed.

**TABLE 7** RECOMMENDED NUTRIENT REQUIREMENTS

---

**Total calories per day:**
2800 for tissue repair
6000 for extensive repair

**Protein:**
50 to 75 g/day early in postoperative period
100 to 200 g/day if needed for new tissue synthesis

**Carbohydrates:**
Sufficient in quantity to meet calorie needs and allow protein to be used for tissue repair

**Fat:**
Not excessive as it leads to poor tissue healing and susceptibility to infection

**Vitamins:**
Vitamin C—up to 1 g/day for tissue repair
Vitamin B—increased above normal for stress management
Vitamin A—adjuncts autommune system
Vitamin E—increases $O_2$ to tissues

**Minerals:**
Zinc—tissue repair
Selenium—cell repair
Calcium/magnesium—relaxes nerves and maintains electrical stimulation

---

2. A special postoperative surgical diet is necessary to promote wound healing, avoid shock from decreased plasma proteins and circulating red blood cells, prevent edema, and promote bone healing.
   a. Provide 2800 total calories for tissue repair and 6000 calories for extensive repair.
   b. Fluid intake is 2000 to 3000 cc/day for uncomplicated surgery and 3000 to 4000 cc/day for sepsis or renal damage. Seriously ill patients with drainage can require up to 7000 cc/day.
3. A postoperative diet protocol progresses from nothing by mouth the day of surgery to a general diet within a few days following surgery. Foods allowed in each phase of the progressive diet include:
   a. A clear-liquid diet is 1000 to 1500 cc/day and is comprised of water, tea, broth, jello, and juices (apple, cranberry or 7-up. Avoid juices with pulp).

   b. A full-liquid diet is clear liquids, milk and milk products, custard, puddings, creamed soups, sherbet, ice cream and any fruit juice.
   c. A surgical soft diet is full liquid and, in addition, pureed vegetables, eggs (not fried), milk, cheese, fish, fowl, tender beef, veal, potatoes, and cooked fruit. Do not include gas-formers.
   d. General diet: Take into consideration specific alterations necessary for patient's health status

*Mechanical Soft Diet*

1. A mechanical soft diet is used when patients
   a. Are edentulous.
   b. Have poorly fitted dentures.
   c. Have difficulty chewing.
   d. Do not chew food thoroughly.

2. Any food that can be easily broken down can be included in this diet. It allows patients variations in tastes that are not allowed on a soft diet (chili beans.)

*Puree Diet*

1. A puree diet provides food that has been blenderized to a smooth consistency.
   a. Mainly used for patients with dysphagia or who are unable to chew.
   b. Often used with small babies.
   c. Some hospitals provide this type of diet for gastrostomy feedings.

2. When assisting patients with this type of diet, talk with them about the meal, describing the different foods. **Rationale:** When the texture is all the same, distinguishing between foods is difficult.

3. Do not mix all pureed food together or feed out of one bowl or dish. Try to keep foods separate and feed alternately with dessert last.

**CHARTING** *for Therapeutic Diets*

☐ Daily weight
☐ Appetite
☐ Patient's response to diet
☐ Patient's compliance
☐ Reasons for noncompliance

## CLINICAL PROBLEM SOLVING

| **Potential Problems** | **Suggested Solutions** |
|---|---|

Patient is noncompliant to diet.

- ☐ Elicit patient's feelings to determine exactly what is behind the noncompliance.
- ☐ Check method of diet preparation and administration to see if it is attractive and appealing.
- ☐ Ensure that environment is conducive to eating.
- ☐ Notify dietician to discuss diet with patient.

Diet is not appropriate to disease status.

- ☐ Notify physician to change diet.
- ☐ Meet with dietician to modify diet.
- ☐ Modify diet within prescribed limits to enhance tolerance.

# UNIT THREE   NUTRIENTS VIA TUBE FEEDING

## NURSING PROCESS DATA

### ASSESSMENT   *Data Base*

Assess overall status:
  Weight change/loss.
  Temperature.
  Presence of sepsis.
  Trauma.
  Mental state.
  Other medically related nutritional problems, e.g., diabetes, hyperlipidemia, alcoholism.

Evaluate oral intake. Is it adequate, moderate, or altered?

Assess nutritional requirements. Are they being met or not being met? Does the patient have special needs?

Assess status of GI tract. Is it normal, limited, or obstructed? Is there a fistula or ostomy present?

Assess capacity to chew and swallow.

Check for presence of gag reflex.

Evaluate respiratory or thoracic conditions.

Check for renal complications.

Check for vomiting and/or diarrhea.

With high-protein diets, assess for fluid and electrolyte imbalance.

### PLANNING   *Objectives*

To provide alternate means of ingesting nutrients for patients with functional gastrointestinal tract.

To intervene in preexisting or impending nutritional depletion from debilitation.

To provide aggressive management for certain disease conditions (anorexia).

To provide means of nutrition if there is an inability to swallow or an existing obstruction in upper alimentary canal.

To provide nutrients for patient in comatose or semiconscious state.

To provide increased nutrient requirements above oral consumption.

To provide nutrients for postoperative patients with bowel sounds present.

To maintain fluid and electrolyte balance.

### IMPLEMENTATION  *Procedures*

Inserting a Nasogastric Tube

Irrigating a Nasogastric Tube

Collecting a Gastric Specimen from Nasogastric Tube

Removing a Nasogastric Tube

Giving a Nasogastric Feeding

Giving a Gastrostomy Feeding

Inserting a Silicone Feeding Tube

### EVALUATION  *Expected Outcomes*

Patient tolerates feeding well, and weight is maintained or increased.

Appropriate residual is obtained from aspiration of stomach contents.

Patient complies with feeding procedure.

Intake and output balance is maintained.

Nasogastric tube functions efficiently and remains patent.

## INSERTING A NASOGASTRIC TUBE

### Equipment

Syringes, delivery system, method of delivery (flow control), formula or ordered feeding (prepared daily by dietary department)

Portable suction equipment available

Number 6, 8, 12 Levin tube

Water-soluble lubricant

Feeding equipment, 60-cc asepto syringe or feeding bag

Hypoallergenic tape

Tincture of benzoin

Towel

Emesis basin

Stethoscope

Tongue blade

Normal saline irrigation solution

20-cc syringe or asepto syringe

Disposable irrigation set (optional)

### Preparation

1. Check order and Patient Care Plan for tube feeding.

2. Warm feeding to room temperature.

3. Discuss procedure with patient. **Rationale:** Demonstration and display of items to be used will help to allay patient's fear and to gain cooperation.

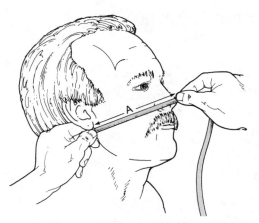

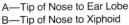

A—Tip of Nose to Ear Lobe
B—Tip of Nose to Xiphoid

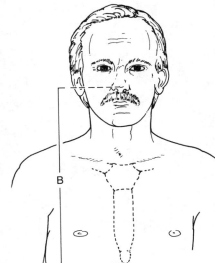

Measure NG tube from the tip of earlobe to tip of nose and then to xiphoid process.

4. Provide privacy.

**Procedure**

1. Wash hands.

2. Position patient at 45-degree angle or higher with head elevated.

3. Examine nostrils and select the most patent nostril by having patient breathe through each one.

4. Measure from earlobe to tip of nose to xiphoid process of sternum to determine appropriate length for tube insertion. If tube is to go below stomach, add an additional 15 to 25 cm. Mark point on tube with tape.

---

**Clinical Alert:**

Nurses never insert or withdraw a nasogastric tube for patients with gastric resections. The suture line could easily be interrupted, and hemorrhage could occur.

---

5. Lubricate first 4 inches of tube with water-soluble lubricant. A stylet may be used to stiffen tube.

6. Insert tube through nostril to back of throat and ask patient to swallow. **Rationale:** Sips of water may aid in pushing tubing past oropharynx.

7. Continue advancing tube until taped mark is reached.

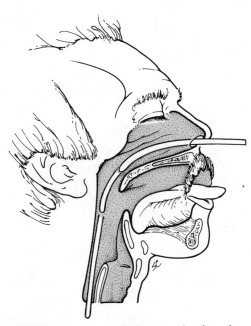

Use flashlight to check NG placement by observing mouth to check if tube is coiled in pharynx.

8. Check position of tube.
   a. Inject 10 cc of air through nasogastric tube and listen with the stethoscope over stomach for a rush of air.
   b. Aspirate gastric contents if still unsure (sometimes difficult with small-bore tubes).

**Clinical Alert:**
It is no longer considered safe practice to hold the proximal end of the N.G. tube in a glass of water while asking the patient to breathe. This was done to observe if bubbling occurred indicating that the tube was in the lung. Air can be trapped in the stomach and cause bubbling to occur when the nasogastric tube is inserted.

c. X-ray confirmation. **Rationale:** If nasoduodenal or nasojejunal feedings are required, patient should have an x-ray to confirm correct placement. Passage through the pylorus may require several days.

d. Tape tube securely to nose and to cheek.

## IRRIGATING A NASOGASTRIC TUBE

### Equipment

Disposable irrigation set

Emesis basin

20 cc syringe

Normal saline irrigation solution

I&O record sheet

### Preparation

1. Check orders and Patient Care Plan.
2. Wash hands.
3. Provide privacy.
4. Explain procedure to patient.

### Procedure

1. Place patient in semi-Fowler's position.
2. Check for nasogastric tube placement by instilling air and listening for "woosh" sound.
3. Draw up 20 cc normal saline into irrigating syringe.
4. Gently instill the normal saline into the nasogastric tube. Do not force the solution.
5. Withdraw the 20 cc irrigation solution and empty into basin.
6. Repeat the procedure twice. **Rationale:** Irrigating the tube once is not sufficient to clear the tube.
7. Record on I&O sheet the irrigation solution that has not been returned.

## COLLECTING GASTRIC SPECIMEN FROM NG TUBE

### Equipment

20 cc syringe

Specimen container

Requisition slip

Label

### Procedure

1. Check physician's orders or Patient Care Plan.
2. Wash your hands.
3. Place patient in supine or left lateral side-lying position. **Rationale:** These positions allow secretions to "pool" near cardiac sphincter.
4. Unclamp or unplug nasogastric tube. Stand plug with flat end down on over-bed table.
5. Attach 20 cc syringe to tube.
6. Pull back on plunger of syringe to aspirate gastric contents.
7. Pinch tube and remove syringe.
8. Reclamp or replug tube.
9. Expel aspirated contents into specimen container.
10. Reposition patient for comfort.
11. Dispose of equipment from bedside.
12. Wash your hands.
13. Label specimen container, affix requisition, and send container to lab.

## REMOVING A NASOGASTRIC TUBE

### Equipment

Tube plug or clamp

Towel

Wash cloth

Paper towel

### Procedure

1. Check physician's orders and Patient Care Plan.
2. Wash your hands.
3. Place towel over patient's chest.
4. Clamp or plug tube.
5. Unpin tube from gown.
6. Loosen tape securing tube.

7. Take paper towel in nondominant hand and place under chin.

8. Pinch tube near nostril and remove with a continuous steady pull. As tube is being removed, hold tube in paper towel. **Rationale:** This action prevents secretions from getting on your hands.

9. Clean patient's face, especially nares.

10. Offer oral hygiene.

11. Assist patient to a comfortable position.

12. Dispose of equipment in trash.

13. Wash your hands.

## GIVING A NASOGASTRIC FEEDING

### Equipment

20 cc syringe

Graduate

Tray

Feeding bag if used

Formula

Water to follow feeding

### Preparation

1. Obtain order from physician for appropriate formula (calories and/or amount).

2. Send requisition for formula to diet kitchen.

3. Check early in shift to ensure adequate formula is available.

4. Warm formula to room temperature using a microwave or set formula in basin of hot water.

5. Assemble feeding equipment. If using bag, fill with ordered amount of formula.

### Procedure

1. Explain procedure to patient and assure privacy.

2. Place patient on right side in high-Fowler's position.

3. Aspirate stomach contents to determine amount of residual. **Rationale:** If residual is over 50–100 cc (according to hospital policy,) you will hold feeding until residual diminishes.

4. Return aspirated contents to stomach to prevent electrolyte imbalance.

5. Pinch the tubing. **Rationale:** This procedure prevents air from entering stomach.

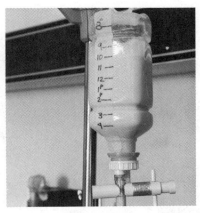

Infuse formula by allowing it to flow, by gravity, over a twenty to thirty minute time period.

6. Remove plunger from barrel of syringe and attach barrel to nasogastric tube.

7. Fill syringe with formula. (If using feeding bag, adjust drip rate to infuse over 30 minutes.) Usually drop factor on feeding bags is 20 drops/cc (most bags do not give you calculated drip factor).

8. Hold container no more than 18 inches above patient.

9. Allow formula to infuse slowly (between 20 to 35 minutes) through the tubing. Do not allow syringe to "run dry." **Rationale:** If syringe runs dry before the addition of more formula, it may cause gas.

10. Follow tube feeding with water in amount ordered.

11. Clamp end of the tube.

12. Wash tray and return it to patient's bedside.

13. Give water in between feedings if tube feeding is the sole source of nutrition.

14. Wash, rinse and dry equipment after each feeding.

## GIVING A GASTROSTOMY FEEDING

### Equipment

20 cc syringe

Graduate or feeding bag

Formula

Clean dressing

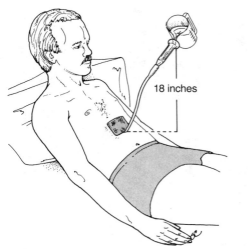

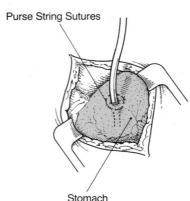

Purse String Sutures

Stomach

Hold gastrostomy tubing straight up from insertion and administer formula through tube.

## Preparation

1. Obtain order from physician for appropriate formula (calories and/or amount).

2. Send requisition for formula to diet kitchen.

3. Check early in shift to ensure adequate formula is available.

4. Warm formula to room temperature using a microwave or set formula in basin of hot water.

5. Assemble feeding equipment. If using bag, fill with ordered amount of formula.

## Procedure

1. Explain procedure to patient and assure privacy.

2. Place patient on right side in high-Fowler's position.

3. Aspirate stomach contents to determine amount of residual. If residual is over 50–100 cc (according to hospital policy) hold feeding until residual diminishes.

4. Return aspirated contents to stomach to prevent electrolyte imbalance.

5. Pinch the tubing to prevent air from entering stomach and detach the syringe.

6. Remove plunger from barrel of syringe and attach barrel to nasogastric tube.

7. Fill syringe with formula. (If using feeding bag, attach bag instead of barrel of syringe, adjust drip rate to infuse over 30 minutes.) Usually drop factor on feeding bags is 20 drops/cc (most bags do not give you calculated drip factor).

8. Hold gastrostomy tubing straight up from insertion. **Rationale:** This position puts less stress on tube.

9. Allow formula to infuse slowly (between 20 to 35 minutes) through the tubing.

10. Clamp end of the tube and remove syringe or feeding bag.

11. Remove dressing around gastrostomy opening.

12. Wash, rinse, and dry skin. Assess skin condition.

13. Apply clean dressing.

14. Wash equipment and return it to patient's bedside.

15. Give water in between feedings if tube feeding is the sole source of nutrition.

16. Wash, rinse and dry equipment after each feeding.

## INSERTING A SILICONE FEEDING TUBE

### Equipment

Silicone rubber feeding tube, size 5 to 8 Fr

Monofilament guide wire

Syringe adapter

### Preparation

1. Check physician's orders.

2. Wash your hands.

3. Gather equipment.

4. Explain procedure to patient.

5. Provide privacy if appropriate.

6. Place in Fowler's position.

**Procedure**

1. Insert guide wire into feeding tube.

2. Explain when tube is to be inserted. **Rationale:** Check hospital policy to determine if only physicians are allowed to insert this tube.

3. Measure tube for placement as you would an NG tube.

4. Insert the tube slowly into the nares. **Rationale:** The tube is small and therefore usually does not cause the gagging that an NG tube causes. Lubricating solutions should not be necessary as the weighted mercury tip and small size of the tube allows for easy passage into the stomach.

5. When the tube has reached the stomach, according to the measurement, remove the guide wire. If placement is in question, do not remove the guidewire but ask the physician for an order to x-ray for tube placement. The tube is radiopaque.

6. Tape the tube in place.

7. The syringe adapter is attached and feeding established by use of bolus, intermittent gravity drip, or continuous infusion. **Rationale:** Aspiration of stomach contents is not done prior to feed-

> These feeding tubes are left in place for long periods of time. They are not repositioned. If necessary, remove and insert a new tube. This tube is used frequently for enteral hyperalimentation.

ing. Once the tube is in place, the weighted tip maintains the correct placement.

8. Observe feedings frequently if intermittent or gravity drip is used, as thick formula or crushed medications can clog the tube.

**CHARTING** *for Tube Feeding*

☐ Weight as ordered

☐ Residual obtained

☐ Nasogastric tube size if inserted

☐ Amount and type of irrigating solution used

☐ Results of nasogastric tube irrigation

☐ Rate and volume of feeding

☐ I and O

☐ Patient's response, behavior, attitude toward feeding

☐ Patient teaching given to encourage self-care

---

## CLINICAL PROBLEM SOLVING

**Potential Problems**

Patient aspirates formula.

Vomiting occurs.

Fluid and electrolyte imbalance occurs.

**Suggested Solutions**

☐ Suction patient. Evaluate respiratory status until normal breathing pattern resumes.

☐ In future feedings, ensure that patient is kept at a 30-degree angle or higher for at least 30 minutes following feeding.

☐ Position patient quickly in high-Fowler's position (if not already) to prevent aspiration.

☐ Suction immediately.

☐ Assess concentration, amount, and rate with which formula was given.

☐ Reduce rate of formula infusion in future feedings.

☐ Reevaluate procedure to make sure stomach contents were replaced after residual was checked.

☐ Reassess formula concentration and amount of water given.

Stress ulcer develops in the GI tract from permanent tube placement.

□ Check to see if the tube can be intermittently placed to avoid constant irritation.
□ Give antacids one hour after feeding.
□ Obtain gastric aspirant to test for blood before each feeding and monitor results.

---

# UNIT FOUR TOTAL PARENTERAL NUTRITION

## NURSING PROCESS DATA

### ASSESSMENT *Data Base*

Assess nutritional needs of patients who are unable to ingest calories normally.

Identify the caloric intake necessary to promote positive nitrogen balance, tissue repair, and growth.

Observe for correct additives in each hyperalimentation bottle.

Check label of solution against physician's orders.

Check rate of infusion on physician's orders.

Assess ability of patient to understand instructions during procedure.

Ensure patency of central venous line following insertion.

Observe catheter insertion site for signs of infection, thrombophlebitis, or possible infiltration.

Inspect dressing over central line to ensure a dry, noncontaminated dressing.

### PLANNING *Objectives*

To provide a nitrogen source for patients unable to ingest protein normally.

To provide adequate calories for patients unable to tolerate oral feedings.

To provide nutrients for patients requiring bypass of the gastrointestinal tract.

To provide increased calories where regular IV solutions are insufficient.

To prevent or correct a deficiency of essential fatty acids.

To provide a contamination-free mode of delivering the hyperalimentation solution.

### IMPLEMENTATION *Procedures*

Assisting with Catheter Insertion

Maintaining Central Vein Infusions

Changing Parenteral Hyperalimentation Dressing and Tubing

Maintaining Hyperalimentation for Children

### EVALUATION *Expected Outcomes*

Catheter is placed correctly with no infiltration.

Solution is infused at prescribed flow rate and tolerated by patient.

Dressing remains dry and intact during interval between changes.

Insertion site remains free of infection and inflammation.

Patient receives nutrients necessary for tissue repair and sustenance.

## ASSISTING WITH CATHETER INSERTION

### Equipment

Intracath (20 cm, 16–gauge, radiopaque, polyvinyl chloride) or peripheral line catheter

Betadine solution

Betadine ointment and swabs

Alcohol sponges

Acetone solution (optional)

Sterile 4″ x 4″ gauze pads

Sterile gloves

Sterile towels or drapes

Sterile gown

Masks (2)

3 cc syringe with 25–gauge needle

Xylocaine or local anesthetic agent

Sterile 00 or 000 black silk suture with needle

IV filter and tubing

Plastic tape/micropore tape or occlusive dressing material

IV extension tubing

500 cc normal saline IV bag or $D_5W$

Hyperalimentation solution from pharmacy

IV infusion pump and cassette (for some equipment)

Bath blanket to provide roll under shoulders

---

**Composition of Hyperalimentation Solutions**

Amino acid—Freamine or Aminosol
Carbohydrates
Vitamins
Minerals
Hypertonic glucose/dextrose (20% to 50%)— calories (1000 to 2000 cal/liter)
Electrolytes
Water
Hyperalimentation solution is prepared in the pharmacy under a laminar flow hood.

---

### Preparation

1. Explain procedure to patient to allay anxiety.

2. Obtain consent from patient and/or family.

3. Teach the Valsalva's maneuver if patient does not have a cardiac disorder. **Rationale:** This maneuver prevents air from entering the catheter during catheter insertion or tubing changes.
   a. Ask patient to take a deep breath and bear down.
   b. Apply gentle pressure to the abdomen.

4. Review physician's order for correct hyperalimentation solution additives. Check solution content with orders. **Rationale:** Incompatible additives could cause a severe reaction or complication.
   a. TPN bottles come directly from the pharmacy and are numbered sequentially.
   b. Each TPN bottle label will include patient's name, room, number, additives, IV number, start time, date, and stop time.

5. Inspect TPN bottle for cracks, turbidity or precipitates.

6. Assemble IV insertion tray or kit, normal saline solution bottle or $D_5W$, IV tubing, extension tubing, and filter.

7. Wash hands, assemble IV equipment, and flush IV tubing with IV solution.

8. Place IV tubing through infusion pump. (IV tubing may be placed through an infusion cassette with some equipment.)

9. Place catheter insertion equipment on bedside stand.

### Procedure

1. Position patient in head-down position with head turned to opposite direction of catheter insertion site. Place a small roll between patient's shoulders to expose insertion site. **Rationale:** This position increases intrathoracic venous pressure and reduces risk of air embolism.

2. Cleanse insertion area with acetone and then Betadine solution. (If allergic to Betadine, use 70

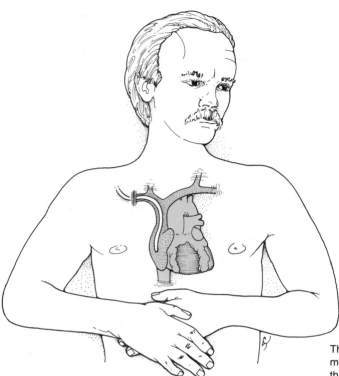

The right subclavian vein is the most common site for catheter placement. Glucose and protein concentrations of over 10% are infused through central lines.

percent isopropyl alcohol and Neosporin ointment.)

  a. Cleanse a large area around insertion site.

  b. Use a circular motion to cleanse from insertion site to periphery.

3. Assist physician to gown, mask, and glove prior to beginning procedure.

4. Don mask and sterile gloves.

5. Assist physician as needed during catheter insertion.

6. Instruct patient in Valsalva's maneuver when stylet is removed from catheter and when IV tubing is connected to catheter. **Rationale:** This procedure reduces the risk of air embolism by preventing air from entering the catheter.

7. After tubing is connected, instruct patient to breathe normally.

8. Tape area between tubing and catheter hub. **Rationale:** Secure taping holds connection together and lessens chance of contamination.

9. Turn on IV infusion pump, using normal saline solution, at slow rate, 10 drops/minute, until x–ray ensures accurate catheter placement.

10. Place Betadine (or Neosporin) ointment over catheter insertion site. Apply 4" x 4" sterile gauze pad over IV site and occlude dressing with micropore or plastic tape.

11. Order portable chest x–ray to verify correct catheter placement.

12. Following confirmation of catheter placement, change IV solution to hyperalimentation solution and adjust flow rate as ordered.

13. Time tape the bottle after adjusting flow rate. Be prepared to document on IV hourly infusion record.

14. Observe for signs of air embolism, subcutaneous bleeding, pneumothorax, or allergic responses to protein (chills, increased temperature, nausea, headache, urticaria, dyspnea).

15. Take vital signs every four hours. **Rationale:** If signs change or temperature rises significantly, the patient may be developing complications.

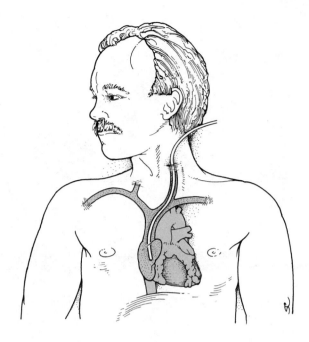

The jugular vein can be used as an alternative to the subclavian site for high concentration IV infusions, although the jugular is more difficult to use for catheter insertion.

## MAINTAINING CENTRAL VEIN INFUSIONS

### Equipment

Hyperalimentation solution (refrigerated)

IV tubing, filter and infusion pump

Extension tubing

Sugar and acetone testing equipment

Specific gravity urometer

I&O record

TPN record sheet

### Procedure

1. Store hyperalimentation solution in refrigerator until 30 minutes before use. (Some pharmacies deliver the solution before each infusion.) **Rationale:** Solution is refrigerated to prevent growth of organisms, but should be warmed to room temperature prior to use.

2. Change IV tubing, filter, and infusion pump cassette (if used) every 24 hours.

3. Change extension tubing every 48 hours. Change should accompany IV fluid bottle change.

4. Maintain IV flow rate at prescribed rate.
   a. If rate is too rapid, hyperosmolar diuresis occurs (excess sugar will be excreted); if severe enough, intractable seizures, coma, and death can occur.
   b. If rate is too slow, little benefit will be derived from the calories and nitrogen.

5. Monitor IV flow rate every 30 to 60 minutes even though you are using an IV pump.

---

**Clinical Alert**

Do not correct an overload or deficit in flow, as doing so could result in complications for the patient. Notify physician if this occurs.

---

6. Change solution every 12 hours if dextrose is used. **Rationale:** Changing the solution prevents growth of bacterial organisms that proliferate in a sugar solution.

7. Check urine specific gravity, sugar, and acetone every four hours.

8. If necessary, administer insulin according to prescribed rainbow coverage.

9. Notify physician of urine sugars of 3+ or 4+ and positive urine acetone. **Rationale:** Most patients will show a sugar level as high as 2+ during the first few days of treatment.

10. Maintain accurate I&O. Record on special total

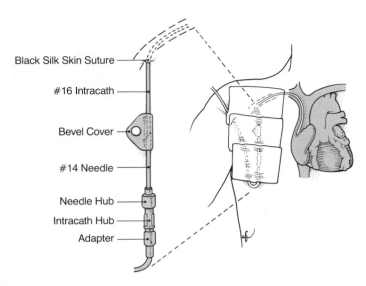

Black Silk Skin Suture
#16 Intracath
Bevel Cover
#14 Needle
Needle Hub
Intracath Hub
Adapter

Tape the dressing securely around the catheter insertion site to maintain an infection-free cannula site. The dressing needs to be occlusive.

parenteral nutrition (TPN) sheet at least every four hours.

11. Weigh daily and record on graphic sheet and TPN sheet.

12. Observe for complications such as air embolus, hyperglycemia, osmotic diuresis, infiltration, or sepsis.

## CHANGING PARENTERAL HYPERALIMENTATION DRESSING AND TUBING

### Equipment

Hyperalimentation dressing tray

Sterile towels or drapes

Sterile gown

Clean and sterile gloves

Masks (2)

IV tubing and filter

TPN solution

4″ x 4″ sterile gauze pads

Betadine swabs and ointment

Micropore tape

Paper bag

Hydrogen peroxide solution

Acetone solution

70% isopropyl alcohol

Tincture of benzoin

### Preparation

1. Gather equipment and wash hands thoroughly.

2. Add IV tubing and filter to parenteral hyperalimentation solution bottle.

3. Flush tubing to force out air.

4. Place IV tubing through IV pump or insert pump cassette into infusion pump and then prime cassette if used.

5. Prepare dressing material: open 4″ x 4″ sterile gauze pads, Betadine swabs and ointment, and tear tape into 4–inch strips.

6. Place the patient in a head-down position with head turned in the opposite direction of the insertion site. Instruct the patient not to talk or cough. (Place mask on patient if patient cannot cooperate.) **Rationale:** These instructions reduce risk of contamination.

### Procedure

1. Place mask over your nose and mouth and put on sterile gloves.

2. Take off old dressing and dispose of it in paper bag. (Do not touch the insertion site.) Remove gloves.

3. Put on new sterile gloves.

4. Cleanse around the insertion site with sterile sa-

line or hydrogen peroxide solution, using a circular movement from inside out. **Rationale:** This action cleanses the site of dried blood or serum.

5. Drape area with sterile towels.

6. Observe insertion site for signs of erythema, drainage, or possible thrombophlebitis.

7. Defat the skin around the catheter site with an acetone solution on a 4" x 4" sterile gauze pad, using a circular, outward motion. Do not allow the solution to touch the plastic tubing. **Rationale:** Acetone reacts with plastic and has a corrosive effect on the catheter.

8. Apply Betadine solution (povidone-iodine) in same circular motion, working outward from catheter site. Allow at least two minutes for drying.

9. Cleanse the area with 70 percent isopropyl alcohol. **Rationale:** This removes Betadine which can cause burning.

10. Apply povidone-iodine ointment directly to the insertion site.

11. Place precut 2– by 2–inch sterile gauze pad under catheter hub and around the insertion site, with the catheter protruding through the center of the pad.

12. Apply tincture of benzoin around the edges. Allow 30 seconds for drying.

---

**Clinical Alert**

When central-line dressings are loose, wet, or soiled, they are considered contaminated and must be changed.

---

13. Change the tubing if hospital policy dictates that tubing is changed at the same time as the dressing.
    a. Remove gloves and wash hands or keep hands gloved.
    b. Loosen the tubing in the catheter hub. Policy may dictate that the hub be wiped with alcohol swab.
    c. Tell the patient to hold breath and bear down while the new tubing is inserted into the hub of the catheter. **Rationale:** This prevents air from entering the catheter during tubing change.
    d. Tape the connection between the tubing and catheter hub.

14. Tape down the dressing around the catheter site. Tape the connection (tubing-catheter hub) to the skin. If a filter is part of the central line tubing, as with a hyperalimentation catheter, secure the filter onto the dressing with tape.

15. Label the dressing with the date and your initials.

16. Answer any questions the patient may have about the procedure and make him comfortable before leaving the room.

## MAINTAINING HYPERALIMENTATION FOR CHILDREN

### Equipment

Same as for adult hyperalimentation with these additions:

Intracath, 22–gauge needle

Microdrip IV tubing administration set

Restraints, if necessary

### Procedure

1. Examine solution. Generally, there is a higher concentration of calcium, phosphorus, magnesium, and vitamins. Usually, a 10 percent solution of dextrose is started. It can be increased to 25 percent if tolerated.

2. Monitor patency of catheter (usually placed through internal or external jugular or scalp veins). Stopcocks are never used. Monitor constant infusion pump and filter.

3. Obtain urine sugar and acetone samples. **Rationale:** Sugar level will rise, but usually exogenous insulin is not required as the pancreas adapts to high-glucose loads.

4. Change the dressing every 48 hours and the tubing every 24 hours using aseptic technique. Stockinette can be used to keep scalp dressing secure. Tight-fitting T-shirt can keep chest site secure.

5. Monitor for accurate rate of infusion. Do not "catch up" if infusion is behind. Positive pressure pumps can be used to maintain infusion rates, particularly when small amounts of solution are being infused.

6. Observe the child when ambulating for accidents such as twisting or kinking the tubing, getting the tubing caught in the crib, or stepping on it.

7. Instruct parents on rationale for treatment and

methods to prevent accidental dislodging of the tubing.

8. Provide play therapy and sources of stimulation to distract the child from thinking about the catheter.

## CHARTING  *for Hyperalimentation*

☐ Special TPN sheet may be used. If so, charting is done directly on the sheet

☐ Catheter insertion site, size, physician's name, and any difficulty in insertion

☐ X–ray, following insertion

☐ Type of hyperalimentation solution and flow rate

☐ Specific gravity

☐ Results of urine sugar and acetone

☐ If insulin administered, type, amount, and site

☐ Time of dressing and/or tubing change date, and condition of catheter insertion site, along with name or initials of person who did the change

☐ Condition of insertion site

☐ Patient's tolerance of procedure

☐ Signs of hypoglycemia or hyperglycemia

☐ Daily weights

☐ Vital signs every four hours

---

## CLINICAL PROBLEM SOLVING

### Potential Problems

Hyperalimentation solution is not infused at the prescribed rate.

### Suggested Solutions

☐ Observe filter to ensure patency. A plugged filter is the most common cause of infusion failure. Replace the plugged filter.

☐ Ensure that the next hyperalimentation bottle is ready to be superimposed. If bottle is not ready, add a bottle of $D_{10}W$ until the hyperalimentation solution can be superimposed.

☐ Observe for signs of hypoglycemia caused by sudden change in dextrose concentration: weakness, trembling, sweating, hunger.

☐ Adjust flow rate to that which was ordered. Do not attempt to "catch up" the amount not infused as this action could lead to osmotic diuresis from hyperglycemia.

Catheter insertion site does not remain free of infection, inflammation, or infiltration.

☐ Notify physician immediately so catheter can be discontinued.

☐ Cut tip of catheter off with sterile scissors and place in sterile container. Send to lab for culture and sensitivity for specific causative organism.

☐ Cleanse site of catheter insertion with Povidone and place sterile dressing over site.

☐ Obtain order for and administer antibiotics as needed.

The dressing does not remain dry and intact during the interval between changes.

☐ Change the dressing as soon as moisture is observed, following aseptic technique.

☐ If the dressing is exposed to moisture or secretions, a plastic, adhesive-like Steridrape or Saran wrap can be applied over sterile dressing.

## UNIT FIVE   INTRALIPID THERAPY

### NURSING PROCESS DATA

#### ASSESSMENT   *Data Base*

Observe for signs of essential fatty acid deficits; rash; eczema; dry, scaly skin; poor wound healing; sparse hair.

Assess pancreatic function.

Assess patient for predisposing factors that could promote fat emboli such as anemia, coagulation disorders, abnormal liver, or pulmonary function.

Check IV site for patency, erythema, and edema before infusing solution.

Assess vital signs to establish baseline.

#### PLANNING   *Objectives*

To spare protein in critically ill patient.

To provide a source of energy for patients with deficient protein intake.

To provide essential fatty acids.

#### IMPLEMENTATION   *Procedure*

Infusing IV Fat

#### EVALUATION   *Expected Outcomes*

Adequate calories and essential fatty acids are provided to patients unable to ingest them by usual means.

No untoward effects or complications are experienced as a result of procedure.

Parenteral nutrients are provided without complications.

---

## INFUSING IV FAT

### Equipment

IV fat solution: Intralipid 10 percent (soybean oil); Liposyn 10 percent (safflower oil)

Nonphthalate IV tubing infusion set (to prevent pooling of fat on IV tubing)

Iodophor sponges

Alcohol swabs

Volume control device

20–gauge needle

Small gauge needle if piggybacking into dual injection site

Micropore tape

### Preparation

1. Explain procedure to patient.

2. Review physician's orders.

3. Obtain Intralipid (refrigerated) from the pharmacy and warm the solution to room temperature or obtain Liposyn (nonrefrigerated) from the pharmacy.

4. Examine bottle for separation of emulsion into

---

### Guidelines for IV Fat Infusion

IV fat solutions are isotonic and provide 1.1 calories/ml of solution. 1 ml of Intralipid equals 0.1 g.

Putting additives into IV bottle is contraindicated as additives might be incompatible.

Use of an IV filter is contraindicated as the particles are large and the infusion will not pass through the filter and it will become plugged.

---

### Clinical Alert

Observe for IV lipid side effects after starting lipid infusion:

chills
fever
flushing
diaphoresis
dyspnea
cyanosis
allergic reactions
chest and back pain
nausea and vomiting
headache
pressure over the eyes
vertigo
sleepiness
thrombophlebitis

---

layers or fat globules or for accumulation of froth. Do not use if any of these appear.

5. Label bottle with correct patient name, room number, date, time, flow rate, bottle number, and start and stop times.

### Procedure

1. Take vital signs for baseline assessment. **Rationale:** Baseline information is needed because an immediate reaction can occur.

2. Wash hands and then swab stopper on IV bottle with iodophor sponge and allow to dry.

3. Attach special IV tubing to bottle, twisting the spike to prevent particles from the stopper falling into the emulsion.

4. Hang IV bottle at least 30 inches above IV site. **Rationale:** Due to the solution viscosity, fat emulsion needs to be higher than other IV solutions. This height prevents backing up into infusion tubing.

5. Fill drip chamber two-thirds full, slightly open clamp on the tubing, and prime the tubing slowly. **Rationale:** Priming more slowly reduces chance of air bubbles with this solution.

6. Attach the tubing to the IV site and tape connectors to prevent dislodging of the tubing.

7. Infuse fat solutions initially at 1.0 ml/min for adults and 0.1 ml/min for children. Time period for initial infusions varies from 15 to 30 minutes for Intralipid to 30 minutes for Liposyn.

8. Monitor vital signs every ten minutes and observe for side effects during first 30 minutes of the infusion. If side effects occur, stop the infusion and notify the physician.

9. Adjust flow to prescribed IV rate if no adverse reactions occur.

10. Monitor and maintain the infusion at the following rates:

*For adults*

Intralipid 10 percent—Up to 500 ml four to six hours on first day to maximum of 2.5 gms/kg body weight per day. Do not exceed 60 percent of patient's total caloric intake per day. Liposyn 10 percent—No more than 500 ml/day in four to six hours.

*For children*

Intralipid 10 percent—Up to 1 g/kg in four hours. Do not exceed 60 percent of total caloric intake.

11. Monitor serum lipids four hours after discontinuing infusion. **Rationale:** If you draw blood too soon after infusion is completed, incorrect blood values will result.

12. Monitor liver function tests for evidence of impaired liver function. **Rationale:** These tests indicate the patient's ability to metabolize the lipids.

13. Discard partially used bottles. **Rationale:** This action prevents contamination.

14. Continue to monitor vital signs and observe patient for adverse reactions during the entire process of infusion.

15. Flush tubing with normal saline when infusion is completed.

16. Answer any questions the patient may have about the prodecure and make patient comfortable before leaving room.

**CHARTING** *for Fat Emulsion Therapy*

☐ Type of solution infused

☐ Initial rate and maintenance rate of infusion

☐ Site of infusion

☐ Adverse clinical manifestations and appropriate nursing intervention

## CLINICAL PROBLEM SOLVING

| **Potential Problems** | **Suggested Solutions** |
|---|---|
| Patient experiences difficulty and cannot continue with lipid infusion. | ☐ Reassess patient's ability to tolerate fat solution. <br> ☐ Notify physician for order to discontinue fat solution and administer hyperalimentation solution. <br> ☐ Observe liver function tests. |
| Patient develops dyspnea, cyanosis, or allergic reaction such as nausea, vomiting, increased temperature or headache. | ☐ Stop infusion immediately and notify physician. |
| Patient's serum triglyceride and liver function tests remain elevated. | ☐ Attach the IV tubing to the Luer adapter. <br> ☐ Hang the solution bottle on an IV standard as you would an IV bottle. <br> ☐ Begin the feeding with a weaker concentration of formula and increase the concentration slowly as ordered. |
| Patient develops hyperlipemia or hypercoagulability. | ☐ Monitor lab results, particularly liver function tests, and notify physician when any abnormality occurs. |

## ━━━ NUTRITIONAL SUPPLEMENT ━━━

### THE BASIC FOUR FOOD GROUPS

#### Milk Group

*Foods Included*

☐ Milk: whole, evaporated, skim, dry, buttermilk

☐ Cheese: cottage, cream, cheddar, natural or processed

☐ Ice cream

*Contribution to Diet*  Milk is a leading source of calcium, which is needed for bones and teeth. It also provides high-quality protein, riboflavin, vitamin A (if milk is whole or fortified), and other nutrients.

*Amounts Recommended*  Some milk every day for everyone. Recommended amounts are given below in terms of whole fluid milk.

| | 237-ml (8-ounce) cups |
|---|---|
| Children under 9 | 2 to 3 |
| Children 9 to 12 | 3 or more |
| Teenagers | 4 or more |
| Adults | 2 or more |
| Pregnant women | 3 or more |
| Nursing mothers | 4 or more |

Part or all of the milk may be fluid skim milk, buttermilk, evaporated milk, or dry milk.

Cheese and ice cream may replace part of the milk. To substitute, figure the amount on the basis of calcium content. Common portions of various kinds of cheese and ice cream and their milk equivalents in calcium are:

| | |
|---|---|
| 16 cc (1-inch cube) cheddar-type cheese | = 1/2 cup milk |
| 1/2 cup cottage cheese | = 1/3 cup milk |
| 2 tablespoons cream cheese | = 1 tablespoon milk |
| 1/2 cup ice cream or ice milk | = 1/3 cup milk |

# DRUG-NUTRIENT INTERACTIONS

| THERAPEUTIC CLASS | DRUG NAME PROPRIETARY EXAMPLES | GENERIC/ ACTIVE COMPOUND | RECOMMENDED DAILY VITAMIN/MINERAL SUPPLEMENT OR RESTRICTION DURING DRUG THERAPY* |
|---|---|---|---|
| Dermatological preparation | Accutane® | isotretinoin | Avoid vitamin A supplement |
| Antibiotics | Panmycin® Achromycin® Other Aureomycin® | tetracycline chlortetracycline | Riboflavin (B$_2$), 5 mg Ascorbic acid, 100-200 mg Calcium, 0.8-1.5 gm** |
| Anticonvulsants | Dilantin® | phenytoin | Vitamin D, 400-800 IU† Vitamin K, 1-5 mg Folic acid, 0.4-1.0 mg (not > 2.0 mg/day) |
|  | Mysoline® | primidone | Vitamin K, 1-5 mg† |
| Anti-inflammatory | Azulfidine® | sulfasalazine | Folic acid, 0.4-1.0 mg |
|  | Bayer aspirin® Bufferin® Other aspirin | aspirin | Ascorbic acid, 50-100 mg Folic acid, 0.4-1.0 mg Iron, 20-50 mg |
|  | Indocin® | indomethacin | Iron, 20-50 mg |
| Antilipemic | Questran® Colestid® | cholestyramine colestipol | Vitamin A, 2000-5000 IU Vitamin D, 200-800 IU Vitamin K, 2-25 mg‡ Folic acid, 0.4-1.0 mg |
| Antituberculous | INH Rifamate® | isoniazid rifampin-isoniazid | Vitamin B$_6$, 25-50 mg Niacin, 15-25 mg Vitamin D, 400-800 IU |
| Anticoagulant | Coumadin® | coumarin anticoagulants | Avoid vitamin K |
| Diuretic | Dyrenium® Dyazide® | triamterene | Folic acid, 0.4-1.0 mg |
| Gastrointestinal | Agoral® | mineral oil | Vitamin A, 5000-10,000[11] IU Vitamin D, 400-800 IU |
|  | Soda mint | antacids | Folic acid, 0.4-0.8 mg |
| Hypotensive | Apresoline® | hydralazine | Vitamin B$_6$, 25-100 mg |
| Oral contraceptives | Norinyl® Demulen® Ovral® Ortho-Novum® Modicon® and others | estrogen/progestin | Vitamin B$_6$, 1.5-5 mg Folic acid, 0.4-1.0 mg Avoid high doses of vitamin C (i.e. ≥ 1000 mg) |
| Tranquilizer | Thorazine® Mellaril® | chlorpromazine thioridazine other phenothiazines | Riboflavin, 2-5 mg |
| Other | Larodopa® | levodopa | Vitamin B$_6$, restrict supplement < 5 mg |
|  | Depen® | penicillamine | Vitamin B$_6$, 25-100 mg |

Pregnant or lactating women should consult their physicians for specific micronutrient recommendations.

*Short-term drug therapy may or may not necessitate specific vitamin/mineral supplementation.

**Calcium-containing foods and supplements should be given ≥ 2 hours away from drug dose.

†If Dilantin (phenytoin)-induced demineralization is identified, give vitamin D 2000 IU/day. Pregnant women on Dilantin or Mysoline should receive vitamin K$_1$, 5 mg/day for 3 days prior to delivery and neonate should receive 1 mg.

‡Routine use of vitamin K$_1$ not required with Questran (cholestyramine) or Colestid (colestipol). Give vitamin K$_1$ I.M. in stated dosage range if hypoprothrombinemia exists.

[11]When daily dose of mineral oil preparation equals or exceeds 30 ml/day, a vitamin supplement is required. Recommended supplement, vitamin A, 5000-10,000 IU/day plus vitamin D, 400-800 IU/day. Mineral oil should be taken at bedtime and never within 2 hours of a meal. Toxic signs of hypervitaminosis A may occur with chronic intake of vitamin A (retinol), ≥ 50,000 IU/day in the adult and ≥ 20,000 IU/day in the infant or child. Hypervitaminosis D may occur with chronic intake of vitamin D ≥ 4000 IU/day or ≥ 1000 IU/day in the infant or child.

 **ROCHE** Prepared by Daphne Roe, M.D., Professor of Nutrition, Cornell University, Ithaca, New York, as a service to the health profession by Hoffmann-La Roche Inc.

## Meat Group

*Foods Included*
☐ Beef; veal; lamb; pork; variety meats, such as liver, heart, kidney
☐ Poultry and eggs
☐ Fish and shellfish
☐ Alternates: dry beans, dry peas, lentils, nuts, peanuts, peanut butter

*Contribution to Diet* Foods in this group are valued for their protein, which is needed for growth and repair of body tissues, muscle, organs, blood, skin and hair. These foods also provide iron, thiamin, riboflavin, and niacin.

*Amounts Recommended* Choose 2 or more servings every day.

Count as a serving: 57 to 85 G (not including bone weight) cooked lean meat, poultry, or fish. Count as alternates for ½ serving meat or fish: 1 egg, ½ cup cooked dry beans, dry peas, or lentils; or 2 tablespoons peanut butter.

## Vegetable-Fruit Group

*Foods Included* All vegetables and fruit. This guide emphasizes those that are valuable as sources of vitamin C and vitamin A.

*Sources of Vitamin C*
Good Sources: Grapefruit or grapefruit juice, orange or orange juice, cantaloupe, guava, mango, papaya, raw strawberries, broccoli, brussel sprouts, green pepper, sweet red pepper.

Fair Sources: Honeydew melon, lemon, tangerine or tangerine juice, watermelon, asparagus tips, raw cabbage, cauliflower, collards, garden cress, kale, kohlrabi, mustard greens, potatoes and sweet potatoes cooked in the jacket, rutabagas, spinach, tomatoes or tomato juice, turnip greens.

*Sources of Vitamin A*
Dark-green and deep-yellow vegetables and a few fruits, namely, apricots, broccoli, cantaloupe, carrots, chard, collards, cress, kale, mango, persimmon, pumpkin, spinach, sweet potatoes, turnip greens and other dark-green leaves, winter squash.

*Contribution to Diet* Fruits and vegetables are valuable chiefly because of the vitamins and minerals they contain. In this plan, this group is counted on to supply nearly all the vitamin C needed and over half the vitamin A.

Vitamin C is needed for healthy gums and body tissues. Vitamin A is needed for growth, normal vision, and healthy condition of skin and other body surfaces.

*Amounts Recommended* Choose 4 or more servings every day, including:
☐ 1 serving of a good source of vitamin C or 2 servings of a fair source.
☐ 1 serving, at least every other day, of a good source of vitamin A. If the food chosen for vitamin C is also a good source of vitamin A, the additional serving of a vitamin A food may be omitted.
☐ The remaining 1 to 3 or more servings may be of any vegetable or fruit, including those that are valuable for vitamin C and vitamin A.

Count as 1 serving: ½ cup of vegetable or fruit; or 1 medium apple, banana, orange, or potato, half a medium grapefruit, a slice of cantaloupe, or the juice of 1 lemon.

## Bread-Cereal Group

*Foods Included* All breads and cereals that are whole grain, enriched, or restored; *check labels to be sure.*

Specifically, this group includes bread, cooked cereal, ready-to-eat cereal, cornmeal, crackers, flour, grits, macaroni and spaghetti, noodles, rice, rolled oats, and quick bread and other baked goods if made with whole-grain or enriched flour. Parboiled rice and wheat also may be included in this group.

## Other Foods

To round out meals and meet energy needs, almost everyone will use some foods not specified in the four food groups. Such foods include unenriched, refined bread, cereal, flour; sugar; butter, margarine, other fats. Often these are ingredients in a recipe, or are added to other foods during preparation or at the table. Include some vegetable oil among the fats used.

---

## TERMINOLOGY

**Alimentary:** of or pertaining to nutrition.
**Anorexia:** loss of appetite for food.
**Aspirate:** to remove fluids or gases by suction.
**Calorie:** the amount of heat necessary to raise the temperature of 1 kilogram of water 1° C.

**Carbohydrates:** a group of chemical substances, including sugars, glycogen, starches, dextrins, and celluloses, that contain only carbon, oxygen, and hydrogen.
**Cardio:** word part that pertains to the heart.

**Cardiovascular:**   term that pertains to the heart and blood vessels as cardiovascular system.

**Diabetic:**   one who has inadequate production and utilization of insulin.

**Diet:**   liquid and solid food substances regularly consumed.

**Digestion:**   the process by which food is broken down mechanically and chemically in the gastrointestinal tract.

**Diverticula:**   a sac or pouch in the walls of a canal.

**Diverticulosis:**   diverticula of the colon without inflammation or symptoms.

**Emaciation:**   a condition characterized by extreme leanness or thinness.

**Emesis:**   the act of vomiting.

**Erythema:**   redness of the skin produced by capillary congestion as in a sunburn.

**Fat:**   substance made up of carbon, hydrogen, and oxygen, occurring naturally in most foods but especially meat and dairy products.

**Food supplement:**   a preparation added to the regular diet that aids nourishment.

**Gastric gavage:**   introduction of nourishment into the stomach by mechanical means.

**Gastrointestinal:**   term that pertains to the stomach and intestines.

**Hematemesis:**   vomitus containing blood.

**Hyperalimentation:**   the process of nourishing the body through parenteral means.

**Hyperglycemia:**   condition characterized by an increase in blood sugar.

**Hypertonic:**   solution having a higher osmotic pressure or tonicity than a solution to which it is compared.

**Hypoglycemia:**   condition characterized by a deficiency of sugar or glucose in the blood.

**Infuse:**   introduce a liquid into a vein.

**Ingest:**   the process of taking material into the gastrointestinal tract or the process by which a cell takes in foreign particles.

**Intralipids:**   fatlike emulsion used to correct fatty acid deficiencies via parenteral nutrition.

**Irrigate:**   to rinse or wash out with a fluid.

**Isotonic:**   a solution that has the same tension or tonicity as another solution to which it is compared.

**Jejunostomy:**   surgical creation of a permanent opening into the jejunum.

**Kwashiorkor:**   a state of extreme malnutrition due to severe protein insufficiency.

**Lumen:**   the inner open space of a tube.

**Malnutrition:**   a condition characterized by a lack of necessary food substances or improper absorption and distribution of food substances in the body.

**Minerals:**   inorganic elements or compounds.

**Nasogastric tube:**   a tube that is passed through the nose and into the stomach.

**Nausea:**   a feeling of sickness accompanied with a desire to vomit.

**Nutrient:**   nourishing; food item that supplies the body with necessary elements.

**Obstruction:**   blocking of a structure that prevents it from functioning normally; obstacle.

**Polyunsaturates:**   a long chain of carbon compounds, especially fats.

**Projectile vomiting:**   the expulsion of vomitus with great force.

**Proteins:**   substances that contain amino acids essential for growth and repair of tissues.

**Protocol:**   description of steps taken.

**Renal:**   term that pertains to the kidney.

**Sepsis:**   pathologic state usually febrile, resulting from the presence of microorganisms or their poisonous products in the blood stream.

**Thrombo:**   a clot of blood; a thrombus.

**Thrombophlebitis:**   inflammation of a vein before the development of a thrombus.

**Trauma:**   an injury or wound.

**Uremia:**   toxic condition associated with renal insufficiency and the retention of nitrogenous substances in the blood.

**Vitamins:**   a group of organic substances essential for life.

**Xiphoid:**   the lowest portion of the sternum.

# Chapter 17

# Physical Assessment

Physical Assessment
Mental-Spiritual Assessment
Maternity Assessment
Newborn and Pediatric Assessment

## LEARNING OBJECTIVES

List the four phases of physical assessment.

Outline the essential elements obtained from a health history.

Describe the abnormal manifestations associated with each specific body system for one patient with whom you are familiar.

List four normal responses that determine the patient's level of consciousness.

Describe four abnormal responses in pupil assessment.

State three assessment components of the skin.

Describe normal and abnormal lung sounds.

Outline the steps of breast assessment.

Identify the four heart sounds by auscultation.

List at least five essential elements included in a mental status assessment.

List the assessment actions in an initial physical assessment for pregnancy.

Describe what is meant by baseline data for pregnancy.

List the characteristics observed in a newborn assessment.

Identify one major abnormality in each system that might be observed during pediatric assessment.

## ASSESSMENT TECHNIQUES

An assessment technique is practical if it can be accomplished easily, with minimal equipment. The techniques discussed in this chapter can be performed in less than ten minutes, using a stethoscope, flashlight, your hands and observational skills. Although you may not be able to perform assessments rapidly at first, you will have many opportunities to practice your skills since every patient needs to be assessed at least once during a shift.

The four phases of assessment are inspection, auscultation, palpation, and percussion. Inspection is an overview of the patient. While interviewing the patient, observe such characteristics as hair, skin, general posture and psychosocial behavior; in other words, the general appearance of the patient. Auscultation is accomplished by using a stethoscope to listen to respiratory, heart, and bowel sounds. Palpation and percussion are performed using fingers and hands to assess abnormalities of sound such as vocal fremitus, enlarged organs, organ displacement, and expansion of the chest or abdomen.

As you conduct the assessment, use your hands for palpation. Using the proper technique will provide you with more complete findings and cause minimal discomfort to the patient. When palpating an area, use the entire surface of all five fingers. Apply pressure slowly but firmly. Sudden pressure or probing with one finger may cause discomfort or cause the patient to tense the area you are palpating.

The two basic physical assessment formats are head-to-toe and body systems. This chapter recommends a modified systems approach. You start at the patient's head and examine the body as you move from head to toe.

To ensure that your assessment is methodical, follow the same format each time. It is not important which of the several formats you choose, only that you follow the same one consistently.

**Types of Equipment**   The primary instrument used during assessment is the stethoscope. As you use this instrument, remember that any movement, such as moving your fingers on the chest piece or tubing or moving the chest piece on the skin, can cause extraneous noise that obliterates the sounds you want to hear. The diaphragm piece should be applied firmly to the skin. The bell piece should be placed on the skin very lightly to pick up low-pitched sounds such as heart murmurs. If the bell is pressed firmly, it stretches the skin and acts like a diaphragm. Other instruments used are the flashlight, tuning fork, ophthalmoscope, and otoscope.

# HEALTH HISTORY

A total physical assessment should include a health history. The patient's past health conditions, current problems, and present needs should be clearly identified in this process.

Information obtained from the interview and the physical assessment comprises the basis for establishing the individualized nursing care plan. A complete health history includes the following elements:

- □ *Biographical information:* age, sex, whether patient is a good historian.

- □ *Chief complaint:* condition that brought patient to health care facility.

- □ *Present health status or illness:* onset of the problem; clinical manifestations, including severity of symptoms; pain characteristics if present, etc.

- □ *Health history:* general state of health, past illnesses, surgeries, hospitilizations, allergies, current medications, and general habits such as smoking.

- □ *Family history:* age and health status of parents, siblings, and children; cause of death for immediate family members.

- □ *Psychosocial factors, lifestyles:* cultural beliefs that influence health management; religious or spiritual beliefs.

- □ *Nutrition:* dietary habits, preferences, or restrictions.

## NEUROLOGICAL ASSESSMENT

The neurological examination is begun with the initial contact with the client. Evaluation of verbal responses, movement, and sensation are carried out throughout the examination. In addition, a general assessment of the function of the cerebrum, cerebellum, cranial nerves, spinal cord, and peripheral nerves is done. The level of consciousness is the most sensitive and reliable index of cerebral function.

| ASSESSMENT | NORMAL | ABNORMAL |
|---|---|---|
| **LEVEL OF CONSCIOUSNESS** | | |
| Evaluate **verbal responses** | Alert | Lethargic |
| If client seems awake and alert but does not respond properly, check to see if client is blind, deaf, or speaks another language | Restless | Drowsy |
| | Responds to verbal command | Hard to awaken |
| | Answers questions appropriately | Unable to give date, month, place |
| | Speaks clearly | Irritable |
| | Oriented to time, person, place | Does not recognize family |
| | | Does not respond to own name |
| Observe and test **motor responses** on both sides of body | Eyes open | Eyes closed |
| | Ability to stick out tongue, squeeze fingers, move extremities | Does not follow directions to stick out tongue, squeeze fingers, or move extremities |

| ASSESSMENT | NORMAL | ABNORMAL |
|---|---|---|
| Exert pressure on nailbed with pen<br>Apply pressure to supraorbital notch<br>Pinch ear lobes or between big toe and second toe | Responds to painful stimuli by reaching out or trying to stop pressure | Does not respond to painful stimuli<br>Assumes *decorticate posturing* (legs extended; feet extended with plantar flexion; arms internally rotated and flexed on chest): due to lesion of corticospinal tract near cerebral hemisphere<br>Assumes *decerebrate posturing* (arms stiffly extended and hands turned outward and flexed; legs extended with plantar flexion): may be due to lesion in diencephalon, pons, or midbrain<br>Assumes *flaccid posturing* (no motor response): may be due to extreme brain injury to motor area of brain |

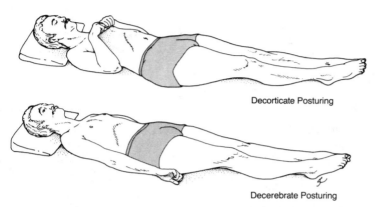

Decorticate Posturing

Decerebrate Posturing

Decorticate and Decerebrate posturing.

*Involuntary movements*

choreiform (jerky and quick): present in Sydenham's chorea

athetoid (twisting and slow): present in cerebral palsy

tremors: hyperthyroid, cerebellar ataxia, parkinsonism

spasms: cord injured clients

convulsions: epilepsy, heat stroke

asterixis: liver disease, uremia

## PUPIL ASSESSMENT

| | | |
|---|---|---|
| Observe **appearance of pupils** by holding eyelids open and checking for: | | |
| **Size of pupils** | Diameter: 1.5 to 6 mm | Unilateral dilation: sign of third cranial nerve involvement<br>Bilateral dilation: sign of upper brainstem damage<br>Dilated and nonreactive: sign of increased intracranial pressure or ipsilateral oculomotor nerve compression from tumor or injury |
| **Shape of pupils** | Round and midposition | Midposition and fixed: sign of midbrain involvement<br>Pinpoint and fixed: sign of pontine involvement |
| **Equality of pupils** | Equal | Unequal: sign that parasympathetic and sympathetic nervous systems are not in synchronization |
| Observe **reaction to light** by using pen light in darkened room<br>  Open eyelid being tested; cover opposite eye<br>  Move light toward client's eye from side position | Pupil constricts promptly | Sluggish reaction: early warning of deteriorating condition<br>Light reflex is the most important sign differentiating structural from metabolic coma |

| ASSESSMENT | NORMAL | ABNORMAL |
|---|---|---|
| Observe consensual **light reflex** <br> Hold both eyelids open <br> Shine light into one eye only <br> Observe opposite eye | Pupil constricts | Pupil does not constrict: sign that connection between brainstem and pupils is not intact |

## MOTOR FUNCTION

| ASSESSMENT | NORMAL | ABNORMAL |
|---|---|---|
| Assess **muscle strength** <br> Test hand grip by asking client to squeeze your fingers | | Absence of motor function: may be sign of hemiplegia (paralysis of one side of the body); paraplegia (paralysis of the legs and/or lower part of the body); quadriplegia (paralysis of arms and legs) |
| Test arm strength by asking client to close eyes and hold arms out in front with palms up | Maintain position for 20 to 30 seconds | Inability to maintain position with both arms: possible sign of hemiplegia |
| Assess **flexion** and **extension** strength in extremities <br> Stand in front of client, place your hand in front of client, and ask client to push your hand away | Equal response in both arms | |
| Place your hand on client's forearm and ask client to pull his or her arm upward | | |
| Position client's leg with knee flexed and foot resting on bed; as you try to extend leg, ask client to keep his or her foot down | Equal response in both legs | |
| Place one hand on client's knee and one hand on client's ankle; ask client to straighten his or her leg as you apply resistant force to knee and ankle | | |
| Assess **muscle tone** <br> Flex and extend client's upper extremities to assess how well client resists your movements <br> Flex and extend client's lower extremities to assess resistance | Client resistance is apparent | Increased resistance: sign of increased muscle tone from muscle rigidity or spasticity <br> Increased in UMN lesions and parkinsonism <br> Decreased resistance: sign of decreased muscle tone from flaccidity <br> Decreased in LMN and cerebellar lesion |
| Assess **coordination** <br> *Hand coordination* <br> Ask client to pat both thighs as rapidly as he or she can | Client able to perform coordinated movements upon request | Uncoordinated movements: may be due to cerebellum or basal ganglia involvement |

| ASSESSMENT | NORMAL | ABNORMAL |
|---|---|---|
| Ask client to turn his or her hands over and back in quick succession<br>Ask client to touch each finger to his or her thumb in rapid succession — repeat with other hand | | |
| *Foot coordination*<br>Place your hands close to client's feet<br>Ask client to tap your hands alternately with the balls of his or her feet | | |
| *Hand positioning coordination*<br>With client's eyes open, extend your hand in front of client's face<br>Ask client to touch his or her nose with index finger several times in rapid succession<br>Repeat test with client's eyes closed | | Inability to perform task with eyes closed: may be due to loss of positioning sense |
| *Leg positioning coordination*<br>Ask client to put heel on opposite knee and to slide heel down leg to foot | | |
| **Assess reflexes** | | |
| *Blink reflex*<br>Hold client's eyelid open<br>Approach client's eye unexpectedly from side of head or brush client's eyelashes | Eyes close immediately | Absence of blink response; eyelid continuously in open position: due to fifth or seventh cranial nerve not being intact |
| *Gag and swallow reflex*<br>Open client's mouth and hold tongue down with tongue blade<br>Touch back of pharynx on each side with applicator stick | | Absense of gag and swallow reflex; inability to swallow food or liquid: due to ninth or tenth cranial nerve not intact |
| *Plantar response (Babinski reflex)*<br>Run top of pen along outer lateral aspect from heel to little toe of client's foot<br>Continue tracing a line across ball of foot toward great toe | Flexion of toes | Great toe dorsiflexes; other toes fan: due to upper motor neuron lesion |

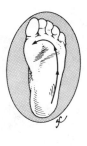
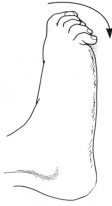
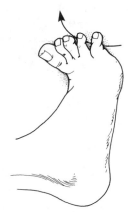

Negative Babinski       Positive Babinski       Negative and positive Babinski response.

| ASSESSMENT | NORMAL | ABNORMAL |
|---|---|---|
| *Deep tendon reflex* | | |
| Ask client to relax | Biceps reflex: flexion at elbow and contracting of biceps muscle | Absent or diminished: sign of $C^5$ or $C^6$ injury |
| Position limb to be assessed so that muscle is somewhat stretched | | |
| Using reflex hammer, strike tendon quickly while applying additional tendon stretch | Triceps reflex: extension at elbow and contraction of triceps muscle | Absent or diminished: $C^7$ or $C^8$ injury |
| Assess according to scale | Knee reflex: extension of knee and contraction of quadriceps | Absent or diminished: $C^2$, $C^3$ or $C^4$ injury |

*Grading Scale*

4+   Hyperactive (indicative of disease state)
3+   More brisk than usual but not indicative of disease state
2+   Average/normal
1+   Slightly diminished, low normal
0    No response

## SENSORY FUNCTION

Assess **superficial sensations**

**Pain**

| | | |
|---|---|---|
| Ask client to close eyes | Ability to distinguish between sharp and dull sensations | Alterations in pain or temperature sensations: indicate lesion in posterior horn of spinal cord or spinothalamic tract of cord |
| Stroke skin with safety pin, alternating blunt end and sharp end of pin | | |
| Ask client to distinguish sharp and dull pain | | |

| ASSESSMENT | NORMAL | ABNORMAL |
|---|---|---|
| **Temperature** | | |
| Fill two test tubes with water, one hot, one cold<br>Ask client to close eyes and touch client's skin with test tubes | Ability to distinguish between hot and cold | |
| **Touch** | | |
| Ask client to close eyes<br>Stroke cotton wisp over client's skin | Ability to identify light touch | |
| **Positioning** | | |
| Ask client to close eyes<br>Grasp client's finger with your thumb and index finger<br>Move client's finger up and down<br>Ask client to identify direction finger is moving | Ability to identify position | Inability to determine direction of movement: may be due to loss or injury of position sense |
| **VITAL SIGNS** | | |
| Assess rate and quality of **respirations** | Regular rate: 12 to 20 | Cheyne-Stokes (rhythmic rising and falling of depth of respiration): may be due to deep cerebral or cerebellar lesion<br>Central neurogenic hyperventilation<br>Apneustic<br>Cluster breathing<br>Ataxis |
| Monitor **arterial blood gases** if signs of respiratory imbalances occur | pH: 7.35 to 7.45<br>$pCO_2$: 35 to 45 mm Hg<br>$HCO_3$: 22 to 26 mEq/l | Alterations in pH and $pCO_2$ values: indicate respiratory imbalances<br>pH below 7.35 and $pCO_2$ above 45: signs of acidosis<br>pH above 7.45 and $pCO_2$ below 35: sign of alkalosis<br>$HCO_3$ altered: indicates compensation |
| Assess **temperature**<br>If client is semi-comatose or comatose, take temperature rectally<br>If rectal temperature contraindicated or if there are signs of increased intracranial pressure, take axillary temperature | Ability to maintain normal body temperature (approximately 98.6° F) | Inability to maintain normal temperature: may be due to damage to hypothalamus<br>No sweating below level of injury: due to spinal cord injury<br>Hypothermia |

| ASSESSMENT | NORMAL | ABNORMAL |
|---|---|---|
| Assess **pulse**<br>   Observe character of pulse<br>   Observe pulse rate | Regular rhythm (rate: 60 to 100) | Premature beats: may be due to hypoxia<br>Slow pulse rate with accompanying widening pulse pressure and bradypnea: sign of increased intracranial pressure |
| Assess **blood pressure**<br>   Position neurological clients in low to semi-Fowler's position | Normal pressure (range 120/80 to 140/90) | Systolic blood pressure rises with diastolic pressure remaining same: sign of increased intracranial pressure<br>Blood pressure over 140/90: sign of hypertension<br>Blood pressure below 95/60: sign of hypotension |

## ASSESSMENT OF SKIN

The skin is the body's first line of defense against disease and injury. It is made up of three layers: the epidermis, the dermis, and the subcutaneous tissues.

The epidermis is divided into two avascular, or bloodless, layers: an outer layer that consists of dead keratinized cells and an inner layer that consists of live cells where keratin and melanin are formed. The dermis contains blood vessels, connective tissue, sebaceous glands and some of the hair follicles. The subcutaneous tissues contain the remainder of the hair follicles, fat, and the sweat glands.

Hair, nails, sweat glands, and sebaceous glands are appendages of the skin. There are two types of sweat glands: eccrine and apocrine. Eccrine glands are distributed over most of the body except for the palms and soles. These glands help control body temperature through their sweat production. The apocrine glands are found mainly in the axillary and genital areas and are stimulated by emotional stress. The decomposition of secretions in these glands causes body odor.

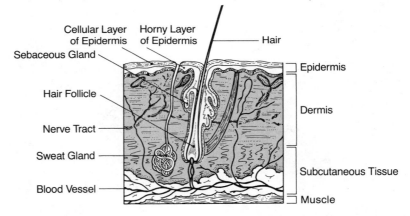

Skin is the first line of defense against disease and injury.

| ASSESSMENT | NORMAL | ABNORMAL |
|---|---|---|
| Note **color** of the skin by assessing the oral mucous membranes, the conjunctiva, and the nail beds | Pink, tan, or brown, depending on the client's basic skin color | Decrease in color or pallor<br>   *Example*: anemia from acute blood loss (hemorrhage), renal failure, dietary deficiencies, or peripheral vascular disorders<br>Vasoconstriction due to smoking, fear, or anger<br>Jaundice (icterus): due to the presence of conjugated or unconjugated bilirubin in the blood and tissues; appears most frequently in the face and trunk; seen best under natural light |

| ASSESSMENT | NORMAL | ABNORMAL |
|---|---|---|
| | | Cyanosis (blue, bluegray, or purple discoloration of the skin and mucous membranes): caused by hypoxia, a result of an increased amount of reduced hemoglobin<br>Peripheral: seen in nail beds and earlobes<br>*Example*: anxiety or hypothermia<br>Central: seen in nail beds, lips (circumoral) and oral mucosa<br>Erythema (redness of the skin): caused by capillary congestion; occurs with inflammation or infection; usually a local finding |
| Note **pigmentation** | | Hyperpigmentation<br>*Example*: use of oral contraceptives, pregnancy, Addison's disease, and hyperthyroidism |
| Note **turgor** and **mobility** | Smooth and elastic | Tight or stretched and difficult to move: due to local or generalized edema |
| Pinch skin on an extremity<br>If the fold persists, skin turgor is poor | Resilient and supple | Wrinkled: due to dehydration caused by rapid weight loss; appears as folds of skin on upper arms or abdomen<br>Thin and translucent (parchment)<br>*Example*: chronic steroid use<br>Thin, shiny, and smooth with alopecia on lower extremities<br>*Example*: chronic arterial insufficiency |
| Press finger into skin on ankle bone; grade amount of fluid from 1 to 4+ | Resilient and no evidence of fluid retention | Pitting edema: excess intracellular fluid<br>*Example*: congestive heart failure, renal failure, cirrhosis of the liver |
| Note **moistness** and **temperature** of the skin | Warm and dry | Warm (hot) and moist due to hyperthermia<br>Cool and moist (cold and clammy): may be due to shock states<br>Abnormally dry: may be due to dehydration, decreased sebaceous gland secretions, or the excessive use of soap |
| Assess for **sensation** — response to external stimuli | Feels touch, sensitive to heat and cold and pressure | Absence of touch or pain sensation<br>*Example*: spinal cord injury or nerve damage<br>Diminished heat and cold sensation<br>*Example*: peripheral vascular disease<br>Itching and tingling<br>*Example*: peripheral vascular disease, drug incompatibility, histamine reaction |
| Note **lesions** on the skin<br>Physical characteristics include color, elevation, shape, mobility, and contents | No lesions present | Macules (localized changes in color without elevation)<br>*Example*: petechiae, first degree burns, purpura<br>Papules, plaques, nodules (solid, elevated, varying in size)<br>*Example*: psoriasis, xanthomas |

| ASSESSMENT | NORMAL | ABNORMAL |
|---|---|---|

Wheals (elevated, circumscribed, transient)
  *Example*: urticaria, insect bites)
Vesicles and bullae (clear, fluid-filled pockets
  between skin layers)
  *Example*: second degree burns
Pustules (vesicles or bullae filled with exudate)
  *Example*: furuncles, acne

## ASSESSMENT OF HEAD AND NECK

The names of the regions of the head are derived from the bones that form the skull. Knowing the names of the bones and regions of the skull can assist in describing the location of the physical findings.

An understanding of the function of each lobe of the brain allows the nurse to be able to identify potential client problems when an injury occurs to that portion of the brain.

The brain is comprised of three segments, the brainstem, cerebrum and the cerebellum. There are twelve cranial nerves, which will be discussed in this chapter, and 31 spinal nerves with the respective dorsal and ventral roots.

The brainstem is divided into four sections. The diencephalon is comprised of the thalamus, which screens and relays sensory impulses to the cortex, and the hypothalamus, which regulates the autonomic nervous system, stress response, sleep, appetite, body temperature, water balance, and emotions. The midbrain is responsible for motor coordination and conjugate eye movements. The pons controls involuntary respiratory reflexes and contains projection tracts between the spinal cord, medulla, and brain. The medulla contains cardiac, respiratory, vomiting, and vasomotor centers. In addition, all afferent and efferent tracts must pass between the spinal cord and brain through the medulla.

The cerebral hemispheres have an outer layer formed by cellular gray matter, called the cerebral cortex. The two cerebral hemispheres are divided

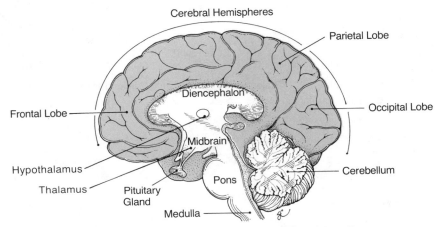

Three segments of brain: brainstem, cerebrum, cerebellum.

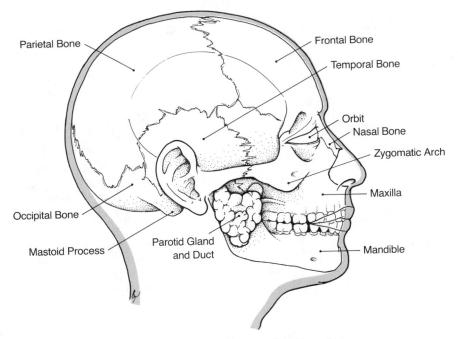

Lobes of brain covered by associated bone layer.

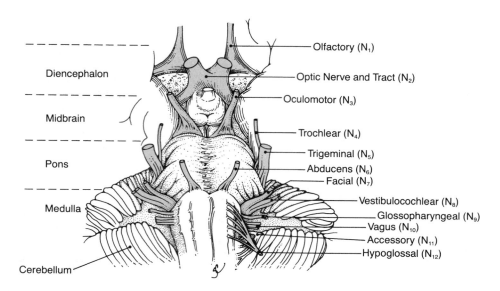

Brainstem and anatomical position of twelve cranial nerves.

into four major lobes. The frontal lobe controls emotions, judgments, motor function and the motor speech area. The parietal lobe integrates general sensations, interprets pain, touch and temperature, and governs discrimination. The temporal lobe contains the auditory center and sensory speech center. The occipital lobe controls the visual area. The cerebellum coordinates muscle movement, posture, equilibrium and muscle tone.

The twelve cranial nerves are summarized below. The second through twelfth nerves arise from the brainstem.

The cranial nerves are 12 pairs of parasympathetic nerves with their nuclei along the brainstem.

First cranial nerve: olfactory. Sensory nerve

Second cranial nerve: optic. Sensory nerve; conducts sensory information from the retina

Third cranial nerve: oculomotor. Motor nerve; controls four of the six extraocular muscles; raises eyelid and controls the constrictor pupillae and ciliary muscles of the eyeball

Fourth cranial nerve: trochlear. Motor nerve; controls the superior oblique eye muscle

Fifth cranial nerve: trigeminal nerve. Mixed nerve with three sensory branches and one motor branch; the ophthalmic branch supplies the corneal reflex

Sixth cranial nerve: abducens. Controls the lateral rectus muscle of the eye

Seventh cranial nerve: facial. Mixed nerve; anterior tongue receives sensory supply; motor supply to glands of nose, palate lacrimal, submaxillary, and sublingual; motor branch supplies hyoid elevators and muscles of expression and closes eyelid

Eighth cranial nerve: acoustic. Sensory nerve with two divisions—hearing and semicircular canals

Ninth cranial nerve: glossopharyngeal. Mixed nerve; motor innervates parotid gland; sensory innervates auditory tube and posterior portion of taste buds

Tenth cranial nerve: vagus. Mixed nerve with motor branches to the pharyngeal and laryngeal muscles and to the viscera of the thorax and abdomen; sensory portion supplies the pinna of the ear, thoracic, and abdominal viscera

Eleventh cranial nerve: accessory. Motor nerve; innervates the sternocleidomastoid and trapezius muscles

Twelfth cranial nerve: hypoglossal. Motor nerve; controls tongue muscles

| ASSESSMENT | NORMAL | ABNORMAL |
|---|---|---|
| **EYE ASSESSMENT** | | |
| Note **visual acuity** by observing client performance of activities of daily living<br>    Factors influencing visual acuity include client's previous status and age | Adequate performance of activities of daily living<br><br>Appropriate responses to environment | Hyperopia (farsightedness)<br>Myopia (nearsightedness)<br><br>Cataract (opacification of the lens)<br>Enucleation (loss of an eye): may have prosthesis in place |
| Note exact location, size, and color of any **external lesions**<br>    Palpate for mobility and firmness | No external lesions | Circumocular ecchymosis: may be sign of basal skull fracture<br>Xanthalasma (small, yellowish, well-circumscribed plaques): may appear on eyelids of clients with lipid disorders<br>*Example*: atherosclerosis |
| Note **equality of eyelid movement** | Eyelids are equal in movement | Ptosis (paralytic drooping of the upper eyelid) |
| Note color, consistency, amount, and origin of **discharge** from eyes | No discharge | Sty, or hordeolum<br>Thick white discharge: may be due to conjunctivitis |
| Note **internal lesions** | No internal lesions | Conjunctival or ciliary injection (dilatation of the blood vessels) |
| Assess differences between **pupil size and reaction**<br>    Note presence of hemorrhage | Both pupils are the same size | Anisocoria (indicates unequal pupil size): may be indicative of neurological trauma or deficit<br>Corneal edema (very soft, movable mass that looks like raw egg white): frequently occurs in clients who have increased intracranial pressure<br>Arcus senilis (partial or complete whitish circle near the outer edge of the cornea): usually due to aging |

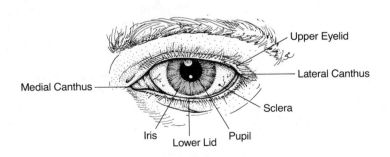

**Eye structures usually assessed for abnormalities.**

| ASSESSMENT | NORMAL | ABNORMAL |
|---|---|---|
| **EAR ASSESSMENT** | | |
| Note **auditory acuity** by asking client to indicate if he or she hears normal sounds as you make them | Adequate responses to normal sounds<br>Auditory changes due to aging | Deafness: may be caused by continued use of antibiotics<br>Abnormal sounds in the ears<br>*Example*: ringing or buzzing |
| Note exact size, color, and location of any **external lesions**<br>Palpate lesions for mobility and firmness | No external lesions | Battle's sign (ecchymosis behind the ear): may be sign of basilar skull fracture |
| Note color, quantity, and consistency of any **discharge** from the ears<br>Test clear fluid for glucose using a Labstix | No discharge | Cerebrospinal fluid leak: may be due to head injury. If drainage is blood and CSF, it will develop a ''halo'' with a reddish area in the center and a whitish circle if placed on white material<br>Perforation of tympanic membrane: serosanguineous or purulent drainage |

Ear structures assessed for abnormalities.

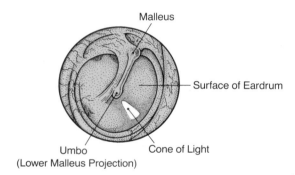

Malleus

Surface of Eardrum

Umbo
(Lower Malleus Projection)

Cone of Light

| **NOSE ASSESSMENT** | | |
|---|---|---|
| Note any **structural changes** in the nose by observing client breathe<br>Gently occlude one nostril at a time; ask client to breathe through the non-occluded nostril | Regular breathing with mouth closed<br><br>Breathing through non-occluded nostril | Breathing through the mouth only: furuncles may occlude breathing<br><br>Obstruction in the nose due to deviated nasal septum, or excessive mucus secretions |
| Note color, quantity, and consistency of any **discharge** from the nose | Minimal discharge | Cerebrospinal fluid leak (Fluid tests positive for glucose with Labstix.)<br>Copious, watery-to-thick, mucopurulent discharge: may be due to acute rhinitis |

| ASSESSMENT | NORMAL | ABNORMAL |
|---|---|---|
| **MOUTH AND LIP ASSESSMENT** | | |
| Note size, color, and location of any **external lesions**<br>    Palpate for mobility and<br>      firmness | No external lesions | Excessive build-up of mucous secretions<br>Dehydrated mouth or lips<br>Fissures<br>Pressure sores<br>Necrosis |
| Note size, color, and location of any **internal lesions**<br>    Palpate for mobility and<br>      firmness | No internal lesions | Moniliasis (a fungal infection indicated by white plaques similar to milk curd) |
| **NECK ASSESSMENT** | | |
| Note any **lesion or swelling** in the neck<br>    Ask client to relax and flex neck<br>      slightly<br>    Palpate the neck, using the<br>      pads of your fingers to move<br>      the skin and underlying<br>      tissues | Occasional small, mobile discrete, nontender lymph nodes | Enlarged, tender immobile nodes |

## ASSESSMENT OF THE CHEST

The chest or thorax area extends from the base of the neck to the diaphragm. The overall shape of the thorax should be elliptical, although deformities such as barrel chest, pigeon chest or funnel chest do occur. Total assessment includes the external aspect: the nurse should observe for movement, posture, shape and symmetry, especially of the breast and axilla area; and the internal components of the lungs and the heart.

The lungs anteriorly extend from 2 – 4 cm above the inner third of the clavicle to the eighth rib at the mid-axillary line and the sixth rib at the midclavicular line.

Posteriorly, the lungs extend from the third thoracic spinous process and descend to the tenth process or, on deep inspiration, to the twelfth process.

Breath sounds of clients will be different due to the depth of breathing, underlying disease, obesity, etc. Be-

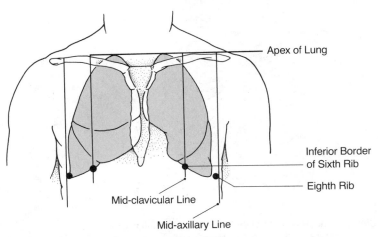

Anatomical relationship of lungs to skeletal structure.

Apex of Lung

Inferior Border of Sixth Rib

Eighth Rib

Mid-clavicular Line

Mid-axillary Line

cause of these differences, it is difficult to compare the breath sounds of one client with another. The basic principle to remember when auscultating the lungs is to do a comparison between the right and left lung. To make these comparisons, begin auscultating at the apices of one lung, alternating sides as you work down through both lungs. By comparing similar areas in both lungs, you will note changes and determine causes for these changes more easily.

Place the client in an upright sitting position with shoulders pulled forward. If the client is lying on his or her

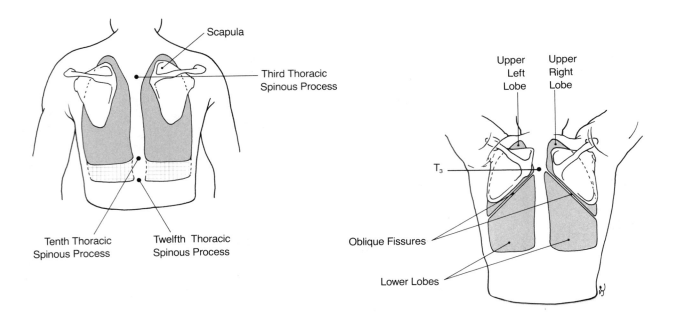

Posterior relationship of lung lobes to skeletal structures.

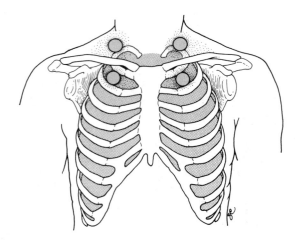

Stethoscope placement sites for anterior auscultation of breath sounds.

side, the lung closest to the bed will be mechanically compressed, and true lung sounds will not be heard.

Ask the client to breathe deeply, through the mouth. Breathing through the nose produces extra sounds that mask true lung sounds.

The heart is located directly behind the sternum, with the left ventricle projecting into the left chest. The heart is usually thought to be in the left chest for two reasons: the left ventricle produces the most movement (ventricular contraction), and three of the valve sound areas are located to the left of the sternum.

The action of the heart should be assessed both proximally and distally. Proximal assessment involves evaluating the heart sounds, the heart rate and the rhythm of the ventricular contractions to obtain information about the mechanical activity of the heart. Distal assessment involves evaluating the peripheral pulses to obtain information about the efficiency of the heart's circulatory effectiveness.

One method for assessing heart sounds is to start at the aortic area, moving slowly across to the pulmonic area, down to the tricuspid area, and over to the mitral area. This same general progression can also be used in reverse, starting at the mitral area and progressing up to the aortic area. Most clinicians begin the assessment at the mitral area, which is the point of maximum intensity and where the apical pulse is the loudest.

The most important point to re- member in heart assessments is to use the same method every time, repeating the same steps in the same sequence. By using one systematic approach, you will learn how to compare the different sounds more easily and not neglect to listen to all areas on the chest.

| ASSESSMENT | NORMAL | ABNORMAL |
|---|---|---|
| **THORAX ASSESSMENT** | | |
| Note the **general appearance** of the chest | | |
| While client is standing or sitting | Straight spine, level shoulders | Breathing possible only when sitting forward with arms on pillows or overbed table |
| While client is in bed in high-Fowler's position | Relaxed breathing; rib cage moves symmetrically with respirations | Uses accessory muscles, i.e., scalene, trapezius, sternocleidomastoid, or pectoralis |
| | Estimate the anterior-posterior diameter (normally 5:7 ratio or as low as 1:2) | Intercostal or sternal retractions (present with obstruction and increased effort with atelectasis) |
| Note **shape of chest** | | Deformities such as scoliosis, kyphosis or kyphoscoliosis |
| Note **shape of ribs** | Normal is downward | Horizontal is common in COPD |
| | | Bulging of interspaces during exhalation (present with asthma and emphysema) |
| | | Chest tilted to one side when client sits or stands: may be due to pain in ribs or chest wall or trauma, i.e., fractured ribs or surgery such as a thoracotomy |

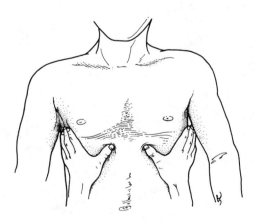
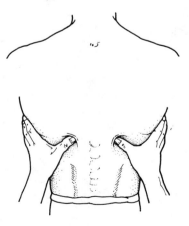

Measure chest excursion while patient takes deep breath.

| ASSESSMENT | NORMAL | ABNORMAL |
|---|---|---|
| Measure **chest excursion**, using your thumbs<br>  Place thumbs on posterior surface at level of and parallel to the tenth ribs<br>  Grasp lateral rib cage with hands<br>  Ask client to inhale<br>  Place thumbs on anterior surface with thumbs along each costal margin and hands along lateral rib cage | On inhalation, the thumbs move equidistant away from spinal cord area | Flail chest: occurs when ribs are broken in two places; rib sections pulled abnormally inward during inhalations, rib sections pushed outward during exhalation<br>Asymmetrical (unequal) chest excursion: occurs when client has a pneumothorax and cannot expand one side of chest; when client has fractured ribs; or when client's chest is splinted due to incisional pain<br>Alteration in the thoracic movement indicates underlying disease of lung or pleura<br>Barrel chest (increased anterior-posterior diameter): usually due to COPD<br>Pigeon breast (congenital; sternum pushed away from spine): due to rickets<br>Funnel breast (congenital; sternum retracted toward spine) |

## BREAST ASSESSMENT

| ASSESSMENT | NORMAL | ABNORMAL |
|---|---|---|
| Inspect **size, symmetry** and **contour** of breasts<br>  Place client in sitting position<br>  Have client remove clothing from waist up<br>  Have client raise arms over her head | Size varies with each client<br>Breasts should be equal in size and symmetrical in position | Masses, dimpling, or flattened areas: indicate possible cancer |
| **Color, edema**, and **venous pattern of skin** | Normal skin color with darker area surrounding nipples<br>No edema or prominent vessels | Erythema: indicates infection or inflammatory carcinoma<br>Edema or increased venous prominence: indicates carcinoma |
| Inspect **size and shape of nipples**<br>  Note direction in which they point, and any **rashes** or **discharge**<br>  To palpate breasts, position client supine or on side<br>  Using three fingers in a circular motion, compress breast tissue gently against chest wall<br>  Examine entire breast<br>  Make frequent checks to assess for changes | Simple inversion of nipples is common<br><br>Soft, elastic tissue with mobile nodules: indicates cystic disease | Flattening, nipple pull, or axis deviation of nipple points: may be due to fibrosis associated with cancer<br>Ulcerations of nipples and areola: may be due to Paget's disease<br>Discharge: may not be malignant but should be observed closely<br>Hard nodules fixed to skin or underlying tissue may indicate cancer<br>When nodules are present<br>  Describe location and quadrant of breast where found<br>  Note size in centimeters<br>  Describe consistency and shape<br>  Note tenderness and mobility of nodule in relationship to underlying tissue |

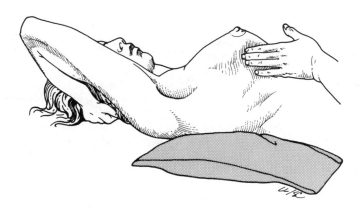

Examine breast systematically using a circular movement to compress breast tissue against chest wall.

| ASSESSMENT | NORMAL | ABNORMAL |
|---|---|---|
| Palpate nipples<br>  Compress nipple between thumb and index finger to inspect for discharge . | No discharge | Bloody discharge: may indicate papilloma |
|   Note **elasticity** | Elastic, no retraction of nipple | Loss of elasticity: indicates possible cancer<br>Inversion, flattening, or retraction: may indicate cancer |
|   Observe for erection of nipple with pal ation | | |

## LUNG ASSESSMENT

Complete a **general assessment** of the lungs

| | | |
|---|---|---|
| *Respiratory rate* | 12 to 20 respirations/minute | Increased respiratory rate: may be due to increased metabolic needs (fever), mechanical injury, surgery, or trauma to chest wall |
| *Respiratory depth* or *volume* | Normal depth is equal to about 500 ml<br>A normal or increased rate does not assume a normal tidal volume | Clients may have an increased rate to compensate for decreased tidal volume, but the resultant minute volume is still not sufficient. (Normal minute volume is 6 to 8 liters/minute.)<br>Increased depth: due to neurological disease, ICP from trauma, drug overdose, exertion, fear, or anxiety<br>Decreased depth: due to neurological disease, ICP from trauma, drug overdose, respiratory disease, or pneumothorax |

Auscultate breath sounds bilaterally.

| ASSESSMENT | NORMAL | ABNORMAL |
|---|---|---|
| Note location and quality of **lung sounds** | | |
| *Vesicular breath sounds* Heard over lung parenchyma (Heart will mask breath sounds on the left side) Lungs extended anteriorly to the sixth intercostal space Lungs extended posteriorly to $T_{10}$ on expiration, to $T_{12}$ on deep inspiration | Low to medium pitch, with low amplitude Soft, whooshing quality Inspiration two to three times longer than expiration | Rales: due to passage of air through fluid or mucus-filled airways; more frequently heard during inspiration Fine rales: high pitched, soft, and crackling Coarse rales: low pitched and bubbling |
| *Bronchovesicular breath sounds* Heard over the mainstem bronchi below the clavicles and adjacent to the sternum, between scapulae | Moderate to high pitch, with moderate amplitude Hollow, muffled quality Inspiration and expiration equal in duration | Rhonchi: produced by air passing through airways narrowed by edema, muscle spasms, or tenacious mucus; characterized as musical or sonorous according to pitch of sound (rhonchi in small airways are musical; those in larger airways are sonorous); more frequently heard during expiration |
| *Bronchial breath sounds* Heard over the trachea above the sternal notch Not true lung sounds, but important because they approximate the sounds heard in areas of atelectasis | High pitch and amplitude Harsh, loud, tubular quality Expiration twice as long as inspiration | Wheezes: produced by air passing through airways narrowed by smooth muscle contraction, secretions, or edema; characterized as high-pitched and musical; more frequently heard during expiration, especially in asthmatic clients Pleural friction rub: produced when irritated or inflamed pleura rub together in the absence of normal pleural fluid; characterized as high-pitched, jerky, and scratchy; frequently transient; may become louder if stethoscope pressed firmly to chest wall |

## HEART ASSESSMENT

| | | |
|---|---|---|
| Evaluate **atrioventricular heart sounds** ($S_1$ heart sound) *Mitral valve sounds:* located between the left atrium and left ventricle; heard best at left, fifth intercostal space at, or medial to, the midclavicular line *Tricuspid valve sounds:* located between the right atrium and the right ventricle; heard best at left, fifth intercostal space at the sternal border | $S_1$ (the first heart sound, a combination of the mitral and tricuspid sounds) heard best over the mitral and tricuspid areas Lubb sound | Heart sounds not heard in the area prescribed; e.g., with left ventricular hypertrophy, mitral sound moves laterally Relative strength of heart sounds in each area change, e.g., $S_1$ may be predominant at pulmonic area (left, second intercostal space at the sternal border), rather than $S_2$ |

| ASSESSMENT | NORMAL | ABNORMAL |
|---|---|---|
| Evaluate **semilunar heart sounds** (S$_2$ heart sounds) | | |
| *Aortic valve sounds*: located between the left ventricle and the aorta; heard best at right, second intercostal space at the sternal border | S$_2$ (the second heart sound, a combination of the aortic and pulmonic sounds): heard best over the aortic and pulmonic areas | Sounds altered with aortic stenosis (thrill) and hypertension (accentuated sound) |
| *Pulmonic valve sounds*: located between the right ventricle and the pulmonary artery; heard best at left, second intercostal space at the sternal border | Dubb sound | Pulsations with increased pressure, thrill with pulmonic stenosis and accentuated sound with pulmonary hypertension |
| Evaluate presence of **other heart sounds** Use bell of stethoscope | | |
| S$_3$ *(ventricular gallop)*: heard just after S$_2$, at the apex or at lower, left sternal border; occurs when blood flow changes from rapid to slow during ventricular diastole | Quiet and low pitched May be a physiological finding in some children and young adults | Sounds like ken-TUC-ky     S$_1$   S$_2$   S$_3$ Almost always signifies cardiac decompensation when found in a client who has heart disease |
| S$_4$ *(atrial gallop)*: heard just before S$_1$, at the apex or at lower, left sternal border; occurs when blood flow from atrial contraction meets increased resistance in ventricle | Not usually present | Sounds like TEN-nes-see     S$_4$   S$_1$   S$_2$ Heard in clients with heart disease, especially coronary artery disease or myocardial infarction |
| Assess for **heart murmurs** Produced by atypical flow of blood through the heart, e.g., irregularity or partial obstruction, increased flow in normal area, flow into dilated chamber, flow through abnormal passage; regurgitant flow Occurs during systole (between S$_1$ and S$_2$) or during diastole (between S$_2$ and S$_1$) | Faint sound More common during systole Often found in children and young adults | Faint or loud enough to be heard without a stethoscope Occurs during systole or diastole (diastolic murmurs are almost always pathological) — found in older clients with heart disease or infants and children with congenital heart defects |
| Evaluate the **apical pulse** when assessing for general heart rate and rhythm of contractions Auscultate at the apex of the heart (left, fifth intercostal space at the midclavicular line) Palpate and view pulse, if client's chest wall is thin enough | Regular rhythm Heart rate: 60 to 100 beats/minute Moderate bradycardia common in well-trained athletes Mild tachycardia possible with stress, infection, or fever | Irregular rhythm, i.e., atrial fibrillation (no discernible rhythmic pattern) Abnormal rate Bradycardia (less than 60 beats/minute) Tachycardia (more than 100 beats/minute) |

| ASSESSMENT | NORMAL | ABNORMAL |
|---|---|---|
| **Assess for irregular apical pulse** | | |
| With another nurse, take apical and radial pulses simultaneously | | |
| Compare beats per minute for both pulses | Equal apical and radial pulses | Fewer beats at the radial area may indicate an irregular apical pulse |
| **Palpate peripheral pulses**: radial, brachial, femoral, popliteal, dorsalis pedis, posterior tibial | Easily palpated Equally strong on both sides Posterior tibial pulse usually weaker than femoral | Difficult to palpate Unequal pulses Weak pulses Absent pulses |
| (For special cases, after carotid surgery, palpate temporal pulse also) | | |
| Follow these guidelines for palpating peripheral pulses: | | |
| If pulse is not immediately palpable, examine adjacent area | | |
| Pulse locations differ with clients | | |
| Palpate weak pulses gently so that you do not obliterate pulse with too much pressure | | |
| If you cannot differentiate your pulse from client's pulse, check your radial pulse or observe monitor pattern | | |
| Repeat palpations of same area slowly | | |
| Weak pulses may be difficult to feel | | |

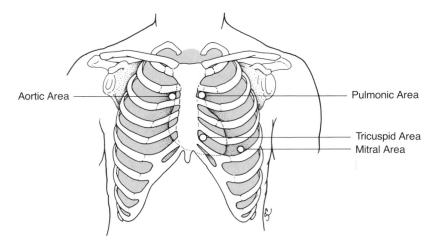

Use diaphragm of stethoscope to hear high-pitched ($S_1$, $S_2$) heart sounds.

## ASSESSMENT OF THE ABDOMEN AND GENITOURINARY TRACT

The abdomen extends from the diaphragm to the pelvis. Generally speaking, there are two body systems present in this area: the gastrointestinal system and the genitourinary system.

The gastrointestinal system begins at the mouth and consists of the stomach, the small and large intestines and associated organs that include the liver, pancreas, and spleen.

The urinary tract consists of the kidneys, ureters, bladder, and the urethra. The urinary tract should be assessed frequently and accurately because changes in the status of the urinary organs can rapidly affect other body systems.

The most common way to assess the urinary tract is to note the quantity and quality of the urinary output. Some medications or foods produce unusual odors and colors in urine, e.g., sulfasalazine (Azulfidine) turns urine a yellow-orange color; asparagus gives urine a musty odor.

External male genitalia include the penis, the scrotum, and the testicles. External female genitalia include the vulva, the urethral orifice, and the vagina.

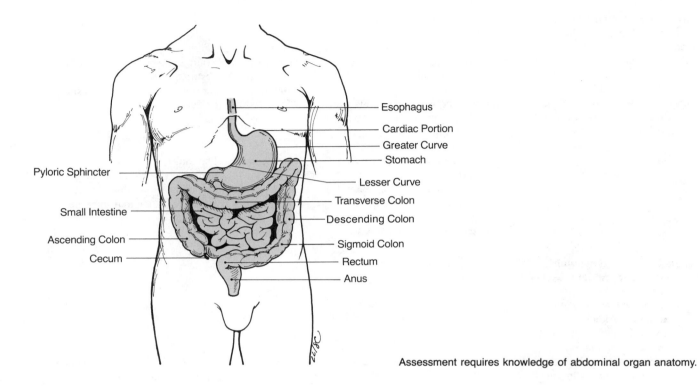

Esophagus

Cardiac Portion

Greater Curve

Stomach

Lesser Curve

Transverse Colon

Descending Colon

Sigmoid Colon

Rectum

Anus

Pyloric Sphincter

Small Intestine

Ascending Colon

Cecum

Assessment requires knowledge of abdominal organ anatomy.

| ASSESSMENT | NORMAL | ABNORMAL |
|---|---|---|
| **ABDOMEN** | | |
| Assess the **general contour** of the abdomen with client lying flat in bed | Abdomen flat between chest and pubis | Scaphoid (concave) abdominal contour: due to inadequate intake of food or IV calories, energy needs which exceed caloric intake, or to inadequate food absorption<br>Protuberant abdomen: caused by hemorrhage after trauma, e.g., auto accident or surgery |
| Assess **circumference** for intra-abdominal hemorrhage by placing a tape measure around the largest circumference of the abdomen and drawing two lines around client's entire abdomen, one line at the top of the tape measure, one line at the bottom of the tape measure; perform measurement when client exhales | No increase in abdominal circumference | Abdominal circumference increases steadily within one to two hours |

| ASSESSMENT | NORMAL | ABNORMAL |
|---|---|---|
| Auscultate abdomen to assess presence and quality of **bowel sounds** | | |
|    Place diaphragm of stethoscope firmly on abdomen, lateral to and below umbilicus<br>   Listen for several minutes since bowel sounds are not continuous like pulses | Bowel sounds similar to fairly frequent gurgle<br><br>Varying frequency of sounds with clients and time of day, i.e., more sounds right before and after eating<br>Decreased or absent bowel sounds after surgery<br>After general anesthesia, normal sounds in one to two days<br>After abdominal surgery, normal sounds in three to five days | Increased bowel sounds: due to diarrhea or to partial bowel obstruction (sounds become high-pitched and tinkling or come in "rushes," followed by silence as obstruction progresses)<br><br>Decreased bowel sounds<br>Absent bowel sounds: may be due to complete bowel obstruction or systemic illness<br>Bowel sounds hypoactive, quiet, and infrequent: may be due to paralytic ileus or no obvious cause |
| Palpate abdomen to determine condition of **abdominal muscles** and organs beneath muscles | | |
|    Tell client to relax, lie flat in bed, and flex knees<br>   Place your hand flat on client's abdomen, holding four of your fingers together and exerting pressure with the flat part of your fingers<br>   Never palpate with one finger or with finger tips<br>   Begin palpation at the pubis, moving upward. Palpate any problem areas last to minimize effects of discomfort<br>   Palpate all quadrants of abdomen to assess organs contained in each quadrant<br>   Superficial palpation: use slight pressure only<br>   Deep palpation: indent the abdominal wall 4 to 5 cm | Soft, pliant musculature when relaxed | Rigid, tender muscles: may be due to presence of inflammation or infection (peritonitis) |

## URINARY TRACT ASSESSMENT

| | | |
|---|---|---|
| Assess the **external urethra** | Orifice is pink and moist; clear, minimal discharge | Burning or pain at urethral orifice: may indicate urinary infection |
| Assess the quantity, color, odor, specific gravity, and pH of **urine output** | Output: 1200 to 1500 ml/24 hours, or 30 to 50 ml/hour | Increased output: may indicate potential diabetes or inappropriate ADH response<br>Decreased output: may indicate dehydration, acute nephritis, cardiac disease, or renal failure |

| ASSESSMENT | NORMAL | ABNORMAL |
|---|---|---|
| | Clear, yellow-amber color (Vegetarians may have slightly cloudy urine) | Cloudy (turbid): may indicate possible urinary tract infection or early signs of hematuria<br><br>Dark amber: may indicate very concentrated urine due to dehydration<br><br>Dark amber to green: may indicate hepatitis or obstructive jaundice |
| | Slight odor (Ammonia-like odor indicates that specimen has been sitting for some time) | Foul-smelling: may indicate urinary tract infection, drug or specific food ingestion<br><br>Sweet odor: may indicate acetone from keto-acidosis |
| | Specific gravity: 1.003 to 1.030 | Specific gravity of more than 1.030: indicates dehydration<br><br>Constant specific gravity of 1.010, regardless of fluid intake: indicates renal failure |
| | pH range from 4.5 to 7.5; average is 6-7 | Acidic pH below 6.0: may indicate starvation or acidosis<br><br>Alkaline pH greater than 7.0: indicates metabolic alkalosis |
| Assess for **blood** in urine using Hemastix or Labstix | No blood present | Mildly pink-tinged to grossly red-colored urine indicates blood in urine<br><br>Sudden decrease or termination of urine output<br><br>*Prerenal* causes affecting urine formation: inadequate intake, acute CHF, diabetes insipidus (large amounts of dilute urine output)<br><br>*Renal* causes affecting quantity or makeup of urine: renal failure, acute tubular necrosis, glomerulonephritis<br><br>*Postrenal* causes resulting in decreased urine output: BPH, blockage of ureters by kidney stones, or plugged catheter |
| Palpate for **bladder distension** | Not normally palpated | Distended bladder (firm, round mass) accompanied by discomfort and urge to void: indicates distention (common following surgery, where catheter is not used) |
| Assess for **pain** | No pain | Severe pain in the flank region (below ribcage posteriorly and lateral to spine): indicates kidney infection or stones |
| | Clear urine | Urine cloudy and odorous |

## GENITAL ASSESSMENT

| | | |
|---|---|---|
| Visually examine the **male genitalia** | Clean<br>No odor<br>No lesions | Unclean<br>Odor<br>Lesions and discharge: may indicate venereal disease |
| Retract the foreskin of the penis to note cleanliness, any **lesions**, and **discharge** | No discharge | Oval and round, dark erosion: may indicate syphilitic chancre |
| | Urethra opens midline of the tip of the glans | Hypospadias: due to congenital displacement of the urethral meatus |

| ASSESSMENT | NORMAL | ABNORMAL |
|---|---|---|
| | Size of the penis and the scrotum vary<br>Two testicles in the scrotum | Indurated nodule or ulcer: may indicate carcinoma<br>Mass in scrotum: indicates possible hernia, hydrocele, testicular tumor, or cyst |
| Visually examine **female genitalia** | Clean<br>No odor | Unclean<br>Odor |
| Assess for **lesions** or **discharge** | Minimal, clear discharge<br>Menstrual flow<br>Lochia (normal discharge after delivery)<br>No lesions | Thick; thin, white, yellowish, or green discharge: may indicate Trichomonas<br>Thick, white, and curdy discharge: may indicate Candida<br>Lesions: could indicate syphilitic chancre, herpes infection, venereal wart, or carcinoma of vulva |

## MENTAL-SPIRITUAL ASSESSMENT

The mental assessment is completed throughout the physical assessment and history-taking time frame. It is not generally considered a separate entity. Mood, memory, orientation, and thought processes can be evaluated while obtaining the health history. A spiritual assessment can be obtained as a part of the health history, although specific sociocultural beliefs may need to be ascertained separately. Nutritional preferences and restrictions can be accomplished as a part of a client care plan and may or may not be included in the general client assessment.

The purpose of a spiritual assessment is to facilitate the client adapting to the hospital environment and help the staff understand stressors the client may be experiencing as a result of belief systems.

The purpose of a mental status assessment is to evaluate the present state of psychological functioning. It is not designed to make a diagnosis; rather, it should yield data that will contribute to the total picture of the client as he or she is functioning at the time the assessment is made.

The specific rationale for completing a mental status assessment is:

- To collect baseline data to aid in establishing the etiology, diagnosis, and prognosis.
- To evaluate the present state of psychological functioning.
- To evaluate changes in the individual's emotional, intellectual, motor, and perceptual responses.
- To determine the guidelines of the treatment plan.
- To ascertain if some seemingly psychopathological response is, in fact, a disorder of a sensory organ (i.e., a deaf person appearing hostile, depressed, or suspicious).

- To document altered mental status for legal records.

The initial factors that the nurse must consider in completing a mental status assessment are to correctly identify the client, the reason for admission, record of previous mental illness, present complaint, any personal history that is relevant, (living arrangements, role in family, interactional experience), family history if appropriate, significant others and available support systems, assets, and interests.

The actual assessment process begins with an initial evaluation of the appropriateness of the client's behavior and orientation to reality. The assessment continues by noting any abnormal behavior and ascertaining the client's chief verbalized complaint. Finally, the evaluation determines if the client is in contact with reality enough to answer particular questions that will further assess the client's condition.

# MENTAL STATUS ASSESSMENT

| ASSESSMENT | NORMAL | ABNORMAL |
|---|---|---|
| **GENERAL APPEARANCE, MANNER AND ATTITUDE** | | |
| Assess **physical appearance** | General body characteristics, energy level, sleep patterns | Inappropriate physical appearance, high or low extremes of energy, poor sleep patterns |
| Note **grooming**, mode of dress, and **personal hygiene** | Grooming and dress appropriate to situation, client's age, and social circumstance<br>Clean | Poor grooming<br>Inappropriate or bizarre dress or combination of clothes<br>Unclean |
| Note **posture** | Upright, straight, and appropriate | Slumped, tipped, or stooped<br>Tremors |
| Note speed, pressure, pace, quantity, volume, and diction of **speech** | Moderated speed, volume, and quantity<br>Appropriate diction | Accelerated or retarded speech and high quantity<br>Poor or inappropriate diction |
| Note relevance, content, and organization of **responses** | Questions answered directly, accurately, and with relevance | Inappropriate responses, unorganized pattern of speech<br>Tangential, circumstantial or out-of-context replies |
| **EXPRESSIVE ASPECTS OF BEHAVIOR** | | |
| Note **general motor activity** | Calm, ordered movement appropriate to situation | Overactive, e.g., restless, agitated, impulsive<br>Underactive, e.g., slow to initiate or execute actions |
| Assess **purposeful movements** and **gestures** | Reasonably responsive with purposeful movements, appropriate gestures | Repetitious activities, e.g., rituals or compulsions<br>Command automation<br>Parkinsonian movements |
| Assess style of **gait** | | Ataxic, shuffling, off-balance gait |
| **CONSCIOUSNESS** | | |
| Assess **level of consciousness** | Alert, attentive, and responsive<br>Knowledgeable about time, place, and person | Disordered attention; distracted, cloudy consciousness<br>Delirious<br>Stuporous<br>Disoriented in time, place, and person |

| ASSESSMENT | NORMAL | ABNORMAL |
|---|---|---|
| **THOUGHT PROCESSES AND PERCEPTION** | | |
| Assess **coherency**, **logic**, and **relevance** of thought processes by asking questions about personal history, e.g., "Where were you born?" "What kind of work do you do?" | Clear, understandable responses to questions<br>Attentiveness | Disordered thought forms<br>Autistic or dereistic (absorbed with self and withdrawn); abstract (absent-mindedness); concrete thinking (dogmatic, preaching) |
| Assess **reality orientation**: time, place, and person awareness | Orderly progression of thoughts based in reality<br>Awareness of time, place, and person | Disorders of progression of thought: looseness, circumstantial, incoherent, irrelevant conversation, blocking<br>Delusions of grandeur or persecution: neologisms, use of words whose meaning is known only to the client<br>Echolalia (automatic repeating of questions)<br>No awareness of day, time, place, or person |
| Assess **perceptions** and reactions to personal experiences by asking questions such as "How do you see yourself now that you are in the hospital?" "What do you think about when you're in a situation like this?" | Thoughtful, clear responses expressed with understanding of self | Altered, narrowed, or expanded perception<br>Illusions<br>Depersonalization |
| **THOUGHT CONTENT AND MENTAL TREND** | | |
| Ask questions to determine general themes that identify **degree of anxiety**, e.g., "How are you feeling right now?" "What kinds of things make you afraid?" | Mild or 1+ level of anxiety in which individual is alert, motivated, and attentive | Moderate to severe (2+ to 4+) levels of anxiety |
| Assess **ideation** and **concentration** | Ideas based in reality<br>Able to concentrate | Ideas of reference<br>Hypochondria (abnormal concerns about health)<br>Obsessional<br>Phobias (irrational fears)<br>Poor or shortened concentration |
| **MOOD OR AFFECT** | | |
| Assess prevailing or **variability in mood** by observing behavior and asking questions such as "How are you feeling right now?" Check for presence of abnormal **euphoria** | Appropriate, even mood without wide variations high to low | Cyclothymic mood swings; euphoria, elation, ecstasy, depressed, withdrawn |

| ASSESSMENT | NORMAL | ABNORMAL |
|---|---|---|
| If you suspect **depression**, continue questioning to determine depth and significance of mood, e.g., "How badly do you feel?" "Have you ever thought of suicide?" | May be sad or grieving but mood does not persist indefinitely | Flat or dampened responses<br>Inappropriate responses<br>Ambivalence |

## MEMORY

| ASSESSMENT | NORMAL | ABNORMAL |
|---|---|---|
| Assess **past and present memory** and **retention** (ability to listen and respond with understanding or knowledge); ask client to repeat a phrase, e.g., an address | Alert, accurate responses<br>Able to complete digit span<br>Past and present memory appropriate | Hyperamnesia (excessive loss of memory); amnesia; paramnesia (belief in events that never occurred)<br>Preoccupied<br>Unable to follow directions |
| Assess **recall** (recent and remote) by asking questions such as "When is your birthday?" "What year were you born?" "How old are you?" | Good recall of immediate and past events | Poor recall of immediate or past events |

## JUDGMENT

| ASSESSMENT | NORMAL | ABNORMAL |
|---|---|---|
| Assess **judgment, decision-making ability** and interpretations by asking questions such as "What should you do if you hear a siren while you're driving?" "If you lost a library book, what would you do?" | Ability to make accurate decisions<br>Realistic interpretation of events | Poor judgment, poor decision-making ability, poor choice<br>Inappropriate interpretation of events or situations |

## AWARENESS

| ASSESSMENT | NORMAL | ABNORMAL |
|---|---|---|
| Assess **insight**, the ability to understand the inner nature of events or problems, by asking questions such as "If you saw someone dressed in a fur coat on a hot day, what would you think?" | Thoughtful responses indicating an understanding of the inner nature of an event or problem | Lack of insight or understanding of problems or situations<br>Distorted view of situation |

## INTELLIGENCE

| ASSESSMENT | NORMAL | ABNORMAL |
|---|---|---|
| Assess **intelligence** by asking client to define or use words in sentences, e.g., recede, join, plural | Correct responses to majority of questions | Incorrect responses to majority of questions indicates possible severe psychiatric disorders |

| ASSESSMENT | NORMAL | ABNORMAL |
|---|---|---|
| Assess **fund of information** by asking questions such as "Who is President of the United States?" "Who was the President before him?" "When is Memorial Day?" "What is a thermometer?" (Consider client's cultural and educational background) | Correct responses to majority of questions | Deteriorated or impaired cognitive processes |

**SENSORY ABILITY**

| | | |
|---|---|---|
| Assess the **five senses**, e.g., vision, hearing, tasting, feeling, and smelling abilities | Able to perceive, hear, feel, touch appropriate to stimulus | Lack of response<br>Suspicious, hostile, depressed<br>Kinesthetic imbalance |

**DEVELOPMENTAL LEVEL**

| | | |
|---|---|---|
| Assess client's **developmental level** as compared to normal | Behavior and thought processes appropriate to age level | Wide span between chronological and developmental age<br>Mentally retarded |

**LIFE-STYLE PATTERNS**

| | | |
|---|---|---|
| Identify **addictive patterns** and effect on individual's overall health | Normal amount of alcohol ingested<br>Smoking habits<br>Prescriptive medications<br>Adequate food intake for physical characteristics | High quantity of alcohol taken frequently<br>Heavy smoker<br>Addicted to illegal drugs<br>Habituative medication; user of over-the-counter or legal medications<br>Anorexic eating patterns<br>Obese or overindulgence of food |

**COPING DEVICES**

| | | |
|---|---|---|
| Identify **defense-coping mechanisms** and their effect on individual | Conscious coping mechanisms used appropriately such as compensation, fantasy, rationalization, suppression, sublimation or displacement<br>Mechanisms effective, appropriate, and useful | Unconscious mechanisms used frequently such as repression, regression, projection, reaction-formation, insulation or denial<br><br>Mechanisms inappropriate, ineffective, and not useful |

## MATERNITY ASSESSMENT

This section outlines the essential assessment data that is required throughout pregnancy. Information obtained from this assessment assists the clinician in determining the progression of the pregnancy as well as identifying potential complications. When complications are identified early in the pregnancy, interventions may be planned that will preserve the fetus and protect the mother.

Initial physical findings will vary depending in what week of the pregnancy the examination is done. The information obtained from this assessment will provide baseline data in order to evaluate changes throughout the pregnancy. Clients are assessed monthly during the first seven months of gestation. In the seventh and eighth months assessments are done twice a month. In the ninth month weekly assessments are done.

A total assessment of the obstetrical client requires a complete health history. The health history includes personal medical history, family medical history, social history, menstrual history, contraceptive/sexual history, and previous obstetrical history.

The expected date of confinement (EDC) is determined during the first health care visit. The date of the last menstrual period (LMP) is needed to determine the EDC. Nägele's rule is generally used for determining the due date. To obtain the EDC, take the first day of the LMP, minus three months, and add seven days. If the date of the LMP is unknown, the EDC can be estimated when the first fetal heart tone (FHT) is audible using the doptone. This occurs about 11 to 12 weeks after conception. The fetoscope picks up the FHT at about 18-20 weeks gestation. When quickening (the first sign of life) occurs, the fetus is about 17 to 19 weeks gestation.

An important aspect of the maternal assessment involves identifying the client's knowledge of nutrition and physical care during pregnancy. A healthy client generally has fewer complications and a healthier infant. It is important that each obstetrical client be provided prenatal teaching.

A supplement containing nutritional aspects and recommendations for prenatal and postpartum clients is found at the end of this section to assist in providing the necessary information for client teaching. In addition, signs of pregnancy, major discomforts and relief measures, and the stages and phases of labor are outlined.

## OBSTETRICAL ASSESSMENT

| ASSESSMENT | NORMAL | ABNORMAL |
|---|---|---|
| **INITIAL PHYSICAL ASSESSMENT** | | |
| Assess **breasts** and **nipples** | | |
| Contour and size | | |
| Presence of lumps | No lumps | Lumps |
| Secretions | Colostrum secretions in late first trimester or early second trimester | Secretions, other than colostrum |
| Assess **abdomen** | | |
| Contour and size | | |
| Changes in skin color | Linea nigra (black line of pregnancy along midline abdomen) Primiparas: coincidentally with growth of fundus Multiparas: after 13 to 15 weeks gestation | |

| ASSESSMENT | NORMAL | ABNORMAL |
|---|---|---|
| Striae (reddish-purple lines) | On breasts, hips, and thighs during pregnancy<br>After pregnancy, faint silvery-grey | |
| Scars, rashes, or other skin disturbances | Usually none present | |
| **Fundal height** in centimeters (fingerbreadths less accurate): measure from symphysis pubis to top of fundus | Fundus palpable just above symphysis at 8 – 10 weeks<br>Halfway between symphysis and umbilicus at 16 weeks<br>Umbilicus at 20 – 22 weeks | Large measurements: EDC is incorrect; tumor; ascites; multiple pregnancy; and poly-hydramnios<br>Less than normal enlargement: fetal abnormality, oligohydramnios, placental dysmaturity, missed abortion, fetal death |
| **Perineum**: scars, moles, rashes, warts, discharge | | |

## BASELINE DATA

Evaluate **weight**

Take **vital signs**, **blood pressure** (BP), **temperature**, **pulse**, and **respiration** (TPR)

| Evaluate **lab findings** | | |
|---|---|---|
| Urine: sugar, protein, albumin | Negative for sugar, protein, and albumin throughout pregnancy | Positive for sugar, protein, and/or albumin |
| Human calcitonin (HCT)<br>Hemoglobin (Hgb)<br>Blood type and Rh factor | 38% to 47%<br>12% to 16% | If Rh negative, father's blood should be typed<br>If Rh positive, titers should be followed; possible RhoGAM at termination of pregnancy |
| Pap smear<br>VD smears and screening | | |

## ANTEPARTUM ASSESSMENT

| Evaluate **weight** to assess maternal health and nutritional status and growth of fetus | 1st trimester: 3 to 4 lbs<br>2nd trimester: 12 to 14 lbs<br>3rd trimester: 8 to 10 lbs<br>Minimum weight gain during pregnancy: 24 lbs (2 lbs/week or 5 lbs/month) | Inadequate weight gain: possible maternal malnutrition<br><br>Excessive weight gain: if sudden at onset, may indicate preeclampsia; if gradual and continual, may indicate overeating |
|---|---|---|
| Evaluate **blood pressure** | Fairly constant with baseline data throughout pregnancy | Increased: possible anxiety (Client should rest 20 to 30 minutes before you take BP again)<br>Rise of 30/15 above baseline data: sign of pre-eclampsia<br>Decreased: sign of supine hypotensive syndrome. If lying on back, turn client on left side and take BP again |

| ASSESSMENT | NORMAL | ABNORMAL |
|---|---|---|
| Evaluate **fundal height** | Drop around 38th week: sign of fetus engaging in birth canal<br>Primipara: sudden drop<br>Multipara: slower, sometimes not until onset of labor | Large fundal growth: may indicate wrong dates, multiple pregnancy, hydatidiform mole, poly-hydramnios, tumors<br>Small fundal growth: may indicate fetal demise, fetal anomaly, retarded fetal growth, abnormal presentation or lie, decreased amniotic fluid |
| Determine **fundal position**, using Leopold's maneuvers. Complete external palpations of the pregnant abdomen to determine fetal position, lie, presentation and engagement<br>    First maneuver: to determine part of fetus presenting into pelvis<br>    Second maneuver: to locate the back, arms, and legs; fetal heart heard best over fetal back<br>    Third maneuver: to determine part of fetus in fundus<br>    Fourth maneuver: to determine degree of cephalic flexion and engagement | Vertex presentation | Breech presentation or transverse lie |

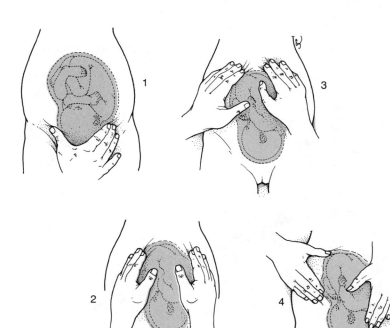

Steps of Leopold's maneuvers.

| ASSESSMENT | NORMAL | ABNORMAL |
|---|---|---|
| Evaluate **fetal heart rate** by quadrant, location, and rate | 120 to 160 beats/minute | More than 160 or less than 120: may indicate fetal distress. *Notify physician* |
| Check for presence of **edema** | In lower extremities towards end of pregnancy | In upper extremities and face: may indicate preeclampsia |
| Evaluate **urine** (clean catch midstream) | Negative for sugar, protein, and albumin | Positive for sugar: may indicate subclinical or gestational diabetes<br>Positive for protein and/or albumin: may indicate preeclampsia |
| Evaluate **levels of discomfort** (See Obstetrical Supplement at end of this section) | | |

## INTRAPARTUM ASSESSMENT

| | | |
|---|---|---|
| Assess for **lightening** and **dropping** (the descent of the presenting part into the pelvis) | Several days to two weeks before onset of labor<br>Multipara: may not occur until onset of labor<br>Relief of shortness of breath and increase in urinary frequency | No lightening or dropping: may indicate disproportion between fetal presenting part and maternal pelvis |
| Check if **mucous plug** has been expelled from cervix | Usually expelled prior to onset of labor | |
| Assess for **"bloody show"** | Clear, pinkish, or blood-tinged vaginal discharge that occurs as cervix begins to dilate and efface | |
| Assess for **ruptured membranes** | | |
| Time water breaks | Before, during, or after onset of labor | Breech presentation: frank meconium or meconium staining |
| Color of **amniotic fluid** | Clear, straw color | Greenish-brown: indicates meconium has passed from fetus, possible fetal distress<br>Yellow-stained: fetal hypoxia 36 hours or more prior to rupture of membrane or hemolytic disease |
| Quantity of amniotic fluid | 500 to 1000 ml of amniotic fluid, rarely expelled at one time | Polyhydramnios: excessive fluid over 2000 cc<br>Observe newborn for congenital anomalies: craniospinal malformation, orogastrointestinal anomalies, Down's syndrome and congenital heart defects<br>Oligohydramnios: minimal fluid, less than 1000 cc<br>Observe newborn for malformation of ear, genitourinary tract anomalies, and renal agenesis |
| Odor of fluid | No odor | Odor: may indicate infection; deliver within 24 hours |

| ASSESSMENT | NORMAL | ABNORMAL |
|---|---|---|
| **Fetal heart rate** | 120 to 160 beats/minute<br>Regular rhythm | Decreased: indicates fetal distress with possible cord prolapse or cord compression<br>Accelerated heart rate: initial sign of fetal hypoxia<br>Absent: may indicate fetal demise |
| Evaluate **contractions**<br>*Frequency*: from start of one contraction to start of next | 3 to 5 minutes between contractions | Irregular contractions with long intervals between: indicates false labor |
| *Duration*: from beginning of contraction to time uterus begins to relax | 50 to 90 seconds | Over 90 seconds: uterine tetany; stop pitocin if running |
| *Intensity* (strength of contraction): measured with monitoring device | Peak 25 mm Hg<br>End of labor may reach 50-75 mm Hg | Over 75 mm Hg: uterine tetany or uterine rupture |

## LABOR AND DELIVERY ASSESSMENT

| | | |
|---|---|---|
| **First stage**<br>*Latent phase* (0 to 10 cm dilatation) | 0 to 5 cm over 6 to 10 hours | Prolonged time in any phase: may indicate poor fetal position, incomplete fetal flexion, CPD, or poor uterine contractions |
| *Active phase* (5 to 7 cm) | | |
| *Transition phase* (8 to 10 cm) | Progresses from 8 to 10 cm in 1 to 2 hours | Labor less than 3 hours: indicates precipitous labor, increasing risk of fetal complications, or maternal lacerations and tears |
| Assess for **bloody show** | | |
| Observe for presence of **nausea or vomiting** | | |
| Assess **perineum** | Beginning to bulge | |
| Evaluate **urge to bear down** | | Often uncontrolled<br>Multipara: can cause precipitous delivery<br>"Panting" (can be controlled until safe delivery area established) |
| **Second stage** (10 cm to delivery) | Primipara: up to 2 hours<br>Multipara: several minutes to 2 hours | Over 2 hours: increased risk of fetal brain damage and maternal exhaustion |
| Assess for **presenting part** | Vertex with ROA or LOA presentation | Occiput posterior, breech, face or transverse lie |
| Assess **caput** (infant head)<br>Multipara: move to delivery room when caput size of dime<br>Primipara: move to delivery room when caput size of half dollar | Visible when bearing down during contraction | "Crowns" in room other than delivery room: delivery imminent (Do not move client) |

| ASSESSMENT | NORMAL | ABNORMAL |
|---|---|---|
| Assess **fetal heart rate** | 120 to 160/minute | Decreased: may indicate supine hypotensive syndrome (Turn client on side and take again.) Hemorrhage (Check for other signs of bleeding; notify physician.) Increased or decreased: may indicate fetal distress secondary to cord progression or compression (Place client in Trendelenburg's or knee-chest position; give oxygen if necessary; inform physician.) |
| Evaluate **breathing** | Controlled with contractions | Heavy or excessive: may lead to hyperventilation and/or dehydration |
| Evaluate **pain** and **anxiety** | Medication required after dilated 4 to 5 cm unless using natural childbirth methods | Severe pain early in first stage of labor: inadequate prenatal teaching, backache due to position in bed, uterine tetany |
| **Third stage** (from delivery of baby to delivery of placenta) | Placental separation occurs within 30 minutes (usually 3-5 minutes) | Failure of placental separation Abnormality of uterus or cervix, weak, ineffectual uterine contraction, tetanic contractions causing closure of cervix Over 3 hours: indicates retained placenta |
| **Fourth stage** (first hour postpartum) | | Mother in unstable condition (hemorrhage usual cause) Highest risk of hemorrhage in first postpartum hour |
| Temperature | 36.5° to 37.5°C | Over 37.5°C: may indicate infection Slight elevation: due to dehydration from mouth breathing and NPO |
| Pulse | Pulse: 60 to 100 | Increased: may indicate pain or hemorrhage |
| Respiration | Respirations: 12-22 | |
| Blood pressure | Blood pressure: 140-120/80 | Increased: may indicate anxiety, pain or posteclamptic condition Decreased: hemorrhage |

## POSTPARTUM ASSESSMENT

| | | |
|---|---|---|
| Assess **vital signs** every 15 minutes for 1 hour, every 30 minutes for 1 hour, every hour for 4 hours, every 8 hours, and as needed | Pulse may be 45-60/minute in stage 4 Pulse to normal range about third day | Decreased BP and increased P: probably postpartum hemorrhage; elevated temperature above 38°C: indicates possible infection Temperature elevates when lactation occurs |
| Assess **fundus** every 15 minutes for 1 hour, every 8 hours for 48 hours, then daily | Firm (Like a grapefruit) in midline and at or slightly above umbilicus Return to prepregnant size in 6 weeks: descending at rate of 1 fingerbreadth/day | Boggy fundus: immediately massage gently until firm; report to physician and observe closely; empty bladder; medicate with pitocin if ordered Fundus misplaced 1 to 2 fingerbreadths from midline: indicates full bladder (Client must void or be catheterized.) |

| ASSESSMENT | NORMAL | ABNORMAL |
|---|---|---|
| Assess **lochia** every 15 minutes for 1 hour, every 8 hours for 48 hours, then daily | | |
| Color | 3 days postpartum: dark red (rubra)<br>4 to 10 days postpartum: clear pink (serosa)<br>10 to 21 days postpartum: white, yellow brown (alba) | Heavy, bright-red: indicates hemorrhage (Massage fundus, give medication on order, notify physician.)<br>Spurts: may indicate cervical tear<br>No lochia: may indicate clot occluding cervical opening (Support fundus; express clot.) |
| Quantity | Moderate amount, steadily decreases | |
| Odor | Minimal | Foul: may indicate infection |
| Assess **breasts** and **nipples** daily | Day 1 to 2: soft, intact, secreting colostrum<br>Day 2 to 3: engorged, tender, full, tight, painful<br>Day 3+: secreting milk<br>Increased pains as baby sucks: common in multiparas | Sore or cracked (Clean and dry nipples; decrease breast feeding time; apply breast shield between feeding.)<br>Milk does not "let down": help client relax and decrease anxiety; give glass of wine or beer |
| Assess **perineum** daily | Episiotomy intact, no swelling, no discoloration | Swelling or bruising: may indicate hematoma |
| Assess **bladder** every four hours | Voiding regularly with no pain | Not voiding: bladder may be full and displaced to one side, leading to increased lochia (Catheterization may be necessary.) |
| Assess **bowels** | Spontaneous bowel movement 2 to 3 days after delivery | Fear associated with pain from hemorrhoids |
| Assess mother-infant **bonding** | Touching infant, talking to infant, talking about infant | Refuses to touch or hold infant |
| Evaluate **Rh-negative status** | Client does not require RhoGAM | RhoGAM administered |

## OBSTETRICAL GUIDELINES

This supplement contains pertinent information regarding recommendations for prenatal and postpartum clients; signs of pregnancy, major discomforts and relief measures; and the stages and phases of labor.

| ASSESSMENT | NORMAL | ABNORMAL |
|---|---|---|
| **RECOMMENDATIONS FOR PRENATAL CLIENTS** | | |
| Instruct about **nutrition** | | |
| Instruct about intake of **sodium**, which is essential for maintaining increased body fluids needed for adequate placental flow, increased tissue requirements, and adequate renal blood flow | | |
| Instruct about **exercise**<br>Exercise is beneficial in moderation<br>Continued exercise in familiar sports throughout pregnancy is recommended<br>Participation in new or unfamiliar sports is not recommended | Fatigue in early pregnancy: may need to decrease exercise | Excessive fatigue: may indicate too much exercise |
| Instruct about **rest**<br>Frequent rest periods are necessary to prevent fatigue<br>Legs should be elevated to promote venous return<br>Crossing legs at knees should be avoided to prevent pressure on veins | Venous stasis in legs and feet late in pregnancy: may occur due to weight of fetus on femoral plexus | |
| Instruct about **clothing**<br>Bras should support with wide shoulder straps<br>Client may need several sizes during pregnancy<br>Shoes should be supportive, with low heels<br>Clothing should be loose and comfortable. Client should avoid constrictive clothing, especially on legs | | |
| Instruct about **bathing**<br>Tub baths are acceptable if membranes intact and no bleeding<br>Client should be helped when getting in and out of the tub | | Tub baths avoided: client large and unstable on feet; signs of bleeding, onset of labor |

| ASSESSMENT | NORMAL | ABNORMAL |
|---|---|---|
| Instruct about **drugs** and **tobacco**<br>  Tobacco should be eliminated<br>   or decreased<br>  Alcohol should be eliminated | | Alcohol use associated with small-for-gestational-age infants (SGA)<br>If mother is allergic to alcohol: fetal alcohol syndrome |
| Instruct about **sexual relations** | Continuation if no bleeding, ruptured membranes, or premature contractions | |
| Instruct about **preparations for labor and delivery** at about 30th to 32nd week of gestation | | |
| Instruct about **major discomforts** and **relief measures** | | |

## RECOMMENDATIONS FOR POSTPARTUM CLIENTS

| | | |
|---|---|---|
| Instruct about **nutrition** | | |
| Instruct about **exercise** | Return to previous level of activity slowly, progressively, with physician's approval | Early, strenuous exercise: may lead to fatigue and hemorrhage |
| Encourage adequate **rest** | | |
| Inform about **care of baby**<br>  Bathing/skin care<br>  Diapering/dressing<br>  Feeding/burping<br>  Sleeping/positioning<br>  Temperature/signs of illness<br>  Medical check-ups/<br>    immunizations<br>  Safety<br>  Growth and development | | |
| Instruct about **contraceptives** if necessary | Nursing: use condom, gel, foam for first 6 weeks then method of choice may be used<br>Nonnursing: may use oral contraceptives after delivery | |
| Instruct about **sexual relations** | Resume when episiotomy healed and lochia stopped | Pain with intercourse: may need water-based jelly for lubrication for four to six months; episiotomy may not be healed |

## THEORIES OF CHILDBIRTH

### Factors that influence pain in labor

1. Preconditioning by "old wives' tales," fantasies, and fears. Accurate information about the childbirth process can often alleviate effects of preconditiong.
2. Pain produces stress, which in turn affects the body's functioning. Interpretations of and reactions to pain can be altered by a refocusing of attention and by conditioning.
3. Feelings of isolation. Social expectations and tension may also increase feelings of pain.

### Childbirth education

1. Each method varies somewhat but basic underlying concepts are similar. Birth is viewed as a natural occurrence. Knowledge about the birth experience dispels fears and tension, and distraction and concentration during labor and delivery modify the pain experience.
2. Purpose is to promote relaxation enabling the mother to work with the labor process. Allows parents to take an active part in the birth process, thereby increasing self-esteem and satisfaction.
3. Goals are accomplished by means of:
   *Education*: anatomy and physiology of reproductive system, and the labor and delivery process; replacement of misinformation and superstition with facts. May include classes on nutrition, discomforts of pregnancy, breast-feeding, infant care, etc.
   *Training*: controlled breathing and neuromuscular exercises.
   *Presence of father*, or significant other, in labor and delivery rooms to serve as coach and lend support.
4. Common methods presently available:
   *Read method (Natural Childbirth)* introduced by Grantly Dick-Read in England. Believed pain in childbirth was psychological rather than physiological. Pain brought about by fear and tension.
   *Lamaze method.*
   *Bradley method.*
   *Scientific relaxation for childbirth.*
5. *LeBoyer technique*: used in delivery room to reduce stress of birth upon infant.
   Includes increasing room temperature to one comfortable for infant, reducing external stimuli by dimming lights, keeping noise level to a minimum.
   Infant is placed in skin-to-skin contact on mother's abdomen and gently stroked; cord clamping is delayed until pulsation stops.
   Infant is submerged up to head in a bath of warm water until it appears relaxed, then is dried and wrapped snugly in a warm blanket.
6. Classes for parents expecting delivery by C-section are now being given.

## MAJOR DISCOMFORTS AND RELIEF MEASURES

| DISCOMFORT | TRIMESTER MOST PROMINENT | RELIEF MEASURES |
| --- | --- | --- |
| Nausea and vomiting | 1st | Eat five or six small, frequent meals. In between meals, have crackers without fluid<br>Avoid foods high in carbohydrates, fried and greasy, or with a strong odor<br>Take antinausea drug if prescribed |
| Frequency | 1st and 3rd | Wear perineal pads if there is leakage |
| Heartburn | 2nd and 3rd | Avoid fatty, fried, and highly spiced foods<br>Have small frequent feedings<br>Use an antacid; *avoid* sodium bicarbonate |
| Abdominal distress | 1st, 2nd, and 3rd | Eat slowly, chew food thoroughly, take smaller helpings of food |
| Flatulence | 2nd and 3rd | Maintain daily bowel movement<br>Avoid gas-forming foods. Take antiflatulents as prescribed by physician |

| DISCOMFORT | TRIMESTER MOST PROMINENT | RELIEF MEASURES |
|---|---|---|
| Constipation | 2nd and 3rd | Drink sufficient fluids. Eat fruit and foods high in roughage<br>Exercise moderately<br>Take stool softener if prescribed by physician. Do *not* use mineral oil |
| Hemorrhoids | 3rd | Apply ointments, suppositories, warm compresses<br>Avoid constipation and get adequate rest |
| Insomnia | 3rd | Exercise moderately to promote relaxation and fatigue<br>Change position while sleeping<br>If severe, take medication as prescribed by physician |
| Backaches | 3rd | Rest and improve posture — use a firm mattress<br>Use a good abdominal support, wear comfortable shoes<br>Do exercises such as squatting, sitting, and pelvic rock |
| Varicosities of legs and vulva | 3rd | Avoid long periods of standing or sitting with legs crossed<br>Sit or lie with feet and hips elevated<br>Move about while standing to improve circulation<br>Wear support hose; *avoid* tight garters |
| Edema of legs and feet | 3rd | Elevate feet while sitting or lying down<br>Avoid standing or sitting in one position for long periods |
| Cramps in legs | 3rd | Extend cramped leg and flex ankles, pushing foot upward with toes pointed toward knee<br>Increase calcium intake |
| Pain in thighs or aching of perineum | 3rd | Alternate periods of sitting and standing<br>Rest |
| Shortness of breath | 3rd | Sit up<br>Lie on back with arms extended above head |
| Breast soreness | 1st, 2nd, and 3rd | Wear brassiere with wide adjustable straps that fits well |
| Supine hypotensive syndrome | 3rd | Change position to left side to relieve pressure of uterus on inferior vena cava |
| Vaginal discharge | 3rd | Practice proper cleansing and hygiene. Avoid douche unless recommended by physician<br>Observe for signs of vaginal infection common in pregnancy |

## NEWBORN AND PEDIATRIC PHYSICAL ASSESSMENT

The basic methods of pediatric assessment are similar to those used for assessing adults. However, the pediatric nurse should be cognizant of some specific differences in techniques, observations, and findings. For example, physical examination findings must be placed within the context of the child's growth and development continuum. Normal and abnormal development of the child's body systems and the child's cognitive processes should also be considered.

Because children are generally not as compliant as adults during physical examinations, it is important to plan your approach before any examination. Knowledge of a child's growth and developmental level, as well as a child's fears and level of understanding, is essential for a successful examination.

Before touching an infant, make sure your hands are warm. Start with the nonintrusive portions of the examination, such as observing muscle tone and body symmetry. Progress to the more intrusive portions, such as adducting

hips for dislocation. When a child is quiet, listen to the heart rate and rhythm and respirations. An active or crying child makes auscultation difficult.

When you are assessing toddlers allow the child to sit on his or her mother's lap for security. Use simple terms to explain what you are about to do. Before using a stethoscope or tongue blade, let the child examine it. Begin the examination with the least threatening procedures; gradually proceed to the more threatening ones. For example, observe the child's hands and feet, chest and abdomen; then auscultate and percuss these areas. Observe the child's genital area; examine the child's head, eyes, face, neck, mouth, ears, nose, and throat. (Toddlers do not like anyone holding their heads!)

When assessing school-age children you will be aware that the school-age child is generally more cooperative than a younger one. During the examination, let the client manipulate the instruments and listen to the stethoscope.

Allow the child to keep on underwear until you assess the genitalia. Begin the examination by assessing the child's vital signs, moving from head to toe. Examine the genitalia last. When you conduct this part of the examination, allow the child adequate privacy. Also during the examination, talk with the child about his or her daily activities. This will serve two purposes: it distracts the child from the task at hand; and it gives you an opportunity to assess the child's activities and determine if they are appropriate to the child's age.

The assessment of the adolescent should proceed with the physical examination as with an adult. Use your discretion to determine whether the parent should be present. Respect the wishes of the young adult in this matter. As you conduct the examination, explain every procedure. Pay particular attention to the adjustment the young adult is making to physical and emotional changes in his or her life.

## NEWBORN ASSESSMENT

| ASSESSMENT | NORMAL | ABNORMAL |
|---|---|---|
| **SKIN ASSESSMENT** | | |
| Note skin **color** and **lesions** | Pink | Cyanosis, pallor, beefy red |
| | Mongolian spots | Petechiae, ecchymoses, or purpuric spots: signs of possible hematologic disorder |
| | Capillary hemangiomas on face or neck | Cafe au lait spots (patches of brown discoloration): possible sign of congenital neurological disorder |
| | | Raised capillary hemangiomas on areas other than face or neck |

| ASSESSMENT | NORMAL | ABNORMAL |
|---|---|---|
| | Localized edema in presenting part | Edema of peritoneal wall |
| | Cheesy white vernix | Poor skin turgor: indicates dehydration |
| | Desquamation (peeling off) | Yellow discolored vernix (meconium stained) |
| | Milia (small white pustules over nose and chin) | Impetigo neonatorum (small pustules with surrounding red areas) |
| | Jaundice after 24 hours; gone by second week | Jaundice at birth or within 12 hours |
| | | Dermal sinuses (opening to brain) |
| | | Holes along spinal column |
| | | Low hairline posteriorly: possible chromosomal abnormality |
| | | Sparse or spotty hair: congenital goiter or chromosomal abnormality |
| Note color of **nails** | Pink | Yellowing of nail beds (meconium stained) |
| Note **skin tone** | Strong, tremulous | Flaccid, convulsions |
| | | Muscular twitching, hypertonicity |

## HEAD AND NECK ASSESSMENT

| ASSESSMENT | NORMAL | ABNORMAL |
|---|---|---|
| Note **shape of head** | Fontanels: anterior open until 18 months; posterior closed shortly after birth | Depressed, tense, bulging, or absent fontanels: indicates hydrocephalus or dehydration |
| | | Cephalohematoma that crosses the midline |
| | | Microcephaly and macrocephaly |
| Assess **eyes** | Slight edema of lids | Purulent discharge |
| | | Lateral upward slope of eye with an inner epicanthal fold in infants not of Oriental descent |
| | | Exophthalmos (bulging of eyeball): may be congenital anomaly, sign of congenital glaucoma or thyroid abnormality |
| | | Enophthalmos (recession of eyeball): may indicate damage to brain or cervical spine |
| | Pupils equal and reactive to light by three weeks of age | Constricted pupil, unilateral dilated fixed pupil, nystagmus (rhythmic nonpurposeful movement of eyeball): continuous strabismus |
| | Intermittent strabismus (occasional crossing of eyes) | |
| | Conjunctival or sclera hemorrhages | Haziness of cornea |
| | Symmetrical light reflex (light reflects off each eye in the same quadrant): sign of conjugate gaze | Absence of red reflex; asymmetrical light reflex |
| Note **placement of ears**, shape and position | | Low set ears: may indicate Down's syndrome |
| Assess **nose** | Discharge, sneezing | Thick, bloody nasal discharge |

| ASSESSMENT | NORMAL | ABNORMAL |
|---|---|---|
| Assess **mouth** | Sucking, rooting reflexes<br>Retention cysts (pears)<br>Occasional vomiting | Cleft lip, palate<br>Flat, white nonremovable spots (thrush)<br>Frequent vomiting: may indicate pyloric stenosis<br>Vomitus with bile: fecal vomiting<br>Profuse salivation: may indicate tracheo-esophageal fistula |
| Assess **neck** | Tonic neck reflex (Fencer's position) | Distended neck veins<br>Fractured clavicle<br>Unusually short neck<br>Excess posterior cervical skin<br>Resistance to neck flexion |
| Assess **cry** | Lusty cry | Weak, groaning cry: possible neurological abnormality<br>High-pitched cry; hoarse or crowing inspirations; cat-like cry: possible neurological or chromosomal abnormality |

## CHEST AND LUNG ASSESSMENT

| ASSESSMENT | NORMAL | ABNORMAL |
|---|---|---|
| Assess the **chest** | Circular<br>Enlargement of breasts<br>Milky discharge from breasts | Depressed sternum<br>Retractions, asymmetry of chest movements: indicates respiratory distress and possible pneumothorax |
| Assess the **lungs** | Abdominal respirations<br><br>Respiration rate: 30 to 50<br>Respiration movement irregular in rate and depth<br>Resonant chest (hollow sound on percussion) | Thoracic breathing, unequal motion of chest, rapid grasping or grunting respirations, flaring nares<br>Deep sighing respirations<br>Grunt on expiration: possible respiratory distress<br>Hyper-resonance of chest or decreased resonance |

## HEART ASSESSMENT

| ASSESSMENT | NORMAL | ABNORMAL |
|---|---|---|
| Assess the **rate**, **rhythm**, and **murmurs** of the heart | Rate: 100 to 180 at birth; stabilizes at 120 to 140<br>Regular rhythm<br>Murmurs: significance cannot usually be determined in newborn | Heart rate above 200 or less than 100<br><br>Irregular rhythm<br>Dextrocardia, enlarged heart |

## ABDOMEN AND GASTRO-INTESTINAL TRACT ASSESSMENT

| ASSESSMENT | NORMAL | ABNORMAL |
|---|---|---|
| Assess the **abdomen** | Prominent | Distention of abdominal veins: possible portal vein obstruction |

| ASSESSMENT | NORMAL | ABNORMAL |
|---|---|---|
| Assess the **gastrointestinal tract** | Bowel sounds present | Visible peristaltic waves<br>Increased pitch or frequency: intestinal obstruction<br>Decreased sounds: paralytic ileus<br>Distention of abdomen |
| | Liver 2 to 3 cm below right costal margin<br>Spleen tip palpable<br>May be able to palpate kidneys<br>Bladder percussed 1 to 4 cm above symphysis pubis<br>Umbilical cord with one vein and two arteries<br>Soft granulation tissue at umbilicus | Enlarged liver or spleen<br>Midline suprapubic mass: may indicate Hirschsprung's disease<br>Enlarged kidney<br>Distended bladder; presence of any masses<br><br>One artery present in umbilical cord: may indicate other anomalies<br>Wet umbilical stump or fetid odor from stump |

**GENITOURINARY TRACT ASSESSMENT**

| | | |
|---|---|---|
| Assess the **genitalia** | Edema and bruising after delivery<br>Unusually large clitoris in females a short time after birth<br>Vaginal mucoid or bloody discharge may be present in the first week | Inguinal hernia |
| Urethra orifice | Urethra opens on ventral surface of penile shaft | Hypospadias (urethra opens on the inferior surface of the penis)<br>Epispadias (urethra opens on the dorsal surface of the penis)<br>Ulceration of urethral orifice |
| Testes | Testes in scrotal sac or inguinal canal | Hydroceles in males |

**SPINE AND EXTREMITIES ASSESSMENT**

| | | |
|---|---|---|
| Assess the **spine** | Straight spine | Spina bifida, pilonidal sinus; scoliosis |
| Assess **extremities** | Soft click with thigh rotation | Asymmetry of movement<br>Sharp click with thigh rotation: indicates possible congenital hip<br>Uneven major gluteal folds: indicates possible congenital hip<br>Polydactyly (extra digits on a hand or foot); syndactyly (webbing or fusion of fingers or toes) |
| Assess **anus and rectum** | Patent anus | Closed anus: no meconium |

| ASSESSMENT | NORMAL | ABNORMAL |
|---|---|---|

## PEDIATRIC ASSESSMENT

### MEASUREMENTS

| ASSESSMENT | NORMAL | ABNORMAL |
|---|---|---|
| Measure **height** and **weight** and plot on a standardized growth chart | Height/weight proportional Sequential measurements: pattern follows normal growth curves | Height/weight below third percentile Sudden drop in percentile range of height and/or weight: possible sign of disease process or congenital problem |
| Assess **temperature** (axillary until six years of age) | Axillary 97° F; 36.4° C Elevations following eating or playing not unusual | Temperature of 104° to 105° F: corresponds roughly with 101° to 102° F in an adult Large daily temperature variations Hypothermia: usually result of chilling |
| Measure **circumference of head and chest** Examine or check circumferences when child is less than two years old Compare measurements with standardized charts | Head at birth: about 2 cm greater than chest During first year: equalization of head and chest After two years: rapid growth of chest; slight increases in size of head | Increase in head circumference greater than 2.5 cm per month: sign of hydrocephalus |

### VITAL SIGNS

| ASSESSMENT | NORMAL | ABNORMAL |
|---|---|---|
| Assess **pulse** apically | Birth to one year: 120 to 140 One year: 80 to 160 Two years: 80 to 130 Three years: 80 to 120 Over three years: 70 to 115 | Pulse over 180 after first month of life: cardiac or respiratory condition Inability to palpate femoral pulses: possible coarctation of the aorta |
| Assess **respirations** | Birth: 30 to 50 Six years: 20 to 25 Puberty: 14 to 16 (Young children have abnormally high respiration rate with even slight excitement) | Consistent tachypnea: usually a sign of respiratory disease Respiratory rate over 100: lower respiratory tract obstruction Slow rate: may be sign of CNS depression |
| Assess **blood pressure** | Birth: 60 to 90 mm Hg systolic 20 to 60 mm Hg diastolic Rise in both pressures: 2 to 3 mm Hg per year of age Adult level reached at puberty | Elevated blood pressure in upper extremities: coarctation of aorta Narrowed pulse pressure (normal or elevated diastolic with lowered systolic; less than 30 mm Hg difference between systolic and diastolic readings): possible sign of aortic or subaortic stenosis or hypothyroidism Widened pulse pressure: possible sign of hyperthyroidism |

| ASSESSMENT | NORMAL | ABNORMAL |
|---|---|---|
| **APPEARANCE** | | |
| Observe **general appearance** | Alert, well-nourished comfortable, responsive | Lethargic, uncomfortable, malnourished, gross anomalies, dull |
| Listen to **voice and cry** | Strong, lusty cry | Weak cry, low- or high-pitched cry: may indicate neurological problem or chromosomal abnormality |
| | Facial expression animated | Expressionless, unresponsive |
| | No indications of pain | Doubling over, rubbing a body part, general fretfulness |
| | No odor | Musty odor: sign of phenylketonuria, diphtheria |
| | | Odor of maple syrup: may be maple syrup urine disease |
| | | Odor of sweaty feet: one type of acidemia |
| | | Fishy odor: may be metabolic disorder |
| | | Acetone odor: acidosis, particularly diabetic ketoacidosis |
| **SKIN ASSESSMENT** | | |
| Assess **pigmentation** | Usually even | Multiple cafe au lait spots: possible neurofibromatosis |
| | Pigmented nevi common | Cyanosis |
| | Large, flat, black and blue areas over sacrum, buttocks (Mongolian spots) | Jaundice |
| | | Pallor |
| Assess **lesions** | Usually none | Erythematous lesions |
| | Adolescence: acne | Multiple macules, papules, or vesicles |
| | | Petechiae and ecchymoses: may indicate coagulation disorder |
| | | Hives |
| | | Subcutaneous nodules: may indicate juvenile rheumatoid arthritis |
| Note **consistency of skin** | Good turgor | Poor turgor |
| | Smooth and firm | Dryness |
| | | Edema |
| | | Lack or excess of subcutaneous fat: sign of malnutrition or excess nutrition |
| Assess **nails** | Nail beds: normally pigmented | Cyanosis |
| | Good nail growth | Pallor |
| | | Capillary pulsations |
| | | Pitting of the nails: possible sign of fungal disease or psoriasis |
| | | Broad nail beds: possible sign of Down's syndrome or other chromosomal abnormality |

| ASSESSMENT | NORMAL | ABNORMAL |
|---|---|---|
| Assess **hair** (consistency appropriate to ethnic group) | No excessive breaking | Dry, coarse, brittle hair: possible sign of hypothyroidism<br>Alopecia (loss of hair): may be psychosomatic or due to drug therapy<br>Unusual hairiness in places other than scalp, eyebrows, and lashes: may indicate hypothyroidism, vitamin A poisoning, chronic infections, reaction to Dilantin therapy<br>Tufts of hair over spine or sacrum: may indicate site of spina bifida occulta or spina bifida<br>Absence of the start of pubic hair during adolescence: possible hypothyroidism, hypopituitarism, gonadal deficiency, or Addison's disease |
| Assess **lymph nodes** | Nontender, movable, discrete nodes up to 3 mm in diameter in occipital, postauricular, parotid, submaxillary, sublingual, axillary, and epitrochlear nodes<br>Up to 1 mm in diameter inguinal and cervical nodes | Tender or enlarged nodes: may be sign of systemic infection |

## HEAD AND NECK ASSESSMENT

| ASSESSMENT | NORMAL | ABNORMAL |
|---|---|---|
| Assess **scalp** | Usually without lesions | Ringworm, lice |
| Assess frontal and maxillary **sinuses** | Nontender | Tenderness: indicative of inflammatory process |
| Assess **face** | Symmetrical movement | Signs of facial paralysis<br>Twitching: could be due to psychosomatic causes |
| Evaluate the **eyes**<br>  Gross screening of vision with Snellen chart | With younger child, ability to follow movement and to see objects placed a few feet away | Inability to follow movement or to see objects placed a few feet away |
|   Sclerae | Completely white | Yellow sclera: sign of jaundice<br>Blue sclera: may be normal or indicative of osteogenesis imperfecta |
|   Placement in eye socket | Normally placed | Exophthalmos (protrusion of eyeball)<br>Enophthalmos (deeply placed eyeball) |
|   Iris | At rest: upper and lower margins of iris visible between the lids | Setting sun sign (iris appears to be beneath lower lid): if marked, may be sign of increased intracranial pressure |
|   Movement | In newborn, intermittent strabismus | Fixed strabismus or intermittent strabismus continuing after six months of age: indication of muscle paralysis or weakness<br>Nystagmus (constant motion of eye): characteristic of cerebellar lesions and brain tumors |

| ASSESSMENT | NORMAL | ABNORMAL |
|---|---|---|
| Eyelids | Fully covers eye<br>Fully raised on opening | Ptosis of eyelid: may be an early sign of a neurological disorder<br>Sty |
| Conjunctiva | Clear | Inflammation<br>Conjunctivitis<br>Hemorrhage<br>Stimson's lines (small red transverse lines on conjunctiva) |
| Cornea | Clear | Opacity: sign of ulceration<br>Inflammation<br>Redness |
| Discharge | Tears | Purulent discharges: note amount, color, consistency |
| Pupils | Round, regular<br>Clear, equal<br>Brisk reaction to light<br>Accommodation reflex (pupil contraction as object is brought near the eye) | Sluggish or asymmetrical reaction to light: indicates intracranial disease<br><br>Lack of accommodation reflex |
| Lens | Clear | Opacities (cataracts) |
| Evaluate the **ears**<br>Sinuses | None present | Small holes or pits anterior to ear: may be superficial but could indicate the presence of a sinus leading into brain |
| Position | Top of ear above level of eye | Top of ear below level of eye: congenital defects |
| Discharge | None | Discharge: note color, odor, and amount |
| Hearing | In infant: turning to sound<br>In older child: response to whispered command | Diminished hearing in one or both ears |
| Assess the **nose** | No secretions<br><br>Breathing through nose | Secretions: note characteristics<br>Any unusual shape or flaring of nostrils<br>Breathing through mouth |
| Assess the **mouth** | <br><br><br><br>Intact palate<br>Teeth in good condition<br>In older child, presence of permanent teeth | Circumoral pallor: possible sign of cyanotic heart disease, scarlet fever, rheumatic fever, hypoglycemia; also seen in other febrile diseases<br>Asymmetry of lips: seen in nerve paralysis<br>Cleft palate<br>Delayed appearance of deciduous teeth: may indicate cretinism, rickets, congenital syphilis, or Down's syndrome; may be normal<br>Poor tooth formation: may be seen with systemic diseases<br>Green or black teeth: seen after iron ingestion or death of tooth<br>Stained teeth: may be seen after prolonged use of tetracyclines |
| Assess the **gums** | Retention cysts in newborn | Inflammation, abnormal color, drooling, pus, tenderness<br>Black line along gums: may indicate lead poisoning |

| ASSESSMENT | NORMAL | ABNORMAL |
|---|---|---|
| Assess the **tongue** | Moves freely | Tremors on protrusion: may indicate chorea, hyperthyroidism<br>White spots (thrush)<br>Tongue-tie |
| Assess the **throat** | Tonsils normally enlarged in childhood | White membrane over tonsils<br>White pus on sacs, erythema |
| Assess the **larynx** | Normal vocal tones | Hoarseness or stridor: possible respiratory tract obstruction |
| Assess the **neck** | Short in infancy<br>Lengthens at two to three years<br>Trachea slightly right midline | Trachea deviated to left or right: may indicate shift with atelectasis |
| Thyroid | Not enlarged | Enlarged: may be due to hyperactive thyroid, malignancy, goiter |
| Motion | Full lateral and upward/downward motion | Limited movement with pain: may indicate meningeal irritation, lymph node enlargement, rheumatoid arthritis, or other diseases |

## LUNGS AND THORAX ASSESSMENT

| ASSESSMENT | NORMAL | ABNORMAL |
|---|---|---|
| Assess the **lungs** | Normally clear breath sounds bilaterally | Presence of rhonchi, rales or wheezes<br>Diminished breath sounds heard over parts of lung |
| | No retractions | Mild or severe intercostal or sternal retractions |
| | Symmetry of diaphragmatic movement | Asymmetry of movement |
| Assess the **sputum** | None or small amount of clear sputum in morning | Thick, tenacious sputum with foul odor<br>Blood-tinged or green sputum |
| Assess the **breasts** | Slightly enlarged in infancy<br>Generally slightly asymmetrical at puberty | Discharge or growth in male |

## HEART ASSESSMENT

| ASSESSMENT | NORMAL | ABNORMAL |
|---|---|---|
| Assess **heart sounds** | $S_1$, $S_2$, $S_3$ | $S_4$: indicates congestive heart failure |
| Assess **femoral pulses** | Strong | Weak |
| Note **edema** | None present | Edema: note location (initially periorbital) and duration |
| Note **clubbing** of fingers | None present | Clubbing: note location and duration |
| Note **murmurs** | | Murmur grade three or higher |
| Note **cyanosis** | None normally present | Circumoral or peripheral cyanosis: indicates respiratory or cardiac disease<br>Abnormal pulse rate for age |

| ASSESSMENT | NORMAL | ABNORMAL |
|---|---|---|
| **ABDOMEN ASSESSMENT** | | |
| Assess **skin condition** | Soft | Hard, rigid, tender |
| Assess for **peristaltic motion** | Not visible | Visible peristalsis: may indicate pyloric stenosis |
| Assess **shape** | Slightly protuberant in standing adolescent | Large protruding abdomen: may indicate pancreatic fibrosis, hypokalemia, rickets, hypothyroidism, bowel destruction, constipation |
| | | Inguinal hernias, unilateral or bilateral: observe for reducibility |
| | Umbilical protrusion | Umbilical hernia |
| **GENITOURINARY TRACT ASSESSMENT** | | |
| Assess **female genitalia** | | |
| Discharge | Mucoid | Foul or copious discharge; any bleeding prior to puberty |
| Assess **male genitalia** | | |
| Presence of urethral orifice | Orifice on distal end of penis | Hypospadias or epispadias (urethral orifice along inferior or dorsal surface) |
| Urethral opening | Normal size | Stenosis of urethral opening |
| Foreskin | Covers glans completely | Foreskin incompletely formed ventrally when hypospadias present |
| Placement of testes | Descended testes | Undescended testes |
| | | Enlarged scrotum |
| Assess **urine output** | Full, steady stream of urine | Urine with pus, blood, or odor |
| | | Excessive urination or nocturia: possible sign of diabetes |
| Check **anus and rectum** | No masses or fissures present | Hemorrhoids, fissures, prolapse, pinworms |
| | | Dark ring around rectal mucosa: may be sign of lead poisoning |
| **MUSCULOSKELETAL ASSESSMENT** | | |
| Assess **extremities** | Coloration of fingers and toes consistent with rest of body | Cyanosis: can indicate hypothermia, respiratory, or cardiac disease |
| | | Clubbing of fingers and toes: indicates cardiac or respiratory disease |
| | Quick capillary refill on blanching | Sluggish blood return on blanching: indicates poor circulation |
| | Temperature same as rest of body | Temperature variation between extremities and rest of body: indicates neurological or vascular anomalies |
| | Presence of pedal pulses | Absence of pedal pulses indicates circulatory difficulties |
| | No pain or tenderness | Presence of localized or generalized pain |
| | Straight legs after two years of age | Any bowing after two years of age: may be hereditary or indicate rickets |

| ASSESSMENT | NORMAL | ABNORMAL |
|---|---|---|
| | Broad-based gait until four years of age; feet straight ahead afterwards | Scissoring gait: indicates spastic cerebral palsy<br>Persistence of broad-based gait after four years of age: possible abnormalities of legs and feet or balance disturbance<br>Any limp or ataxia |
| Assess **spine** | No dimples | Presence of dimple or tufts of hair: possible spina bifida |
| | Flexible | Limited flexion: indicates central nervous system infections<br>Hyperextension (opisthotonos): indicates brainstem irritation, hemorrhage, or intracranial infection |
| | No lateral curvature or excessive anterior posterior curvature | Presence of lordosis, kyphosis, or scoliosis |
| Assess **joints** | Full range of motion without pain, edema, or tenderness | Pain, edema, or tenderness: indicates tissue injury |
| Assess **muscles** | Good tone and purposeful movement | Decreased or increased tone |
| | Ability to perform motor skills approximate to developmental level | Spasm or tremors: may indicate cerebral palsy<br>Atrophy or contractures |

**NEUROLOGICAL ASSESSMENT**

| | | |
|---|---|---|
| Refer to adult section on neurological assessment for complete overview | | |
| Assess **fine motor movements** | Presence of fine motor activity approximate to age | Continued presence of primitive reflexes after fading of reflex should normally occur: may indicate brain damage |
| Assess presence of **reflexes** | | Any asymmetry of movement |

---

## TERMINOLOGY

**Anisocoria:** inequality of the diameter of the pupils; may be normal or congenital.

**Anorexia:** lack or loss of appetite for food.

**Apical:** pertinent to apex, as in apex of the heart.

**Assessment:** the act of assessing or evaluating.

**Ataxia:** disorder or irregularity; muscular incoordination.

**Auscultation:** listening for sounds produced in some of the body's cavities.

**Autonomic:** spontaneous; self-controlling; independent.

**Bronchi:** primary divisions of the trachea, penetrating the lungs on the right and left.

**Cerebral:** pertaining to the brain.

**Clubbing:** a rounding, as clubbed fingers; a rounding and swelling of fingers in children with congenital heart disease and adults with pulmonary disease.

**Comatose:** in coma or an abnormally deep stupor from which the patient cannot be aroused.

**Conjunctiva:** the mucous membrane that lines the eyelids and covers the exposed surface of the sclera.

**Contraction:** a drawing together; a reduction in size; a shortening or tightening.

**Cranial nerves:** twelve pairs of nerves, which have their origin in the brain.

**Cyanosis:** a slightly bluish or grayish discoloration

of the skin due to reduced oxygenation of the blood.

**Dereistic:** overexercising the imagination to the extent of ignoring reality.

**Ecchymosis:** a form of macula appearing in large irregularly formed hemorrhagic areas of the skin.

**Edema:** a localized or generalized condition in which the body tissues contain an excessive amount of fluid.

**Epidermis:** the outer layer of skin; cuticle.

**Erythema:** a form of macula showing diffuse redness all over the skin.

**Extensor:** a muscle that extends a part.

**Flexor:** a muscle that bends a part in a generally proximal direction.

**Fremitus:** vibratory tremors, especially those felt through the walls of the chest by palpation.

**Furuncles:** boils.

**Hemangioma:** a benign tumor of dilated blood vessels.

**Hemorrhage:** abnormal internal or external discharge of blood.

**Hyperventilation:** increase in rate or depth of respiration or both.

**Hypotension:** decrease of systolic and diastolic blood pressure below normal.

**Intracranial:** within the skull.

**Lochia:** the discharge from the uterus of blood, mucous, and tissue during the puerperal period.

**Mucous membranes:** the lining in passages and cavities communicating with air.

**Multipara:** a woman who has borne more than one offspring.

**Occiput:** the back part of the head.

**Opthalmoscope:** an instrument for examining the interior of the eye.

**Otoscope:** a device for examining the ear.

**Palpation:** the process of examining by using the hands and or fingers.

**Perineum:** the structures occupying the pelvic outlet and comprising the pelvic floor.

**Peristalsis:** a progressive wavelike motion that occurs involuntarily in hollow tubes in the body.

**Petechiae:** small, purplish hemorrhagic spots on the skin.

**Pneumothorax:** a collection of air or gas in the pleural cavity.

**Ptosis:** the dropping or drooping of an organ or part, such as the upper eyelid from paralysis.

**Puerpera:** a woman who has just given birth to an infant.

**Puerperium:** the six-week period following delivery.

**Purulent:** suppurative; forming or containing pus.

**Rales:** an abnormal sound heard on auscultation of the chest, either on inspiration or expiration.

**Rhonchi:** a rale or rattling in the bronchial tube.

**Turgor:** normal tension in a cell; distension or swelling.

**Urethra:** a canal for the discharge of urine from the bladder to the outside.

**Urticaria:** a vascular reaction of the skin characterized by the eruption of pale evanescent wheals, which are associated with severe itching.

**Vasoconstriction:** constriction or a closing down of blood vessels.

**Vertex:** the top of the head.

**Vesicular:** pertinent to vesicles or small blisters.

# Chapter 18

# Specimen Collection

## LEARNING OBJECTIVES

Discuss the nursing responsibilities for reporting abnormal laboratory values.

Describe the major patient instructions that ensure a midstream urine specimen is not contaminated.

State two objectives for obtaining a stool specimen.

List four precautions that must be carried out when obtaining a stool specimen for parasite identification.

Demonstrate the procedure when you test for occult blood.

Write charting information necessary to include in a patient's record when collecting a stool specimen.

Explain the objectives for collecting a sputum specimen.

Outline the steps of collecting a sputum specimen from a Lukin's trap.

Compare and contrast obtaining an aerobic and anaerobic culture.

State the purpose for using an autolet.

Demonstrate the use of the autolet to obtain a blood specimen.

Write two nursing diagnoses which are relevant for specimen collection.

Demonstrate the removal of blood using a vacutainer.

State two suggested solutions for the problem of blood not flowing into the syringe when withdrawing blood.

State the nursing action when a hematoma occurs at the puncture site.

State the purpose for sending IV cannula tips to the laboratory.

## LABORATORY TESTS

Laboratory tests are used as an adjunct to diagnose health care problems and assess the health status of patients. Test findings can reveal occult problems, determine the stage of disease, estimate the activity of the disease process, and measure the effect of therapy. Multiple laboratory tests are usually ordered not only to assist in diagnosing problems but also to "rule out" certain disease states.

Laboratory tests can be analyzed individually or as a part of a screening panel. For example, a routine urinalysis screens for the chemical makeup of the urine as well as color, clarity, and presence of abnormal cells. Blood chemistry components can be tested individually as well as in combination through a multiparameter test. These tests provide data on 8, 12, or 16 different elements of blood, depending on the laboratory equipment. It is more cost effective when all the tests are run simultaneously with one blood specimen. For example, a "panel 12" will analyze the following tests: total protein, albumin, calcium, inorganic phosphorous, cholesterol, glucose, BUN, uric acid, creatinine, total bilirubin, alkaline phosphatase, SGOT.

Every laboratory establishes its own normal values for each test. The normal values are generally printed on each laboratory slip to facilitate comparisons with the patient's findings. Healthy patients do not always fall within the calculated laboratory norms. The physician, considering other variables, will have to judge the value and diagnostic implications of these tests.

**Nursing Responsibility**  Nursing responsibilities associated with the collection of specimens range from patient education to the reporting of abnormal laboratory findings to the appropriate health team member. When specimens are ordered, it is essential that the patient understands the full impact of "how" and "why" the specimen will be obtained. If sterile or clean technique is required, patient teaching can provide an understanding of the process. If the patient is involved with obtaining the specimen, he should be given precise instructions.

To prevent unnecessary lost time and cost to the patient, the nurse must be well-informed of the correct procedure for obtaining, handling, and processing each specimen. If the nurse is unfamiliar with the procedure, she should refer to the laboratory manual for the health care facility. Specific directions are written for most tests performed by the laboratory. If there is any question about the procedure, the laboratory should be called for directions before obtaining the specimen.

The physician should be notified immediately of any abnormal laboratory findings which could be potentially life-threatening. Verbal communication is the most appropriate and efficacious method. When the nurse leaves written messages on the chart, several hours may elapse before the physician sees the findings.

All patients admitted to a health care facility will have at least one laboratory specimen collected during their hospitalization. The most frequent laboratory tests ordered are those involving the urine and blood.

**Urine Tests**   Nursing responsibilities include collecting, temporarily storing, and performing tests on the urine specimen. Timed urine specimens are usually left in the nursing unit until completion of the test. When urine specimens are retained in the nursing unit, the nurse must take special care in the storing and handling of the specimen to ensure reliable results. Generally, urine specimens collected over a period of hours must be refrigerated or have preservatives added to the specimen to ensure accurate results. Preservatives, such as hydrochloric acid or thymol, prevent deterioration of the specimen.

Most urine specimens are collected and sent directly to the laboratory. Single urine specimens are obtained through random sampling, voiding into a clean receptacle and then transferring the urine into a specimen bottle, or by using the clean catch or midstream method. The midstream method necessitates that proper instructions in cleansing the genitalia and obtaining the specimen be given to the patient.

When timed specimens are ordered, the nursing role encompasses not only the handling of the urine specimen but also precise instructions to the patient for collecting the specimen. The collection of urine needs to start and finish at the designated time. A 24-hour urine specimen that is started at 9 A.M. must be finished at 9 A.M. the next day in order to obtain accurate results. Instructions to the patient include having the patient void at 9 A.M., discard that urine specimen, and collect the rest of the urine at 9 A.M. the next morning.

The clinitest, acetest, and test for specific gravity are usually performed by the nurse and are not done by the laboratory. Nurses should follow the specific procedures for each test to obtain accurate results.

**Blood tests**   Even though blood studies are carried out on venous, capillary, or arterial blood, the usual sample is obtained from venous blood. Capillary blood is used to check for RBCs, WBCs, and differential counts. Arterial samples are obtained for blood gas determination and cultures.

Blood specimens are placed in specific blood tubes according to the type of test ordered and sent to the laboratory for analysis. Each health care facility has a list of blood tests that are analyzed from blood in a specific color-top test tube. The colored top on the test tube indicates whether or not the tube contains a preservative. When whole blood is required for the test, an anticoagulant, such as heparin or trisodium citrate, is placed in the test tube to keep the blood from clotting. When serum is needed for the laboratory test, no preservative is added to the blood as the clot is used for the test. If the test tube contains a preservative, the tube should be gently agitated to prevent the blood from clotting.

---

**Test Tube Identification**

| *Color of Top* | *Blood Test* |
|---|---|
| Striped red with preservative | Chemical panels, drug assays, serology, cold agglutins, isoenzymes |
| Solid red | Blood type and cross match |
| Lavender | Coagulation studies |
| Purple | Hemoglobin, hematocrit |
| Green | Ammonia, glucose, electrolytes |

---

Some blood tests require that the patient fast for several hours prior to obtaining the specimens. Other blood tests have no special requirements for collection. Blood studies requiring a fasting specimen for accuracy include fasting blood sugar, lipid panels, glucose tolerance tests, and insulin levels.

If a needle and syringe are used for drawing blood, the top should be removed from the blood tube. After removing the top, slowly inject the blood into the test tube. When blood is ejected through both the needle and the rubber stopper, hemolysis occurs and the specimen is destroyed.

**Cultures**  Cultures are ordered from the throat, eyes, nose, vagina, wounds, sputum, stool, urine, and blood. Special tubes or containers with culture media are used for organism growth. The culture is prepared in the laboratory according to the type of test ordered. It is essential that the proper technique be used to place the culture in the appropriate container to ensure accurate results. Specimens obtained for culture and sensitivity require immediate processing and must be sent directly to the laboratory after they are obtained. If a time lapse occurs, the specimen may need to be discarded and a new one obtained. If the specimen is allowed to dry before the examination, the organism will not transfer to the slide and, thus, the culture medium.

**NURSING DIAGNOSES**

The following nursing diagnoses may be appropriate to include in a Patient Care Plan when the components are related to collecting specimens.

| **Nursing Diagnosis** (Potential) | **Defining Characteristics; Etiology** (Examples) |
|---|---|
| ☐ Comfort, Alterations in: Pain, *related to* | Fear of procedure, e.g., IV puncture for wound culture. |

☐ Anxiety, *related to*   Dread of unknown outcome, e.g., results of specimen tests.

☐ Coping, Ineffective Individual, *related to*   Poor adjustment to procedure or specimen collection, e.g., pain, stress.

☐ Noncompliance, *related to*   Inadequate understanding of the purpose or value of diagnostic test, e.g., language and/or cultural barriers.

## UNIT ONE   URINE SPECIMENS

### NURSING PROCESS DATA

#### ASSESSMENT   *Data Base*

Assess patient's ability to understand instructions and to obtain specimens properly.

Identify if signs and symptoms of urinary tract infections are present; frequency, urgency, dysuria, hematuria, flank pain, fever, and cloudy urine with sediment.

#### PLANNING   *Objectives*

To instruct the patient in the method for obtaining a specimen.

To obtain a noncontaminated urine specimen for culture and sensitivity.

To maintain the collection of urine for 24 hours.

#### IMPLEMENTATION   *Procedures*

Collecting Midstream Urine

Collecting 24-Hour Urine Specimen

#### EVALUATION   *Expected Outcomes*

Patient is able to obtain urine specimen.

Noncontaminated urine specimen is obtained.

24-hour urine specimen completed appropriately.

## COLLECTING MIDSTREAM URINE

### Equipment

Cleaning swab or bactericidal soap

Sterile specimen container

Label for container

### Procedure

1. Gather equipment.

2. Wash your hands.

3. Identify patient by checking identaband.

4. Explain procedure to patient.

**Clinical Alert:**

A contaminated specimen is the single most common reason for inaccurate reporting on urinary cultures and sensitivities. To prevent contamination, place cap of container with sterile side up while collecting specimen and do not touch inside of container.

5. Instruct patient to clean the urinary meatus and obtain urine specimen.

*For a male:*

a. Wash hands and open container.

b. Cleanse end of penis with cleansing swab using circular motion and moving from middle toward outside. **Rationale:** Always swab from clean to dirty area to decrease bacteria levels.

c. Initiate urine stream.

d. After single stream achieved, pass specimen bottle into stream and obtain urine sample. **Rationale:** The microorganisms which accumulate at the urinary meatus have been flushed out with the original stream of urine and will not be collected in the specimen.

*For a female:*

a. Wash hands and open container.

b. Spread labia minora with nondominant hand.

c. Cleanse area with disinfectant swab, beginning above the urethral orifice and moving posteriorly.

d. Initiate urine stream. Holding labia open *throughout* the voiding process.

e. After single stream achieved, pass specimen bottle into the stream and obtain sample.

6. To prevent contamination of specimen with skin flora, instruct the patient to remove the bottle *before* the flow of urine stops and *before* releasing the labia or penis.

7. Wipe off outside of container after replacing cap.

8. Wash your hands.

9. Label the specimen and take it to the laboratory within 15 minutes. If this is not possible, refrigerate the specimen.

24-hour urine specimens must be collected for the entire time ordered. To obtain accurate finding, the laboratory needs the whole urine specimen.

## COLLECTING 24-HOUR URINE SPECIMEN

### Equipment

Urine specimen container

Additive, if required

Requisition slip

Label for specimen

Sign that urine collection is in progress

### Procedure

1. Explain procedure to patient. Stress the importance of saving all urine for 24 hours.

2. Place sign in patient's bathroom stating that 24-hour urine specimen is in progress with date and time.

3. Collect urine specimen and discard it. **Rationale:** The first specimen is considered "old urine" or urine that was in the bladder before test began.

4. Record date and time of first specimen on label and place bottle in appropriate area. Depending on hospital protocol, specimens may be refrigerated or left in the patient's bathroom.

5. Post sign in appropriate place.

6. Place all urine voided in specimen container.

7. Request patient to void exactly 24 hours after first specimen was obtained. Place voided urine in container.

8. After the last voided specimen is placed in the container, cover and send entire specimen to the lab with the proper requisition.

9. Remove sign and remind patient that the test is completed.

10. If a specimen is accidently discarded, obtain a new container, note the new date and time, and restart the procedure.

### CHARTING  *for Urine Specimens*

☐  Method used to obtain specimen

☐  Color, consistency, and odor of urine

☐  Amount of urine obtained (record this amount on the intake and output record also)

☐  Time specimen sent to laboratory

☐  Refrigeration, if required

☐  Exact time for 24-hour specimen

# CLINICAL PROBLEM SOLVING

| Potential Problem | Suggested Solutions |
|---|---|
| Patient is unable to assist with obtaining a sterile specimen. | □ Place female patient in bed and, after cleaning perineum thoroughly, place on sterile or clean bedpan. Cleanse perineal area with swab and obtain specimen according to procedure.<br>□ Assist patient into bathroom. Assist patient to cleanse perineum, instruct to start urine stream, and place the sterile specimen container under the stream to collect specimen.<br>□ For male patients, cleanse the penis and place a sterile or clean urinal under the patient. Instruct to start stream of urine and then place sterile container under stream. |
| Urine specimen contaminated with feces or toilet paper. | □ Instruct patient on need for accuracy and compliance to urine collection. |
| Patient cannot void on command at completion of test. | □ Instruct patient to void as close to time as possible.<br>□ Chart exact time when last specimen collected on both urine bottle and lab slip. Notify lab of findings. |
| Urine specimen discarded before 24-hour sample collected. | □ If time period is close to 24 hours, call laboratory to determine if test can be completed on sample collected.<br>□ If 24-hour sample must be started again, instruct patient of necessity to save all urine.<br>□ Place signs indicating 24-hour test collection in progress on bathroom door and patient's bedside stand.<br>□ Mark in bold or underlined print in Kardex indicating 24-hour urine collection in progress. |

# UNIT TWO   INFANT URINE SPECIMEN

## NURSING PROCESS DATA

### ASSESSMENT   *Data Base*

Determine the purpose for which the specimen is being obtained.

Determine how the collection is to be obtained.

Assess parents' understanding of the purpose for the procedure.

### PLANNING   *Objectives*

To obtain a clean urine specimen for urinary system diagnosis tests.

To obtain urine specimen for routine hospital admission or as a preoperative urine sample.

To provide a method for ensuring collection of all urine when a 24-hour urine collection is ordered.

**IMPLEMENTATION** *Procedure*

Collecting a Specimen from an Infant

**EVALUATION** *Expected Outcomes*

A noncontaminated urine specimen is obtained.

Family is able to assist in collecting urine from small children.

## COLLECTING A SPECIMEN FROM AN INFANT

### Equipment

Cleansing solution

Towel

Restraints

Pediatric urine collector

Diaper

Appropriate specimen containers

### Procedure

1. Gather equipment.
2. Wash your hands.
3. Identify correct child by checking identaband.
4. Cleanse and dry child's perineum.
5. Remove paper backing from the adhesive on the urine collector.
6. Apply urine collector to child's perineum, avoiding extension over anus to prevent contamination.
   a. *Male:* Place child's penis through the opening of the collector.
   b. *Female:* Place the opening of the collection bag over the child's urinary meatus.
7. Place a diaper on the child to help hold the collector in place.
8. Restrain an active child, if necessary.
9. Wash your hands.
10. Check the collector every 15 minutes until a specimen is obtained.

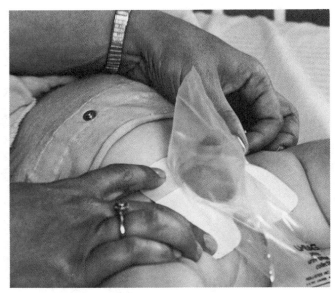

Apply urine collection bag over child's perineum not allowing it to extend over anus.

11. Remove the collector and place a clean diaper on the child.
12. Wash your hands.
13. Send the urine specimen to the lab either by placing the urine collection bag in a urine container or pouring urine from collection bag into the urine container.

### CHARTING *for Collecting a Specimen*

☐ Amount, color, character, and odor of urine

☐ Time specimen obtained and sent to laboratory

☐ Condition of perineum

## CLINICAL PROBLEM SOLVING

| Potential Problems | Suggested Solutions |
|---|---|
| Specimen is lost because collector does not adhere. | ☐ Obtain a new collection bag and repeat the procedure.<br>☐ Tape bag in place with nonallergenic paper tape if necessary. |
| Specimen is lost because collection bag is the wrong size. | ☐ Obtain appropriate size bag and repeat the procedure. |
| Specimen cannot be obtained with a collection bag. | ☐ Notify the physician that you are unable to obtain urine specimen.<br>☐ If possible keep diapers off and observe when infant urinates; attempt to obtain specimen. |

# UNIT THREE   STOOL SPECIMENS

## NURSING PROCESS DATA

### ASSESSMENT   *Data Base*

Determine the purpose for the test.

Check whether the specimen must be sent to the laboratory immediately.

Determine the eliminatory status of the patient, i.e., liquid vs. formed stools, etc.

Assess gastrointestinal tract dysfunction.

### PLANNING   *Objectives*

To obtain stool specimens for diagnosing dysfunction in bowel elimination.

To assess for perforation or bleeding from a gastric ulcer.

To detect presence of parasites.

To determine presence of pinworms.

### IMPLEMENTATION   *Procedures*

Collecting Adult Stool Specimen

Collecting Stool for Parasites

Collecting Infant Stool Specimen

Testing for Occult Blood

Collecting Stool for Bacteria

Testing for Pinworms

### EVALUATION   *Expected Outcomes*

Specimen meets laboratory requirements for diagnostic testing.

Patient does not experience undue discomfort or embarrassment during procedure.

Cellophane tape test completed.

## COLLECTING ADULT STOOL SPECIMEN

### Equipment

Waxed cardboard container with cover

Tongue blade

Label for container

Clean bedpan or bedside commode

### Procedure

1. Check the patient's identaband and explain the procedure to the patient.
2. Before collecting stool specimen, ask the patient to void. Tell patient not to void on the specimen.
3. Clean out all urine from the bedpan or bedside commode.
4. Raise the head of the bed so that patient can assume a squatting position on the bedpan, or help patient sit on the bedside commode.
5. Provide privacy until patient has passed a stool.
6. Remove the bedpan or bedside commode. If necessary, help the patient clean perineum.
7. Use tongue blade to obtain and place a small portion of the formed stool in a container. (For some tests you may need to collect the entire specimen.)
8. Clean bedpan or bedside commode.
9. Wash your hands.
10. Label container with patient's name.
11. Fill out laboratory request for appropriate test.
12. Take specimen to laboratory immediately.

## COLLECTING STOOL FOR PARASITES

### Equipment

Waxed cardboard container with cover

Tongue blade

Label for container

Clean bedpan or bedside commode

### Procedure

1. Follow the steps for Collecting Adult Stool Specimen.
2. Collect exudate, mucus, and blood with all specimens.
3. Keep specimens at body temperature to be examined within 30 minutes. **Rationale:** Organisms must be seen in their active stages, as loose, fluid stools are likely to contain trophozoites or intestinal amoebas and flagellates.
4. There is usually no need to maintain well-formed or semiformed stool specimens at body temperature or to examine them quickly even though they may contain ova or cystic form of parasites.
5. Collect complete stools after purgative medications are administered.
6. When the presence of tapeworms is suspected, all stools must be examined in their entirety in order to find the head of the parasite.
7. Do not give barium, oil, and laxatives containing heavy metals that interfere with the extraction process for seven days prior to stool examination. **Rationale:** Ova or cysts will not be revealed.
8. Use only normal saline solution or tap water if an enema must be administered to collect specimens. Do not use soap suds or other substances.
9. Do not contaminate the specimen with urine as it kills amoeba.
10. Collect three random, normally-passed stool specimens to ensure accurate test results.

## COLLECTING INFANT STOOL SPECIMEN

### Equipment

Diaper

Plastic diaper liner

Waxed cardboard container with cover

Cotton swabs

Label for container

## Procedure

1. Place a clean, disposable diaper on the child or infant.

2. Check diaper frequently so that you obtain a specimen that is not contaminated with urine.

3. If child is passing liquid stools, place a plastic liner inside the diaper.

4. Use cotton swabs to procure the specimen.

5. Place specimen in stool container, wash hands, label, and send to lab immediately.

## TESTING FOR OCCULT BLOOD

### Equipment

Clean bedpan or bedside commode

Tongue blade

Filter paper or packet

Guaiac solution

Glacial acetic acid

Hydrogen peroxide

### Procedure

1. Explain need for stool specimen to patient.

2. Provide privacy for patient.

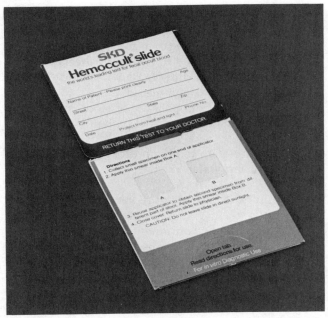

Place small amount of stool on slide packet and complete steps for determining presence of occult blood in stool.

3. Position patient on bedpan or commode.

4. Take stool specimen to bathroom or utility room.

5. Smear small amount of stool on a filter paper or an individualized Hemoccult slide packet.

6. Place two drops of each of the following solutions, in order stated, on the stool smear:
   a. Guaiac solution.
   b. Glacial acetic acid.
   c. Hydrogen peroxide.

7. Observe for blue or green color change within 30 seconds. **Rationale:** Color indicates a positive reaction.

8. Discard filter paper or packet.

9. Wash your hands.

10. Document findings in nurses' notes.

---

**Clinical Alert**

Bleeding from a gastric ulcer or the intestinal tract may be a slow process. If you suspect gastrointestinal bleeding, a guaiac test for occult blood is indicated. Steps for testing occult blood must be followed in sequence.

---

## COLLECTING STOOL FOR BACTERIA

### Equipment

Waxed cardboard container with cover, or sterile test tube with cap

Tongue blade

Label for container

Clean bedpan or bedside commode

### Procedure

1. Follow steps for Collecting Adult Stool Specimen.

2. Collect exudate, mucus, and blood with all specimens.

3. Place a small amount of feces in a sterile test tube (if entire specimen is not needed) wash hands and send entire specimen to the laboratory immediately after collection. If there is any delay, the specimen must be iced.

4. Report and calculate on the basis of daily output any stool specimens that are to undergo chemical analysis.

# TESTING FOR PINWORMS

## Equipment

Clear cellophane tape

Tongue depressor

Glass slide

## Procedure

1. Explain procedure to child and/or parent.
2. Obtain equipment.
3. Provide privacy.
4. Place sticky side of tape over the end of tongue depressor.
5. Place sticky side of cellophane tape over perineal region. **Rationale:** The pinworms are expelled through the anus and adhere to the tape.
6. Leave in place for several seconds.
7. Remove tape from perineal region and place sticky side of tape onto a glass slide for microscopic examination.

> ### Clinical Alert
> For better results the tape test should be done in the morning, before the patient has defecated or bathed.

8. Wash and dry the perineal region.
9. Wash your hands.
10. Label specimen and transport to lab immediately.

## CHARTING  *for Stool Specimens*

☐  Time specimens collected

☐  Time specimens sent to laboratory

☐  Number of specimens sent to laboratory

☐  Description of stool: color, amount, odor, and any purulent patches or blood noted

☐  Condition of perianal skin, if patient is having diarrhea

☐  If serial stool specimens are needed, record each specimen on the Kardex card as well as the chart

---

## CLINICAL PROBLEM SOLVING

### Potential Problems

Patient is embarrassed by having to give stool specimen.

Patient is unable to pass adequate stool for specimen collection.

Patient passes liquid stools.

### Suggested Solutions

☐  Place a bedpan or other collection device under the toilet seat in bathroom to obtain specimen.

☐  If patient is confined to bed, pull sheets over patient's legs and draw curtains around the bed until procedure is completed.

☐  If odor occurs from passage of stool, spray room with air freshener to dispel patient's anxiety.

☐  Notify physician to obtain order to give a normal saline or tap water enema.

☐  Determine if part or entire specimen is required for test.

☐  Obtain a plastic container with a cover and several large cotton swabs. Dip cotton swabs into the liquid stool. Place swabs in plastic container. After procedure, pay close attention to skin care. A protective ointment may be necessary to protect skin from liquid stools.

# UNIT FOUR    VENOUS BLOOD SPECIMENS

## NURSING PROCESS DATA

### ASSESSMENT    *Data Base*

Check order for blood withdrawal in patient's chart.

Note specific requirements for the test, e.g., fasting or administration of medications prior to the test.

Check to see if the test is routine or urgent.

Assess veins for venipuncture site.

### PLANNING    *Objectives*

To obtain an uncontaminated blood specimen.

To obtain a blood sample without complications such as hematoma formation or excessive oozing at the site.

To obtain specimens of blood that can be used to diagnose the patient's illness.

To obtain and transfer specimens without destroying red blood cells.

To ensure accurate test results by making sure the patient follows all requirements for the test, e.g., fasting.

To ensure accurate test results by selecting the right tube for the right test.

To ensure that noncontaminated blood specimen for culture is obtained.

To obtain an accurate blood glucose level.

### IMPLEMENTATION    *Procedures*

Withdrawing Blood

Using Vacutainer System

Collecting a Specimen for Culture

Measuring Glucose with Autolet

### EVALUATION    *Expected Outcomes*

Blood sample is obtained without complications such as hematoma formation or excessive oozing at the site.

Uncontaminated blood specimen is obtained.

Blood samples are sent to the laboratory in the proper tubes.

Blood glucose level obtained.

## WITHDRAWING BLOOD

### Equipment

5-cc or 10-cc syringe

20-gauge one-inch needle(s)

70% alcohol wipe (with blood alcohol specimen, so-lution of benzalkonium will be needed)

Appropriate laboratory tubes

Dry, sterile sponges

### Preparation

1. Check physician's orders for tests to be obtained.
2. Wash your hands.
3. Gather equipment.

### Procedure

1. Identify patient by checking patient's wristband; introduce yourself and explain the procedure.
2. Place a tourniquet above the patient's elbow. (If patient has an IV in place, place the tourniquet on the other arm.) Tighten the tourniquet and tell the patient to open and close his fist.
3. Cleanse the antecubital fossa (inner aspect of el-bow) with an alcohol swab and let the area dry.
4. With needle affixed to the syringe, perform a ven-ipuncture with bevel of the needle pointed up at a 30-degree angle.
5. Pull the syringe plunger back gently and check for placement of the needle in the vein. If place-ment is correct, release the tourniquet, wait a few seconds to allow fresh blood to flow into the vein, and then pull back gently on the plunger.
6. Fill the syringe to the desired amount.
7. Remove the needle from the vein, cover the ven-ipuncture site with a sterile sponge, and press the sponge firmly on the site. (Patient may be able to hold sponge in place.)
8. Remove the top from the laboratory tube. Do not touch the inside of the tube or spill its contents.
9. Remove the needle from the blood-filled syringe and gently eject the blood down the side of the tube. Do not allow the blood to foam or splash. **Rationale:** Red blood cells can be destroyed if the blood sample is not handled carefully.
10. Replace the tube top and rotate the blood gently to mix the blood with the tube contents.
11. Label the tube promptly. Write the patient's name, date, and the time. You may also need to write the initials of the person who drew the specimen if this information is required by hos-pital policy.
12. Check the patient's venipuncture site for oozing. Continue to press the sponge firmly over the site if clots have not begun to form at the site.
13. Take the blood specimens to a designated station or laboratory according to hospital procedure.

## USING VACUTAINER SYSTEM

### Equipment

5-cc or 10-cc syringe

20-gauge one-inch needle(s)

70% alcohol wipe (with blood alcohol specimen, so-lution of benzalkonium will be needed)

Appropriate laboratory tubes

Dry, sterile sponges

Plastic adapter (vacutainer)

Double-ended needle that screws into the adapter

### Procedure

1. Check physician's orders for tests to be obtained.
2. Wash your hands.
3. Obtain plastic adapter, double-ended needle that screws into the adapter, and appropriate vacuum specimen tubes.
4. Screw the double-ended needle into the plastic adapter, with the shorter needle facing the plastic adapter.
5. Prepare the patient by explaining procedure. Tighten the tourniquet above the elbow and cleanse the venipuncture site.
6. Place the vacuum tube inside the plastic adapter, with the top of the tube resting against the short needle.
7. Proceed with the venipuncture. Once the needle is positioned inside the vein, hold the plastic adapter steady and press the vacuum tube firmly into the short needle so that it pierces the top of the tube. Blood should begin to spurt quickly into the tube until the tube is filled.
8. Release the tube and set it aside.
9. Remove the needle from the patient's vein.
10. Wipe and check the site for oozing; press bandaid into place.

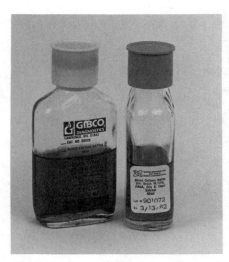

Culture bottle set used for blood cultures.

## COLLECTING A SPECIMEN FOR CULTURE

### Equipment

2 sets of paired culture media bottles

Blood withdrawal equipment e.g. needle and syringe

Povidone-iodine swab

Additional needles

### Procedure

1. Prepare skin with povidone-iodine (alcohol if allergy is present).

2. Withdraw 5 cc blood from a vein without an IV. Do *not* draw specimen through catheter. **Rationale:** Fluid from IV will give altered results.

3. Remove needle used for venipuncture and replace with new sterile needle. **Rationale:** Contamination may result if needle that was used to puncture skin is reused.

4. Swab top of paired blood culture bottles and inject 2½-cc blood into each bottle, changing the needle each time so that a new sterile needle is used for each bottle.

5. In 15 minutes, draw a second sample of blood with a percutaneous stick. (Prepare skin with povidone-iodine solution again.)

6. Place in second set of paired blood culture bottles, using single sterile needle technique.

7. Label bottles and transport to lab immediately. Include site where blood specimens obtained.

## MEASURING GLUCOSE WITH AUTOLET

### Equipment

Autolet wallet with Autolet

Runner of platforms

Lancets

Chemstrip bottle

Soap and water

Cotton ball, sterile sponges

### Preparation

1. Gather autolet wallet and chemstrip bottle and take to bedside.

2. Wash your hands.

3. Take platform runner from wallet and twist off one platform.

4. Face recessed side of platform downwards and insert in slot at bottom of autolet.

5. Pull arm back toward activating button and listen for clicking sound.

6. Insert lancet into socket in the arm and push firmly into place.

### Procedure

1. Wash site on finger (usually second or third finger tip) or heel for infant, with soap and water. **Rationale:** Use soap and water, not alcohol, if repeated sticks will be done as alcohol toughens skin.

2. Gently manipulate finger or heel to determine if good blood supply is available.

3. Place recessed surface of platform against finger or heel to expose tissue through center of platform.

4. Take cover off lancet.

5. Activate the autolet to force the lancet downward by pressing gently on the activating button. The lancet punctures the skin immediately.

6. Gently massage the base of the finger, stroking toward the puncture site. Do not squeeze or apply pressure to site. **Rationale:** Massaging will increase blood flow to the finger tip.

7. Wait a few seconds to allow blood to collect at puncture site.

8. Place a large drop of blood onto both zones of the reagent area on chemstrip.

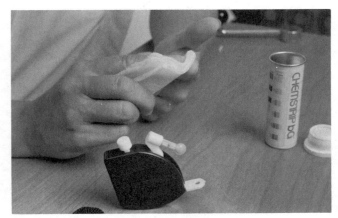

Gently manipulate finger to bring blood to surface.

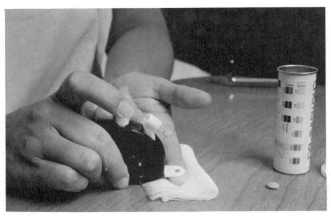

Place autolet platform against finger to expose tissue.

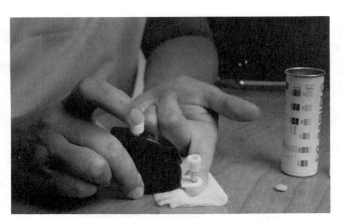

Press button activating autolet to force lancet downward.

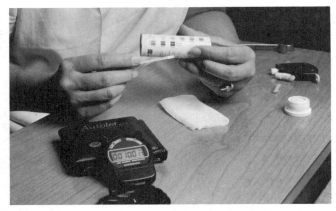

Place blood on chemstrip, wait 60 seconds, then check results.

9. Start the timer simultaneously with dropping blood on strip.

10. Wait 60 seconds, wipe off blood from chemstrip using dry cotton ball.

11. Wait additional 60 seconds and match color chart for results.

12. If color chart indicates reading is darker than 240 mg/dl wait additional 60 seconds and compare chemstrip with color scale.

13. Wipe puncture site with cotton ball to seal site.

14. Wash your hands.

15. Check Kardex or physician's orders for insulin and administer prescribed dose.

16. Document results of blood glucose and insulin dosage on diabetic record and medication sheet.

## CHARTING *for Venous Specimens*

☐ Time of blood withdrawal

☐ Date and name(s) of test(s) for which blood was drawn

☐ Any unusual conditions in either the patient or specimen

☐ Site where blood cultures were obtained

---

## CLINICAL PROBLEM SOLVING

### Potential Problems

Blood does not flow into the syringe.

### Suggested Solutions

☐ Check the position of the needle in the vein.

□ Pull needle back slightly away from the wall of the vein. Rotate needle gently. Do not pull excessively on the plunger, especially if the vein is small, since this movement may cause the vein to collapse.

Blood does not flow into the vacuum tube.

□ Check the position of the needle in the vein. If vacuum in the tube is lost or if the vein is not large enough, discard the tube and get another.
□ If there is pressure on the vein for vacuum pull, select a larger vein or use a syringe and needle instead of the vacutainer method.

Unable to get blood sample with Autolet.

□ Check that fingertip or heel not toughened with over-use of alcohol sponges. Should use soap and water to clean area.
□ Choose an alternate site and repeat the stick.
□ Stroke gently from base of finger toward the tip. Do not apply firm massage as it could interfere with blood flow.

## UNIT FIVE    SPUTUM COLLECTION

### NURSING PROCESS DATA

#### ASSESSMENT    *Data Base*

Check diagnosis which will indicate the advisability of having patient cough.

Observe patient's ability to cough up specimen. You may need to assist the patient while obtaining a specimen, or suction equipment may be necessary.

Determine the degree of pain the patient can tolerate.

Check patient's understanding of procedure so sputum and not saliva is obtained.

#### PLANNING    *Objectives*

To obtain adequate sputum specimen for laboratory examination.

To identify predominant organisms, if respiratory disease is present.

To maintain patient's respiratory status during and after procedure.

#### IMPLEMENTATION    *Procedures*

Obtaining Sputum Specimen

Using Lukin's Trap

Collecting Specimen by Transtrachael Aspiration

#### EVALUATION    *Expected Outcomes*

Adequate sputum specimen is obtained for laboratory examination.

Patient's respiratory status is maintained during and after procedure.

## OBTAINING SPUTUM SPECIMEN

### Equipment

Sterile container and cover for specimen

Label for specimen

Small plastic bag for delivery of specimen to laboratory

Tissues

Laboratory requisition slip

### Preparation

1. Check orders and Patient Care Plan.

2. Gather equipment.

3. Wash your hands.

4. Provide privacy.

### Procedure

1. Explain procedure and rationale to patient.

2. Have patient rinse mouth before coughing to remove any oral contaminants.

---

**Clinical Alert**

Strict asepsis is necessary to obtain an accurate laboratory report.

---

3. Tell patient to take several deep breaths and to cough up sputum (not saliva) directly into sterile container.

4. Obtain 1 to 2 tablespoons of sputum in container; close and seal lid.

5. Assist patient by placing the palms of your hands or a rolled pillow around the incision area if patient is inhibited by pain. **Rationale:** Wrapping a sheet around chest or abdomen will also provide support for body walls during coughing.

6. Evaluate patient's status after procedure.

7. Deliver sputum to the laboratory within 30 minutes after collection. Obtain specimen during treatment if patient is receiving any respiratory treatment (IPPB or PVD).

## USING LUKIN'S TRAP

### Equipment

Suction machine

Sterile catheter and glove

Sterile saline

Sterile sputum trap

Culture tube

### Procedure

1. Set up suction equipment.

2. Attach sputum trap between suction catheter and tubing.

3. Complete suctioning as for naso-oropharyngeal suctioning.

4. Place your thumb on top of sputum trap to monitor; remove your thumb and provide intermittent suction, lifting thumb at intervals until specimen is collected.

5. Suction no more than 15 seconds at a time. **Rationale:** This prevents removal of too much oxygen.

6. Turn off wall suction.

7. Send specimen that was collected in trap to laboratory. (In many hospitals suction tube is also sent to the lab with specimen.)

8. Place patient in a comfortable position.

9. Wash your hands.

## COLLECTING SPECIMEN BY TRANSTRACHEAL ASPIRATION

### Equipment

No. 14 needle with polyethylene tubing or small intracatheter (IV catheter)

Sterile saline and 3–5 cc syringe

Betadine or skin cleansing solution dictated by hospital policy

Xylocaine injection

### Procedure

1. Explain procedure to patient.

2. Collect equipment.

3. Wash your hands.

4. Provide privacy for patient.

5. Position by hyperextending patient's neck and placing a pillow under shoulders.

6. Cleanse cricothyroid area of neck with Betadine solution.

7. Physician will anesthetize area with Xylocaine.

8. Physician will insert 14-gauge needle into cricothyroid area, thread polyethylene tubing through

needle, withdraw needle, and leave tubing in place.

9. Attach syringe (3–5 cc) with 1–2 cc sterile saline into polyethylene tubing.

10. Inject saline into polyethylene tubing to initiate coughing response.

11. To obtain specimen, immediately pull back on barrel of syringe.

12. Withdraw catheter and apply pressure over puncture site.

13. Place sputum secretions in sterile container, label container, and send it to laboratory.

14. Position patient for comfort.

15. Wash your hands.

### CHARTING  *for Sputum Collection*

☐  Amount, color, and consistency of sputum

☐  Mechanical sputum trap used for collection

☐  Patient's tolerance of procedure

---

## CLINICAL PROBLEM SOLVING

**Potential Problems**

Pain inhibits patient from coughing.

**Suggested Solutions**

☐  If diagnosis permits, support painful area with rolled pillows or tight sheets so that external pressure equals internal pressure, thus minimizing pain and discomfort.

☐  Before beginning procedure, ask patient to take several deep breaths. These breaths may trigger the cough reflex and aerate the lungs.

☐  Give patient pain medication as ordered 15 to 30 minutes before obtaining the specimen.

Patient develops coughing spasms during procedure.

☐  Press your third finger lightly over the patient's trachea in the cricoid hollow. This pressure releases the nerve that innervates the coughing reflex.

☐  Report to physician to obtain an order for nebulization.

Unable to obtain sputum specimen.

☐  Notify physician for orders: bronchodilator drugs, nebulization treatment.

☐  Perform PVD to mobilize secretions for expectoration.

☐  Attempt procedure early in the morning when mucus has collected during the night and is more easily expectorated.

---

# UNIT SIX   CULTURES

## NURSING PROCESS DATA

### ASSESSMENT  *Data Base*

Identify appropriate container for culture swabs or material.

Determine time frame for expediting culture to lab.

Assess exact area for culture.

Assess patient's ability to cooperate with procedure.

**PLANNING** *Objectives*

To obtain a non-contaminated culture for study.

To place culture swab or material in container using appropriate techniques.

To send culture to laboratory within specified time frame.

**IMPLEMENTATION** *Procedures*

Obtaining a Throat Culture

Obtaining Aerobic Culture

Obtaining Anaerobic Culture

Obtaining Culture of an IV Cannula

**EVALUATION** *Expected Outcomes*

Non-contaminated cultures obtained.

Cultures placed in appropriate culture medium container.

Cultures sent to laboratory in timely manner.

## OBTAINING A THROAT CULTURE

### Equipment

Tongue depressor

Culture tube with applicator stick

### Preparation

1. Check physician's orders.
2. Wash your hands.
3. Gather equipment.
4. Explain procedure to patient.
5. Position patient in Fowler's position.
6. Place treatment light or face patient toward natural light source to provide good lighting.

### Procedure

1. Remove the sterile applicator from the culture tube.
2. Ask the patient to open his mouth.
3. Use tongue depressor if desired to depress tongue.
4. Swab the back of the throat along the tonsillar area. **Rationale:** Swab only one side of the throat. A second culture of the other side may be taken, check hospital protocol.
5. Remove the applicator stick and place in the culture tube.
6. Push the stick into the tube until the culture media compartment is punctured. **Rationale:** This places the applicator tip into the culture media.
7. Position patient for comfort.
8. Wash your hands.
9. Label culture tube and send to laboratory.

## OBTAINING AEROBIC CULTURE

### Equipment

Culture transport swab with transport medium

Laboratory slip

### Procedure

1. Remove and discard soiled dressing from wound.
2. Remove culture swab and wipe swab in wound. Avoid touching purulent exudate.
3. Swab area of inflamed wound. Avoid touching skin edges or other surfaces that will contaminate the swab.
4. Return swab to container.

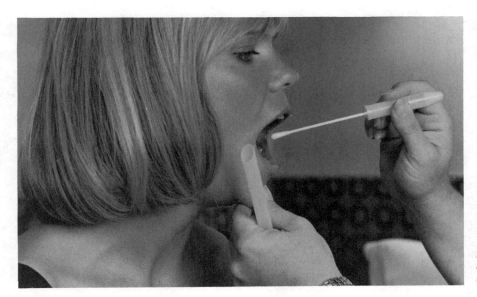

Ask patient to open mouth and swab back of throat along tonsillar area to obtain throat culture.

5. Crush transport medium vial, and push swab tip into contact with transport medium.
6. Replace dressing.
7. Wash your hands.
8. Transport specimen to laboratory within 30 minutes so that organisms are still viable.

> **Clinical Alert**
> Obtain wound culture for both aerobic and anaerobic organisms during scheduled dressing change before any medication or antimicrobial agents have been applied.

## OBTAINING ANAEROBIC CULTURE

### Equipment

Anaerobic transport medium with swab

Laboratory slip

### Procedure

1. Take off and discard dressing from wound.
2. Remove culture swab and wipe in wound as you did with aerobic culturing. Be sure you do not tip anaerobic transport medium tube because it contains carbon dioxide. **Rationale:** Tipping will "spill" the gas out, making it useless to transport anaerobic organisms.

3. Return swab to container.
4. Fill out or affix label to specimen.
5. Have someone transport specimen to laboratory *immediately*.
6. Alternative method:
   a. Draw up exudate in syringe with all air expelled or have a physician aspirate the wound.
   b. Transport specimens to laboratory *immediately*. **Rationale:** Anaerobic organisms may appear on gram stain even though they are not grown in the culture.
7. Replace sterile dressing following protocol.

## OBTAINING CULTURE OF AN IV CANNULA

### Equipment

Blood agar plate or sterile covered test tube

Sterile scissors

Sterile cotton tip applicator

Povidone-iodine swab

Bandaids

### Procedure

1. Wash your hands.
2. Remove catheter, being careful not to touch cath-

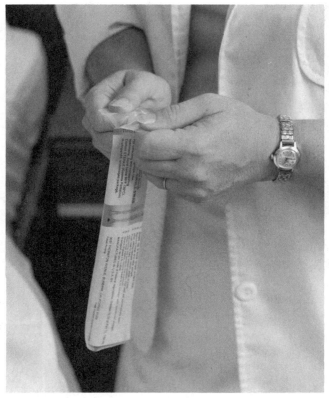

Read directions before removing transport swab and medium from package.

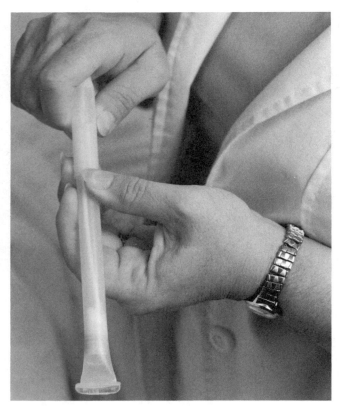

Remove culture swab being careful not to touch edges when removing from container.

eter to any surface as you are removing or once it has been removed.

3. Hold catheter over blood agar plate or test tube. With sterile scissors, cut last one to one-and-a-half inches off catheter and let fall onto blood agar plate or test tube.

4. Roll the catheter across the surface of the blood agar plate with sterile cotton tip applicator.

5. Replace cover of blood agar plate. Label and transport to lab immediately.

6. Cleanse venipuncture site with povidone-iodine solution and apply bandaid.

### CHARTING for Obtaining Culture

□  Exact area where culture obtained

□  Type of culture obtained

□  Characteristics of material sent for culture

□  Time specimen sent to lab

## CLINICAL PROBLEM SOLVING

**Potential Problems**

Inner-surface of collection container contaminated while inserting swab into the culture medium container.

Anaerobic culture not sent to lab immediately.

Anaerobic culture not sent in appropriate container with hydrogen gas.

**Suggested Solutions**

□  Obtain new culture and send to lab.

□  Obtain new culture and send to lab.

□  Obtain appropriate container and send new culture to lab.

# TERMINOLOGY

**Aerobe:** a microorganism that lives and grows in the presence of free oxygen.

**Albuminuria:** the presence of albumin in the urine.

**Anaerobe:** an organism that lives and grows in the absence of molecular oxygen.

**Antimicrobial:** an agent that prevents the multiplication of microorganisms.

**Antimicrobic:** preventing the development or pathogenic action of microbes.

**Asepsis:** prevention of contact with microorganisms.

**Aspiration:** the removal of fluids or gases from a cavity by the application of suction.

**Autolet:** a small instrument with lancet used to obtain a capillary blood specimen; usually used to measure blood glucose level.

**Bacteria:** unicellular plant-like microorganisms lacking chlorophyll.

**Cannula:** a tube for insertion into a duct or cavity.

**Culture:** the growth of microorganisms or living tissue cells in a special media conducive to their growth.

**Dermis:** synonym for corium; the skin layer beneath the epidermis; contains vascular connective tissue.

**Excoriation:** a breakdown of the epidermis.

**Expectorant:** an agent that facilitates the removal of the secretions of the bronchopulmonary mucous membrane.

**Exudate:** material obtained from a wound as the result of the inflammatory process.

**Genitourinary:** pertaining to the genital and urinary systems.

**Glucose:** a monosaccharide, the end product of carbohydrate metabolism; also known as dextrose; found in the normal blood.

**Glycosuria:** the presence of sugar in the urine.

**Granulocytes:** a granular leukocyte.

**Hematuria:** blood in the urine.

**Hemo-:** prefix meaning blood.

**Hypovolemia:** diminished circulating fluid volume.

**Inflammatory process:** localized response when injury or destruction of tissue has occurred; destroys, wards off, or dilutes the causative agent or the injured tissue.

**Intracellular:** inside the cell.

**Micturition:** the process of emptying the urinary bladder; voiding.

**Parasite:** an organism that lives within or upon or at the expense of another organism, known as the host.

**Patency:** the state of being freely open.

**Pathogen:** disease producing organism.

**Peri:** prefix meaning around or about.

**Pinworm:** commonly encountered intestinal parasitic infection; found in children in cosmopolitan areas. Piperazine is drug of choice.

**Polyuria:** the excessive production and elimination of urine.

**Purulent:** containing pus, or caused by pus.

**Pus:** an inflammation containing leukocytes and exudate.

**Septic:** pertinent to pathological organisms or their toxins.

**Septicemia:** presence of pathologic bacteria in the blood.

**Skin turgor:** the tension or fullness of the cells.

**Specific gravity:** weight of a substance compared with an equal volume of water. Water is 1.000.

**Specimen:** a sample taken to show or to determine the character of the whole, as a specimen of urine.

**Sputum:** substance expelled by coughing or clearing the throat.

**Stool:** waste matter discharged from the bowels.

**Transtracheal:** passage of a tube or needle through the wall of the trachea.

**Urinary tract infection (UTI):** an infection of the urinary tract, including all or part of the organs and ducts participating in the secretion and elimination of urine.

**Vacutainer:** a plastic adapter that fits onto a double-ended needle for obtaining a venous blood sample.

**Venipuncture:** puncture of a vein with a needle or catheter.

**Venous:** pertaining to the veins; unoxygenated blood.

**Viscosity:** resistance offered by a fluid; property of a substance that is dependent on the friction of its component molecules as they slide by each other.

Chapter **19**

# Urine Elimination

## LEARNING OBJECTIVES

Describe the process of forming urine as the filtrate passes through the renal tubules.

List four alterations that result in urinary elimination problems.

State two nursing diagnoses that relate to urine elimination.

Complete an intake and output bedside record.

Outline the steps of monitoring specific gravity.

Describe a sugar/acetone test and discuss its purpose.

Outline the steps of inserting a straight catheter.

Describe the major parameters needed to preserve a sterile environment when inserting a Foley catheter.

Explain the cleansing procedure for both a male and female when inserting a Foley catheter.

Demonstrate the clamping protocol used for patients with suprapubic catheters.

Explain how a catheter is attached to a leg bag.

Identify the most important steps to take if infection occurs with a suprapubic catheter.

List the major steps of irrigating by opening a closed urinary system.

Discuss how medications are instilled through a closed urinary system.

Outline the steps necessary to obtain a urine specimen from a closed urinary drainage system.

Outline the steps in applying a urinary diversion pouch.

Compare and contrast nursing interventions for patients on peritoneal dialysis and hemodialysis.

## URINARY SYSTEM

The primary structures of the urinary system are the kidneys, ureters, bladder, and urethra. Each kidney produces urine, which is carried to the bladder by a ureter that is about 25 cm long and 0.6 cm in diameter. Peristaltic waves, pressure, and gravity propel urine through the ureters so that it can be discharged into the bladder.

The bladder serves as a reservoir for urine until the urge to void takes place. When the act of micturition, or urination, occurs, urine passes through two sphincters and is transported from the bladder to the external environment by the urethra.

The anatomical position of the bladder and the structure of the urethra differ in males and females. The bladder in both sexes is posterior to the symphysis pubis. In a female, however, the bladder is anterior to the vagina and the neck of the uterus. In a male the bladder is anterior to the rectum.

The urethra, bladder, ureters, and kidney pelves are lined with a continuous layer of mucous membrane. Because there is no break in the continuity of the lining, bacteria introduced into the normally sterile system can spread rapidly throughout the tract. When the bladder is empty, the lining falls into folds which provide pockets where bacteria can multiply. Since the membrane is highly vascular, bacteria can easily enter the blood stream and septicemia can result.

**Urine Production** Nephrons, the functional units of the kidneys, produce urine. Each nephron consists of a renal corpuscle and a renal tubule, which is surrounded by a capillary bed. Each kidney has approximately a million nephrons.

Urine formed in the renal tubule enters a collecting duct. The collecting ducts from a number of nephrons attach to a single, larger collecting duct, which empties urine into the kidney calyx. The urine collects in the renal pelvis until enough accumulates to flow to the bladder. If movement of urine from the pelvis is interrupted, infection or formation of calculi may occur.

Filtration of blood plasma occurs within the renal corpuscle. Two arterioles circulate blood to and from a capillary network called the glomerulus. Because the inlet to the glomerulus is larger than the outlet, hydrostatic pressure in the capillary network is higher than the pressure in other capillaries of the body. This high pressure causes filtration to occur.

Alterations in pressure change the rate of filtration. The afferent and efferent arterioles control the flow of blood and maintain the appropriate pressure in the glomerulus by constricting and dilating. Other factors that influence the rate of filtration from the glomerulus are the plasma colloidal osmotic pressure and the pressure in the Bowman's capsule into which the filtrate passes.

Due to the pressure in the glomerulus, certain substances are filtered from the blood through the capillary walls into the Bowman's capsule, which surrounds the glomerulus. These substances, which include water, amino acids, electrolytes, glucose, and waste products, form a filtrate that closely resembles blood plasma. This filtrate leaves the Bowman's capsule through the renal tubule.

The renal tubule is comprised of three parts: the proximal convoluted tubule, the loop of Henle, and the distal convoluted tubule. As the filtrate travels through the tubule, some substances are removed through mechanisms such as active transport and osmosis. Other substances are added to the filtrate through excretion. (A summary of the functions of the segments of a tubule appears in Table 1.)

The process of urine formation in all the nephrons of both kidneys reduces 120 ml of filtrate produced each minute to 1 ml of urine. The average daily urine output is, therefore, about 1500 ml. Alterations in the rate of filtration, the filtrate, or functions of the tubule may result in changes in the volume of urine or its constituents.

**TABLE 1**  TUBULAR ALTERATIONS OF FILTRATE

| | |
|---|---|
| Proximal tubule and descending limb | Obligatory water reabsorption, which accounts for about 80% of the absorption of water, occurs in the proximal tube and descending limb. Glucose, amino acids, vitamins, and sodium are actively reabsorbed. Chloride, sulfate, phosphate ions, and urea are passively reabsorbed. Bicarbonate is actively reabsorbed in relation to systemic pH. Water is reabsorbed with these substances, leaving the filtrate osmotic pressure unchanged. |
| Loop of Henle | Sodium is actively transported from the filtrate in the ascending limb into the medullary interstitial fluid, thus raising its osmotic pressure. This rising pressure causes more water to be reabsorbed from the descending limb and the collecting duct and results in the concentration of the urine. |
| Distal tubule and collecting ducts | Facultative or optional reabsorption of water, which accounts for about 10% to 15% of the absorption of water, occurs in the distal tubule and collecting ducts. Sodium is actively reabsorbed in exchange for secreted potassium or hydrogen. As water continues to be reabsorbed, the filtrate becomes more concentrated and its volume is greatly reduced. |

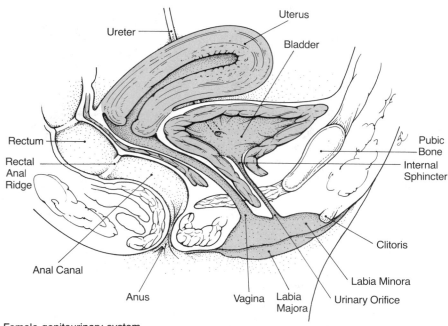

Female genitourinary system.

**Micturition**   Micturition (urination) is a reflex act which occurs in response to pressure changes within the bladder. When urine begins to collect, the muscular walls of the bladder are relaxed, with little change in pressure. After about 300 cc of urine accumulates, the bladder walls tighten, and pressure increases. This rising pressure stimulates receptors in the bladder wall, which send impulses to the spinal cord. After 400 to 500 cc of urine is collected, the bladder walls contract and the internal sphincter relaxes, causing a sense of urgency to void. When urine enters the urethra, the external sphincter relaxes and voiding occurs.

Micturition can occur sooner if the tone of the bladder is increased because of such factors as emotional stress or infection. Micturition can be delayed by voluntary contraction of the external sphincter or contraction of the abdominal muscle. Once the volume of urine reaches about 700 cc, however, most individuals lose their ability to delay micturition.

If an individual is unable to void, as much as 1000 cc of urine can accumulate in the bladder. When a large volume of urine is retained, the bladder's lining and blood vessels can be damaged by the increased stretching and pressure. When this happens, an individual experiences pain, restlessness, chilling, flushing, headache, diaphoresis, and a rise in blood pressure.

## ALTERATIONS IN URINARY ELIMINATION

Alterations in urinary elimination can result from changes in the intake and output of fluids, obstructions to the flow of urine, changes in the secretion of the antidiuretic hormone (ADH), and changes in blood volume.

**Alterations Related to Fluids**   The average person takes in approximately 2600 cc of fluid each day: 1200 cc from drinking, 1100 cc from the water content of food, and 300 cc from changes in metabolism. An increase or decrease in fluid intake will result in a parallel increase or decrease in urine output.

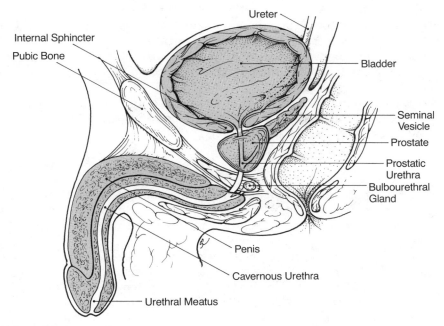

Male genitourinary system.

Healthy individuals rarely experience decreases in urine output because they take in more fluids whenever they are thirsty. Individuals who are ill, however, often experience decreases in urine output because they are unable to respond to the thirst response, their intake is limited due to testing that requires n.p.o. preparations, or their IV fluid intake is not properly maintained.

Fluid is lost from the body not only from urine, but also through respiration, perspiration, and feces. On a daily basis, most individuals lose approximately 2400 cc of fluid: 1500 cc through urine output, 200 cc through respiration, 600 cc through perspiration, and 100 cc through the elimination of feces. Individuals who are ill may also lose fluids through vomiting, bleeding, wound drainage, and suctioning.

**Alterations Related to Obstructions**  A decrease in the output of urine may also be caused by an obstruction to the flow of urine from the bladder. If the obstruction is large enough, the bladder will not empty completely. Instead, it will retain fluid and, over a period of time, become distended. Individuals who have obstructions in the urinary tract experience the need to void more frequently. When they do void, however, they eliminate only very small amounts of urine.

**Alterations Related to Secretion of the Antidiuretic Hormone**  Changes in the rate of secretion of ADH also alter urine output since this hormone controls the amount of water that is reabsorbed in the distal renal tubules and collecting ducts. Common factors that increase the secretion of ADH and reduce urine output include emotional stress, accidental or surgical trauma, pain, hemorrhage, anesthesia, and drugs such as morphine and barbiturates. Factors that reduce the secretion of ADH and thus increase urine output include alcohol, caffeine, cold, and increased carbon dioxide in the blood.

**Alterations Related to Changes in Blood Volume**  Because the production of urine is influenced by the volume of blood filtrate, decreases in this filtrate lead to reductions in the output of urine. Hemorrhage, severe dehydration, and shock reduce the flow of blood through the glomeruli and cause decreases in the filtrate. If the volume of the filtrate is reduced substantially, severe oliguria, or even anuria, may occur.

Other factors that may increase or decrease the output of urine include pathophysiologic states of the kidneys or other body systems, drugs, treatment modalities, diet, and metabolic rate.

## NURSING INTERVENTIONS

The primary purpose for performing nursing interventions associated with urinary elimination is to maintain the integrity of the urinary system, which allows the body to eliminate toxic waste products, and thereby promote homeostasis.

Aseptic technique is essential whenever performing procedures which could introduce bacteria into the urinary tract. Handwashing, using sterile gloves and maintaining a closed urinary collection system decreases the incidence of ascending bladder contamination. Securing catheters to the skin minimizes to-and-fro motion, thus reducing infections of the urinary tract. Retrograde flow of urine must be prevented in order to prevent bladder contamination. Keeping urine collection bags below the level of the bladder helps prevent retrograde flow.

## NURSING DIAGNOSES

The following nursing diagnoses may be appropriate to include in a Patient Care Plan when the components are related to promoting urine elimination.

| Nursing Diagnosis (Potential) | Defining Characteristic; Etiology (Examples) |
| --- | --- |
| □ Self-Concept, Disturbance in: Body Image, *related to* | Alteration in body appearance, e.g., urinary diversion stoma. |
| □ Coping, Ineffective Individual, *related to* | Poor adjustment to prodecure, e.g., inability to tolerate catheter being clamped. |
| □ Fluid Volume, Alteration in: Excess, *related to* | Decreased urine output, e.g., inability to void. |
| □ Noncompliance, *related to* | Unstable glucose level, e.g., inadequate knowledge base, denial of disease state. |
| □ Urinary Elimination, Alteration in: Patterns, *related to* | Retention, e.g., inability to void, bladder atony or surgical repair. |
| | Incontinence, e.g., lack of muscle tone, urinary tract infection. |
| | Infection, e.g., poor insertion technique, contamination of indwelling catheter. |

# UNIT ONE   INTAKE AND OUTPUT

## NURSING PROCESS DATA

### ASSESSMENT   *Data Base*

Assess if strict measurement of intake and output is ordered.

Assess patient's ability to assist in keeping I & O record.

Assess all potential sources of intake (e.g. IV's, oral fluids) and output (e.g. urine, drainage from tubes).

Observe color, clarity, and odor of urine.

Determine all forms where documentation of I & O must occur.

Assess for signs of dehydration or overhydration.

Evaluate weight changes.

### PLANNING   *Objectives*

To accurately measure all sources of fluid intake.

To accurately measure all sources of fluid output.

To identify alterations in fluid balance based on urine and weight assessment.

To record data on appropriate records.

### IMPLEMENTATION   *Procedure*

Measuring Intake and Output

### EVALUATION   *Expected Outcomes*

All sources of intake and output are identified.

Intake and output measurements are accurately maintained.

Signs of fluid imbalance are identified.

Intake and output records are current and accurate.

---

### Methods To Stimulate Voiding

Run water in sink.
Massage the lower abdomen.
Place a hot washcloth on the abdomen.
Pour warm water over the perineum with patient positioned on toilet or bedpan.
Give patient a Sitz bath after obtaining an order.
Put oil of wintergreen on a cotton ball in the bedpan or urinal.

## MEASURING INTAKE AND OUTPUT

### Equipment

Glass or cup

I & O bedside form with fluid conversions

I & O chart record

Graduate for urine and other output measurement

Bedpan/urinal

**TABLE 2**  BEDSIDE INTAKE AND OUTPUT RECORD

| Name _____ | | | Date _____ | | |
| Room # _____ | | | | | |
| Intake | | | Output | | |
| Oral | IV | | Urine | Emesis | Drainage |
| 7 am – 3 pm | | | 7 am – 3 pm | | |
| Total | | | Total | | |
| 3 pm – 11 pm | | | 3 pm – 11 pm | | |
| Total | | | Total | | |
| 11 pm – 7 am | | | 11 pm – 7 am | | |
| Total | | | Total | | |
| 24hr  Total | | | 24hr  Total | | |

Measurements

| Glass 240cc | Ice Cream  100cc |
| Cup 150cc | Jello  100cc |
| Bowl 150cc | Ice Chips  5cc/Cube |
| Juice Glass  100cc | |
| Coffee Pot  240cc | |

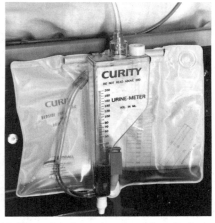

Calibrated drainage bag for a closed urinary drainage system is attached to the bed.

## Preparation

1. Explain purpose of keeping I & O record to patient.
2. Instruct patient to keep record of all fluids taken orally. Keep an I & O record at the bedside for the patient to document intake.
3. Instruct patient to void into bedpan or urinal, not into toilet.
4. Instruct patient not to place toilet tissue in bedpan or defecate in bedpan.

## Procedure

*Oral Intake*

1. Measure all fluids taken orally according to hospital values, e.g. cup 150 cc, glass 240 cc.
2. Record time and amount of oral fluids in the appropriate space on bedside form. Record all IV fluids, NG feedings, etc. on record.
3. Check hospital procedure manual or the bedside I & O record for approximate amounts of oral fluid containers.
4. Transfer 8 hour total fluid intake from bedside I & O record to graphic sheet for 24 hour intake and output record on chart.
5. Record all forms of fluid intake except blood and blood products in the total amount column of the 24 hour record (IV's and oral fluid). These are recorded separately.
6. Complete 24 hour intake record by adding together all three 8 hour totals.

*Output*

1. Empty urinal, bedpan, or Foley drainage bag into

graduate or commode "hat." For accurate record empty urine into graduate. **Rationale:** Measurement is only approximate from Foley drainage bag or "hat."

2. Record time and amount of output on bedside I & O record. Record all urine, drainage from NG tubes, drainage tubes, etc.

3. Transfer 8 hour output totals to graphic sheet or 24 hour I & O record.

4. Complete 24 hour output record by adding together all three output totals and place total on graphic sheet.

**CHARTING** *for Intake and Output*

☐ Time and amount of all oral fluid intake

☐ 8 hour totals of all IV and enteral fluids

☐ 24 hour total of all fluid intake

☐ Time and amount of all urinary output

☐ Time and amount of all drainage, e.g., NG or T-tube

☐ 8 hour total of all fluid output

☐ 24 hour total of all fluid output

---

## CLINICAL PROBLEM SOLVING

**Potential Problems**

Fluid balance is not correct as stated on intake and output record.

**Suggested Solutions**

☐ Report to charge nurse so she can determine if all nurses are keeping accurate records.

☐ Check if patient and/or family can help with keeping the I and O record.

☐ Check the addition on the I and O record to see if an error was made.

Patient does not maintain an intake of at least 1500 cc.

☐ Ensure that the diagnosis allows a 1500-cc intake.

☐ Check if the patient is able to drink fluids by himself, or if he needs assistance.

☐ Ensure that adequate fluids are available for the patient.

---

# UNIT TWO  SPECIFIC GRAVITY AND GLUCOSE

## NURSING PROCESS DATA

### ASSESSMENT  *Data Base*

Assess patient's ability to void when specimens are needed.

Assess color, clarity, and odor of urine.

Assess appropriate time when testing should be done.

Review diagnostic tests and drugs which interfere with test results.

### PLANNING  *Objectives*

To assist the patient to void to obtain urine specimen.

To obtain a nonsterile urine specimen for testing.

To monitor the patient's sugar and acetone levels.

To measure urine specific gravity.

IMPLEMENTATION *Procedures*

Monitoring Specific Gravity

Determining Urine Glucose with Tape

Determining Sugar and Acetone—5 Drop Method

Determining Sugar and Acetone—2 Drop Method

EVALUATION *Expected Outcomes*

Patient able to void when test required.

Accurate specific gravity measured.

Sugar and acetone urine levels monitored.

## MONITORING SPECIFIC GRAVITY

### Equipment

Cylinder

Urinometer

Urine Specimen

### Procedure

1. Fill a cylinder with 20 to 30 cc of urine (about three-fourths full).

2. Place cylinder on a flat surface.

3. Place urinometer into cylinder and spin with your fingers so the urinometer floats freely and does not touch the side of the cylinder. **Rationale:** If urinometer stays against side of cylinder, a false reading occurs.

4. Take the reading just before the spinning stops by checking the curved portion of the urine level to the scale on the urinometer. The scale measures from 0.000 to 0.040 (Normal: 0.003-0.030).

5. Empty and wash the cylinder, and rinse the urinometer with water.

6. Put cylinder and urinometer in appropriate place.

7. Wash your hands.

## DETERMINING URINE GLUCOSE WITH TAPE

### Equipment

Bedpan/urinal

Specimen container

Testape, Urostix or Clinistix

### Procedure

1. Have patient void and take urine specimen to bathroom. Test it and keep results if unable to obtain second urine specimen. **Rationale:** In case second voided specimen cannot be obtained the first specimen will give data and assist in determining actions for care.

2. Obtain second voided specimen approximately 10–20 minutes after first specimen.

3. Take urine specimen to bathroom (bedpan/urinal).

4. Pour small amount of urine into specimen container.

5. Dip test strip into urine.

6. Read color change on test strip container after waiting prescribed amount of time stated on container. Results are read as percent, 1/10-2% or as

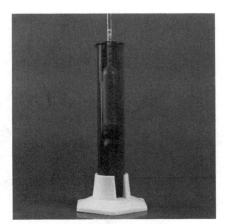

Equipment for measuring specific gravity includes both a cylinder and urinometer.

a plus, one plus (+ or 1+) to four plus (+ + + + or 4+).

7. Replace tape dispenser, away from sink area. **Rationale:** If tape becomes wet it will be ineffective.

8. Return bedpan/urinal to bedside stand or bathroom.

9. Wash hands.

## DETERMINING S/A 5 DROP METHOD

### Equipment

Specimen container

Clinitest tablets

Acetest tablets

Urine testing kit

Color charts

Paper towel

### Procedure

1. Ask patient to void in urinal or bedpan 30 minutes before urine specimen for testing sugar and acetone is needed.

2. Take first voided specimen to utility room or bathroom. Empty small amount of urine from bedpan or urinal and place in specimen container. Test the first voided specimen and record findings if required by facility.

3. Obtain second voided specimen and take to bathroom or utility room.

4. Place 5 drops urine and 10 drops water into test tube.

5. Drop 1 clinitest tablet into test tube.

6. Allow reaction to bubble until it stops.

7. Wait ten seconds, shake gently, and compare results with chart.
   a. Blue indicates negative test.
   b. Orange indicates highly positive test.
   c. Dark greenish-brown preceded by rapid change in color from green to orange indicates urine glucose level above 2%.

8. Place acetest tablet on piece of paper towel.

9. Place one drop of urine on acetest tablet. Wait one minute and compare color of tablet and chart. Dark purple indicates positive results.

10. Clean and replace equipment to proper storage area.

11. Wash your hands.

12. Document findings and determine if insulin needed.

## DETERMINING S/A 2 DROP METHOD

### Equipment

Same as for 5 Drop Method

### Procedure

1. Ask patient to void in urinal or bedpan 30 minutes before urine specimen for testing sugar and acetone is needed.

2. Take first voided specimen to utility room or bathroom. Empty small amount urine from bedpan or urinal and place in specimen container. Test the first voided specimen according to procedure and record findings if required by facility.

3. Obtain second voided specimen and take to bathroom or utility room.

4. Place 2 drops of urine and 10 drops of water into test tube.

5. Drop clinitest tablet into test tube.

6. Allow reaction to bubble until it stops. (Do not shake tube.)

7. Wait 10 seconds, shake test tube, and compare results with chart.
   a. Use only 2 drop method color scale chart.
   b. Seven colors are contained on chart.
   c. Scale ranges from 0–5%.

8. Rinse out test tube and return to container.

9. Wash your hands.

10. Document your findings and determine if insulin is needed.

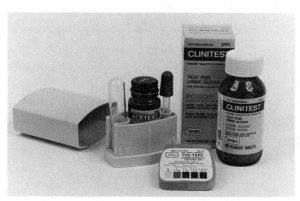

Clinitest tablets and tes-tape test sugar. Acetest tablets test acetone.

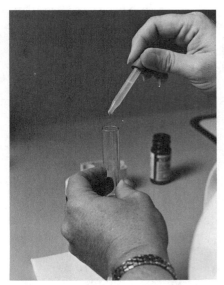

Place 5 drops urine and 10 water into tube.

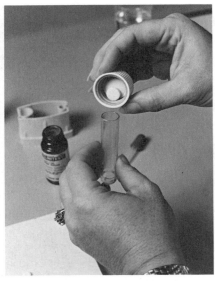

Drop Clinitest into tube without touching.

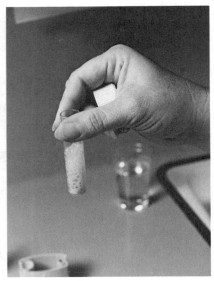

Determine findings when bubbling stops.

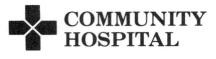

### COMMUNITY HOSPITAL

DIABETIC RECORD

| DIRECTION: Test second voiding whenever possible. | | | | | | | | | | | | |
|---|---|---|---|---|---|---|---|---|---|---|---|---|

| DATE | | | | | | | | | | | | | |
|---|---|---|---|---|---|---|---|---|---|---|---|---|---|
| TIME | 1st void / 2nd void | | | | | | | | | | | | |
| VOLUME | 1st void / 2nd void | | | | | | | | | | | | |
| SUGAR | | | | | | | | | | | | | |
| ACETONE | | | | | | | | | | | | | |
| INSULIN | TYPE | | | | | | | | | | | | |
| | DOSE | | | | | | | | | | | | |
| | TIME | | | | | | | | | | | | |
| | ROUTE | | | | | | | | | | | | |
| | SITE | | | | | | | | | | | | |
| | SIGNATURE | | | | | | | | | | | | |

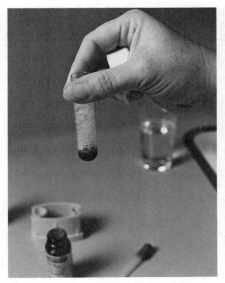
Wait 10 seconds and then shake gently.

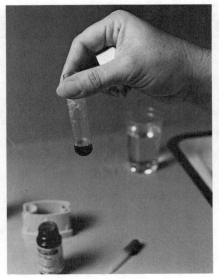
Compare color in test tube to color chart.

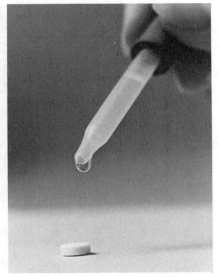
Acetest requires 1 drop of urine on tablet.

**CHARTING**  *Specific Gravity and Glucose*

☐  Amount, color, appearance, and odor of urine

☐  Techniques effective in stimulating voiding

☐  Type of urine testing equipment used, e.g. test tape

☐  Percentage and "plus" readings from urine test

☐  First or second voided specimen

☐  Specific gravity reading

☐  Actions taken based on results

☐  Physician notified, if appropriate

---

## CLINICAL PROBLEM SOLVING

**Potential Problems**

Urine glucose level positive for unknown reason.

Strips or tablets are discolored or moist.

**Suggested Solutions**

☐  Check if new medication contains sugar, e.g. elixirs, cough syrups.

☐  Assess if patient is taking large quantities of ascorbic acid and aspirin. The urine will be positive even though glucose is not present.

☐  Check if patient is taking medications which cause false positive results, e.g. Benamid, levodopa, NegGram, Keflin, etc.

☐  Sensitivity is lost. They need to be disposed of and new strips or tablets used.

☐  Keep tablets and strips away from moisture by keeping them in tightly covered container (original bottle for tablets and baby food jar for tape).

☐  Always check tablet before using to ensure accurate results.

# UNIT THREE   CATHETERIZATION

## NURSING PROCESS DATA

### ASSESSMENT   *Data Base*

Assess the patient's bladder for distention.

Assess purpose of catheterization.

Check physician's orders for method of catheterization to be done.

Assess the patient's physical ability to cooperate with positioning.

Assess urinary meatus and catheter for exudate, edema, inflammation and general cleanliness.

Assess need for perineal care before catheterization procedure.

### PLANNING   *Objectives*

To prevent or relieve discomfort due to bladder distention.

To promote urinary elimination.

To obtain a sterile urine specimen.

To obtain accurate measurements of bladder function.

To provide continual urinary bladder drainage.

To instill medication.

To measure the amount of residual urine.

To monitor the output of a critically ill patient.

To facilitate studies of the urinary system.

To prevent skin breakdown in incontinent bedridden patients.

To prevent urinary tract infections through catheter care.

### IMPLEMENTATION   *Procedures*

Draping a Female Patient

Inserting a Straight (French) Catheter

Inserting a Retention (Foley) Catheter

Providing Catheter Care

Removing a Retention Catheter

### EVALUATION   *Expected Outcomes*

Residual urine measured.

Sterile urine specimen obtained.

Catheterization performed using sterile technique.

Retention catheter inserted without difficulty.

Bladder emptied when patient unable to void.

Urinary tract infections prevented through good catheter care.

Urinary medications instilled using sterile technique.

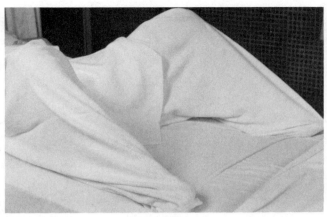

Drape patient's legs and feet before beginning catheterization.

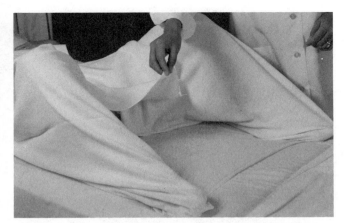

After draping, fold back corner to expose patient's perineal area.

## DRAPING A FEMALE PATIENT

### Equipment

Bath blanket

### Procedure

1. Bring bath blanket to bedside.
2. Identify patient and explain procedure.
3. Provide privacy.
4. Wash your hands.
5. Place bed in HIGH position and lower side rail nearest you.
6. Place bath blanket over patient's top linen so that one corner of the blanket is pointed toward the patient's head to form a diamond shape over the patient.
7. Instruct patient to hold onto bath blanket. Fanfold linen to foot of bed and place on chair.
8. Request that patient flex knees and keep them apart with feet firmly on bed.
9. Wrap lateral corners of bath blanket around feet in a spiral fashion until they are completely covered.
10. The corner of the blanket between knees and extending over perineum can later be folded back over the abdomen.

## INSERTING A STRAIGHT CATHETER

### Equipment

Disposable catheterization tray with straight or French catheter

Bath blanket

Additional light source, if needed

Towel, washcloth

Basin with warm water

Soap

### Preparation

1. Bring equipment to bedside table.
2. Check lighting source.
3. Identify patient and explain procedure and need for patient to keep knees positioned during procedure.
4. Provide privacy.
5. Wash your hands.
6. Place bed in HIGH position and lower side rail on working side.
7. Drape the patient (see Draping Procedure).
8. Have patient bring knees up and out. May need assistance to keep knees in this position. **Rationale:** This position provides for good visualization of urinary meatus.
9. Adjust light source to ensure that exposure is adequate.
10. Fold up bath blanket corner to expose perineum.
11. Provide perineal care with soap and water if needed.
12. Dry perineum thoroughly. Fold bath blanket corner over perineum for privacy.
13. Discard towels, water, and replace basin.
14. Wash your hands.

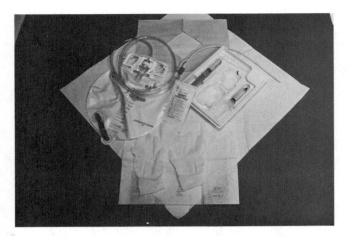

Disposable kit includes equipment for performing a catheterization.

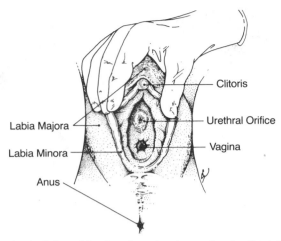

An anatomical view of the female perineal area showing the orifice.

## Procedure

1. Open sterile package by tearing the package on the lined edge of plastic wrap. Place plastic wrap at foot of bed for waste disposal.

2. Place cath tray on bed between patient's legs.

3. Fold back bath blanket to expose perineum.

4. Open white outer wrap away from sterile package with last turn toward patient.

5. Position white wrap under patient's buttocks. **Rationale:** Used for added protection of the bed.

6. Remove sterile absorbent pad and position under patient's buttocks. Have patient lift buttocks if able. Position pad by holding on to corners of pad only.

7. Put on sterile gloves, remove sterile articles from tray and arrange conveniently on sterile field or place tray up close on field.

8. Open package and pour antiseptic solution over cotton balls.

9. Uncap syringe filled with lubricant, or tear open package, pick up catheter tip, and lubricate the tip of the catheter generously. Place catheter back on tray. (May place lubricant on sterile field and put catheter tip on lubricant and leave in place.)

10. If specimen is required, uncap the specimen container.

11. Move the urine collection receptacle close to patient.

12. Place the fenestrated drape over the perineum exposing meatus.

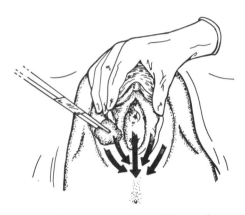

Cleanse meatus with saturated cotton ball in one downward stroke.

13. Cleanse the patient's meatus:
    *For a female:*
    a. Separate the patient's labia minora with your nondominant hand.
    b. With your dominant hand, *use forceps* to pick up an absorbent ball that has been saturated with antiseptic solution.
    c. Cleanse the patient's meatus with one downward stroke of the forceps. Discard the absorbent ball in the plastic cover at foot of bed.
    d. Repeat step C at least three to four times.
    e. Continue to hold the patient's labia apart until you insert the catheter.
    *For a male:*
    a. Hold the patient's penis upright with your nondominant hand. Hold the sides of the penis to prevent closing the urethra.

b. With your dominant hand, *use forceps* to pick up an absorbent ball that has been saturated with antiseptic solution.

c. Cleanse the patient's meatus with one downward stroke of the forceps. Discard the absorbent ball.

d. Repeat step C at least three to four times.

e. Continue to hold the penis until you insert the catheter.

14. Discard the forceps in the plastic bag at the foot of the bed. Using sterile gloved hand, pick up lubricated catheter keeping drainage end in collection container and insert ½ to 2 inches or until urine begins to flow.

15. Move nondominant hand from holding labia open to hold catheter in place.

16. Place the sterile specimen container under the drainage end of the catheter and fill the container with approximately 30cc of urine.

17. Replace catheter drainage end in collection container and allow urine to flow until it ceases.

18. Pinch catheter closed when urine ceases to flow and remove gently and slowly.

19. Remove the drapes, wash and dry the perineum.

20. Position the patient for comfort, put the bed in LOW position with the side rails up.

21. Measure and record urine output on the I & O bedside record.

22. Discard the equipment in the utility room.

23. Wash your hands.

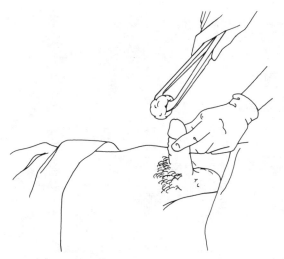

Cleanse tip of penis with forceps holding saturated cotton ball.

## INSERTING A RETENTION CATHETER

### Equipment

Disposable catheter kit with appropriate size catheter (size 8 to 10 for child, size 14 to 16 for adult female, and size 18 to 20 for adult male)

Closed drainage set, if not included in kit

Additional lighting, if needed

Bath blanket

Towels, washcloth

Basin with warm water

Soap

### Preparation

Same as for Inserting a Straight (French) catheter

### Procedure

1. Open sterile package by tearing the package on the lined edge of plastic wrap. Place plastic wrap at foot of bed for waste disposal.

2. Place cath tray on bed between patient's legs.

3. Fold back corner of bath blanket to expose perineum.

4. Open white outer wrap away from package with last turn toward patient.

5. Bring white wrap under patient's buttocks.

6. Remove sterile absorbent pad and position under patient's buttocks. Have patient lift buttocks if able. Position pad by holding on to corners of pad only. **Rationale:** Holding on to the edges will keep the center sterile.

7. Put on sterile gloves and separate the two containers. Place container with cotton balls and lubricant toward patient. Place container with catheter and bag toward foot of bed (next to first container).

8. Open package and pour antiseptic solution over cotton balls.

9. To test Foley catheter bag, remove rubber protector and insert tip of the pre-filled syringe into catheter side arm to inflate balloon. Standard catheters have 5cc balloons. Omit pre-testing step for catheters with pre-filled balloons on drainage end of catheter. **Rationale:** Once pre-filled balloons are opened and fluid forced into balloon at tip of catheter, the fluid cannot be aspirated back into drainage end.

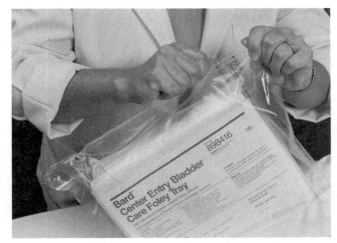

Obtain prepackaged sterile catheterization kit by tearing lined edge.

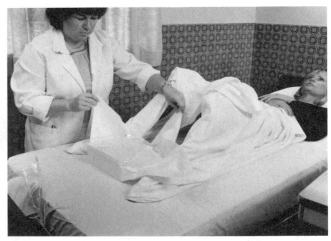

Place kit at end of bed and open wrapper away from sterile package.

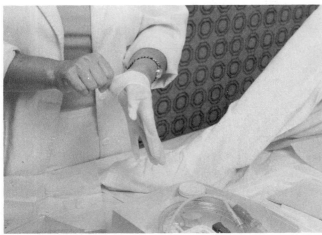

Maintain sterile technique by using gloves throughout procedure.

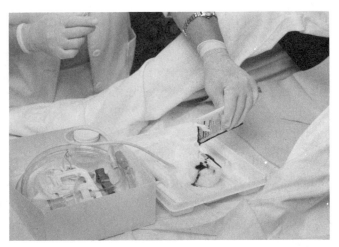

Lift tray from kit and pour antiseptic solution over cotton balls.

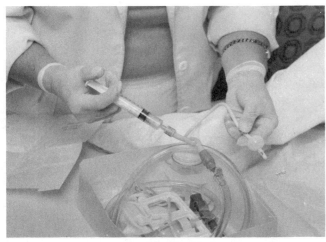

Test balloon by inserting tip of pre-filled syringe into catheter.

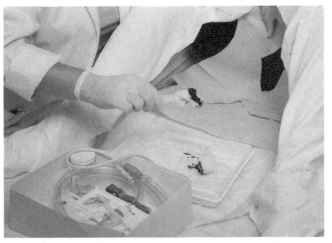

Cleanse meatus with sterile cotton balls and povidone-iodine.

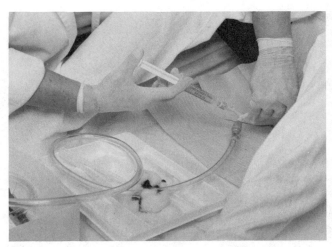

Instill sterile water into balloon after catheter is inserted.

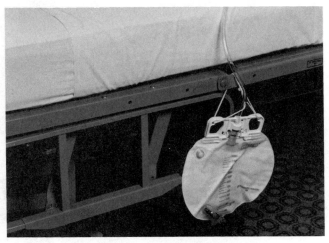

Attach drainage bag to hang freely at patient's bedside.

10. After testing balloon, pull back on syringe to remove fluid. **Rationale:** Testing is done to ensure that balloon is able to be inflated without leaking.

11. Lubricate catheter by uncapping syringe filled with lubricant or open package, and generously lubricate tip in lubricant. Keep catheter on tray. **Rationale:** Lubricating the catheter prevents friction and trauma to the meatus.

12. Position fenestrated drape over the patient to expose the genitalia.

13. Cleanse the patient's meatus:
    *For a female:*
    a. Separate the patient's labia minora with your nondominant hand.
    b. With your dominant hand, *use forceps* to pick up an absorbent ball that has been saturated with antiseptic solution.
    c. Cleanse the patient's meatus with one downward stroke of the forceps. Discard the absorbent ball in plastic bag at foot of bed.
    d. Repeat step C at least three to four times.
    e. Continue to hold the patient's labia apart until you insert the catheter.
    *For a male:*
    a. Hold the patient's penis upright with your nondominant hand. Hold the sides of the penis to prevent closing the urethra.
    b. With your dominant hand, *use forceps* to pick up an absorbent ball that has been saturated with antiseptic solution.
    c. Cleanse the patient's meatus with one downward stroke of the forceps. Discard the absorbent ball.

    d. Repeat step C at least three to four times.
    e. Continue to hold the penis until you insert the catheter.

14. Discard forceps in plastic bag at foot of bed.

15. With uncontaminated hand, take catheter from tray, and insert gently into meatus ½" to 2" or until urine starts to flow.

16. Guide the catheter gently through the urethra until the urine begins to drain. (Insert the catheter 2–3 in beyond the point at which urine begins to flow.) **Rationale:** Inserting the catheter further into bladder ensures it is beyond the neck of the bladder.

17. Inject the entire contents of the pre-filled syringe into the side arm of the catheter used for balloon inflation. If the catheter has a pre-filled balloon at the drainage end of catheter, inflate the retention balloon by releasing the clamp on the pre-filled balloon.

18. Retract the catheter until you feel resistance.

19. Tape the catheter with one-inch tape.
    a. *For a female:* Tape catheter to the side of the leg.
    b. *For a male:* Tape catheter to the abdomen to prevent pressure on the penoscrotal angle.

20. Attach drainage bag to bed frame (not side rails).

21. Cleanse the patient's perineum of the antiseptic solution. Remove drapes.

22. Reposition the patient for comfort; put bed in LOW position with side rails up.

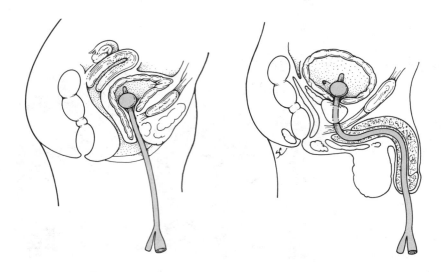

Foley catheter placement is maintained with inflated retention balloon.

23. Remove all equipment and discard disposable trash.
24. Measure and record urine output on I & O bedside record.
25. Wash your hands.

## PROVIDING CATHETER CARE

### Equipment

Commercially prepared kit

*or*

Antiseptic solution

Swabs or cotton balls

Sterile gloves

Paper bag

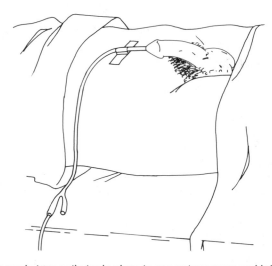

Securely tape catheter in place to prevent pressure and irritation.

### Procedure

1. Check physician's orders and Patient Care Plan.
2. Gather equipment.
3. Identify patient by checking identaband.
4. Provide privacy.
5. Wash hands.
6. Explain procedure to patient.
7. Raise bed and lower side rail on working side.
8. Place patient in supine position and expose perineal area to easily visualize the meatus.
9. Open sterile catheter care kit or assemble equipment on overhead table within easy reach.
10. Put on sterile gloves.
11. Pour antiseptic solution over cotton balls or open package of cleansing swabs.
12. Open antibiotic ointment and place a small amount on sterile swab or cotton ball.
13. Cleanse urinary meatus using circular motion moving from middle toward outside with antiseptic soaked cotton ball or swab. **Rationale:** This motion prevents bacteria from entering the urinary meatus.
14. Gently pull catheter taut and cleanse with new swab or cotton ball from catheter insertion site down catheter tubing approximately 4 to 5 inches toward drainage bag.
15. Place ointment around catheter at the meatus and down catheter tubing about ½ to 1 inch.
16. Position patient for comfort.
17. Lower bed and raise side rail.

18. Discard equipment.

19. Wash hands.

## REMOVING A RETENTION CATHETER

### Equipment

10cc syringe

Paper towel

Catheter clamp

Soap, water

Towel

### Preparation

1. Check physician's orders.

2. Wash your hands.

3. Gather equipment.

4. Explain procedure to patient.

5. Provide privacy.

### Procedure

1. Clamp catheter.

2. Insert syringe into balloon port of catheter. Do not cut the catheter with a scissor. **Rationale:** Balloon may not totally deflate if cut.

3. Withdraw fluid from balloon (usually 5 to 10cc water in balloon).

4. Pull gently on catheter to ensure balloon is deflated before attempting to remove. **Rationale:** Damage to the urethra can occur if balloon is not totally deflated.

5. Hold a paper towel under the catheter with your nondominant hand.

6. If resistance is not met, slowly withdraw the catheter allowing it to fall into paper towel.

7. Disconnect catheter bag from bed frame.

8. Empty catheter bag into graduate and measure output.

9. Record output on I & O bedside record.

10. Dispose of catheter in trash.

11. Wash perineum with soap and water. Dry thoroughly.

12. Position patient for comfort.

13. Wash your hands.

14. Instruct patient to drink oral fluids as tolerated and observe for signs and symptoms of urinary tract infections (burning, frequency, urgency).

15. Offer bedpan or urinal at least every 2 to 4 hours after removing catheter, until voiding occurs. Keep accurate I&O record.

### CHARTING  *for Catheterizations*

☐ Type of catheterization

☐ Amount, color, and odor of urine obtained

☐ Size of catheter used

☐ Patient's tolerance of procedure

☐ Specimen sent to lab (if ordered)

☐ Catheter care provided

☐ Condition of urinary meatus

☐ Catheter removed

☐ Voiding: Time and amount after catheter removal

☐ Intake and output

---

## CLINICAL PROBLEM SOLVING

### Potential Problems

Catheter is inserted in the vagina of a female patient.

### Suggested Solutions

☐ Leave the catheter in place and follow these actions:
   a. Reposition your fingers to assist in visualizing the urethral meatus.
   b. Have someone obtain a new catheter and new gloves. You may need a whole new kit if contamination of the sterile field has occurred.
   c. Locate the patient's urinary meatus before inserting the catheter.
   d. Repeat the catheterization procedure.

Catheter is contaminated when attempting to insert.

- ☐ Obtain a new catheter and repeat the catheterization.
- ☐ If the sterile field has been contaminated, obtain a new catheter kit. Repeat the catheterization procedure.

Unable to insert catheter into a female patient.

- ☐ Repeat the procedure following these actions:
  a. Ask patient to hold her legs apart or ask for assistance from another health team member so you have better access to the urethral meatus.
  b. Before cleansing the patient, identify the area of the urethral meatus.
  c. When cleansing with antiseptic solution, observe the urethral opening for movement when pressure is applied to meatus.
  d. Repeat the catheterization procedure using a new catheter kit or new gloves and a new catheter if the kit has not been contaminated.

Unable to insert catheter into male patient.

- ☐ Obtain a new catheter kit and follow these actions:
  a. Hold penis vertical to patient's body.
  b. Insert catheter while applying slight traction by gently pulling upward on the shaft of the penis.
  c. If you encounter resistance, rotate the catheter, increase the traction, and change the angle of the penis slightly.
  d. When urine begins to flow, lower the patient's penis.

Urine exceeds 1000cc with catheterization.

- ☐ If Foley catheter inserted, clamp catheter for 20–30 minutes and then unclamp.
- ☐ If bladder appears to be grossly distended when palpated, insert Foley catheter instead of straight catheter.
  a. If urine exceeds 1000cc inflate balloon and clamp for 30 min.
  b. Open clamp and drain remaining urine and deflate balloon.
  c. Remove catheter after urine flow ceases or notify physician of results and ask if Foley should be left in place.

Catheter comes out with balloon still inserted.

- ☐ Assess patient for signs of urethral trauma, e.g., bleeding, pain.
- ☐ Obtain a new catheter and repeat the catheterization procedure, making sure that the balloon is inflated with at least 10 cc water.
- ☐ Monitor urine output for bleeding.
- ☐ Notify physician to determine if a Foley with a 30cc balloon should be inserted.

# UNIT FOUR   EXTERNAL CATHETER SYSTEM

## NURSING PROCESS DATA

### ASSESSMENT   *Data Base*

Assess the genital area for signs of irritation and edema during the use of condom catheter.

Assess activity level of patient to determine when a leg bag or a continuous drainage system is necessary.

### PLANNING   *Objectives*

To provide a means for preventing incontinency.

To provide a means of collecting urine in a system which allows patient ambulation.

To prevent urinary tract infections in patients who are at risk but require a method of urine collection to maintain continency.

### IMPLEMENTATION   *Procedures*

Applying a Condom

Attaching Catheter to Leg Bag

### EVALUATION   *Expected Outcomes*

Urinary tract infection is prevented.

Patient remains continent.

Genital area remains free of inflammation.

Patient is able to ambulate without a catheter drainage bag.

## APPLYING A CONDOM

### Equipment

Soap, water, towel

Commercial condom catheter

Leg bag or continuous drainage system

Alcohol wipes

### Preparation

1. Check physician's orders and Patient Care Plan.

2. Gather equipment, condom catheter, soap, towel, and basin with warm water.

3. Explain procedure to patient.

4. Wash your hands and provide privacy.

5. Raise bed and lower side rail on working side of bed.

6. Wash genital area with soap and water and dry area thoroughly.

### Procedure

1. When commercial condom catheters are used, apply protective coating to skin on penile shaft and allow to dry completely (30 seconds).

2. Peel off paper from both sides of the adhesive liner that accompanies the commercial product.

3. Spirally wrap the adhesive liner around the penile shaft behind the glans.

4. Take the latex condom catheter and place the prerolled latex sheath so the funnel is against the glans.

5. Unroll the latex sheath up the penis until it is completely over the adhesive liner.

6. Gently squeeze the condom against the liner to seal it after the sheath is completely rolled over the penis. Do not wrinkle the latex as wrinkles cause urine to leak through the catheter.

7. Attach the condom to a drainage system. The drainage system can be a leg bag or a continuous drainage system depending on the activity level and condition of the patient.

8. Lower bed and raise side rail or assist patient out of bed if he is to be ambulated.

9. Wash your hands.

## ATTACHING CATHETER TO LEG BAG

### Equipment

Leg bag

Alcohol swab

### Procedure

1. Obtain order for leg bag from physician.

2. Gather leg bag and alcohol wipe.

3. Wash your hands and provide privacy.

4. Raise bed and lower side rail on working side of bed.

5. Disconnect drainage tubing from indwelling or condom catheter.

6. Wipe the leg bag and catheter connectors with alcohol.

7. Connect the tip of the leg bag into the catheter.

8. Place the cap from the leg bag tip on the collection tubing.

9. Secure the leg bag to the lower leg by placing the rubber strap through the bag and around the leg. Secure the strap by placing the button through the opening in the strap.

10. When removing leg bag, disconnect the catheter from the leg bag and wipe each connection end with alcohol wipes.

11. Take leg bag cap off the drainage tubing and replace it on the leg bag.

12. Connect the catheter to the drainage tubing.

13. Lower bed and raise side rail.

14. Rinse the leg bag in warm soap and water and place in bathroom to dry.

15. Wash your hands.

### CHARTING   *for External Catheter*

☐  Condom catheter applied

☐  Size of catheter used

☐  Condition of genital area

☐  Type of protective coating applied to skin

☐  Whether catheter connected to leg bag or continuous drainage

☐  Amount, color, and odor of urine obtained

☐  Patient's tolerance of procedure

---

## CLINICAL PROBLEM SOLVING

### Potential Problems

Incontinency continues even with use of condom catheter.

Condom falls off.

### Suggested Solutions

☐  Improvise ways in which catheter can be placed to provide wrinkle-free application.

☐  Assess need for a smaller size condom catheter (pediatric size may be indicated for adult patient).

☐  Use additional adhesive, such as tincture of benzoin evenly spread around penile shaft.

Penis becomes reddened and excoriated.

- □ Remove condom catheter as much as possible to allow air to reach penile shaft.
- □ Notify physician for topical medication order.
- □ Diaper the patient, and change frequently. Keep condom off penis until area is healed.
- □ Wash perineal area frequently.

## UNIT FIVE  SUPRAPUBIC CATHETER CARE

### NURSING PROCESS DATA

#### ASSESSMENT  *Data Base*

Observe for urine flow through catheter.

Observe for excessive bleeding through catheter or at insertion site.

Check that suture site is clean, dry and intact.

Check that straight drainage is maintained.

Assess that fluid intake is at least 2000cc daily.

Assess patient for pain, bladder distention, or spasms.

Assess patient's ability to assist with clamping procedure.

Assess ability to tolerate catheter being clamped.

#### PLANNING  *Objectives*

To prevent urinary tract infection when a suprapubic catheter is inserted.

To maintain a patent suprapubic catheter.

To monitor the suprapubic clamping procedure.

To prevent infection at catheter insertion site.

To provide discharge teaching if catheter is to remain in place when patient is discharged.

#### IMPLEMENTATION  *Procedure*

Providing Suprapubic Catheter Care

#### EVALUATION  *Expected Outcomes*

Catheter remains patent; bladder drains completely.

Patient voids spontaneously after routine clamping.

Patient remains free of urinary tract infections.

Insertion site is clean and dry.

## PROVIDING SUPRAPUBIC CATHETER CARE

### Equipment

Closed drainage system, including Foley catheter tubing and bag

Catheter clamp

Dry sterile dressing and tape if ordered

### Preparation

1. Check physician's orders and Patient Care Plan.
2. Explain purpose of catheter.
3. Describe procedure for monitoring and clamping suprapubic catheter.
4. Wash your hands.
5. Provide privacy.

### Procedure

1. Observe catheter for patency.
   a. First 24 hours: check the catheter every hour to detect possible obstruction. Urine output should be in excess of 30 cc/hour.
   b. Second day: check the catheter every eight hours.
   c. Third day: check the catheter when the catheter is unclamped.
2. Maintain a closed drainage system. Do not open system to irrigate or obtain urine sample.
3. Observe for signs and symptoms of urinary tract infection (color, odor, presence of sediment).
4. Keep the dressing dry around site of insertion. Apply a new dressing every morning and as necessary at other times.
5. Monitor clamping protocol after the third postoperative day. Use this protocol or clamp according to physician's orders.
   a. Explain the clamping procedure and ask patient to help you monitor the clamping.
   b. Instruct patient to notify you if he feels fullness in the bladder during clamping.
   c. Clamp the catheter.
   d. Empty the drainage bag. Record urine output on I & O bedside record.
   e. Leave the catheter clamped for three to four hours depending on patient's level of comfort and physician's orders.
   f. At 3–4 hour intervals, or when patient feels fullness in bladder, ask patient to void nor-

mally. Measure the urine and record output on I & O bedside record.
   g. Immediately after patient voids, unclamp catheter and leave unclamped for five minutes, collecting the residual urine.
   h. Measure the residual urine following unclamping of the catheter.
   i. Reclamp catheter.
   j. Send a urine specimen to laboratory after the first clamping. **Rationale:** To check for presence of microorganisms.

6. Continue clamping protocol every three to four hours. (For the first few days of the clamping procedure the catheter may be open to drainage from bedtime until six in the morning.)
7. When the patient is voiding normally, clamp the catheter throughout the night in preparation for its removal.
8. When the patient's residual urine output is less than 100 cc on two successive checks, notify the physician for removal of the catheter.
9. Apply a bandaid or small two- by two-inch dressing over the insertion site (if ordered by physician.)
10. Dispose of the catheter in the utility room.
11. If the patient is discharged from the hospital with the catheter, provide the following teaching for home care:
    a. Instruct the patient to drink one glass of fluid every hour while awake.
    b. Instruct patient to follow clamping procedure when awake or as instructed by physician.
    c. Instruct the patient to leave the catheter open to the drainage system at night. (Drainage

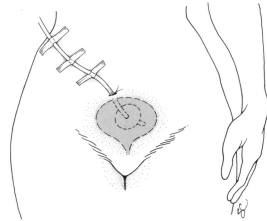

Tape catheter and connect to a closed system.

system may be urinary tubing and bag or leg bag.)

d. Tell patient to notify physician if dysuria occurs when voiding or if urine becomes cloudy, odorous, or full of sediment.

## CHARTING *for Catheter Care*

☐ Time catheter clamped

☐ Length of time clamped

☐ Patient's ability to void spontaneously

☐ Patient's feelings of fullness

☐ Time specimen sent to laboratory

☐ Color, amount, and odor of urine obtained

☐ Color, amount, and odor of residual urine

---

## CLINICAL PROBLEM SOLVING

### Potential Problems

Suprapubic catheter was not sutured in place and becomes dislodged.

Patient develops urinary tract infection.

Patient unable to void spontaneously through urethra.

### Suggested Solutions

☐ Place sterile dressing over puncture site. Do not attempt to replace the catheter.
☐ Notify physician immediately.
☐ Have new suprapubic catheter ready for insertion by physician.

☐ Observe patient for signs and symptoms of urinary tract infection: temperature; cloudy, foul-smelling urine with sediment present; bladder spasms.
☐ Inform physician of possible urinary tract infection and obtain order for urinary antibiotic.
☐ Force fluids to at least 2000 cc per day unless contraindicated by diagnosis. Give cranberry juice or fluids that acidify urine.
☐ Clarify physician's order for protocol regarding clamping catheter or keeping the catheter open to straight drainage while evidence of infection is present.

☐ Notify physician for orders.

---

# UNIT SIX  BLADDER IRRIGATION AND INSTILLATION

## NURSING PROCESS DATA

### ASSESSMENT  *Data Base*

Determine presence of active bleeding, i.e., dense, dark red drainage.

Note rate of urine flow from bladder.

Assess for distended bladder.

Assess for bladder discomfort.

**PLANNING** *Objectives*

To remove blood clots from patient's bladder.

To instill medications into patient's bladder.

To ensure patency of drainage system.

To relieve bladder spasms.

**IMPLEMENTATION** *Procedures*

Irrigating by Opening a Closed System

Irrigating a Closed System

Instilling Medications

Maintaining Continuous Irrigation

**EVALUATION** *Expected Outcomes*

Blood clots are removed from patient's bladder.

Medications are instilled easily into patient's bladder.

Continuous flow of antibacterial solution is instilled into patient's bladder to prevent or treat a urinary tract infection.

Continuous flow of solution is maintained to evacuate clots and prevent catheter obstruction.

Catheter remains patent and unobstructed by sediment.

## IRRIGATING BY OPENING A CLOSED SYSTEM

### Equipment

Sterile irrigation set (new set for each irrigation)

Sterile gloves if required

Sterile normal saline irrigant (or solution as ordered)

### Procedure

1. Check physician's order and Patient Care Plan.
2. Gather equipment.
3. Check patient's identaband.
4. Explain procedure and rationale to patient.
5. Wash your hands.
6. Provide privacy and place the patient in a comfortable position. The dorsal-recumbent position is the most convenient if patient can tolerate this position. Raise bed and lower side rails if needed.
7. Palpate patient's bladder to check for distention.
8. Open sterile container on bed or on the over-bed table. Maintain sterility of the inside of the container.
9. Place an absorbent pad under the end of the catheter to form a working field.
10. Pour irrigant into solution container.
11. Place syringe in container. Do not contaminate the syringe tip.
12. Place catch basin on pad to form the working field. (Always keep syringe tip and irrigant uncontaminated.)
13. Put on gloves if hospital protocol requires.
14. Disconnect catheter from drainage tube. Place the sterile protective cap over the end of the drainage tube.
15. Place catheter over the edge of the catch basin. Do not allow end of catheter to touch covers, underpad, exposed skin surfaces, or drainage tube.
16. Instill 30 to 50 cc of irrigant into the patient's bladder with a gentle but firm pressure.

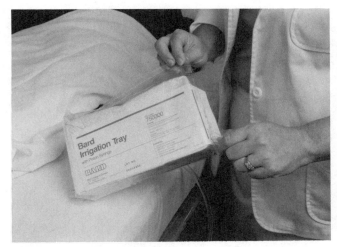

Obtain a new sterile irrigation kit for every bladder irrigation.

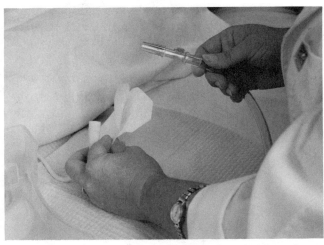

Place a sterile protective cap over the end of the drainage tube.

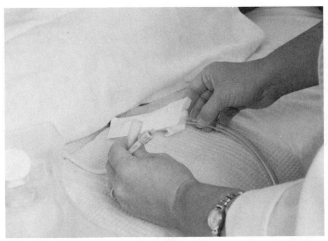

Prevent contamination by keeping the catheter off the bed linens.

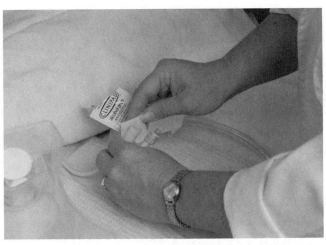

Wipe end of catheter with alcohol and connect to the drainage tube.

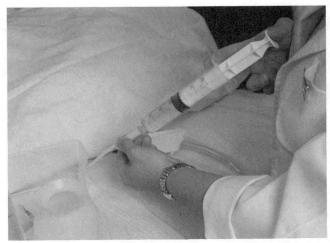

Instill 30 to 50 cc irrigant with firm pressure into patient's bladder.

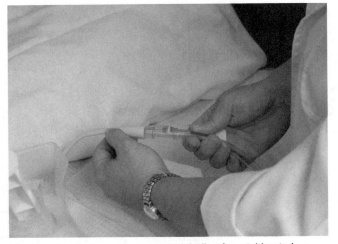

Reconnect catheter and ensure straight line from tubing to bag.

a. Remove syringe and allow solution to drain.

b. Continue to irrigate patient's bladder with 30 to 50 cc of irrigant until fluid returns are clear or clots removed.

17. Remove the protective top from the drainage tube and wipe it with an alcohol sponge.

18. Wipe the end of the catheter with an alcohol sponge and connect the catheter to the drainage tube.

19. Ensure straight line from tubing to drainage bag. Curl excess tubing loosely on the bed and secure the tubing to the linen.

20. Tape catheter to the inner thigh for a female and to the abdomen for a male.

21. Lower bed and raise side rails.

22. Remove and discard equipment.

23. Make sure the patient is clean and comfortable. Place the call light within easy reach.

24. Wash your hands.

25. Subtract any irrigating solution still remaining in the urinary drainage system from the patient's intake and output record.

## IRRIGATING A CLOSED SYSTEM

### Equipment

Irrigation set

Leur-Lok syringe and 25-gauge needle

Alcohol or Betadine swab

Irrigating solution

Catheter clamp

### Procedure

1. Check physician's order and Patient Care Plan.

2. Gather equipment.

3. Check patient's identaband. Explain procedure and rationale to patient.

4. Wash hands.

5. Provide privacy and place patient in dorsal-recumbent position, if tolerated.

6. Raise bed and lower side rail on working side of bed.

7. Open sterile container. Maintain sterility on the inside of the container.

8. Place absorbent pad under the end of the catheter to form a working field.

9. Pour irrigant into solution container.

10. Fill large Luer-Lok syringe with the amount of irrigating solution ordered.

11. Place the needle onto the syringe.

12. Clamp tubing just distal to injection port.

13. Swab the injection port of catheter with alcohol or Betadine solution.

14. Insert the needle into the injection port.

15. Inject solution slowly to prevent back pressure in urinary drainage system.

16. Remove syringe and needle from the injection port.

17. Unclamp drainage tube.

18. Lower bed and raise side rail.

19. Remove equipment from room.

20. Wash your hands.

21. Subtract the irrigating solution from the patient's intake and output record.

## INSTILLING MEDICATIONS

### Equipment

Syringe with Luer-Lok and 25-gauge needle

Alcohol or Betadine solution and swabs

Appropriate medication for irrigation or instillation

Clamp for catheter

### Procedure

1. Check physician's order and Patient Care Plan.

2. Explain procedure to patient.

3. Provide privacy.

4. Wash your hands.

5. Assemble equipment and draw up ordered medication in syringe.

6. Scrub port site on Foley catheter tubing with alcohol or Betadine solution.

7. Clamp drainage tubing so that medication will be retained in the patient's bladder.

8. Insert the needle at an angle into the injection port.

9. Instill medication slowly.

10. Withdraw the needle and cleanse the port site with an alcohol or Betadine swab.

11. Keep tubing clamped for 15 to 20 minutes.

12. Wash your hands.

13. Observe for bladder distention or spasms while catheter is clamped.

14. Unclamp tube after 15 to 20 minutes.

## MAINTAINING CONTINUOUS IRRIGATION

### Equipment

Irrigating solution and container

Tubing

Alcohol or Betadine swab

### Procedure

1. Check physician's orders and Patient Care Plan.

2. Obtain irrigating solution (from pharmacy or central supply).

3. Identify patient by checking identaband.

4. Explain procedure to patient and provide privacy.

5. Wash your hands.

6. Connect tubing to irrigating solution container, using aseptic technique.

7. Place irrigating solution container on IV pole and prime tubing by running solution through tubing and clearing out all air. **Rationale:** To prevent air from entering bladder and causing discomfort.

8. Cleanse the third lumen of the three-way indwelling catheter with an alcohol or Betadine swab.

9. Connect tubing to third lumen using aseptic technique.

10. Adjust drip rate of the solution by adjusting the clamp on the tubing to deliver prescribed hourly rate of irrigant.

    a. With clear drainage, drip rate should be approximately 40 to 60 drops per minute.

    b. With drainage that is bright red or contains blood clots, the drip rate should be increased to clear the drainage and flush out clots.

    c. Change irrigation solution bottle using aseptic technique.

    d. Tubing should be changed at a minimum of every 24 hours.

11. Monitor urine output at least every hour to observe patency of system.

12. Wash your hands.

### CHARTING   *for Irrigation and Instillation*

☐ Type and amount of medications administered

☐ Type and amount of solution administered for irrigation

☐ Rate of administration of irrigating solution

☐ Description of urinary output, including color and presence of clots

☐ Any signs of discomfort or cramping

☐ Amount of actual urine output (total urine output minus amount of irrigant instilled)

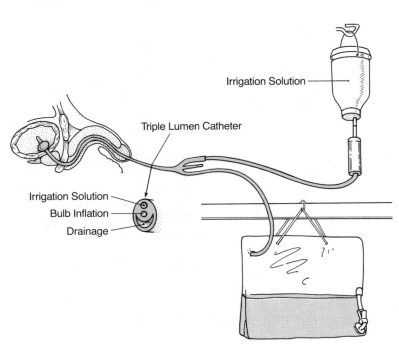

Irrigation Solution

Triple Lumen Catheter

Irrigation Solution
Bulb Inflation
Drainage

Maintain continuous bladder irrigation by using a triple lumen catheter for procedure.

# CLINICAL PROBLEM SOLVING

| **Potential Problems** | **Suggested Solutions** |
|---|---|
| Irrigation flow is not infusing at prescribed rate. | ☐ May need to raise or lower IV standard with attached irrigation bag to assist in regulating flow using gravity. <br> ☐ Move the flow adjuster clamp to a new site on the tubing if flow is slower than ordered. Tubing may be collapsed due to constant pressure from clamp. <br> ☐ If infusion rate slows, may indicate clots are blocking flow. Irrigate catheter following physician's orders. |
| Irrigation solution is not returned because of an obstruction in the system. | ☐ Follow these steps to obtain irrigation solution: <br>   a. Aspirate the solution from the catheter, using moderate "pull back" pressure. <br>   b. If the irrigant does not return, palpate the patient's bladder and instill 30 to 50 cc of irrigating solution to agitate and clear any clots. <br>   c. If irrigant does not return, reconnect urinary system and observe for 30 minutes. Bladder spasms can block the flow of urine through the system. <br>   d. If irrigant does not return, cleanse patient's urinary meatus and the catheter tubing with Betadine solution. Gently insert the Foley catheter further into the patient's bladder. If the lumen opening of the catheter is against the wall of the bladder, it will obstruct the flow of urine. <br>   e. If irrigant still does not return after performing the above procedures, notify physician for further orders. |
| Patient's pain and anxiety causes "clamping down" and creates an obstruction in the outflow opening to the catheter thus irrigation solution is not returned. | ☐ Help patient practice relaxation techniques. <br> ☐ Place a warm towel over patient's abdomen to ease bladder spasms. <br> ☐ Reposition patient to reduce pressure on the catheter. <br> ☐ If patient is unable to expel the irrigant, administer medications to relieve patient's pain and/or bladder spasms. |
| Patient experiences excessive bladder spasms. | ☐ Notify physician of bladder spasms in order to obtain an order to place a heating pad on the patient's abdomen. <br> ☐ Follow physician's order and administer urinary antispasmodic. |
| Bright red drainage continues even when solution flow rate is increased. | ☐ Notify physician. <br> ☐ Continue to infuse solution at a rapid rate to |

cleanse patient's bladder until you obtain physician's orders.

☐ Assess patient for signs of anemia and/or significant blood loss. Take vital signs, observe capillary filling pressure, and observe mucous membranes for signs of anemia.

# UNIT SEVEN  SPECIMENS FROM CLOSED SYSTEMS

## NURSING PROCESS DATA

### ASSESSMENT  *Data Base*

Assess the type of specimen needed: sterile specimens for culture and sensitivity tests; clean specimens for urinalysis.

Check to see if the closed urinary system has a port for obtaining a specimen or catheter is made of self-sealing material (not silastic or silicone).

Identify amount of urine needed for specimen.

### PLANNING  *Objectives*

To prevent urinary infection by obtaining a urine specimen without interrupting a closed urinary drainage system.

To determine the specific microorganism causing a urinary tract infection.

To obtain a urine specimen for use in a diagnostic urinary workup.

### IMPLEMENTATION  *Procedure*

Collecting Specimen from a Closed System

### EVALUATION  *Expected Outcomes*

Noncontaminated urine specimen is obtained from the closed urinary drainage system.

Catheter does not develop a leak from improper puncture for urine specimen.

## COLLECTING SPECIMEN FROM A CLOSED SYSTEM

### Equipment

Syringe with 25-gauge needle

Sterile specimen container

Antimicrobial swab

### Procedure

1. Gather equipment.

2. Wash your hands.

3. Identify patient by checking identaband.

4. Explain the procedure and rationale to the patient.

5. Wipe the aspiration port of the drainage tubing with the antimicrobial swab.

6. Insert the needle into the aspiration port. Allow urine to accumulate in the tubing. (2 cc of urine is sufficient for a specimen.)

7. Aspirate the urine sample by gently pulling back

on the syringe plunger, and then remove the needle.

8. Wipe the aspiration port with the antimicrobial swab.

9. Empty the syringe into the sterile urine container. (Sometimes the urine is sent to the laboratory in the syringe.)

10. Wash your hands.

11. Label the container and take it to the laboratory within 15 minutes. If this is not possible, refrigerate specimen.

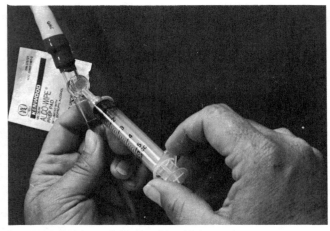

Insert needle into aspiration port to obtain specimen.

### CHARTING for Collecting Specimen

☐ Type of specimen obtained

☐ Mode of obtaining specimen from port

☐ Color, consistency, and odor of urine

☐ Time of urine collection

☐ Time specimen sent to laboratory

## CLINICAL PROBLEM SOLVING

| Potential Problems | Suggested Solutions |
|---|---|
| Signs and symptoms of urinary tract infection occur. | ☐ Notify the physician of signs and symptoms the patient experiences.<br>☐ Make sure there are no kinks in urinary system tubing or that the system is not clamped off. This ensures that the urine will drain into the catheter bag and not stagnate in bladder.<br>☐ Give ordered antibiotics on correct time schedule.<br>☐ Do not interrupt the closed urinary drainage system. |
| Bacteremia develops secondary to urinary tract infection. | ☐ Administer antibiotics as ordered.<br>☐ Encourage patient to force fluids to flush out bladder.<br>☐ Use cranberry juice or other acid-producing (non-citric) juices.<br>☐ Obtain frequent vital signs and assessment data.<br>☐ Observe color and clarity of urine for further infectious problems. |

## UNIT EIGHT   URINARY DIVERSION

### NURSING PROCESS DATA

#### ASSESSMENT   Data Base

Assess location of stoma on patient's abdomen.

Check abdomen for folds, contour, incision line.

Observe stoma color (same color as mucous membrane lining the mouth).

Assess skin for erythema and excoriation.

Ascultate bowel sounds.

Assess most appropriate pouching system for patient. (System depends on patient's age, manual dexterity, and size of stoma.)

Assess patient's ability to manage self-care.

### PLANNING    *Objectives*

To provide a pouching system that prevents skin irritation.

To instruct the patient in self-care.

To monitor stoma for viability.

To obtain a sterile urine specimen.

### IMPLEMENTATION    *Procedures*

Obtaining Specimen from an Ileal Conduit

Applying a Urinary Diversion Pouch

### EVALUATION    *Expected Outcomes*

Patient demonstrates self-care skills.

Pouching system fits tightly and skin remains free of irritation.

Sterile urine specimen obtained.

Stoma remains viable.

## OBTAINING SPECIMEN FROM AN ILEAL CONDUIT

### Equipment

Sterile drape

Sterile gloves

Sterile lubricant

#14 Robinson or Foley catheter

Prep solution

Sterile saline or water

Underpad

Sterile specimen container with label

New urinary pouch

Supplies to apply new pouch

Plastic bag for used supplies

### Preparation

1. Check physician's orders and Patient Care Plan.
2. Gather equipment.
3. Wash your hands.
4. Explain procedure to patient.
5. Provide privacy.
6. Place bath blanket over chest and position top covers over lower abdomen.

### Procedure

1. Place sterile drape over stoma.
2. Put on gloves.
3. Apply lubricant to catheter. Remove pouch.
4. Prep stoma with solution and then rinse.
5. Remove top from specimen container and place end of catheter into container.

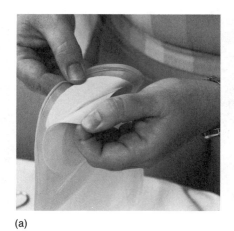

(a)

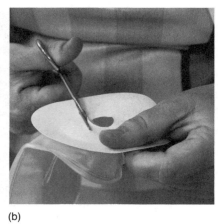

(b)

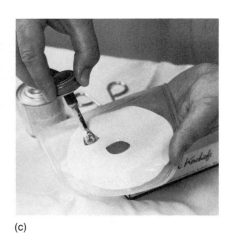

(c)

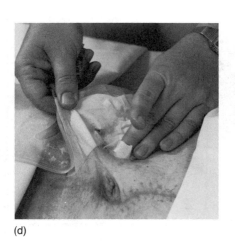

(d)

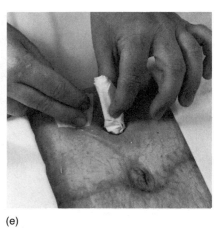

(e)

Specific steps of stoma care for patient with a urinary diversion. Steps include preparing a new urinary pouch, removing the old urinary pouch, wicking the stoma, preparing the skin, and applying new pouch.

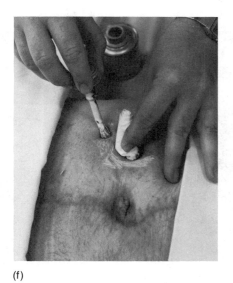

(f)

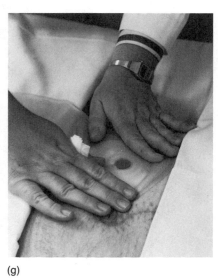

(g)

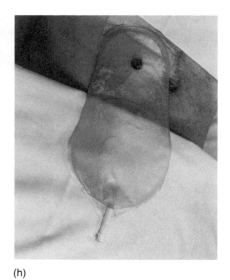

(h)

6. Insert tip of catheter into stoma 2 to 2½ inches.

7. When flow of urine completed (usually not more than 20 to 40 cc), clamp catheter with fingers and remove.

8. Return lid to specimen container, apply label, and send to lab.

9. Remove completely any residual prep solution and lubricant.

10. Continue with pouching procedure.

## APPLYING A URINARY DIVERSION POUCH

### Equipment

Clean pouch with spigot at bottom to empty urine

Night drainage bag

Items to clean stoma, e.g., soft cloth or gauze sponges.

Plastic bag for disposal of used equipment

Tissue for drying skin

Tissue or tampon for wicking stoma

Underpad to protect bedding from leakage

Scissors with sharp point

Protective barriers such as skin prep, skin gel, or protective barrier film (If excoriation or insensitivity is present, a skin barrier such as Stomahesive, Reliaseal, or Holliseal is needed.)

Skin bond cement

Stoma measuring guide

Micropore or dermicel tape

### Preparation

Same as Using a Catheter to Obtain a Specimen from an Ileal Conduit

### Procedure

1. Place underpad under patient.

2. Prepare new urinary pouch for application at conclusion.

3. Remove old pouch and discard in plastic bag.

4. Wash skin with warm water. If large residual of cement on skin, remove with solvent.

5. Measure stoma site with measuring guide.

6. Trace size of stoma on adhesive backing on pouch.

7. Cut panel ⅛ to ¼ inch larger than stoma.

8. Remove paper from adhesive on pouch. Apply thin coat of skin bond cement to adhesive area. Set aside.

9. Wicking stoma with tissue or tampon, apply protective barrier to healthy skin. If skin is excoriated, apply skin barrier. **Rationale:** Protective barriers on excoriated skin contain alcohol and will cause burning and pain.

10. Let dry thoroughly.

11. Wick stoma to keep urine off skin; then apply thin coat of skin bond cement to the skin.

12. Let dry thoroughly.

13. Center and apply pouch to dry skin.

14. Smooth tape to skin.

15. "Picture-frame" sides of pouch with 1 inch tape.

16. Attach to gravity drainage bag.

17. Wash your hands.

18. Give patient written set of instructions.

### CHARTING  *for Urinary Diversion Care*

☐ Color and amount of urine obtained from catheterization

☐ Amount of residual urine

☐ Catheter size used for catheterization

☐ Peristomal skin condition

☐ Patient's acceptance of stoma

☐ Type and method of drainage pouch applied

## CLINICAL PROBLEM SOLVING

**Potential Problems**

Urinary tract infection is suspected.

**Suggested Solutions**

☐ Ensure that catheterized specimen is not contaminated before sending to lab.

Excess of 50cc urine present in ileal conduit when catheterized.

Pouch does not keep patient dry.

Patient unable to manage own urinary diversion.

Unable to insert catheter into conduit.

No urine obtained from conduit.

Odor in pouch.

☐ Force fluid to eight glasses per day. Encourage use of cranberry juice to acidify urine.

☐ Notify physician as stasis of urine could be caused by urine remaining in conduit.

☐ Check area for crease or dip in skin which allows urine to pool and leak out.
☐ Fill in area with Karaya paste to prevent pooling.
☐ Belt may be applied to minimize leak if it appears on one side only.
☐ If leak due to dissolving of skin barrier, change product.

☐ Simplify pouch procedure if possible. Provide detailed instruction in a more simplified manner if possible.
☐ Include family in teaching to enable them to support and assist the patient.
☐ May need referral to home health care facility for follow-up care.

☐ Insert catheter into stoma but do not force it. Wait for a few seconds to see if abdominal muscles relax enough to allow catheter to slide in. If not, notify physician.

☐ Rotate catheter or position patient on side to allow urine to flow into catheter. As little as 1–3cc is needed for culture and sensitivity.

☐ Odor usually due to alkaline urine in pouch turning to ammonia. Keep urine acidic by taking vitamin C, 500 mg b.i.d. to t.i.d., and drinking cranberry juice. Other citrus juices should be avoided, as they form an alkaline ash.
☐ Wash urinary equipment clean with mild soap and water and rinse in vinegar weekly.
☐ Inform patient that certain foods and drugs, such as asparagus and vitamin B complex, give an odor to the urine. The pouch should be emptied frequently if these substances are ingested.
☐ Cloudy and strong odor to urine may be due to urinary tract infection. Advise physician and collect sterile urine specimen.

# UNIT NINE   PERITONEAL DIALYSIS

## NURSING PROCESS DATA

### ASSESSMENT   *Data Base*

Obtain baseline measurements of vital signs (especially blood pressure).

Assess for edema; measure abdominal girth.

Check patient's weight.

Review renal function tests.

Examine dietary regimen: Prior to dialysis, a low protein diet is prescribed to reduce end products of protein metabolism. During dialysis, protein restriction may not be necessary. Provide diet that is high calorie, with limited sodium and potassium.

Evaluate patient's abdomen for signs of infection or distention. Report any abnormalities to the physician.

Assess for signs of shock.

Auscultate breath sounds for rales and possible atelectasis.

Assess results of stool analysis for occult blood.

Assess condition of skin.

Review orders for solution to be used, number of cycles, and inflow, diffusion, and outflow times.

Verify signed consent form.

## PLANNING  *Objectives*

To remove end products of metabolism when the kidneys are nonfunctional.

To provide an effective method of reducing symptoms of renal failure.

To remove excess fluid and reestablish fluid balance.

To remove toxic substances that kidneys are unable to process from patients who have taken an overdose of drugs.

To control blood pressure, creatinine and BUN levels.

To manage peritoneal dialysis procedure and provide external shunt care.

## INTERVENTION  *Procedures*

Assisting with Catheter Insertion

Managing Peritoneal Dialysis

Maintaining Peritoneal Dialysis

Providing Catheter Site Care

## EVALUATION  *Expected Outcomes*

Specific symptoms decrease, and manifestations of renal failure diminish.

Excessive fluid is reduced through use of peritoneal dialysis, and fluid balance is regulated.

Creatinine and BUN levels are reduced.

Asepsis is maintained throughout the procedure.

Complications are detected early and treatment initiated promptly.

Catheter site remains free of infection.

## ASSISTING WITH CATHETER INSERTION

### Equipment

Sterile gowns, caps, masks, and gloves

Razor and blade

Povidone-iodine solution

Catheter insertion tray, with sterile drapes, catheter, trocar, connector, syringes, needles, sterile dressings, and sutures

Local anesthetic, usually 1 percent Xylocaine without epinephrine

Antimicrobial ointment

Tape

Dialysis inflow tubing

### Preparation

1. Explain procedure to patient, reinforcing the physician's explanation and correcting any misconceptions.
2. Have patient empty bladder to lessen the risk of bladder perforation.
3. Prime dialysate delivery system.
   a. Check bottle or bag labels against orders.
   b. Check bottle or bag for signs of contamination.
   c. Connect dialysate bottle or bag to administration set.
   d. Clear air from inflow tubing and clamp line. If using an automated delivery system, set controls according to the manufacturer's directions.

### Procedure

1. Wash your hands.
2. Provide privacy.
3. Remove top linens and place bath blanket over patient's lower extremeties.
4. Place patient in supine position.
5. Shave abdomen between umbilicus and symphysis pubis.
6. Perform surgical scrub of shaved area.
7. Don sterile attire.
8. Hold bottle of local anesthetic so that physician can withdraw desired amount.

   *Physician's Actions*
   a. Physician dons sterile gown and gloves.

   b. Abdomen is draped with sterile towels.
   c. Local anesthetic is withdrawn and administered.
   d. Insertion area is infiltrated and catheter inserted.
   e. Trocar is removed.
   f. Catheter is sutured in place.

9. Assess patient's level of comfort during procedure and relieve patient's anxiety as necessary.
10. After physician has removed the trocar, connect the inflow tubing to the catheter.
11. Apply a sterile dressing around the catheter site following suturing of catheter.

## MANAGING PERITONEAL DIALYSIS

### Equipment

Dialysis machine (if available)

Dialysis administration set

Sterile, prewarmed dialysis solution

Dialysis log

### Procedure

1. Inject admixtures if ordered (e.g., potassium, heparin).
2. Connect inflow tubing to dialysate bottle or bag.
3. Infuse dialysate solution by following protocol for inflow phase.
   a. Open all clamps between the bottle of dialysate and the catheter.
   b. Check that all clamps between the catheter and the drainage bottle are closed.
   c. Make sure that the tubing is not kinked.
   d. Note the time required to infuse the amount of solution ordered. Usually, it takes 5 to 10 minutes to infuse 1500 to 2000 ml.
   e. Observe the patient's breathing pattern and level of comfort.
   f. Inspect the catheter insertion site for leakage or bleeding.
4. Shut off the inflow line. Allow dialysate to dwell in abdomen 20 minutes (diffusion or dwell period).
5. Complete dialysis cycle by following protocol for outflow phase:
   a. Place the patient in semi-Fowler's position.
   b. Place bed in high position.
   c. Open clamps between catheter and outflow bottle.

d. Provide an airway in bottle by inserting needle into air vent. **Rationale:** This assists in drainage of fluid into bottle.

e. Allow dialysate to drain by gravity for 30 to 35 minutes.

f. Observe appearance of outflow fluid.

6. Calculate fluid balance at end of cycle:
   a. Subtract the amount drained from the amount infused.
   b. Describe the results as positive or negative in relation to the peritoneal cavity.
   c. If the number is positive, fluid was retained in the cavity. If the number is negative, more fluid was drained out than instilled.

7. Throughout the cycle, monitor patient status by assessing:
   a. Vital signs.
   b. Abdominal distention.
   c. Mental status.
   d. Blood pressure and pulse every 15 minutes during the first cycle and every hour thereafter.
   e. Temperature every four hours.
   f. Color of dialysate solution.
   g. Area surrounding catheter site.

8. Culture the outflow fluid from the first cycle and one cycle a day thereafter.

9. Weigh patient daily with abdomen empty.

## MAINTAINING PERITONEAL DIALYSIS

### Procedure

1. Monitor hydration status.
   a. Check intake and output daily.
   b. Record daily weight.
   c. Check for edema.
   d. Auscultate lungs for rales.

2. Evaluate electrolyte balance.
   a. Check for leg cramping and diarrhea (signs of hyperkalemia).
   b. Monitor ECG for tall, peaked T-waves and widening QRS segment (evidence of hyperkalemia).
   c. Check potassium levels frequently.

3. Evaluate lung status at least every shift.
   a. Perform deep breathing and coughing to prevent pulmonary complications.
   b. Check for signs of pulmonary edema (dyspnea, restlessness, rales).

4. Examine site for possible infection (high temperature, leukocytosis, lethargy).

5. Monitor for any seizure activity: have padded side rails and tongue blade at bedside.

6. Check Chvostek's and Trousseau's signs frequently for indications of low calcium level.

7. Monitor diet: low potassium and sodium, high calorie, high bulk, and adjusted protein to complete amino acids (necessary to maintain positive nitrogen balance and replace protein lost through dialysis).

8. Maintain good skin care to prevent skin breakdown and pruritus.

9. Evaluate for signs of bleeding at catheter site, in stools, and in urine; check hemoglobin and hematocrit frequently.

10. Monitor any medications. If iron is given as a supplement, have patient take iron with meals.

## PROVIDING CATHETER SITE CARE

### Equipment

4″ × 4″ gauze pads

ABD pad

Tape

Povidone-iodine swab or solution

Applicator sticks

Hydrogen peroxide

Sterile saline

Mask

Sterile gloves (two pair)

Forceps (optional)

### Procedure

1. Explain procedure to patient.

2. Wash hands.

3. Provide privacy.

4. Put on mask and gloves.

5. Remove old dressing with forceps or sterile gloves.

6. Inspect site for infection or bleeding.

7. Use hydrogen peroxide to remove any dried blood or drainage.

8. Rinse area with normal saline.

9. Dry area thoroughly.

10. Change gloves.
11. Cleanse area surrounding catheter with povidone-iodine swab or applicator sticks.
12. Apply sterile pads around catheter at exit site and on top of catheter.
13. Remove gloves.
14. Tape dressing nonocclusively.

## CHARTING  *for Peritoneal Dialysis*

☐ Predialysis weight and baseline assessment
☐ Time of catheter insertion
☐ Composition of dialysis solution
☐ Time of onset and termination of each cycle
☐ Number of cycles
☐ Amount of solution infused for each cycle
☐ Amount of fluid recovered for each cycle
☐ Cumulative fluid balance
☐ Appearance of outflow
☐ Postdialysis weight and clinical status
☐ Signs or symptoms of complications
☐ Nursing interventions to prevent or treat complications

---

# CLINICAL PROBLEM SOLVING

**Potential Problems**

**Suggested Solutions**

Pain occurs during procedure.

☐ Evaluate characteristics to differentiate dialysis-related pain from other types (for example, myocardial infarction).
☐ If on inflow, reassure patient that pain sometimes occurs.
☐ Check that dialysate is at body temperature.
☐ Promote effective fluid drainage.
☐ Provide diversionary activities.
☐ If persistent, consult with physician about decreasing infusion volume or instilling a local anesthetic through the catheter.
☐ If accompanied by signs of peritonitis (abdominal rigidity, rebound tenderness, cloudy outflow fluid or fever), alert physician immediately.

Dialysate return is not clear.

☐ If dialysate is cloudy, culture solution immediately and send to laboratory for culture and sensitivity.
☐ Monitor patient for signs of abdominal wall rigidity, abdominal palpation tenderness, cloudy dialysate outflow, and increased temperature.
☐ Notify physician.
☐ If dialysate contains blood, this is usual following catheter insertion. If condition persists, reassess catheter insertion.
☐ Observe for signs of bleeding: petechiae, ecchymosis, or signs of blood in stool and urine.
☐ Monitor hemoglobin and hematocrit to determine extent of bleeding.

The amount of fluid return is less than desired.

☐ Increase dialysate glucose concentration according to physician's orders. The higher glucose level will "pull" more fluid across the semipermeable membrane (peritoneal cavity).

Creatinine and BUN levels are not reduced.

☐ Make sure dialysate is body temperature when infusing. Cold fluid can promote vasoconstriction and increase fluid loss.

☐ Make sure each dialysis cycle is only one hour long. To increase diffusion of BUN and creatinine across the peritoneal membrane, make sure the dialysate is allowed to stay in the abdomen no more than 20 minutes. Longer time periods cause equilibration of the BUN and creatinine on either side of the membrane so that BUN and creatinine are not reduced as necessary.

☐ Warm the dialysate to body temperature to increase urea clearance.

☐ Increase glucose, as ordered, in dialysate solution to increase urea clearance.

During catheter insertion, patient experiences sudden pressure in bladder, rectum, or epigastrium.

☐ Alert physician immediately, as these signs indicate malposition of catheter and require repositioning.

Inflow is slower than normal.

☐ Check inflow tubing for kinks.
☐ Lower bed position.

Outflow is slow or absent.

☐ Check that outflow clamps are open.
☐ Check for kinks in outflow tubing.
☐ Check for and eliminate any air in drainage tubing.
☐ Turn patient from side to side.
☐ Raise the head of the bed to a higher position.
☐ Gently massage the abdomen.
☐ Consult physician about possible blockage of catheter. He may probe catheter to dislodge fibrin plugs or reposition it to release a subcutaneous kink.

There is negative fluid balance at end of cycle.

☐ Repeat outflow phase.
☐ If negative balance is within limits specified by physician (usually 250 ml maximum), continue with next cycle.

Patient experiences dyspnea.

☐ Elevate head of bed.
☐ Institute deep breathing and coughing exercises to prevent atelectasis.
☐ If acute respiratory distress, immediately drain the fluid and notify the physician.

Patient appears confused or lethargic; other signs of hyperglycemia are present during dialysis; signs of hypoglycemia are present after dialysis.

☐ Check that dialysate glucose concentration on bottle label matches ordered concentration of glucose.
☐ Be sure that dialysate is drained promptly at the end of the diffusion period.
☐ Place diabetics on routine urine glucose and acetone tests.
☐ Consult with physician about discontinuing dialysis slowly, giving the body time to readjust blood glucose and insulin levels.

Fecal-colored drainage or decreased drainage and diarrhea are present.

☐ Notify physician as these signs indicate possible bowel perforation. Surgical repair may be necessary.

Patient experiences bladder fullness and increased urinary output, and there is decreased drainage.

☐ Notify physician as these signs indicate possible bladder perforation; surgical repair may be necessary.

Patient on high glucose dialysate develops tachycardia or hypotension.

☐ Alert physician and implement changes in orders. A dialysate with lower glucose concentration will usually be ordered for future cycles to minimize recurrence of these signs.

There is leakage around catheter site.

☐ Change dressing as needed.
☐ Apply sterile plastic drape over skin.
☐ Weigh dressings to estimate fluid loss (1 gram = 1 ml).

## UNIT TEN  HEMODIALYSIS

### ASSESSMENT  *Data Base*

Review dialysis orders.

Evaluate type of vascular access.

a. Femoral vein catheter: used for immediate vascular access in life-threatening situations.

b. Arteriovenous cannula (shunt): an external connection between an artery and vein.

c. Arteriovenous fistula: an internal anastomosis between an artery and vein, present only in clients undergoing chronic hemodialysis.

Review chart and laboratory reports for factors that may alter management of dialysis.

Assess vital signs.

a. Observe for shock and hypovolemia.

b. Assess causes of hypotension: fluid loss; decreased blood volume, especially if hematocrit is low; or use of antihypertensive drugs between dialysis.

Check serum electrolytes frequently (pre-, mid-, and post-dialysis).

Weigh patient before and after dialysis to determine fluid loss.

Complete physical examination for signs of fluid and electrolyte imbalances, e.g., edema.

Establish date of last HAA and results (Australian antigen).

### PLANNING  *Objectives*

To remove byproducts of protein metabolism: urea, creatinine, and uric acid.

To remove excessive fluid by changing osmotic pressure (this is done by adding high concentrations of dextrose to dialysate).

To maintain or restore body buffer system.

To maintain or restore level of electrolytes in the body.

To maintain a patent access site for hemodialysis.

To instruct the patient in self care.

To maintain patent femoral catheter.

**INTERVENTION** *Procedures*

Initiating Hemodialysis

Managing Hemodialysis

Terminating Hemodialysis

Providing Cannula Site Care

Maintaining Femoral Catheter Patency

**EVALUATION** *Expected Outcomes*

Asepsis is maintained throughout the procedure.

Creatinine and BUN levels are reduced, and electrolyte balance remains in a satisfactory state.

Excessive fluid is reduced.

Toxic substances are removed, and patient's health status is improved.

Access site remains patent.

Patient is able to care for self following patient teaching.

Femoral catheters remain patent.

## INITIATING HEMODIALYSIS

### Equipment

Dialyzer (types are hollow fiber, parallel plate, and coil)

1000 ml bag of normal saline IV solution

Macrodrop administration set

Fistula needles 15/16 gauge or 1 or 1–¼ inch (for internal shunt)

Sterile masks and gloves

Sterile gauze pads and alcohol swabs

Hemostats, cannula ("bulldog") clamps

Cannula separator, cannula Teflon connectors, and infusion T connector (for external shunt)

Tape

Sterile bowl and air pump

Syringes and needles

Heparin clotting rack and glass tubes

Stop watch

Hemastix

Dialysis log

Actin

Gelfoam (optional)

### Preparation

1. Prepare dialysate bath composition as ordered.

2. Set up 1000-ml IV of normal saline, macrodrop tubing, and large gauge needle on pole near bedside.

3. Set up heparin infusion pump on arterial line if constant heparinization is ordered.

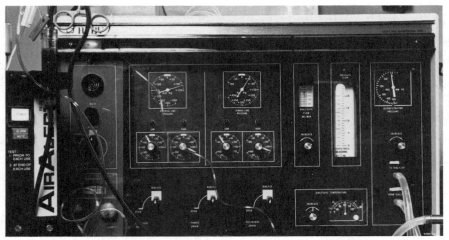
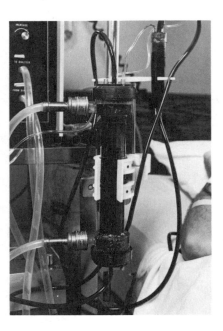

After priming the dialyzer with saline, the patient is connected to the machine. Dialysis is accomplished by the action of blood flowing down the hollow fiber dialyzer through small cellulose tubes utilizing a counter-current flow for removing the exogenous waste materials. The dialysate fluid is pumped into the bottom of the coil and moves upward against the blood flow.

4. Check location of nearest emergency power outlet in case routine power fails.

5. Prime the dialyzer and blood lines with saline.

6. Hang additional IV solution of saline. **Rationale:** The saline infusion must be available immediately in case of need for rapid reversal of hypotension or discontinuation of dialysis.

## Procedure

1. Place blood lines at the same level as the bed.

2. Mask and wash your hands.

3. Unwrap the cannula dressing and discard it.

4. Put on sterile gloves.

5. Place sterile gauze pads under cannula connection to create a sterile field.

6. Clean cannula connection with an alcohol swab.

7. Clamp arterial cannula with a cannula ("bulldog") clamp.

8. Clamp venous cannula with a bulldog clamp.

9. Use a cannula separator to disconnect the cannulae.

10. Draw blood for predialysis blood samples as ordered by the physician. (These usually consist of electrolytes, BUN, hematocrit, clotting time, and any others necessary for the specific patient, e.g., HAA for first acute dialysis treatment.)

11. After blood is drawn for lab work, heparin load should be given to patient according to baseline whole blood partial thromboplastin time, (WBPTT) and patient's weight.

12. Insert sterile connectors into the disconnected cannulae.

13. Prime the extracorporeal circuit with blood.
    a. Connect the dialyzer's arterial blood line to the arterial cannula.
    b. Place the end of the venous line into a sterile basin. (The blood entering the extracorporeal circuit will displace the saline in the dialyzer into the bowl.)
    c. Remove the venous blood line clamp.
    d. Remove the arterial blood line clamp.
    e. Remove the arterial cannula clamp. Do not remove the venous cannula clamp yet.
    f. As blood enters the arterial drip chamber on the arterial line, add the prescribed dose of heparin prime.
    g. Allow blood to circulate through the system until the saline in the venous drip bulb chamber is pink.
    h. Clamp the venous blood line.

14. After priming the extracorporeal circuit, complete the circuit.
    a. Wipe the venous cannula end with an alcohol swab.
    b. Attach the venous blood line to the venous cannula.

c. Remove the venous blood line clamp.

d. Remove the venous cannula clamp.

15. Note the time of dialysis initiation.

16. Tape all connections securely; tape the tubing to the pateint's limb.

17. Add air to each drip chamber so that blood is about 1.2 cm below the top of the chamber.

18. Connect the pressure monitor lines to each drip bulb.

19. Set the alarm pressures—high and low.

20. Connect the air leak detector to the venous drip chamber.

21. Establish the specified blood flow rate (usually 200 to 250 ml/minute).

22. Test the dialysate outflow with a Hemastix. (Testing the outflow provides a double-check against the blood leak detector.)

23. Perform and record machine checks.

24. Check the patient's blood pressure and pulse every two to five minutes while the dialyzer is filled and the blood flow rate is increased.

25. Increase the blood flow rate slowly to the specified rate. (The rate usually is 200 to 250 ml/minute.)

26. Maintain ordered clotting times of patient and dialyzer.

   a. Take clotting time about one hour before patient comes off the machine. If less than thirty minutes, do not give protamine (heparin antagonist).

   b. Follow protocol for heparin administration to keep clotting time at appropriate level for patient's condition.

27. Assess patient at least hourly for vital signs and potential complications.

28. Perform and record machine checks hourly.

29. Administer any ordered medications via the venous line.

---

**Protocol to maintain clotting times with heparin**

20 × dry weight* = 90—110 sec. = low dose

30 × dry weight = 120—135 sec. = midrange

35 × dry weight = 140—160 sec. = high range

   * Equals the amount of heparin administered to keep the clotting time at the appropriate level.

---

30. Maintain dialysate temperature near body temperature (99°F).

31. After establishing transmembrane pressure increase negative pressure if ordered to establish ultrafiltration. **Rationale:** This action is necessary to obtain required fluid loss.

## MANAGING HEMODIALYSIS

**Procedure**

1. Limit fluid intake (400 cc over previous day's output); provide accurate intake and output.

2. Maintain diet: low sodium (20 to 40 g), low protein, high carbohydrate, high fat, and foods low in potassium and sodium.

3. Check vital signs for hypovolemia; check temperature for infection.

4. Auscultate lungs for signs of pulmonary edema.

5. Provide shunt care.

6. Observe level of consciousness—indicative of electrolyte imbalance or thrombus.

7. Administer antihypertensive drugs between dialysis if ordered.

8. Administer diuretics if ordered.

9. Administer blood if ordered (cellular portion only is needed because of low hematocrit).

10. Weigh daily to assess fluid accumulation.

11. Prevent use of soap (urea causes dryness and itching, and soap will just add to this problem.)

12. Provide continued emotional support.

   a. Allow for expression of feelings about change in body image.

   b. Encourage expression of fears of death especially during dialysis.

   c. Encourage family cooperation.

   d. Give support for required change in life style.

## TERMINATING HEMODIALYSIS

**Procedure**

1. Reduce negative pressure to zero. Discontinue alarms.

2. Put on mask.

3. Remove tape and dressing to visualize cannula connectors.

4. Put on sterile gloves.

**DIALYSIS ACTIONS FOR INTERNAL SHUNTS**

INITIATING DIALYSIS

    Place sterile drape under shunt site.

    Put on sterile gloves.

    Cleanse area with alcohol swab or povidone-iodine swab.

    Insert 15 or 16 gauge fistula needles into shunt site.

    Attach arterial and venous tubing to needles, using extension tubing.

TERMINATING DIALYSIS

    Infuse blood via venous site.

    Rinse access site tubing with normal saline.

    Apply pressure to AV fistula site following needle removal.

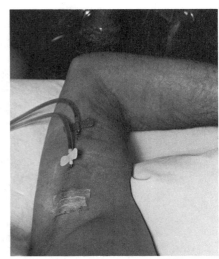

Needle placement for internal AV Shunt.

5. Place sterile pads under connectors.

6. Clamp arterial cannula and arterial blood line.

7. Separate cannula and tubing with cannula separator.

8. Connect IV of normal saline to arterial tubing.

9. Release arterial line clamp and infuse about 150 ml to rinse tubing if hollow fiber kidney used.

10. Clamp saline and arterial line.

11. Using saline infusion, return blood remaining in extracorporeal circuit to patient.

12. Separate venous line from venous cannula.

13. Insert cannula T connector into venous and arterial cannulae. Tape connections securely.

14. Remove venous cannula clamp and then arterial cannula clamp.

15. Perform site care, as explained in following intervention.

16. Measure and record postdialysis vital signs and weight.

## PROVIDING CANNULA SITE CARE

### Equipment

Masks

Soap, water, and washcloth

Hydrogen peroxide

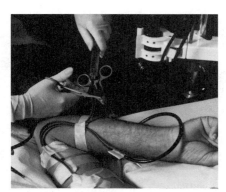

When taking patient off hemodialysis, return as much blood from machine as possible.

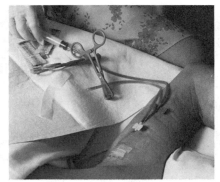

Rinse the access site tubing with normal saline before taking patient off dialysis.

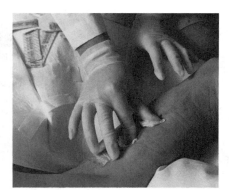

Apply pressure for at least five minutes to AV fistula site after needles are removed.

Sterile cotton applicators and alcohol swabs

Antiseptic ointment

Telfa pads

Sterile gauze pads, tape, and flexible gauze roll

**Procedure**

1. Don mask and wash your hands.
2. Remove and discard old dressing.
3. Examine site for infection, bleeding, security of connections, and alignment of tubing.
4. Wash and dry skin under dressing area, except for immediate area of exit sites.
5. Using sterile cotton applicators and hydrogen peroxide, cleanse exit sites. Start at point closest to tubing exit from skin and work outward.
6. Use dry cotton applicators to dry exit sites.
7. Clean tubing with alcohol swabs, working from sites to connections.
8. Apply antimicrobial ointment if ordered.
9. Apply nonadherent gauze over sites if there is any bleeding or drainage; otherwise, apply sterile gauze pads.
10. Cover most of cannula tubing with gauze pad but leave a small loop visible for inspection.
11. Tape dressing to skin.
12. Use flexible gauze to wrap extremity securely but without constriction.
13. Tape end of gauze roll.
14. Place tape on dressing with the date, time, and your initials.
15. Attach bulldog clamps to dressing. **Rationale:** Used to clamp cannula if separation occurs.
16. Do not allow nursing staff to use T connector to draw lab work.

---

**Safety Precautions for Shunts**

Do not measure blood pressure on cannulated extremity.
Do not apply tourniquet on cannulated extremity.
Do not perform venipuncture above cannulation site.
Inspect, palpate, and auscultate the cannula every two hours or more often if the shunt is new or flow is poor.
Palpate pulses distal to the shunt, and observe skin temperature and color every two hours at least.

---

**Acceptable Lab Values Following Dialysis**

Sodium 134–145
Potassium less than 6.2
Chlorine 94–104
Hydrochloric acid 18–24
BUN greater than 60, less than 85
Creatinine less than 13
Uric acid less than 10
Glucose 100
Calcium greater than 9.5, less than 11
Phosphorus 5.0–6.0
Alkaline Phosphorus less than 90
Magnesium less than 3.0
Albumin greater than 3.5

---

17. Perform site care at least every 24 hours or whenever dressing is wet or contaminated or whenever sites have been exposed for observation or dialysis.

## MAINTAINING FEMORAL CATHETER PATENCY

**Equipment**

Heparin 500 units (2)

500 cc IV normal saline (2)

IV controller (2)

Rubber-tipped clamps or dialysis clamps (2)

IV microdrop tubing (2)

Povidone-iodine swabs

4″ × 4″ gauze pads

Tape

**Procedure**

1. Wash your hands.
2. Inject 500 units of heparin into each of the IV normal saline solutions.
3. Insert IV tubing into solution bottles or bags.
4. Clear tubing of air.
5. Plug IV controllers into electrical outlet.
6. Place IV tubing through IV controllers.
7. Set controllers to keep-open rate according to directions on controllers. Usually administer IV at 5 to 10 gtts/min.
8. After infusing as much blood as possible from the

dialysis machine into the patient, clamp the catheters.

9. Insert the IV tubing into the catheters. An adapter may be required to provide a secure fit between the IV tubing and catheters. .

10. Cleanse area surrounding catheters with povidone-iodine swab.

11. Place 4″ × 4″ gauze pads over catheter site and tape securely.

12. Turn on power to IV controllers.

13. Press start button.

14. Evaluate IV system to ensure proper function and that IV infusion rate is between 5 to 10 gtts/min.

15. Provide catheter site care every day and as needed.

### CHARTING  *for Hemodialysis*

☐  Predialysis assessment

☐  Time dialysis begun

☐  Dialysate used

☐  Any complications during procedure and actions taken

☐  Time dialysis terminated

☐  Postdialysis assessment

---

## CLINICAL PROBLEM SOLVING

### Potential Problems

Decreased pulse, thrill, or bruit in shunt; blood in shunt very dark or separated into serum and red blood cells.

Hemorrhage is observed from the shunt.

Hypotension occurs during dialysis.

Bleeding occurs during dialysis.

### Suggested Solutions

☐  Notify physician promptly of potential shunt clotting. Shunt will need to be aspirated, irrigated with heparin, or possibly vessel stripped of clots. (Success of declotting depends on speed with which it is instituted.)

☐  Unwrap the dressing and examine the shunt. If cannulae have disconnected, immediately clamp with bulldog clamps. Then clean cannula tip, reconnect the cannulae, release the clamps, and notify the physician.

☐  If cannula has fallen out of vessel, stop bleeding with direct pressure or tourniquet above shunt. Summon physician immediately.

☐  Teach patient how to control bleeding in case he is alone when bleeding occurs.

☐  Anticipate possibility if antihypertensive or diuretic drugs were not omitted before dialysis.

☐  Prime line with 1 unit albumin.

☐  Administer normal saline into the venous line.

☐  Reduce pressure gradient if the client is on ultrafiltration.

☐  If hypotension is severe, consult physician about use of albumin, blood, or vasopressors.

☐  Before future dialyses, consult with physician about using smaller-volume dialyzer, less ultrafiltration, or intermittent normal saline doses to maintain blood pressure.

☐  Administer protamine sulfate as ordered to return clotting time to desired range.

☐  If blood leak alarm sounds, observe dialysate. If no blood is apparent, check dialysate with

Alarms sound during dialysis.

Hemastix since air bubbles can cause false alarms.

☐ If bleeding or blood leak is present, discontinue dialysis.

☐ Before dialysis, thoroughly familiarize yourself with alarm sounds, functions, and troubleshooting maneuvers.

☐ When alarms sound, quickly check for possible causes, such as obstructions or separations of tubing.

☐ In an emergency such as clots, air emboli in venous line, or failure of bypass mode, clamp venous blood line tubing immediately.

Near the end of or following dialysis, dialysis disequilibrium syndrome develops.

☐ Suspect dialysis disequilibrium if patient develops confusion, seizures, headache, nausea, vomiting, and/or hypertension.

☐ If these signs appear during dialysis, consult physician and implement possible orders to slow blood flow rate or discontinue dialysis.

☐ Administer medications as ordered to control symptoms, for example, dilantin for seizures.

☐ For future dialyses, consult with physician about possible orders regarding prevention, such as early dialysis before BUN rises excessively, shorter dialysis, or a change or the less-efficient peritoneal dialysis.

Signs and symptoms of fluid overload and/or electrolyte imbalance occurs during dialysis.

☐ Increase ultrafiltration.

☐ Check serum electrolyte values on fresh blood sample.

☐ Consult physician about possible changes in orders.

## TERMINOLOGY

**Albuminuria:**   the presence of albumin in the urine.

**Anemia:**   a condition where there is a reduction in the number of circulating red blood cells or hemoglobin.

**Antibiotic:**   a substance which has the power to inhibit or destroy other organisms, especially bacteria.

**Antidiuretic:**   decreasing the rate of urine secretion; an agent having such an action.

**Anuria:**   a total suppression or lack of production of urine.

**Bactericidal:**   able to destroy bacteria.

**Calyx:**   any cuplike division of the kidney pelvis.

**Catheterization:**   a sterile tube insertion for the injection of or removal of fluids from a vessel or body cavity.

**Dehydration:**   the process of losing water as in depriving the body tissues of water.

**Distention:**   stretching out or inflating of an organ such as the bladder.

**Diuresis:**   the excessive production and elimination of urine.

**Dorsal:**   pertaining to the back.

**Dysuria:**   difficult or painful urination.

**Edema:**   a condition in which body tissues contain an excessive amount of fluid.

**Electrolyte:**   composed of acids, bases, and salts; a compound that dissociates into ions when placed into solution and becomes a conductor of electricity.

**Excoriation:**   a breakdown of the epidermis.

**Foley catheter:**   a type of indwelling tube that is inserted through the urethra into the bladder to provide continuous urinary drainage.

**Genitourinary:**   pertaining to the genital and urinary systems.

**Glycosuria:**   the presence of sugar in the urine.

**Hematuria:**   blood in the urine.

**Hemorrhage:**   abnormal internal or external escape of blood from the vessels.

**Hydrometer:**   instrument used to determine the specific gravity of urine.

**Incontinence:**   inability to retain urine, semen, or feces through loss of sphincter control.

**Indwelling urethral catheter:**   synonym for retention, or Foley catheter.

**Infection:**   condition in which the body or a part is invaded by a pathogenic agent.

**Irrigation:**   the flushing of a tube, canal, or area with solution.

**Malpighian corpuscle:**   a spherical body consisting of a glomerulus and Bowman's capsule found in the cortex of a kidney.

**Micturition:**   the process of emptying the urinary bladder; voiding.

**Nocturia:**   excessive urination during the night.

**Oliguria:**   the diminished production of urine by the kidneys.

**Patency:**   the state of being freely open.

**Peri:**   prefix meaning around or about.

**Peristalsis:**   a progressive wavelike movement that occurs involuntarily in hollow tubes in the body, especially the alimentary tract.

**Polyuria:**   the excessive production and elimination of urine.

**Pyuria:**   the presence of pus in the urine.

**Renal:**   pertaining to the kidney.

**Sediment:**   a substance settling at the bottom of a liquid.

**Septic:**   pertinent to pathological organisms or their toxins.

**Septicemia:**   presence of pathologic bacteria in the blood.

**Shock:**   a state of collapse resulting from acute peripheral circulatory failure.

**Specific gravity:**   weight of a substance compared with an equal volume of water. Water is 1.000.

**Stoma:**   artificially created opening in the abdominal wall.

**Suction:**   the act of sucking up by reduction of air pressure over part of the surface of a substance.

**Urethra:**   a canal for the discharge of urine from the bladder to the outside.

**Urinary diversion:**   an interruption in normal flow of urine through the urinary system by surgical intervention.

**Urinary tract infection (UTI):**   an infection of the urinary tract, including all or part of the organs and ducts participating in the secretion and elimination of urine.

# Chapter 20

# Bowel Elimination

## LEARNING OBJECTIVES

Explain both the mechanical and chemical aspects of digestion.

Compare and contrast hypermotility with hypomotility.

Discuss what is meant by obstruction of the bowel.

Describe the anatomical locations where an ileostomy, cecostomy, or colostomy would be placed.

List the components of a good bowel training program.

Outline the essential steps in administering a tap water or saline enema to an adult patient.

Describe the precautions necessary when performing digital stimulation to remove a fecal impaction.

Compare and contrast stoma care of an ileostomy and a colostomy.

Outline the steps for performing a colostomy irrigation.

State the conditions under which ostomy irrigations are contraindicated.

Describe at least three potential problems you could encounter when irrigating a colostomy.

Describe at least three precautions necessary when applying a fecal ostomy pouch.

Discuss the corking and intubation procedure for patients with a continent ileostomy.

---

**ANATOMY AND PHYSIOLOGY**

The gastrointestinal system converts food into products that can be used as nutrients on the cellular level and disposes of wastes incurred in the process. The primary structures in this system include the mouth, esophagus, stomach, small intestine, and large intestine.

The mouth, esophagus, and stomach are the structures of the upper gastrointestinal tract, where the process of digestion begins. The small intestine, where digestion is completed and most absorption takes place, is a 12-foot tube composed of the duodenum, jejunum, and ileum. The large intestine is made up of the cecum, colon, and rectum. The cecum contains the ileocecal valve and the appendix. The colon is divided into the ascending, transverse, descending, and sigmoid colon. The rectum extends from the sigmoid colon to the anus. The terminal end of the rectum is called the anal canal and is guarded by the internal and external sphincter muscles. The chief functions of the colon are to reabsorb water and sodium and to store wastes.

Digestion is accomplished mechanically and chemically. Food is mechanically churned through the intestinal tract by sharp contractions, or peristaltic waves, of the circular and longitudinal muscles of the intestinal wall. Muscular sphincters and valves are located at strategic points throughout the intestinal tract. These structures help propel the food bolus or feces at appropriately timed intervals in a process called rhythmic segmentation. The sphincters and valves, when functioning properly, prevent reflux of contents. Peristaltic waves, coupled with rhythmic segmentation, allow maximal contact between food and the bowel wall so that chemical reactions can accomplish digestion and absorption can take place.

The chemical aspects of digestion in the small intestine begin in the duodenum with the introduction of pancreatic juices and bile. Pancreatic juices

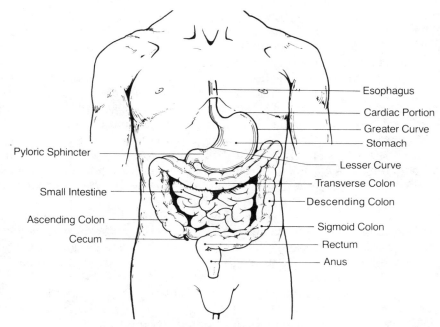

Anatomy of the gastrointestinal tract.

are rich in enzymes, which work to break down proteins and fats and to complete the transformation of starch to sugar. Bile, secreted by the liver, aids in the emulsification and absorption of fats. These substances work in an alkaline medium that combines with the acidity of chyme to provide a neutral pH in the duodenum, thereby protecting the duodenal mucosa.

In the 20 feet of jejunum and ileum approximately 3000 cc of digestive enzymes are secreted. These enzymes, which are secreted by the mucus glands of the intestines, complete the digestive processing of food prior to absorption. Again, the alkaline nature of these secretions works to protect the mucous membrane of the intestinal tract.

The peristaltic activity of the gastrointestinal tract, as well as its secretory functions, is governed, to a large degree, by parasympathetic and sympathetic nerve fibers. Stimulation of the parasympathetic system increases the activity of the intestinal tract, while stimulation of the sympathetic nervous system inhibits activity in the tract. The internal anal sphincter, however, is activated by sympathetic stimulation, while the external anal sphincter is under voluntary control.

Absorption, another primary function of the small bowel, is the passage of prepared materials from the gastrointestinal lumen to the blood and cells. Most absorption in the small intestine results from the churning action of the bowel. Chyme is continually exposed to the circular folds of the mucosal surface, which is lined with threadlike projections called villi. Villi serve as the sites of absorption of fluid and nutrients. The duration of contact between chyme and the mucosal surface of the bowel is very important in absorption. Hypermotility in the small intestine can result in decreased contact with the mucosal wall and deficient absorption; hypomotility can result in increased absorption of fluids as well as problems with elimination.

The circulatory system delivers nutrients to tissue cells and transports the waste products of metabolism. The small bowel and colon are supplied by the superior and inferior mesenteric arteries. Blood that contains absorbed nutrients is carried from the gastrointestinal tract by the superior and inferior mesenteric veins, which become a part of the portal system delivering blood to the liver. Each villus on the intestinal wall contains a network of small capillaries, which absorb sugar and amino acids, and a central lymph channel, which absorbs fatty acids and glycerol. When circulation is compromised, absorption is decreased and cells are lost.

By the time chyme reaches the ileocecal valve—the junction between the small and large intestines—most nutrients have been absorbed. While three liters of fluid pass through the small bowel, only 500 cc actually pass through the ileocecal valve. The semiliquid material received by the large intestine consists of living and dead bacteria, undigested food and residue, and cell debris. As residue is slowly passed along the colon by peristaltic-like mass movements, fluid is absorbed. These movements occur relatively infrequently (perhaps two or three times per day) and are stimulated by the entrance of food into the stomach by the gastrocolic reflex.

Absorption of fluid in the colon takes place primarily in the ascending and transverse colon. Fecal masses are stored in the sigmoid colon and move into the rectum with mass peristaltic movement. When the rectum fills and becomes sufficiently distended, centers in the sacral area of the spinal cord facilitate a defecation reflex, which contracts the rectum and relaxes the internal and external anal sphincters. The resulting urge, facilitated by higher centers, leads to contraction of the abdominal, perineal, and diaphragmatic muscles. Willful defecation is a coordinated, learned habit. Voluntary inhibition of the act returns the stool to the sigmoid colon.

## ALTERATIONS IN ELIMINATION

By-products of digestion must be continually eliminated to maintain normal body function. Alterations in normal elimination can result from changes in motility, obstruction of the lumen of the bowel, circulatory deficiencies, and surgically-induced alterations to the structures of the intestinal tract.

**Changes in Motility**  Motility in the gastrointestinal system is the ability to move spontaneously. Normal motility of the bowel provides peristaltic activity which pushes and churns food and chyme through the upper tract and feces through the lower tract at timed intervals.

Hypermotility may be caused by direct stimulation or irritation of the autonomic nervous system, as well as by inflammatory processes in the gastrointestinal tract. Stimulation of parasympathetic nerves promotes peristalsis and increases bowel muscle tone. Increased peristalsis speeds the propulsion of chyme through the upper tract, resulting in deficient absorption of nutrients. When increased peristalsis speeds the propulsion of feces through the lower tract, diarrhea occurs.

Stimulation of the autonomic nervous system may be psychic in origin. Anxiety, for example, may be mediated through either parasympathetic nerves with resultant diarrhea or through sympathetic nerves with resultant constipation. The action on the parasympathetic nervous system of certain drugs may also cause hypermotility of the intestine. Antihypertensive drugs, such as reserpine, and cholinergic drugs can cause diarrhea by their stimulation of parasympathetic nerves.

Hypermotility caused by the stimulating effect of an irritant on intestinal peristalsis may arise from infectious agents, chemical agents, or inflammatory disease processes. The most common intestinal irritants are the products of certain bacteria which release toxins in the digestive tract. Chemical agents which irritate the intestinal mucosa include cytotoxic drugs, castor oil, and quinidine. Ulcerative and inflammatory disease processes include diverticulitis, tuberculous lesions, ulcerative colitis, and Crohn's disease.

Hypomotility may be caused by direct stimulation or blockage of the autonomic nervous system, intestinal muscle weakness, and chemical agents which inhibit peristalsis and induce flaccidity in the intestinal tract. Decreased peristalsis causes chyme to move sluggishly through the upper tract so that fluids are overabsorbed. Decreased peristalsis also slows the propulsion of feces through the lower tract and causes constipation, fecal impaction, and obstruction.

Stimulation or blockage of the autonomic nervous system may be congenital in origin, as is the case in Hirschsprung's disease, where the absence of parasympathetic nerve ganglia results in failure of peristalsis of the affected portion of the bowel. The effects of trauma or toxins on autonomic innervation of the intestine, which occur with paralytic (adynamic) ileus, inhibit motility to the point of obstruction.

Intestinal muscle weakness which results from disease processes, old age, or a lack of essential vitamins (notably the B group) or electrolytes (particularly potassium) may all contribute to hypomotility. Certain drugs, such as codeine and morphine, can also cause hypomotility by relaxing the smooth muscles of the digestive tract and by increasing spasms of the intestinal sphincters.

**Obstruction of the Lumen of the Bowel**   Obstruction of the lumen of the bowel may be partial or complete. The severity of the obstruction depends on the region of the bowel that is affected, the degree to which the lumen is occluded, and the degree to which the circulation in the bowel wall is disturbed.

A small bowel obstruction which occurs as a consequence of persistent vomiting (reverse peristalsis) can cause severe disturbances in the electrolyte balance of the body. Large bowel obstructions, even if complete, are not as dramatic, provided that the blood supply to the colon is not disturbed.

The causes of intestinal obstruction are varied. In rare instances, obstruction may result when a foreign body, such as a large fruit stone or a mass of parasitic worms, becomes lodged in the bowel. More frequently, intestinal obstructions are caused by strictures, adhesions, hernia, volvulus, intussusception, polyps, neoplasms, and fecal impactions.

The physiology of an obstruction in the lumen of the bowel is generally the same, regardless of the cause. As the lumen of the bowel is blocked, the body attempts to overcome the obstruction by increasing peristalsis. During this process, liquid feces move past the site of obstruction and cause diarrhea and increased obstruction which leads to obstipation. Within several hours peristalsis is reduced and the bowel becomes flaccid. As intraluminal pressure builds up, fluid is retained and absorption decreases. The increased intraluminal pressure then leads to the compression of the bowel wall and its capillaries which causes necrosis of the bowel wall.

**Circulatory Deficiencies**   An adequate circulatory flow is essential for maintaining the structure of the bowel and for carrying on cellular nutrition. Any interruption of the arterial blood supply inhibits the bowel function. An occlusion of the circulatory flow, also called an intestinal infarction, results in gangrene of the bowel unless surgical intervention is carried out. A partial occlusion of the mesenteric arteries due to atherosclerosis can cause abdominal angina, a condition that occurs when the blood supply is increasingly interrupted.

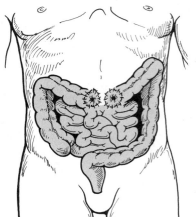

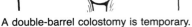

A double-barrel colostomy is temporary.

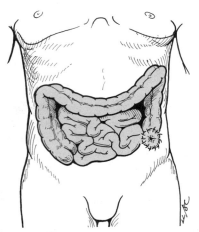

A sigmoid colostomy is permanent.

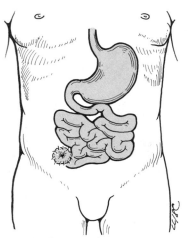

An ileostomy is permanent.

**Surgically-Induced Alterations in the Structure of the Bowel**   When alterations in bowel elimination become life-threatening and medical management fails, surgical intervention becomes necessary. Diversionary surgical procedures of the bowel include ileostomy, cecostomy, and colostomy.

An ileostomy is a surgically created opening from the ileum through the abdominal wall. The entire large intestine is bypassed and/or removed and the distal ileum is brought through the abdominal wall to form a stoma. The discharge from an ileostomy contains water and many digestive enzymes which have not yet been absorbed by intestinal villi. Strict attention should be paid to skin protection around the ileostomy stoma to prevent breakdown caused by the digestive enzymes.

A cecostomy is a surgically created opening from the cecum through the abdominal wall. This procedure is generally a temporary method of decompressing the bowel to relieve obstruction. Frequently, a catheter is left in the opening. This catheter requires frequent irrigation to ensure a patent lumen. If a catheter is not left in the opening, the cecostomy opening should be pouched in the same manner as an ileostomy.

A colostomy is a surgically created opening from the colon through the abdominal wall. In a colostomy the diseased portion of the colon is bypassed and/or removed and a portion of healthy colon is brought to the outside of the abdomen to form a stoma. Colostomies are named after the section of the colon surgically altered. The location of the colostomy dictates the type of drainage as well as the proper method of management.

An ascending colostomy will probably have liquid to semisoft effluent, which may flow throughout the day and night. The discharge from an ascending colostomy will contain some digestive enzymes caused by this portion of the colon's proximity to the small intestine. It will also contain a great deal of water, since much of the water-absorbing portions of the colon are bypassed. The stoma is usually located on the right lower quadrant of the abdomen. A drainable pouch with good skin protection is required for management of an ascending colostomy.

The discharge from a descending or sigmoid colostomy is formed and firm, since most of the water has been absorbed by the time the feces reaches these portions of the colon. The flow of output from a descending or sigmoid

**TABLE 1**  COMPARISON CHART FOR OSTOMIES

| COLOSTOMY | ILEOSTOMY |
| --- | --- |
| *Etiologic Factors* | |
| Cancer of colon—Permanent | Ulcerative colitis |
| Traumatic or congenital disruption of intestinal tract—Permanent or temporary | Crohn's disease (regional ileitis) |
| | Birth defects |
| Diverticulitis (double barrel)—Can be reanastomosed after inflammatory process healed | Trauma |
| | Cancer |
| *Surgical Procedure* | |
| Portion of colon brought through abdominal wall | Portion of ileum brought through abdominal wall |
| *Bowel Control* | |
| Sigmoid—Yes | None |
| Ascending—No | |
| *Stool Consistency* | |
| Sigmoid—Formed | Liquid to semiliquid |
| Ascending—Semiformed | |
| *Irrigation for Bowel Control* | |
| Sigmoid—Not usually irrigated | No |
| Ascending—Can irrigate | |
| *Use of Appliance* | |
| Sigmoid—Not usually | Yes |
| Ascending—Yes | |
| *Nursing Care Priorities* | |
| Control bowel evacuation | Control not possible |
|   a. Diet | |
|   b. Irrigation (ascending) | |
| Maintain skin integrity | Maintain skin integrity |
|   a. Wash stoma area |   a. Wash stoma area |
|   b. Provide skin barrier |   b. Provide skin barrier |
|   c. Ensure proper fit of appliance, if used |   c. Ensure proper fit of appliance |
| *Fluid Requirement* | |
| Sigmoid—Usual | Increased |
| Ascending—Increased | |
| *Diet Control* | |
| Avoid gas-forming foods | Low residue |
| | High calorie |
| | Avoid gas-forming foods |
| *Medications* | |
| Sigmoid—Stool softeners | Electrolyte replacement: |
| Ascending—Electrolyte replacement: $K$  $Na$  $NaHCO_3$ |   $K$  $Na$  $NaHCO_3$  $Mg$  $Ca$ |
| | Vitamins, especially K Minerals |
| *Psychosocial* | |
| Promote self-image | Promote self-image |
| Refer to Ostomy Club | Refer to Ostomy Club |

colostomy may be controlled by diet, the careful use of stool softeners, or colostomy irrigations.

Colostomy irrigations can establish regularity of bowel elimination when the stool is formed as it is evacuated from the colostomy. Irrigations are always contraindicated if peristalsis is absent, if perforation is suspected, or in cases of persistent diarrhea. Once control has been gained, a small, closed-ended pouch may be used to cover the stoma. Not everyone with a descending or sigmoid colostomy is a candidate for regulation. A drainable pouch with appropriate skin barriers is necessary for a nonregulated descending or sigmoid colostomy.

A loop colostomy is often performed in the transverse or ascending colon to allow the remaining portion of the colon to rest. This type of colostomy is usually temporary. The surgical procedure for a loop colostomy requires the surgeon to lift a loop of healthy bowel through the abdominal wall and to place a rod of some type behind the loop to stabilize the bowel on the abdomen. During the surgery or shortly afterward, the surgeon opens the loop to allow fecal elimination. When the bowel adheres to the abdominal wall, usually five to seven days after the operation, the surgeon removes the rod.

A double-barrel colostomy, which may also be temporary, is one in which there are two stomas. The proximal stoma, which connects to the rest of the digestive tract, is the functioning part of the colostomy. The distal stoma, which connects to the rectum, is the nonfunctioning part of the colostomy. The proximal stoma discharges fecal material, while the distal stoma discharges mucus. Irrigation procedures are not usually taught to patients with a temporary colostomy.

An end colostomy means the rectum has been removed. This type of colostomy is always permanent and may occur anywhere along the colon, although it is usually located in the sigmoid or descending colon.

## NURSING DIAGNOSES

The following nursing diagnoses may be appropriate to include in a Patient Care Plan when the components are related to alterations in bowel elimination.

| Nursing Diagnosis (Potential) | Defining Characteristic; Etiology (Examples) |
| --- | --- |
| ☐ Bowel Elimination, Alteration in: Constipation, *related to* | Decreased bowel motility, e.g., improper diet (low roughage), decreased exercise, disease states, medications. |
| ☐ Grieving, Anticipatory, *related to* | Loss of body contiguity, e.g., operative procedure (colostomy, ileostomy). |
| ☐ Self-Concept, Disturbance in: Body Image, *related to* | Altered body integrity, e.g., stoma. |
| | Decreased self-confidence, e.g., odor or flatus. |
| ☐ Skin Integrity, Impairment of, *related to* | Skin irritation or breakdown, e.g., poor pouching techniques. |
| ☐ Health Maintenance Deficit, *related to* | Inability to manage own disease treatment or health promotion activities, e.g., cognitive impairment, depression, immobility. |

# UNIT ONE   RECTAL TUBE INSERTION

## NURSING PROCESS DATA

### ASSESSMENT   *Data Base*

Palpate patient's abdomen to determine the degree of abdominal distention.
May need to measure abdominal girth.

Assess discomfort caused by flatulence.

Note quality and rate of respirations.

Note the presence or absence of hemorrhoids.

### PLANNING   *Objectives*

To promote removal of flatulence in the digestive tract following abdominal
surgery.

To promote removal of flatulence that occurs with excessive swallowing of air.

To stimulate expulsion of flatus in the lower digestive tract.

To prevent abdominal distention caused by flatulence, which can interfere
with diaphragmatic muscle contraction and cause dyspnea.

### IMPLEMENTATION   *Procedure*

Inserting a Rectal Tube

### EVALUATION   *Expected Outcomes*

Relief of abdominal distention and increased comfort.

Relief from dyspnea if flatulence has caused respiratory distress.

Flatus is removed from lower gastrointestinal tract.

## INSERTING A RECTAL TUBE

### Equipment

Rectal tube: size 22 to 24 French for adults and size
12 to 18 French for children

Small plastic bag or stool specimen container

Hypoallergenic paper tape

Water-soluble lubricant

Bed protector

### Procedure

1. Check physician's orders and Patient Care Plan.

2. Gather equipment.

3. Identify the correct patient and explain the procedure to the patient.

4. Provide privacy. Place patient on left side, in a recumbent position.

5. Tape the plastic bag around the distal end of the rectal tube or insert the tube into the stool specimen container.

6. Vent the upper side of the plastic bag to prevent inflation.

7. Lubricate the proximal end of the rectal tube with water-soluble lubricant.

8. Gently insert the tube into the patient's rectum, past the external and internal anal sphincters

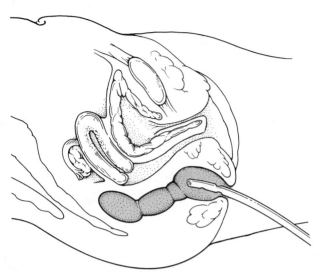

Insert rectal tube past the external and internal anal sphincters.

(two to four inches in adults, one to three inches in children).

9. With adults, gently tape the tube in place, using hypoallergenic paper tape. With children, hold the tube in place manually.

10. Leave the tube in place no longer than 20 minutes. **Rationale:** Prolonged stimulation of the anal sphincter may result in a loss of the neuro-muscular response. The prolonged presence of a catheter may cause pressure necrosis of the mucosal surface.

11. Remove the tube and provide perianal care as needed.

12. Help the patient assume a comfortable position.

13. Clean the tubing and replace in bathroom if to be reused. Remove and discard the plastic bag.

14. Instruct patient that chewing gum, sucking on candy, drinking liquids through a straw, and smoking tend to promote the swallowing of air and increase abdominal distention.

15. Wash your hands.

## CHARTING *for Rectal Tube Insertion*

☐ Time rectal tube inserted

☐ Amount, color, and consistency of feces collected

☐ Time rectal tube removed

☐ Presence, absence, or change in abdominal distention

☐ Patient's reaction to procedure

☐ Any unexpected outcomes and measures taken to treat these outcomes

---

## CLINICAL PROBLEM SOLVING

**Potential Problems**

No relief of abdominal distention.

**Suggested Solutions**

☐ Reposition patient at an angle that raises the lower part of his body, e.g., in a prone position with the foot of the bed raised.

☐ Instruct patient to circle, raise, and lower his legs.

☐ Reinsert the tube after two or three hours.

☐ Remove the tube and check for feces that may be clogging the outlet. Clean tube and reinsert.

Fecal impaction lower in rectum prevents insertion of rectal tube.

☐ Perform digital examination with gloved finger and water-soluble lubricant. Break up impaction if present.

☐ Position patient on left side in Fowler's position.

☐ Reinsert the rectal tube.

## UNIT TWO   REGULAR BOWEL EVACUATION

### NURSING PROCESS DATA

#### ASSESSMENT   *Data Base*

Evaluate patient's diet.
> Amount of high-bulk foods.
> Amount of fluid intake daily.

Evaluate patient's physical status.
> Ability to ambulate, i.e., spinal cord injury, CVA.
> Ability to perform bed exercises, abdominal exercises.
> Extent of disease process.

Assess effectiveness of drugs such as stool softeners, bulk formers, suppositories.

Assess time of day patient usually evacuates bowels.

Identify patient's ability to adapt and psychological readiness for the above program.

Identify position most effective for bowel evacuation.

Assess consistency of stool for abnormal findings (diarrhea or fecal impaction).

Assess when patient had last bowel movement.

Assess for abdominal distention.

#### PLANNING   *Objectives*

To promote regular bowel evacuation.

To prevent constipation.

To remove a fecal impaction.

To establish a bowel program to which the patient can easily adapt.

To develop a bowel program that the patient can perform him or herself.

#### IMPLEMENTATION   *Procedures*

Removing a Fecal Impaction

Providing Digital Stimulation

Developing a Regular Bowel Routine

Administering a Suppository

#### EVALUATION   *Expected Outcomes*

Patient establishes regular bowel evacuation program.

Fecal impaction is removed.

Patient is able to evacuate bowels at a convenient time.

# REMOVING A FECAL IMPACTION

## Equipment

Nonsterile gloves

Lubricant

Absorbent pad

Washcloth and towel

Bedpan

## Preparation

1. Check physician's order for impaction removal if the patient is at risk for possible complications from vagal stimulation (i.e., cardiac or spinal cord injured patient). **Rationale:** Vagal stimulation can result from manual removal of feces. It should be used only as a last resort and with specific physician's order. It causes a decreased pulse rate by decreasing conductivity at the S-A node and decreasing the rate of impulse firing at the node.

2. Gather equipment.

3. Identify the correct patient and explain procedure to patient.

4. Provide privacy.

5. Wash your hands.

## Procedure

1. Obtain baseline pulse and blood pressure.

2. Place patient on left side.

3. Place absorbent pad on bed.

4. Place bedpan next to patient's buttocks.

5. Place glove on hand and lubricate fingers well.

6. Ask patient to take a deep breath and exhale slowly as your index finger is gently inserted into rectum.

7. Gently remove the hardened stool.

8. Allow patient to rest between digital removal if any untoward effects such as palpitations, faint feeling, etc., are exhibited.

9. Obtain vital signs if patient complains of any discomfort.

10. When stool is removed wash and dry buttocks thoroughly.

11. Dispose of equipment.

12. Wash your hands.

13. Position patient for comfort.

14. Send stool specimen to lab if ordered; otherwise, dispose of stool in toilet.

15. Wash your hands.

# PROVIDING DIGITAL STIMULATION

## Equipment

Nonsterile gloves

Lubricant

Bedpan or commode

Absorbent pad

Washcloth and towel

Medication if ordered

## Procedure

1. Check physician's order and Patient Care Plan.

2. Gather equipment.

3. Identify the correct patient and explain procedure to patient.

4. Provide privacy.

5. Place patient in position for bowel evacuation (bedpan, commode, toilet).

6. Place glove on hand or finger cot on index finger and lubricate well.

7. Insert finger into rectum 1½ to 2 inches.

8. Move your finger from side to side in a circular motion to slightly stretch the rectal wall. Move toward the spine and not the bladder to prevent injury to the bladder.

9. Continue stretching the rectal wall for one to three minutes until the internal sphincter muscle relaxes.

10. Work with patient to discover an associated stimulus to help establish a good bowel routine. **Rationale:** Abdominal massage, coughing, deep inhalations, and tightening of abdominal muscles, in conjunction with digital stimulation, assists in bowel evacuation.

11. Repeat digital stimulation for one to three minutes at five minute intervals up to 20 minutes if a bowel movement does not occur.

> **Clinical Alert**
> Digital stimulation, given one-half hour after dinner or breakfast, is usually required for spinal cord injured patients.

12. After bowel evacuation occurs, assist the patient with cleaning and drying perineum.

13. Remove equipment from room.

14. Position the patient for comfort.

15. Wash your hands.

## DEVELOPING A REGULAR BOWEL ROUTINE

### Equipment

Nonsterile gloves

Lubricant

Bedpan or commode

Absorbent pad

Specific enema if ordered

Washcloth and towel

### Preparation

1. Check physician's order and Patient Care Plan.

2. Identify the correct patient and explain procedure to patient.

3. Identify time of day patient usually evacuates bowels.

4. Evaluate diet, exercise, former use of medications for bowel evacuation.

5. Administer the following drugs as ordered:
   a. Stool softener (Colace or Parlax) daily.
   b. Bulk former (Metamucil), q.d. to t.i.d.
   c. Mild laxative (Senokot, Doxidan) eight hours before program.
   d. Suppository (glycerin or Dulcolax) just before digital stimulation.

### Procedure

1. Perform digital stimulation one-half hour after dinner or breakfast. (See previous intervention.)

2. Place patient on toilet or commode. (Use bedpan if patient is on bed rest.)

3. Provide privacy and sufficient time for evacuation.

4. Wash and dry perineal area if patient unable to do so.

5. Place patient in wheelchair or bed and position for comfort.

6. Wash your hands.

7. Wean patient away from suppositories and laxatives when spontaneous bowel movements occur with digital stimulation.

Good bowel training programs include:
1. Initiation of defecation on demand with digital stimulation and abdominal massage
2. Evacuation at same time each day
3. Proper diet
4. Daily physical exercise regime
5. Patient and family education

## ADMINISTERING A SUPPOSITORY

### Equipment

Nonsterile gloves

Lubricant

Bedpan or commode

Absorbent pad

Suppository as ordered

Washcloth and towel

### Procedure

1. Check physician's order and Patient Care Plan.

2. Wash your hands.

3. Gather equipment.

4. Identify the correct patient and explain procedure to patient.

5. Provide privacy.

6. Place glove on hand or use finger cot and lubricate well.

7. Insert suppository (usually glycerin) with pointed end first, and place high in rectum beyond external and internal sphincters.

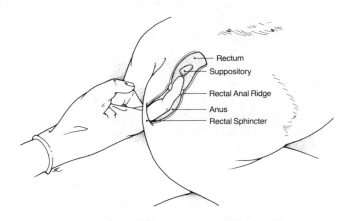

Rectum
Suppository
Rectal Anal Ridge
Anus
Rectal Sphincter

Insert rectal suppositories beyond the anal-rectal ridge for retention.

**Clinical Alert**

If patient has a spinal cord injury, observe for signs of autonomic hyperreflexia (goose pimples, pounding headache, hypertension, perspiration above level of spinal cord injury).

If signs and symptoms of autonomic hyperreflexia occur, discontinue digital stimulation, apply Nupercainal and Xylocaine Ointment around anus and rectum as ordered. This will anesthetize the area and decrease the stimulation that caused the response. Wait ten minutes for symptoms to decrease and then gently remove the feces.

8. Push the suppository against the side of the rectal wall. Ensure it is not placed into fecal mass as it will be ineffective.

9. Place patient on toilet or commode.

10. If bowel movement does not occur, in 20 minutes perform digital stimulation.

11. Repeat with stronger suppository if ordered (Dulcolax) after 20 minutes if there are no results.

12. Allow patient to retain Dulcolax suppository for 20 minutes. If no results, do digital stimulation again.

13. Following bowel evacuation, cleanse and dry perineal area.

14. Wash your hands.

15. Position patient in wheelchair or bed.

## CHARTING *for Regular Bowel Evacuation*

- ☐ Type and number of suppositories used
- ☐ Digital stimulation used
- ☐ Approximate time used for digital stimulation
- ☐ Amount, consistency, characteristics of stool
- ☐ Protocol for bowel evacuation for patient
- ☐ Untoward complications of bowel training
- ☐ Nursing interventions needed to correct complications

---

## CLINICAL PROBLEM SOLVING

### Potential Problems

When digital stimulation is performed, patient exhibits reflex spasm that prevents stool expulsion.

Patient develops diarrhea.

Patient exhibits signs and symptoms of vagal response during removal of fecal impaction.

### Suggested Solutions

- ☐ Apply local anesthetic around rectum and anus, if ordered.
- ☐ Wait for spasm to relax and then proceed with stimulation.

- ☐ Identify possible cause of diarrhea.
- ☐ Observe dietary intake for possible cause. Provide for bulk.
- ☐ Hold the laxatives and stool softeners temporarily.
- ☐ Instruct patient to eat yogurt and drink milk if not contraindicated by condition.
- ☐ Inform physician of diarrhea and obtain orders for Kaopectate. Administer 2 teaspoons after each loose stool for 24 hours.
- ☐ Check with physician if medications should be readjusted for bowel training as needed.

- ☐ Immediately discontinue procedure.
- ☐ Place patient in shock position.
- ☐ Monitor vital signs every five to fifteen minutes until condition is stable.
- ☐ Notify physician of findings and request medication order such as Atropine.
- ☐ Be prepared for "Code" situation, even though it is not likely to occur.

Effective bowel evacuation program is not established.

□ Ask dietician for altered diet (including more fruits and vegetables).
□ Check if patient can have fluids increased to 3000 cc daily.
□ Obtain order from the physician to administer stool softeners and bulk formers in greater quantity.
□ Have patient increase physical activity, especially exercise of the abdominal muscles if not contraindicated by condition.
□ Ensure that patient begins bowel training program one-half hour after a meal.

# UNIT THREE   ENEMA ADMINISTRATION

## NURSING PROCESS DATA

### ASSESSMENT   *Data Base*

Review patient's present and past eliminatory status.

Assess the need for an enema.

Evaluate amount of solution a patient can tolerate.

Assess if fecal impaction is present.

Assess the degree of abdominal distention.

Assess degree of sphincter control.

### PLANNING   *Objectives*

To relieve constipation.

To relieve fecal impactions.

To cleanse the bowel prior to surgery, childbirth, or diagnostic examination.

To evacuate the bowel in patients with neurologic dysfunction.

To provide nutrients.

To introduce an exchange resin.

### IMPLEMENTATION   *Procedures*

Administering an Enema

Administering an Enema to a Child

Administering a Disposable Enema

Administering a Retention Enema

### EVALUATION   *Expected Outcomes*

Increased comfort and relief from abdominal distention.

Clear returns if preparing patient for diagnostic examination or surgery.

Relief obtained from fecal impaction.

Complete return of solution plus formed, soft feces.

## Types of Enemas

**Cleansing:** Stimulates peristalsis through irritation of colon and rectum and by distention. Agents: soap suds, tap water and saline.

*Soap suds:* Mild soap solutions stimulate and irritate intestinal mucosa. Strong soap solutions can cause severe irritation of the mucous membrane of the colon. Dilute 5 ml of castile soap in 1000 ml of water.

*Tap water:* Give with caution to infants or to adults with altered cardiac and renal reserve. Tap water is a hypotonic solution.

*Saline:* For normal saline enemas, use a smaller volume of solution. Hypertonic solutions draw fluid into the colon from the body tissues. These solutions are mildly irritating to the mucous membrane of the colon.

**Oil:** Lubricates the rectum and colon and softens feces. Agents: mineral oil, salad oil, liquid petrolatum.

**Carminative:** Promotes expulsion of flatus. Agents: 1-2-3 enema (30 gm of magnesium sulfate, 60 gm of glycerin, and 90 cc of warm water); milk and molasses (180 ml to 240 cc of equal amounts).

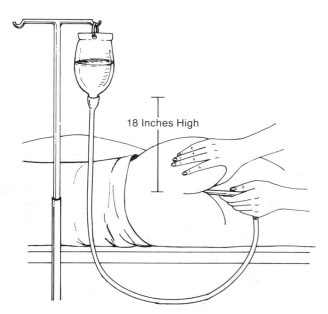

18 Inches High

Place enema solution container no more than 18 inches above rectum for safety.

## ADMINISTERING AN ENEMA

### Equipment

Fluid container with attached rectal tube (size 22 to 32 French for adults)

Normal saline, tap water, soap solution

Water-soluble lubricant

Clean bedpan with cover

Bed protector

Skin care items, e.g., soap, water, towels

### Preparation

1. Check physician's order and Patient Care Plan.
2. Gather equipment.
3. Provide privacy.
4. Wash your hands.
5. Identify correct patient and explain the procedure to the patient. Explain the benefits of relaxing and taking periodic deep breaths.

### Procedure

1. Raise bed to HIGH position and lower side rails.
2. Place bed protector under patient.

3. Place patient on left side in a Sims' position.
4. Fill water container with 750 to 1000 cc of lukewarm solution, 105° to 110° F. **Rationale:** Solutions that are too hot or too cold or solutions that are instilled too quickly can cause cramping, damage to rectal tissues, and extreme shock.
5. Allow solution to run through the tubing so that air is removed. **Rationale:** If air is instilled during the procedure, the patient will experience discomfort.
6. Lubricate the tip of the tubing with water-soluble lubricant.
7. Gently insert tubing three to four inches into patient's rectum, past the external and internal sphincters. Avoid traumatizing hemorrhoids during insertion. **Rationale:** Vagal nerve stimulation from enemas, digital examination, or rectal tube placement may cause cardiac arrhythmias.
8. Raise the water container to a maximum height of 18 inches.
9. Allow solution to flow slowly. **Rationale:** If the flow is slow, the patient will experience fewer cramps. The patient will also be able to tolerate and retain a greater volume of solution.

10. Hold the tubing in place in the patient's rectum at all times. Keep a bedpan nearby.

11. After you have instilled the solution, gently remove the tubing. Instruct patient to hold solution for 10 to 15 minutes.

12. Elevate the head of the bed so that the patient can assume a squatting position on the bedpan or assist to bathroom.

13. Provide privacy until the patient has expelled the total volume of the instilled solution.

14. Remove and cover bedpan.

15. Assist patient with perineal care and help patient to assume a comfortable position.

16. If patient is on strict I & O measure returns to make sure total volume of the solution is expelled.

17. Clean all equipment and replace in bathroom or appropriate location.

18. Wash your hands.

## ADMINISTERING AN ENEMA TO A CHILD

### Equipment

Water container with attached rectal tube (size 14 to 18 French for children, and size 12 French or infant enema syringe with bulb for infants)

Normal saline, tap water, soap solution

Water-soluble lubricant

Clean potty chair for children

Bed protector

Skin care items, e.g., soap, water, towels

### Preparation

1. Check physician's orders and Patient Care Plan.

2. Gather equipment.

3. Provide privacy for child.

4. Wash your hands.

5. Identify correct patient and explain procedure to child and/or family. Take time to calm a frightened child and to answer the child's questions.

### Procedure

1. Place bed protector under child.

2. Place child on left side or in knee-chest position.

3. Fill water container with 100° F solution (500 cc or less for child, 250 cc for an infant).

4. Allow solution to run through the tubing so that air is removed.

5. Lubricate tip of tubing or infant enema syringe with bulb.

6. Gently insert catheter or syringe into child's rectum (one to one and one-half inches for infants, two to three inches for children).

7. Elevate water container no more than 12 to 18 inches. **Rationale:** Height increases pressure of solution entering colon—too much pressure may damage colon.

8. Allow solution to flow slowly for 10 to 15 minutes.

9. After you have instilled the solution, gently remove the tubing or syringe.

10. Retain solution 10 to 15 minutes for cleansing enemas.

11. Hold child's buttocks together or tape them with hypo-allergenic paper tape. If child is toilet trained, place a potty chair nearby.

12. Place the child on a potty chair or bedpan.

13. If there are no contraindications, you may gently massage child's abdomen to help child expel returns.

14. If the child wants to be left alone while expelling returns, provide privacy. Child should expel the total volume of the instilled solution.

15. Remove and cover the potty chair or bedpan.

16. Clean the child's perineal area and help child assume a comfortable position.

17. Estimate returns to determine that the child expelled the total volume of the solution.

18. Clean all equipment and replace in appropriate area.

19. Wash your hands.

## ADMINISTERING A DISPOSABLE ENEMA

### Equipment

Commercially prepared enema

Water soluble lubricant

Bedpan or commode

Bed protector

Skin care items, e.g., soap, water, towels

## Preparation

1. Check physician's orders and Patient Care Plan.
2. Gather equipment.
3. Wash your hands.
4. Identify correct patient and explain the procedure to the patient. Explain the benefits of relaxing and taking periodic deep breaths.
5. Place bed protector under patient.
6. Place patient on left side in a Sims' position.
7. Provide privacy.

## Procedure

1. Read directions on enema container.
2. Lubricate with water-soluble lubricant if necessary. (Usually rectal tube is self-lubricated.)
3. Expose the anal opening to assist you in inserting the tube without traumatizing the tissue.
4. After inserting rectal tube, squeeze the container and empty entire 120 cc of hypertonic solution.
5. Instruct patient to hold solution five to seven minutes.
6. When ready to expel solution elevate the head of the bed so that the patient can assume a squatting position on the bedpan. If able, may expel solution in toilet.
7. Provide privacy until the patient has expelled the total volume of the instilled solution.
8. Remove and cover bedpan.
9. Assist patient with perineal care and help patient to assume a comfortable position.
10. Measure returns if on strict I & O.
11. Dispose of equipment.
12. Wash your hands.
11. Dispose of equipment.
12. Wash you hands.

## ADMINISTERING A RETENTION ENEMA

### Equipment

Commercially prepared disposable oil retention enema

Oil: adult 150–200 cc, child 75–100 cc, 91° F

Water soluble lubricant

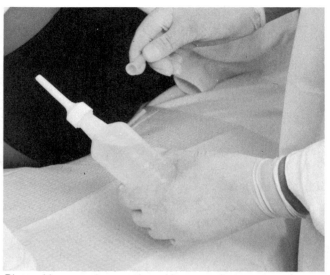

Disposable enema is prepackaged for convenient use.

Bedpan or commode

Bed protector

Skin care items, e.g., soap, water, towels

### Procedure

1. Identify and prepare patient as for any enema.
2. Disposable oil retention enema is administered like a disposable Fleet's enema. Read directions on enema container.
3. Expose anal opening and insert rectal tube tip of container 3–4 inches.
4. Squeeze contents slowly and empty entire amount into rectum.
5. Remove rectal tube gently.
6. Explain to patient that oil should be retained for one to three hours before it is expelled. **Rationale:** Purpose of enema is to soften stool.
7. A cleansing enema may need to be given to remove oil and stimulate defecation.

### CHARTING *for Administering an Enema*

☐ Time enema given
☐ Volume and type of solution used
☐ Results obtained: amount, consistency, and color
☐ Any unexpected outcomes and measures taken to remedy problems
☐ Patient's reactions to procedure

## CLINICAL PROBLEM SOLVING

**Potential Problems**

**Suggested Solutions**

Patient expels solution prematurely.

- Calm and ease patient's distress by reassuring him as you clean the equipment.
- Place bedpan under patient. Place patient in semi-Fowler's position with knees flexed.
- Hold the rectal tube in patient's rectum between thighs. Slow the water flow and continue with the enema.

Patient complains of severe and sudden abdominal pain, nausea, and distention.

- Remove tubing and notify physician immediately of possible perforation.
- Assess vital signs. If you suspect cardiac dysrhythmias, remove bedpan and notify physician immediately.
- Be prepared to administer emergency drugs such as atropine.
- If an IV is not in place, start an IV of $D_5W$ using a large bore needle for emergency use.

The flow of water is impeded or an obstruction is felt.

- Open clamp on tubing. Allow a small amount of solution to flow. (The warm solution may help relax the internal sphincter.)
- Withdraw tube slightly and reinsert.
- Gently perform a digital examination for the possibility of fecal impaction. Break up impaction if present. Ask physician for order to give a retention enema, followed by a cleansing enema two to three hours later.

Patient cannot return enema solution.

- Gently massage patient's abdomen if not contraindicated.
- Replace rectal tube. Lower the enema bag below the level of the bed.
- If patient is not uncomfortable, do nothing. If patient complains of discomfort or pain, notify physician.

Enema returns are not clear prior to surgery or diagnostic testing.

- Repeat enema. If, after three enemas, returns are still not clear, notify physician of findings.
- May need to give an enema with a stronger solution.

Fecal impaction is not relieved.

- Check orders for oil retention enema.
- Check catheter size needed.
- Obtain order for and utilize digital stimulation and manual extraction of feces if not contraindicated by diagnosis of cardiac or neurological involvement.

# UNIT FOUR COLOSTOMY IRRIGATIONS

## NURSING PROCESS DATA

### ASSESSMENT *Data Base*

Assess the permanence of the colostomy and patient's prognosis.

Identify the location of the colostomy along the large intestine.

Assess bowel sounds.

Check abdomen for distention.

Assess for stomal complications, i.e., peristomal hernia, stenosed stoma, or prolapsed stoma.

Note any presence of disease in the patient's bowel.

Assess the patient's ability to sit for a prolonged period of time.

Note patient's age and bowel habits prior to surgery.

Assess patient's feelings about colostomy management.

Assess the patient's mental alertness and ability to learn.

### PLANNING *Objectives*

To establish regular bowel elimination.

To evacuate stool from the colon.

To assist patient to develop a positive attitude toward living with a colostomy.

To assist patient to become proficient in colostomy care.

### IMPLEMENTATION *Procedures*

Performing a Colostomy Irrigation

Performing Irrigation in Bed

### EVALUATION *Expected Outcomes*

Complete return of solution plus soft or formed feces.

Bowel elimination is regulated.

Patient develops positive attitude toward living with a colostomy.

Patient becomes proficient in colostomy care.

## PERFORMING A COLOSTOMY IRRIGATION

### Equipment

Water container with cone or size 18 French catheter

Water at 105° to 110° F (500 cc for the first irrigation; 1000 cc thereafter)

Belt and irrigating sleeve cut long enough to reach the water level of the toilet

Items to clean skin and stoma, e.g., wash cloths or gauze sponges

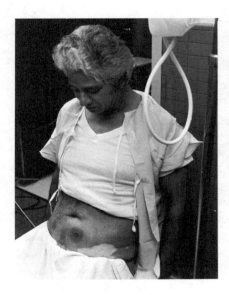 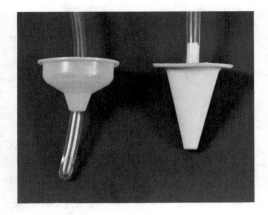

Colostomy irrigation is done with cone or catheter.

### Clinical Alert
The danger of perforation of the colon is much greater when irrigating a colostomy with a catheter. The use of an irrigation cone usually results in safer administration and better water flow.

Plastic bag for disposal of old pouch

Clean pouch and closure device

Skin barriers

Water-soluble lubricant

IV pole

### Preparation

1. Check physician's orders and Patient Care Plan.
2. Gather equipment.
3. Wash hands.
4. Provide privacy.

### Procedure

1. Identify and explain procedure to patient. Explain the benefits of relaxing and taking periodic deep breaths.
2. Remove and dispose of old pouch.
3. Clean stoma and skin with warm water and soft cloth.
4. Apply irrigation sleeve and belt.
5. Fill container with 1000 ml lukewarm water.
6. Remove air from tubing by allowing solution to run through tubing.
7. Suspend container on bathroom hook or IV pole.
8. Lubricate cone tip or tip of catheter.
9. Help patient sit on toilet or on chair in front of toilet.
10. Hang sleeve between patient's thighs.
11. Insert cone into stoma, parallel to floor. (Insert catheter two to four inches into stoma. Never force catheter insertion.)
12. Start water slowly and allow to run into stoma. (Peristomal hernias may increase the difficulty of an irrigation.)
13. Place container at level of patient's shoulder. Instill solution (1000 cc) over 10 to 15 minutes. **Rationale:** The height of the water container and the rate of water flow can affect the results obtained by an irrigation when the patient is in a sitting position.
14. Close off or fold over the top of the sleeve.
15. Allow patient to remain seated while patient returns the majority of the stool and solution.
16. Rinse sleeve with water. Dry bottom and close end of sleeve.
17. Ask patient to wear sleeve in this manner for 30 to 45 minutes. Patient may return to bed, walk around, or proceed with other activities during this time.
18. Remove sleeve and set aside for rinsing.

19. Clean patient's skin and stoma with warm water.

20. Assemble and apply skin barriers and clean pouch.

21. Rinse irrigation sleeve and hang to dry.

22. Wash your hands.

23. Put away all supplies and reorder as needed.

## PERFORMING IRRIGATION IN BED

### Equipment

Water container with cone or size 18 French catheter

Water at 105° to 110° F (500 cc for the first irrigation; 1000 cc thereafter)

A belt and an irrigating sleeve cut long enough to reach bedpan on chair at bedside.

Items to clean skin and stoma, e.g., wash cloths or gauze sponges

Plastic bag for disposal of old pouch

Clean pouch and closure device

Skin barriers

Water-soluble lubricant

IV pole

Bedpan

Chair

### Preparation

1. Check physician's orders and Patient Care Plan.

2. Gather equipment.

3. Wash hands.

4. Provide privacy.

### Procedure

1. Identify and explain procedure to patient.

2. Position patient comfortably in bed.

3. Close off the bottom of the irrigation sleeve and allow it to rest in a bedpan at the patient's side.

4. Remove and dispose of old pouch.

5. Clean stoma and skin with warm water and soft cloth.

6. Apply irrigation sleeve and belt.

7. Fill container with 1000 cc lukewarm water. **Rationale:** Water that is too hot can cause vertigo.

8. Remove air from tubing.

9. Suspend container on IV pole.

10. Lubricate cone tip or tip of catheter.

11. Place bedpan on chair by the bedside. Place sleeve in the bedpan.

12. Insert cone into stoma, parallel to floor. (Insert catheter two to four inches into stoma. Never force catheter insertion.)

13. Start water slowly and allow to run into stoma. **Rationale:** Water that flows too rapidly can cause vertigo.

14. Raise the container even with patient's shoulder if sitting. Raise 18 inches above stoma if in supine position. It should take 10 to 15 minutes for 1000 cc of fluid to be instilled in a colostomy. **Rationale:** Too little water does not provide complete elimination. Too much water causes the bowel to become flaccid and work poorly.

15. Close off or fold over the top of the sleeve.

16. Wait about 30 to 35 minutes to allow most of the irrigation fluid to return.

17. Open the bottom of sleeve into the bedpan.

18. Remove sleeve and set aside for cleansing.

19. Clean patient's skin and stoma with warm water.

20. Apply appropriate pouch and skin barriers.

21. Place patient in a comfortable position.

22. Rinse sleeve and hang to dry.

23. Wash your hands.

24. Put away all supplies and reorder as necessary.

### CHARTING *for Colostomy Irrigation*

☐ Time irrigation administered

☐ Amount and type of solution used

☐ Results obtained; amount, color, and consistency of returns

☐ Condition and color of stoma (it should be healthy red)

☐ Condition of peristomal skin

☐ Extent of patient participation

☐ Patient's reaction to procedure

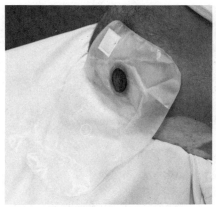

Remove old pouch gently to protect skin.

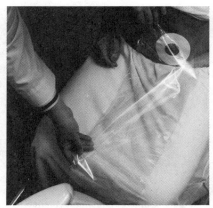

Position sleeve opening around stoma.

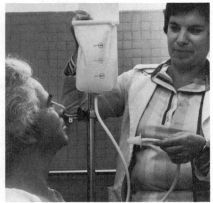

Run solution through tubing to clear air.

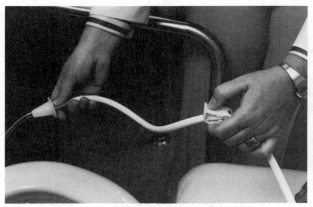

Allow irrigating solution to flow from bag through tubing to cone.

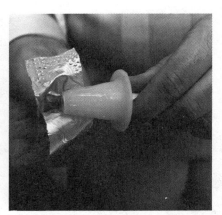

Lubricate tip with water soluble lubricant.

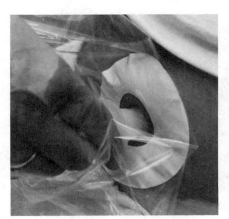

Gently insert cone 2 to 4 inches into stoma.

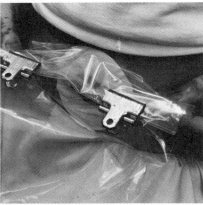

Fold sleeve over and close with clamp.

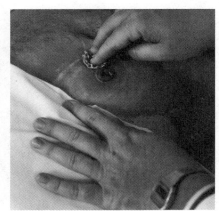

Clean patient's skin following irrigation.

# CLINICAL PROBLEM SOLVING

| Potential Problems | Suggested Solutions |
|---|---|

**Potential Problems**

Stool leaks out under irrigation sleeve.

Water does not flow easily into colostomy stoma.

Patient experiences cramping, nausea, or dizziness during irrigation.

Inability to run water into colostomy.

No return of stool or water from irrigation.

Continual spillage of stool between irrigations.

Poor returns due to constipation and/or fecal impaction.

**Suggested Solutions**

- ☐ Apply dampened Karaya washer around the faceplate at the opening of the irrigation sleeve.
- ☐ Tighten belt slightly.

- ☐ Change angle or position of cone slightly.
- ☐ Check for kinks in tubing from container.
- ☐ Check height of water container.
- ☐ Ask patient to relax and to take deep breaths.
- ☐ Instill small amounts of water to loosen stool.

- ☐ Stop flow of water, leaving cone or catheter in place.
- ☐ Do not resume until cramping has passed.
- ☐ Check water temperature. Water that is too hot can cause vertigo.
- ☐ Check height of water bag. Water that flows too rapidly can also cause vertigo.

- ☐ Perform digital exam to assess construction of stoma, since cone or catheter is probably against wall of bowel.
- ☐ Rotate cone or catheter to different position to start flow.

- ☐ Apply drainable pouch.
- ☐ Have patient increase fluid intake. Patient may be dehydrated.
- ☐ Repeat irrigation next day.

- ☐ Reassess type of colostomy—only those in descending or sigmoid colon are to be irrigated.
- ☐ Be sure patient uses and retains 1000 cc of tap water.
- ☐ Assess the patient's past bowel habits prior to surgery. Patients who have had very irregular bowel habits or frequent stools may not be candidates for irrigation.

- ☐ Assess the patient's diet. The dietician may need to be notified to provide more bulk foods.
- ☐ Assess medications patient is taking. (Drugs such as codeine, iron, and vincristine can be very constipating.)
- ☐ Stool softeners and/or mild laxative may be needed.
- ☐ Assess patient's fluid intake. Increasing the amount of fluids may be necessary.
- ☐ Perform a digital exam to check for impaction. If impaction or severe constipation persists, colostomy may be irrigated with 30 cc soap, 60 cc oil and 500 cc water. (Warn patient that this can

| | |
|---|---|
| | cause severe cramping.) This procedure requires physician's order. |
| | ☐ Obtain physician's order to add liquid Colace or mineral oil to irrigating solution. A soft rubber catheter may be used to put the liquid medication nearer to the obstruction. |
| Diarrhea occurs. | ☐ Do not irrigate colostomy. Apply drainable pouch. |
| | ☐ If patient is receiving radiation therapy, which usually causes diarrhea, check with physician about stopping irrigations until therapy is completed. |
| | ☐ Assess patient's medications. (Antibiotics or chemotherapy drugs can cause diarrhea.) |
| | ☐ If diarrhea is excessive and/or prolonged, alert the physician as patient may need to be monitored for potassium loss, and have diet adjusted accordingly. |
| Patient does not develop a positive attitude toward living with a colostomy. | ☐ Arrange visit between ostomy visitor and patient to demonstrate the rehabilitation possible following surgery. |
| | ☐ Ask physician to refer patient to health specialist skilled in teaching ostomy management. |
| | ☐ Ask physician to refer patient to ostomy club. |
| | ☐ Ask physician if referral to psychologist for support would be advisable. |
| | ☐ Allow patient to grieve over change in body image. |

## UNIT FIVE    FECAL OSTOMY POUCH APPLICATION

### NURSING PROCESS DATA

#### ASSESSMENT    *Data Base*

Observe stoma color.

Inspect patient's abdomen for creasing, firmness, softness, contour, scars, folds, and incisions.

Inspect patient's peristomal skin for signs of erythema, excoriation, ulceration, and fistula formation.

Assess patient's learning abilities, age, and manual dexterity.

---

**Clinical Alert**

Usually stoma color is dark pink to red. Blanching or lightening of the color may indicate circulation problems. Dark red color indicates alterations in stoma's blood supply.

---

**PLANNING** *Objectives*

To collect effluent for accurate assessment of output in the hospital.

To collect effluent for the comfort of the patient.

To contain drainage and odors so that the patient feels that he is socially acceptable.

To protect peristomal skin from erythema, excoriation, infection, and fistula formation.

To protect the patient's clothing.

**IMPLEMENTATION** *Procedure*

Applying a Fecal Ostomy Pouch

**EVALUATION** *Expected Outcomes*

Pouch remains intact without leakage for three to five days.

Pouching system provides maximal skin protection.

Pouching system remains odorproof for three to five days.

Patient gradually assumes an active role in applying the pouch.

Patient's skin remains free of erythema or excoriation.

## APPLYING A FECAL OSTOMY POUCH

### Equipment

Clean pouch (a drainable pouch should be used for all fecal ostomies except regulated descending or sigmoid ostomies)

Skin barriers, e.g., Skin Gel, or Skin Prep (an occlusive skin barrier with the correct sized opening should be used for patients with a history of allergic responses or for patients who have an ileostomy, cecostomy, ascending colostomy, or transverse colostomy)

Warm water

Soft cloths

Plastic bag for disposal of old pouch

Tail closure for drainable pouch

Deodorant (optional if pouch is odorproof)

Hypoallergenic paper tape (optional)

### Preparation

1. Check physician's orders and Patient Care Plan.
2. Gather equipment.

3. Explain procedure to patient.
4. Provide privacy for procedure.
5. Wash hands. Pouch application is not a sterile procedure. Gloves are not needed unless infection is present and their use may contribute to the patient's feelings of non-acceptance.
6. Raise bed to HIGH position and lower side rails on working side of the bed.

### Procedure

1. Place bath blanket over patient and fold top linen to bottom of bed.
2. Prepare the clean pouch.
   a. Measure the stoma with a measuring guide.
   b. Trace a circle one-sixth to one-eighth inch larger than stoma on the paper covering the adhesive backing.
   c. Cut the stoma pattern, and apply cement or double-faced adhesive disc according to the type of pouch being applied. Pouches applied with adhesive can be left in place for seven days unless leakage or skin irritation occurs.
3. Prepare occlusive skin barrier. Make sure the opening of the barrier is the same size as the

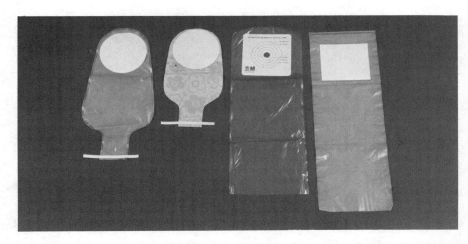

Styles of ileostomy pouches.

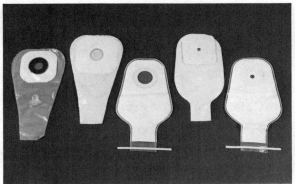

Open-ended or drainable pouches for colostomies.

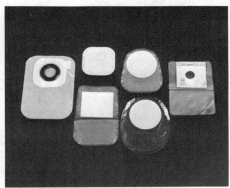

Non-drainable pouches for colostomies.

stoma to prevent contact between the stoma and the skin. If using a Karaya ring, rub moisture into ring until the ring turns sticky. If using Stomahesive or Reliaseal, cut opening to fit stoma as was done for the pouch. **Rationale:** Chemical composition and consistency of effluent play a large role in the selection of skin barriers and pouches to be used in ostomy care.

4. Empty the old pouch. **Rationale:** Pouches should be emptied when one-third to one-half full of feces or flatus to prevent destruction of the pouch seal.

5. Gently remove old pouch. If it is disposable, discard it. If it is reusable, set it aside for cleaning.

6. Clean the patient's skin and stoma gently with warm water and a soft cloth. **Rationale:** Oily substances should be kept away from areas of pouch application as they interfere with the adhesive.

7. Dry patient's skin well with a soft cloth.

8. Observe skin and stoma for changes in size, ul-

cerations, or color. (Skin should be a healthy red.) **Rationale:** Breakdown of peristomal skin may be caused by improperly fitting pouches, leakage of stool on the skin, hair follicle irritation, misuse of skin barriers, bacterial or fungal infections, perspiration, or allergic reactions.

9. If *not* using occlusive skin barrier, spray the skin with skin prep, allow it to dry, and spray again.

10. Apply a skin barrier such as Stomahesive, Hollihesive, Crixiline, Reliaseal, or Karaya washer or rings.

11. Center and apply clean pouch. Pouch should be applied away from fresh incision lines to decrease infection. The pouch is applied either directly on the skin or on the Karaya ring if used. **Rationale:** The opening of the faceplate of the pouch should be one-eighth inch larger than the stoma to prevent rubbing, cutting, or trauma to the stoma.

12. Press the adhesive around the stoma to form a seal. Do not allow adhesive to wrinkle in order to prevent leakage.

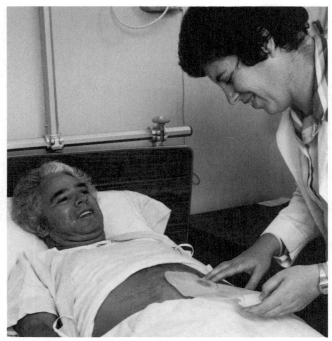

A trusting nurse-patient relationship assists the patient to accept a colostomy and learn the required care.

The surgical construction of the stoma, the contour of the abdomen, and the firmness of the abdomen dictate the types of skin barriers and pouches used.
- □ If the stoma is flush with the peristomal skin, a thin, occlusive skin barrier and a thin faceplate is needed to prevent leakage. Peristomal skin is skin that surrounds the stoma for an area between two and five inches.
- □ If the stoma protrudes nicely above the skin, a broader range of skin barriers and pouches may be applied.
- □ If the abdomen is very soft and large, a convex faceplate may be needed to prevent leakage.
- □ If the abdomen is firm and small, a flat faceplate may be used.

20. Position patient for comfort.
21. Lower bed and raise side rails.

13. Insert deodorant, either liquid or tablet, if bag is not odorproof.
14. Close and secure the end of the pouch with tail closure.
15. "Picture-frame" the faceplate of the pouch with hypoallergenic paper tape (optional).
16. Attach belt to faceplate of pouch (optional).
17. Wash your hands.
18. Check supplies and reorder as necessary.
19. Clean and store all reusable items.

### CHARTING   *for Applying a Fecal Ostomy Pouch*

- □ Type of pouch and skin barrier used
- □ Time pouch applied
- □ Time pouch emptied
- □ Amount, color, and consistency of stool emptied from pouch
- □ Presence or absence of flatus through the stoma
- □ Patient participation in pouch application
- □ Condition of peristomal skin and stoma
- □ Condition of incision line, i.e., any redness or swelling
- □ Condition of abdomen, e.g., distention, etc.

## CLINICAL PROBLEM SOLVING

**Potential Problems**

The stoma appears dark, dusky-colored, or black.

The stoma becomes ulcerated or cut.

**Suggested Solutions**

- □ Notify physician of findings immediately.
- □ Keep the ostomy pouch off the skin until the physician assesses the stoma.

- □ Examine the pouching system to see if the faceplate of the pouch may be rubbing or cutting into the stoma.
- □ Slightly enlarge the opening of the faceplate to the pouch to avoid traumatizing the stoma.
- □ Notify the physician, since this outcome may indicate a recurrence of disease.

The pouching system does not provide skin protection.

☐ Reassess the abdomen and the pouching system for weak points.
☐ Apply an occlusive skin barrier to allow the peristomal skin to heal.
☐ Change the pouch a little more frequently (once per day or every other day) until the peristomal skin is healed.

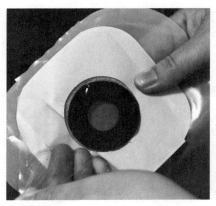

Prepare Karaya ring by taking off the protective cover.

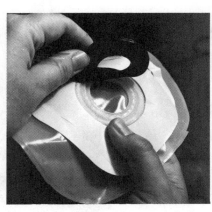

Remove Karaya ring from pouch before applying to patient's skin.

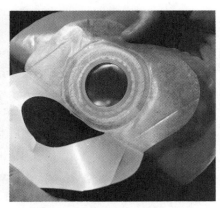

Remove paper from adhesive backing in preparation for application.

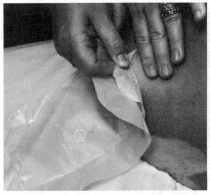

Remove old pouch that is adhered to the skin. Pull gently to protect skin.

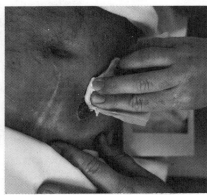

Clean periostomal area and dry thoroughly before applying pouch.

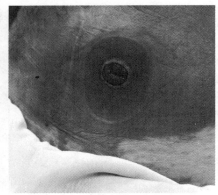

Observe stoma and periostomal area for color and ulceration.

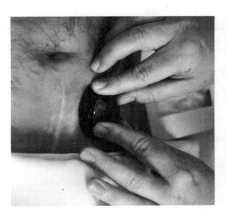

Apply Karaya ring, a skin barrier, flush to stoma before placing pouch.

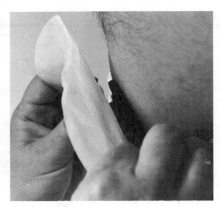

Place pouch on Karaya ring. Ring is cut ⅛ to ¼″ larger than stoma to protect it.

# UNIT SIX   MILLER-ABBOTT TUBE INSERTION

## NURSING PROCESS DATA

### ASSESSMENT  *Data Base*

Determine patient's level of consciousness.

Assess patient's knowledge of the procedure.

Auscultate the patient's abdomen for presence of bowel sounds.

Palpate abdomen for distention.

Assess amount, color and odor of drainage.

### PLANNING  *Objectives*

To decompress the bowel proximal to an obstruction.

To stimulate peristalsis.

To assess gastrointestinal bleeding (infrequent).

To relieve abdominal distention through tube placement.

To prevent muscosal damage upon removal of the tube.

### IMPLEMENTATION  *Procedures*

Assisting in Miller-Abbott Intubation

Removing a Miller-Abbott Tube

### EVALUATION  *Expected Outcomes*

Tube is properly placed and advanced.

A clear tube lumen is maintained throughout the intubation.

Relief of abdominal distention occurs through suction.

Bowel is compressed proximal to obstruction.

Peristalsis is reestablished.

Tube is removed without trauma to the intestinal mucosa.

## ASSISTING IN MILLER-ABBOTT INTUBATION

### Equipment

Water-soluble lubricant

Ice in basin

Miller-Abbott tube (double-lumen, 6–10 feet in length)

Stethoscope

Piston syringes: 5 ml, 10 ml, 50 ml

Emesis basin

Tissues or wash cloth

Towel

2–5 ml mercury

Normal saline solution

Items for oral hygiene

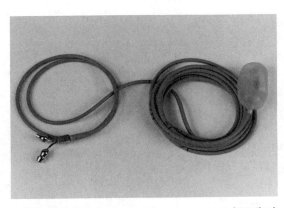

A Miller-Abbott tube is used for assessment, intestinal decompression, and to stimulate peristalsis.

## Preparation

1. Check physician's orders and Patient Care Plan.
2. Gather necessary equipment.

> The Miller-Abbott tube is a double-lumen tube six to ten feet in length. One lumen drains secretions. A balloon containing air and/or mercury is attached to the end of the other lumen to stimulate peristalsis. The tube progresses through the duodenum, jejunum, and ileum by gravity and peristalsis.

3. Notify physician that you are ready to assist with insertion.
4. Wash your hands.
5. Take equipment to patient's room.
6. Identify patient via identaband.
7. Inform patient about procedure and tell the patient what he can expect during and after insertion.
8. Explain how the patient can help with tube insertion.
9. Agree on a signal that the patient can use to stop the procedure for a moment or two.
10. Test the patency of the balloon and measure the capacity by filling it with air (20 to 50 ml of air used). Then completely deflate the balloon.
11. Label the adapters at the proximal end of the tube. One adapter should be labeled for suction; the other should be labeled Balloon.

## Procedure

1. Place the patient in a high-Fowler's position with neck flexed.

2. Spread the towel "bib-fashion" over the chest.
3. Measure the tubing, using the distance from the earlobe to the tip of the nose, plus the distance from the tip of the nose to the bottom of the sternum.
4. Wrap a piece of tape around the tube and mark the distance you measured.
5. Chill the tube; then lubricate the distal end sparingly.
6. Remove dentures. Instruct the patient to breathe through his mouth.
7. Observe physician as he inserts the tube into the patient's nostril. The tube is gently but firmly advanced. The patient is instructed to swallow as the tubing is advanced past the pharynx. **Rationale:** The tube is not secured to the nose until tube has been advanced to the desired position. This will halt the progress of the tube and may lead to bowel injury or intussusception.
8. The tube is advanced to the premarked area on the tube. Observe for aspiration of secretions. **Rationale:** Advancement of the tube more than two to four inches at a time can create knots and kinks in the tubing which may prevent relief from the obstruction or cause intussusception of the bowel.
9. Assist with determining the placement of the tube in stomach using either one of the following measures:

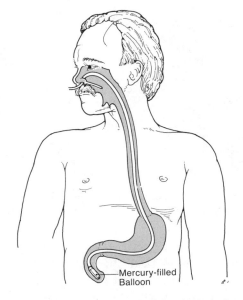

The tube is advanced in increments of one to two inches every hour. Suction is applied only after balloon passes pyloric valve.

a. Instill 5 ml of air in the suction portion of the tube while you listen with a stethoscope over the stomach area. If you hear a "whooosh" sound, the tube is in the stomach.

b. Using a syringe, aspirate for stomach contents through the suction portion of the tube.

10. Once in the duodenum, 2–5 cc of mercury is instilled into the balloon portion of the tube. **Rationale:** Mercury helps the balloon through the pyloric valve.

11. Reposition the patient on right side. **Rationale:** This position facilitates passage of the tube.

12. A fluoroscopy determines if the balloon has passed the pyloric valve. When the balloon has passed the pyloric valve, air is injected into the balloon portion of the tube.

13. Reposition the patient every two hours, turning from right to left side and back to high-Fowler's positon. Encourage ambulation. **Rationale:** Repositioning and ambulation will help the balloon through the gastrointestinal tract.

14. Attach the tube to suction any time after the balloon has passed the pyloric valve.

15. Advance the tube as ordered—one to two inches every hour, or two to four inches every two hours. When the patient is in bed, coil and pin extra tubing to the bed. When the patient is standing, coil and pin tubing to the gown.

16. When the tube reaches the desired position, secure it with tape to the patient's nose or forehead. Make sure that the tubing is not putting pressure on the lumen of the nostril.

17. Administer oral hygiene at least once every four hours. **Rationale:** Colonic bacteria travel to the patient's mouth by "wick action."

18. Assess amount, color and odor of drainage.

---

**Clinical Alert**

If the patient is suffering from a small bowel obstruction, the drainage from the tube will be yellow and fecal-smelling. If the patient is suffering from a complete bowel obstruction the drainage will be clear and may approach 3000 ml per day.

---

19. To irrigate, slowly instill 30 to 60 cc normal saline in the suction portion of the tube and then aspirate contents of the tube.

20. Advance tube according to schedule.

21. Notify physician if unable to advance or if any untoward effects occur.

22. Observe patient frequently and note relevant changes.

## REMOVING A MILLER-ABBOTT TUBE

### Procedure

1. Removing a tube that has not reached the ileocecal valve.
   a. Explain what the patient should expect as you remove the tube. **Rationale:** Patient may experience nausea as tube is removed.
   b. Insert 5 cc syringe in tube balloon port, aspirate and ensure that the mercury and air are removed from balloon portion of the tube.
   c. Gradually remove the tube a few inches every five to ten minutes.
   d. Give patient oral hygiene immediately.

2. Removing a tube that has passed the ileocecal valve.
   a. Explain what the patient should expect as you remove the tube.
   b. Cut the tubing at the nose.
   c. Allow the tube to advance through the rectum.
   d. Remove the remaining portion of the tube from the rectum with the aid of peristalsis.
   e. Provide perineal care.

3. Reposition patient for comfort.

### CHARTING *for Miller-Abbott Insertion*

- ☐ Time and date tube inserted
- ☐ Time intervals of advancement of tube
- ☐ Amount, consistency, color, and odor of drainage obtained from suction
- ☐ Oral care given
- ☐ Records of intake and output
- ☐ Dates and times irrigated
- ☐ Amount of irrigant used
- ☐ Time intervals tubing is pulled during removal
- ☐ Number of inches tubing is pulled during removal
- ☐ Patient's reactions to all phases of nursing intervention

## CLINICAL PROBLEM SOLVING

**Potential Problems**

Proper placement and advancement of the tube does not occur.

**Suggested Solutions**

☐ Assess that tube is not kinked or coiled by pulling back on the tube and then allowing it to advance again.
☐ Ensure that the tube is not pinned to gown or bed in such a way as to prevent advancement.
☐ Reposition patient to aid in advancement of the tube. If not contraindicated, ambulate patient to assist in advancement of tube.

There is no relief of abdominal distention through suction.

☐ Irrigate the tube through the suction portion of the tube.
☐ Insert rectal tube for 20 minutes as ordered.

Clear tube lumen is not maintained throughout intubation period.

☐ Irrigate tube.
☐ Notify the physician for additional orders.

Removal of tube is traumatizing to intestinal mucosa.

☐ Observe stool for occult blood and notify physician.

## TERMINOLOGY

**Anal fissure:** a small linear ulcerated area in the anal area.

**Bacteria:** unicellular plant-like microorganisms lacking chlorophyll.

**Bowel:** the intestine.

**Bowel movement:** the emptying of the intestinal tract.

**Carminative:** an agent that will remove gases from the gastrointestinal tract.

**Cathartic:** a drug to induce emptying of the intestinal tract; a laxative.

**Colitis:** inflammation of the colon.

**Colon:** the large intestine, which extends from the cecum to the anus.

**Colostomy:** an artificially created opening from the colon to the abdominal surface for the elimination of waste.

**Constipation:** difficult defecation; the passage of dry, hard fecal material.

**Defecation:** emptying of the intestinal tract; bowel movement.

**Diarrhea:** the passage of unformed liquid stools.

**Digestion:** the process by which food is broken down, mechanically and chemically, in the gastrointestinal tract.

**Diverticulitis:** inflammation of diverticuli in the intestinal tract causing stagnation of feces in the small distended sacs (diverticula).

**Diverticulum:** an outpouching of the mucous membrane of the intestine.

**Emulsification:** the breaking down of large fat globules in the intestine to smaller, uniformly distributed particles.

**Enema:** the introduction of fluid through a tube into the lower intestinal tract.

**Feces:** intestinal waste products consisting of bacteria and secretions of the liver, in addition to a small amount of food residue.

**Fistula:** an abnormal tube-like passage from a normal cavity or tube to a free surface or another cavity.

**Flaccid:** relaxed, flabby; having defective or absent muscle tone.

**Flatulence:** excessive gas in the stomach and intestines.

**Gastro:** pertaining to the stomach.

**Gastrointestinal:** having to do with the stomach and intestines.

**Guaiac:** test for blood in stool.

**Hemorrhoids:** abnormally distended rectal veins due to a constant increase in venous pressure.

**Hypermotility:** unusually quick motility in the gastrointestinal tract.

**Hyperreflexia:** increased action of reflexes.

**Hypertonic:** having a higher osmotic pressure than normal body fluid.

**Hypomotility:** unusually slow motility of the gastrointestinal tract.

**Ileostomy:** an artificially created opening from the ileum to the abdominal surface for the elimination of wastes.

**Impaction:** condition of being tightly wedged into a part; as of feces in the bowel.

**Integumentary:** relative to a covering, as the skin.

**Laxative:** a mild-acting drug to induce emptying of the intestinal tract.

**Mucosa:** mucous membrane.

**Necrosis:** death of areas of tissue or bone caused by enzymatic action or lack of circulation.

**Obstipation:** the act or condition of obstructing; extreme constipation due to obstruction.

**Occlude:** to block off, obstruct.

**Occult Blood:** blood in such minute quantities that it can only be detected by a microscope or chemical means.

**Ostomy:** a surgically formed artificial opening that serves as an exit site for the bowel or intestine.

**Parasite:** an organism that lives within or upon or at the expense of another organism, known as the host.

**Perforation:** the act or process of making a hole, such as that caused by an ulcer.

**Peristalsis:** a progressive wave-like movement that occurs involuntarily as in the gastrointestinal tract.

**Reflux:** a return of or backward flow.

**Sphincter:** circular band of muscle fiber constricting a natural orifice.

**Stoma:** an artificially created opening between two passages or between a passage and the body surface.

**Stool:** waste matter discharged from the bowels.

**Suppositories:** semisolid substances for introduction into the rectum, vagina, or urethra where they dissolve; serves as a vehicle for medicines to be absorbed.

**Villi:** short filamentous processes found on certain membraneous surfaces.

# Chapter *21*

# *Heat and Cold Therapy*

## LEARNING OBJECTIVES

Describe the mechanisms responsible for the body's heat loss and heat production.

Discuss the role of the hypothalamus in the body.

List at least three adaptive processes that maintain the body temperature within a normal range.

Discuss how heat transmission occurs.

Outline the steps necessary to prepare for the administration of hot, moist applications.

List four safety factors to consider when applying heat and cold treatments.

Compare and contrast the application of three types of warm soaks.

Explain the steps of providing a sitz bath.

State at least three precautions for providing dry heat treatments.

List two safety factors utilized to prevent skin irritation for infants in a radiant warmer.

Demonstrate preparation of the infant radiant warmer.

Explain the use of an aquathermic pad.

Discuss the safety factors that need to be assessed while administering a tepid sponge bath or ice application.

List the steps in preparing a cooling blanket.

Describe major nursing interventions performed for patients requiring a cooling blanket.

State two nursing diagnoses related to thermic treatments.

## TEMPERATURE CONTROL

The temperature of the human body is regulated and maintained by a group of interrelated feedback systems. When these homeostatic mechanisms are altered by disease or environmental conditions, the body may need assistance to regain its normal temperature.

Temperature control of the body is a homeostatic function that balances heat production and loss to maintain body temperature within a fairly constant range. The body uses neuronal pathways to collect, organize, and transmit temperature information. These pathways also transmit physiological responses to produce temperature adjustments. The main integrative function is carried out by the hypothalamus.

The hypothalamus is the body's thermostat, and it functions to maintain the body as close as possible to a constant or "set point" temperature. Information reaches the hypothalamus by indirect and direct means; that is, indirectly through receptors and directly by circulating blood. The hypothalamus triggers body response in the tissues and vasomotor tone in the organs to produce shivering, sweating, and changes in convection, conduction, and evaporation. The body uses these physiological processes to alter temperature.

The body continuously strives to maintain a constant optimal temperature. As heat is gained through metabolism, exercise, or environmental factors, the body throws off excess warmth through convection, conduction, and/or evaporation. In contrast, upon sensing a loss of heat (cold), the body triggers one or more processes to produce heat (thermogenesis), conserve it, or dissipate it. Although these dynamic processes cannot be observed, their resulting effects, such as violent shivering, are readily evident. The hypothal-

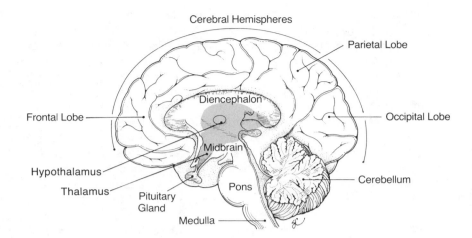

Cerebral Hemispheres

Parietal Lobe

Diencephalon

Frontal Lobe

Occipital Lobe

Midbrain

Hypothalamus

Cerebellum

Thalamus

Pons

Pituitary
Gland

Medulla

The hypothalamus is located in the diencephalon portion of the brain. It controls the
body's thermostat.

amus continuously makes adjustments, varying in intensity, to maintain the
core body temperature.

Our body works to maintain a neutral thermal environment. We consciously and unconsciously alter levels of activity in response to the physiological stimulus from the body's thermostat, the hypothalamus. When we
sense cold, we huddle or curl up to decrease heat lost from the body surface.
When warm, we extend our bodies and separate our limbs. There are sensors
in the hypothalamus and in the dermis that are distributed widely over the
body surface. These sensors react to changes in temperature. In fact, the
hypothalamus is sensitive to very minute changes, as slight as 0.01° C in the
circulating blood.

**Adjustment Processes**    An important adjustment process is heat conservation. When the body perceives a cooling sensation, heat conserving and
heat producing mechanisms are activated. Vasomotor constriction, a heat
conserving mechanism, removes warmed blood from the surface area of the
skin. This reduces heat loss to the cooler exterior through conduction.
Sweating removes heat from the body through the process of evaporation.
The piloerector muscles contract, raising all the body hairs, to create an insu-
lating (nonconductive) layer of air around the body. The latter reaction
produces "goose flesh" and may lead to the behavioral response of huddling,
curling up, or adding clothing to modify the microenvironment.

An emotional reaction can also produce a vasomotor response. Psychological perception of danger triggers the body's alarm system causing epinephrine
to be released. This results in vasoconstriction on the periphery of the body,
piloerection, and increased respiratory rate.

Heat production, or thermogenesis, is a progressive adaptive process. A
mild cold stimulus causes an increase in respiratory rate. This is the result
of the increased oxidative process going on in muscles as they are tensing.
More oxygen is consumed, shivering begins as muscle tension increases, and
heat is produced. This process continues until the temperature, as sensed
by the thermostat hypothalamus, is high enough or has reached the "set
point."

A second kind of thermogenesis, nonshivering thermogenesis, also
activates metabolic processes. Production of norepinephrine, mediated
through neuroendocrine control, stimulates the metabolism of brown fat.
Oxygen consumption is raised during this process, heat is produced, and

body temperature increases. Brown adipose tissue has a special kind of cell structure and is normally present in newborns. Newborns, incapable of shivering, still are able to produce body heat through metabolic processes. Brown adipose tissue reserves are felt to decrease with age, which perhaps explains why we feel extremes of cold more severely as we grow older.

In contrast, when the body perceives excess heat, opposite measures are activated. Sources of excess body heat may be internal (excessive muscle activity) or external (a very warm environment). The adaptability of the multiple systems to maintain temperature within the critical range is again demonstrated when mechanisms are activated to dissipate heat. The thermostat of the hypothalamus and the peripherally situated warmth receptors provide neurologic information to set the cooling mechanisms in motion. Peripheral vasodilatation occurs and warmed blood is brought to the surface of the body. Surface vessels dilate, promoting radiation of heat away from the body. Behavioral responses are to remove insulative layers and to extend our body to increase the surface area for greater heat conduction. Heat conservation mechanisms are reduced, muscle activity is decreased, and heat production is minimized.

When mild thermoregulatory activities are ineffective, sweating will begin. Sweating is stimulated by thermal signals from circulatory and integumentary receptors. Sweat glands are innervated by the cholinergic sympathetic nervous system. Thus, emotions such as anxiety and fear can trigger sweating.

One of the most effective mechanisms for heat loss is evaporation. As internal temperature increases, the sweating and vasodilator responses work together. Behavioral responses to heat include a decrease in activity manifested by apathy and inertia, and decreased hunger sensations. Heat dissipation processes become more efficient as the heat load persists. Then, as the body approaches normal temperature, the activities decrease and the dynamic process for thermoregulation continues.

Some processes associated with heat production may also promote heat loss, and vice versa. For example, physical exercise produces heat, but it also allows a larger body area to be exposed for heat dissipation. Exercise also disturbs the insulative thin-air layer around the body.

All thermoregulatory activities require functional pathways for receptors and effectors. Physiological systems must be healthy and intact to respond to the constant adjustments. The behavioral/intellectual systems must also function effectively to be able to manipulate the immediate environment to maintain body temperature. Our ability to adapt to alterations in temperature is affected by many external factors, such as pathogens, medications, physical disorders, and general health conditions related to age, circulation, physical fitness, and nutrition, etc.

**Conditions That Affect Adaptive Processes**   Pathogens in the form of viruses and bacteria can produce fever, generally a temperature of over 38.3° C, or 101° F. Fever caused by a pathogenic process is a thermoregulation disorder in which the "set point" is displaced upward. In response, the body perceives it is cold and seeks to conserve heat (i.e., shivering). The basal metabolic rate increases approximately 7% to 8% for every half degree centigrade of temperature elevation. Age, the duration and amount of temperature increase, and the overall disease condition are variables influencing the body's reaction.

Medications can alter the "set point" of the hypothalamus as well as affect one's ability to shiver or to exert vasomotor control. Drugs such as Thorazine,

Demerol, or Phenergan may suppress the brain's temperature regulatory center.

Disorders of or damage to a major adaptive system can make it more difficult for the body to cope with even small changes. For example, the skin is a major organ in the cooling and heating of the body. A severe inflammation or skin infection may render this system unresponsive to temperature fluctuations.

Other health conditions that affect the adaptive processes are poor circulation to the skin, which makes heat dissipation difficult; dermatitis, which decreases the ability of temperature sensors and circulation to respond; and an insufficient amount of muscle mass, which decreases thermogenesis. A very thin person or one with a muscle-wasting disease may not have sufficient muscle mass to be able to shiver. Neurological systems of elderly persons may not be able to transmit or process sensory information. Patients with a pathologic condition of the thyroid may be over or under normal levels yet not be euthermic. A person whose immune responses are deficient may not be able to adequately exhibit a febrile response. Interruptions of the hypothalamus through increased intracranial pressure grossly alter body temperature itself as well as the ability to thermoregulate. Finally, patients with decreased or absent body functions, underdeveloped, or very aged systems, would also have difficulty responding to alterations.

In addition to these internal sources, the environment itself influences the body's ability to adapt to alterations in temperature. For example, a person undergoing a surgical procedure may suffer extreme exposure in a cold operating room. The patient may be without covering for an extended period of time and have the abdomen opened to this environment, causing loss of core body heat. Other external conditions may cause cooling problems even if the cooling is mostly peripheral or surface. Peripheral cooling produces vasomotor changes or vasoconstriction. Continued cool blood from the periphery can eventually reduce the core to subnormal temperature. This cooling process will cause alterations of activity in most organ systems. With extended cooling stress, the thyroid is stimulated and produces an increase in metabolic rate.

In conclusion, alterations in body temperature are influenced by the body systems' integrity, age, particular disease process, and temperature stresses that a healthy person in a moderately neutral environment may experience. Many of these alterations can have temporary as well as chronic qualities. Persons may need assistance for a relatively short time or for the rest of their lives. It is apparent that assistance is often needed to maintain body temperature. Nursing attention and action can make a difference in many situations vital to the patient's comfort, healing, and coping.

Supportive and preventive measures are also therapeutic. When administering thermic applications, keep in mind that heat applications produce widespread effects. Warm applications of short duration produce vasodilation of peripheral vessels, a decrease in general heat production, and an increase in mobility of leukocytes. The application of heat to one body area will produce heat over other body parts and intermittent warmth to an area allows warmth receptors to fully respond with each treatment.

The following principles of patient safety are important to consider when you are applying heat and cold treatments.

☐   In most hospitals, the water temperature is controlled at a temperature not to exceed 110°F (43.3°C) to prevent patient injury.

☐ When a heating pad is used with warm, moist applications, temperature should not exceed 105°F (40.5°C) in order to prevent burning.

☐ A protective layer of Vaseline will assist in preventing tissue damage when hot packs are applied.

☐ Place hot pack on patient's skin for a few seconds, then remove and check condition of skin before leaving pack on the prescribed length of time.

☐ Monitor vital signs frequently when cold applications are applied.

☐ Observe skin for purplish color and check patient for numb feeling after cold applications are removed.

**NURSING DIAGNOSES**

The following nursing diagnoses are appropriate to utilize on Patient Care Plans when the components are related to thermic treatments.

| Nursing Diagnosis (Potential) | Defining Characteristic; Etiology (Examples) |
|---|---|
| ☐ Comfort, Alteration in: Pain, *related to* | Intolerance to treatments, e.g., low pain threshold, tissue damage. |
| ☐ Noncompliance, *related to* | Inadequate knowledge base, e.g., lack of explanation, misinterpretation. |
| ☐ Skin Integrity, Impairment of, *related to* | Burning or irritation of the skin, e.g., prolonged use of cold or hot treatment, excessive temperature of treatments. |
| | Impaired sensation, e.g., paralysis. |
| | Altered tissue perfusion, e.g., extreme temperature and/or prolonged time of treatment. |

---

## UNIT ONE   MOIST HEAT

### NURSING PROCESS DATA

**ASSESSMENT**  *Data Base*

Assess skin condition for possible complications such as redness, burns, and blisters related to previous applications of moist heat.

Determine if sterile technique is required.

Check for length of time heat treatment is ordered.

Assess vital signs, especially respirations on debilitated patients before applying heat.

**PLANNING**  *Objectives*

To conduct heat through moist application.

To produce local vasodilation.

To improve tissue metabolism in an infected area.

To increase circulation to the affected area.

To promote comfort for an injured area.

To increase mobility of leukocytes.

To decrease heat loss due to evaporation by using waterproof materials (moisture barriers).

To apply medications to a specific area.

To hasten suppuration and soften exudate from a wound.

To assist in redistribution of heat to other body parts.

### IMPLEMENTATION *Procedures*

Applying Hot Moist Pack

Applying Warm Sterile Soaks

Applying Clean Moist Compress

Applying Hot Sterile Moist Compress

Providing a Sitz Bath

### EVALUATION *Expected Outcomes*

Increased circulation occurs to the affected area.

Increased warmth occurs to area of application.

Suppuration progresses.

Pain is decreased with heat application.

## APPLYING HOT MOIST PACK

### Equipment

Terry towel or wool pieces for hot packs

Plastic drape or absorbent pad for moisture barrier

Container for warming solution

Petroleum jelly for skin protection

Safety pins

Bath blanket or terry towel for securing pack

Heating pad

Bath thermometer

Kerlix

### Preparation

1. Check orders for type of hot moist treatment ordered, length of treatment, and time interval between treatments.

2. Gather specific equipment for type of hot moist pack ordered.

3. Place material in a warming solution (usually water).

4. Determine amount of time elapsed since last application.

5. Considering age of patient, body part involved, and type of treatment, determine safe temperature of application to prevent burning. **Rationale:** Water temperature in hospitals is usually controlled at 110°F, but the individual patient may require altered temperature.

6. Identify correct patient and explain treatment to the patient.

7. Determine if patient is able to identify alterations in sensation if they were to occur.

8. Inspect skin surface for possible complications associated with heat treatments.

9. Take baseline vital signs.

10. Bring equipment to bedside.

11. Wash your hands.

12. Provide privacy and position patient for application of moist pack.

**Procedure**

1. Lubricate skin with petroleum jelly.

2. Place moisture-proof pad under affected area. **Rationale:** This pad keeps bed linens dry as well as allowing the pack to totally cover body area.

3. Wring out towel or wool pieces as dry as possible.

4. Place towel or wool pieces over affected area for several seconds.

5. Remove material and check skin for redness.

6. Ask patient if temperature of pack is comfortable.

7. Replace moist pack over affected area.

8. Wrap entire surface involved with plastic drape.

9. Place towel or bath blanket over plastic wrap.

10. Place heating pad or Aqua K-pad over plastic drape (optional).

11. Secure blanket or towel with safety pins or kerlix.

12. Take pulse to determine response to heat treatment.

13. Assess patient for possible complications of heat treatment, e.g., diaphoresis, flushed face, palpitations.

14. Time the treatment (usually 20 minutes).

---

**Clinical Alert**

Unless physician orders continuous heat application, treatment time is usually 20 minutes.

---

15. When treatment is completed, remove pack, inspect area for redness or tissue damage, remove petroleum jelly, dry patient, and apply dressing if ordered.

16. Reposition patient in comfortable position and determine any side effects from treatment.

## APPLYING WARM STERILE SOAKS

### Equipment

Plastic drape or absorbent pad for moisture barrier

Sterile basin

Sterile solution

Sterile towel

Sterile dressing (if needed)

### Preparation

1. Check orders for type of hot moist treatment ordered, length of treatment, and time interval between treatments.

2. Gather specific equipment for type of hot moist pack ordered.

3. Determine amount of time elapsed since last application.

4. Considering age of patient, body part involved, and type of treatment, determine safe temperature of application to prevent burning.

5. Identify correct patient and explain treatment to the patient.

6. Determine if patient is able to identify alterations in sensation if they were to occur.

7. Inspect skin surface for possible complications associated with heat treatments.

8. Take baseline vital signs.

9. Bring equipment to bedside and provide privacy.

10. Wash your hands.

### Procedure

1. Open sterile basin, maintaining sterility and keeping basin positioned on sterile wrapper.

2. Pour warmed, sterile solution into basin. Temperature of solution should be from 105° to 110°F (40.5° to 43.3°C) unless otherwise specified. **Rationale:** Temperature should be within this range to prevent tissue damage. (Test it by pouring small amount in another container and checking with your hands.)

3. Remove old dressing.

4. Slowly immerse body part into basin, checking the patient's reaction to temperature of solution before fully immersing.

5. During treatment, keep solution temperature constant by adding warm solution every five minutes. You may need to discard some solution by dipping it out with a sterile graduate.

6. Continue soak for 20 minutes.

7. Remove body part from solution, assess alterations in condition, and dry area with sterile towel.

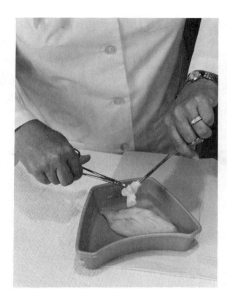
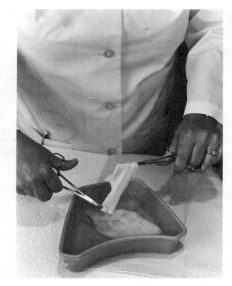
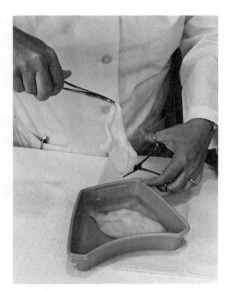
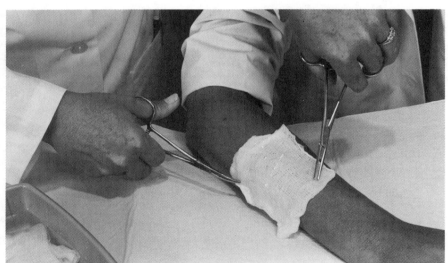

Apply sterile dressing to wound area, maintaining sterility in the application.

8. Apply dressing if ordered, using sterile technique.

9. Position patient for comfort and determine any reactions associated with heat application.

## APPLYING CLEAN MOIST COMPRESS

### Equipment

Terry towel or wool pieces for hot packs

Plastic drape or absorbent pad for moisture barrier

Container for warming solution

Petroleum jelly for skin protection

Safety pins

Bath blanket or terry towel for securing pack

Heating pad or Aqua K-pad

Bath thermomter

Forceps in container

### Preparation

1. Check orders for type of hot moist treatment ordered, length of treatment, and time interval between treatments.

2. Gather specific equipment for type of hot moist pack ordered.

3. Place material in a warming solution (usually water).

4. Determine amount of time elapsed since last application.

5. Considering age of patient, body part involved, and type of treatment, determine safe temperature of application to prevent burning.

6. Identify correct patient and explain treatment to the patient.

7. Determine if patient is able to identify alterations in sensation if they were to occur.

8. Inspect skin surface for possible complications associated with heat treatments.

9. Take baseline vital signs.

10. Bring equipment to bedside and provide privacy.

11. Wash your hands.

12. Lubricate skin with petroleum jelly.

### Procedure

1. Wring out compress with forceps. **Rationale:** Solution is hot, usually 110°F.
   a. Grasp forceps by handles, keeping tips down.
   b. Using forceps, pick up gauze dressing by edges.
   c. Keeping one forcep stable, wind the gauze dressing around the tip of the forcep.
   d. When dressing is dry, unwind and place over the wound.

2. Place compress on skin surface for a few seconds and then lift up to inspect skin.

3. Change compress frequently to ensure warmth.

4. Apply heating pad or Aqua K-pad over compress. Secure with a towel or bath blanket. **Rationale:** Pad maintains temperature and prevents need for constant compress changes.

---

**Clinical Alert**

When heating pad is used with warm, moist applications, temperature should not exceed 105°F in order to prevent burning.

---

5. Maintain treatment for specified time.

6. Remove compress, dry skin, and observe for changes in condition.

7. Reposition patient for comfort.

## APPLYING HOT STERILE MOIST COMPRESS

### Equipment

Terry towel or wool pieces for hot packs

Plastic drape or absorbent pad for moisture barrier

Sterile container for warming solution

Bath blanket or terry towel for securing pack

Heating pad or Aqua K-pad

Sterile solution

Sterile 4 x 4 absorbent pads or cloth

Sterile forceps or gloves

Sterile towel or ABD pad for covering compress

### Preparation

1. Check orders for type of hot moist treatment ordered, length of treatment, and time interval between treatments.

2. Gather specific equipment for type of hot moist pack ordered.

3. Determine amount of time elapsed since last application.

4. Considering age of patient, body part involved, and type of treatment, determine safe temperature of application to prevent burning.

5. Identify correct patient and explain treatment to the patient.

6. Determine if patient is able to identify alterations in sensation if they were to occur.

7. Inspect skin surface for possible complications associated with heat treatments.

8. Take baseline vital signs.

9. Bring equipment to bedside and provide privacy.

10. Wash your hands.

### Procedure

1. Warm sterile solution.

2. Place sterile gauze dressing in sterile basin maintaining sterile technique. Pour warm solution over the gauze.

3. Remove old dressings and cleanse wound of exudate.

4. Wring out gauze dressing, using sterile forceps.

5. Place gauze dressing over wound.

6. Wrap sterile towel around dressing.

7. Place plastic drapes over towel.

8. Apply heating pad or Aqua K-pad (105 to 110°F)(40.5 to 43.3°C).

9. Wrap towel over heating pad and secure with tape.

10. Change compress every one to two hours.

11. Remove compress and discard gauze dressing using the double-bagged technique.

12. Apply sterile dressing to wound between treatments of moist compresses if indicated.

13. Reposition patient for comfort.

## PROVIDING A SITZ BATH

### Equipment

Available bathroom with appropriate size tub for patient

Towels and bathmat

Inflatable ring

Bath blanket

Patient's clean clothes

### Procedure

1. Check physician's order for sitz bath.

2. Taken linen to bathroom.

3. Fill clean tub about one-third full with warm water.

4. Check with your hand to determine that temperature of water is between 105° and 110°F or 40.5° to 43.3°C.

5. Place towel or inflatable ring, if appropriate, on tub bottom and bathmat on floor beside tub.

6. Explain purpose and procedure to patient.

7. Instruct patient to undress.

8. Assist patient into tub, supporting back with rolled towels. Put towel or bath blanket around shoulders for warmth.

9. Check water temperature to see that it is comfortable.

10. Remain with patient during sitz bath or check frequently. Procedure takes 20 minutes.

11. Assess patient for any untoward reactions. **Rationale:** If patient feels dizzy, faint, or weak, remove him immediately. Ring for assistance if necessary.

12. When sitz bath is completed, assist patient from tub.

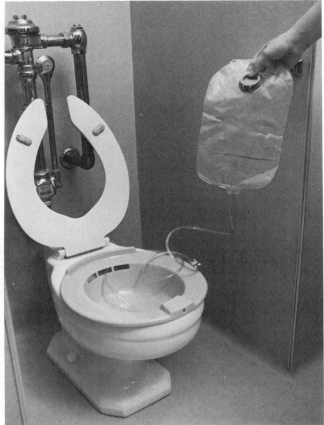

The portable sitz bath, brought into the patient's bathroom, is used to promote healing of the perineal area, especially after surgery.

13. Assist with drying and dressing and accompany patient to room.

14. Discard soiled linen, clean tub, and record procedure on patient's chart.

Portable sitz bath tubs are available and can be brought into the patient's room or placed in the bathroom. Small disposable sitz bath containers can fit under the toilet seat to provide a portable sitz treatment.

### CHARTING  *for Applying Moist Heat*

☐  Type of solution

☐  Length of time of application

☐  Type of heat application

☐  Condition and appearance of wound

☐  Comfort of patient

## CLINICAL PROBLEM SOLVING

| Potential Problems | Suggested Solutions |
|---|---|
| Affected extremity throbs with increased circulation. | ☐ Elevate the extremity above the level of the heart to increase venous return.<br>☐ Determine if application material is too heavy and is putting too much pressure on wound.<br>☐ Check for presence of peripheral pulses. |
| Pain in affected area is increased. | ☐ Assess if application is too hot.<br>☐ Ensure that temperature is not over 110°F (43.3°C) if a heating pad is used.<br>☐ Observe surrounding skin for erythema or burning. |
| Patient refuses to keep application intact. | ☐ Elicit reason for uncooperative behavior. Determine if patient is uncomfortable.<br>☐ Explain rationale for treatment. |
| Pack is difficult to secure due to affected area and/or activity of patient. | ☐ Use a roll of kerlix (wide gauze) to wrap and mold the pack to the body.<br>☐ Use a small sheet to wrap around the trunk.<br>☐ Have a person (parent for child) hold the pack in place only if absolutely necessary. |
| Vasoconstriction occurs due to heat treatment being on too long. | ☐ Observe the treatment time carefully and remove the heat on time.<br>☐ Observe the skin for possible damage due to prolonged heat. Report to physician. |

# UNIT TWO   WARM DRY HEAT

## NURSING PROCESS DATA

### ASSESSMENT   *Data Base*

Observe patient's skin for possible reaction to previous heat treatments.

Assess vital signs, especially temperature, to determine if overheating occurs.

Observe for and remove ointments and creams, which are non-heat-conductive materials.

Assess pain relief obtained from heat treatment.

Check cast for dampness.

### PLANNING   *Objectives*

To increase circulation to compromised area of the body.

To provide comfort and relaxation.

To promote drying of wound or cast.

To warm a body part.

To promote healing.

## IMPLEMENTATION  *Procedures*

Using a Heat Lamp

Using a Heat Cradle

Using the Infant Radiant Warmer

Applying Hot Water Bottle

Applying an Aquathermic Pad

## EVALUATION  *Expected Outcomes*

Body part is warmed.

Drying of cast is accomplished.

Relaxation of muscle spasms occurs.

Healing is accomplished.

Circulation is increased to compromised body area.

## USING A HEAT LAMP

### Equipment

Heat lamp with 60-watt bulb or infrared lamp

Pillows to ensure patient comfort and alignment during treatment

### Preparation

1. Review physician's order to determine treatment area, type of application, temperature of treatment and length of time.

2. Gather equipment and check it for safety factors, i.e., frayed cords, bulb in place.

3. Bring lamp to patient's room.

4. Explain procedure to patient.

### Procedure

1. Ensure that no more than a 60-watt bulb is used for heat lamp or the infrared element is in place for infrared treatment.

2. Wash your hands.

3. Identify patient by checking name band before beginning procedure.

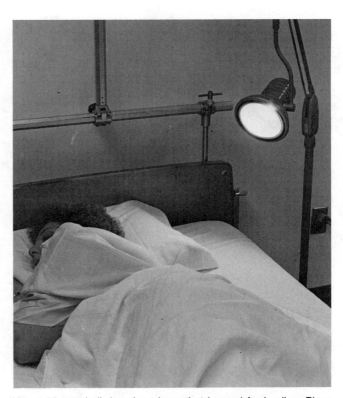

Use a 60-watt bulb in a heat lamp that is used for healing. Place heat lamp at arm's length from the patient to prevent burning.

4. Position cast or cleanse the affected body area well and dry thoroughly. **Rationale:** Drying prevents burning.

5. Place lamp 18–24 inches from patient. **Rationale:** If lamp is any closer, it could burn the patient.

6. Check for any discomfort, burning reaction, or other untoward reaction. **Rationale:** Frequent checking will prevent complications. Do not leave child or irrational adult alone.

7. Instruct patient not to change position nor touch lamp.

8. Remove lamp after 20 minutes and check area for redness, burning, or untoward reaction.

9. Reposition patient for comfort.

10. Return equipment to proper storage area.

## USING A HEAT CRADLE

### Equipment

Heat cradle with 25-watt bulb

Pillows to ensure patient comfort and alignment during treatment

### Preparation

1. Review physician's order to determine treatment area, type of application, and length of treatment.

2. Gather equipment and check it for safety factors, i.e., frayed cords, water leaks, etc.

3. Bring equipment to patient's room.

4. Explain procedure to patient.

### Procedure

1. Ensure that 25-watt bulbs are used.

2. Place cradle over affected area, 18–24 inches from the patient.

3. Cover patient and cradle with bath blanket to prevent exposure and chilling.

4. Remove heat cradle after 10 to 15 minutes.

5. Observe skin for erythema, burning, or untoward effects.

6. Reposition patient for comfort.

7. Return equipment to proper storage area.

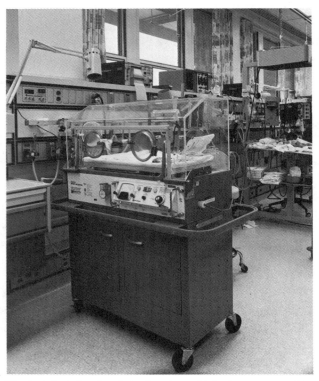

The Isolette Infant Incubator is a type of infant warmer used to maintain optimal body temperature, especially for prematures.

## USING THE INFANT RADIANT WARMER

### Equipment

Radiant warmer with skin or rectal probe

Bedding appropriate for warmer

### Preparation

1. There are several different radiant warmers, or infant care centers, available. Follow the manufacturer's operating instructions for safety and to determine if a manual or proportional controller is used. (General operating instructions and protocols are presented here.)

2. Check caster locks to make certain that each caster is in locked position.

3. Adjust procedure table to desired position.

4. Plug line cord into a three-wire receptacle.

5. Turn power switch ON; the red pilot light and the alarm indicator should glow. Turn alarm switch ON to test alarm system.

6. Turn manual knob to automatic.

**TABLE 1** DRY HEAT APPLICATION

| APPLICATION | USE | PRECAUTIONS |
|---|---|---|
| Heat Lamp | Provide heat to skin surface or mucous membrane | Use only 60-watt bulb |
| | May be used in drying casts | When used to dry casts, be aware that cast may be dry on outside only |
| Infrared Lamp | Provide heat to skin surface or mucous membrane | Be aware that heat penetrates only 3 mm of body tissue |
| Heat Cradle | Supply heat to abdomen, perineum, or chest | Use only 25-watt bulbs |
| | | Ensure that temperature inside cradle does not exceed 125° F |
| Aquathermic Pad | Supply heat to small body part or to portions of back | Ensure that temperature does not exceed 105° F |
| | | Do not secure with safety pins |
| Heating Pad* | Supply heat to any body surface | Do not secure with safety pins as could cause shock if wire were hit |
| | | Set temperature control on medium |
| Hot Water Bottle* | Supply heat to small surfaces Molds easily to area | Do not use water over 110° F |

*Generally not used in hospitals due to safety problems, i.e., burns and electrical malfunctions.

7. Install skin or rectal probe in controller and set switch to either rectal or skin, depending on which probe is being used.

8. Warm unit for seven minutes.

9. Adjust temperature to degree ordered by physician; temperature is dialed on digital temperature set switch.

## Procedure

1. Place infant in warmer.

2. Attach skin probe.
   a. Place 1-cm skin probe with polished surface touching skin to left of the umbilicus.
   b. Use a rectal probe if hospital protocol permits.

3. Monitor placement of skin probe.
   a. Inspect infant's skin under probe at regular intervals. **Rationale:** Infant's skin is delicate and irritates easily.
   b. Change the probe location if irritation begins to appear.
   c. Do not use adhesive tape or pads. **Rationale:** These may cause skin irritation or allergic reactions.

4. Allow three to five minutes for probe to reach infant's temperature.

5. Activate audible alarm by setting switch to ON. **Rationale:** If the infant's temperature exceeds 102° F (38.8° C), the audible alarm sounds and the visible alarm light flashes.

6. When the infant is removed from the warmer, provide preventive maintenance of warmer, such as cleaning thoroughly and inspecting all parts.

## APPLYING HOT WATER BOTTLE

### Equipment

Hot water bottle

Coverings for hot water bottle

Bedding to ensure patient comfort and alignment during treatment

### Preparation

1. Review physician's order to determine treatment area, type of application, and temperature of treatment.

2. Gather equipment and check it for water leaks, etc.

3. Bring equipment to patient's room.

4. Explain procedure to patient.

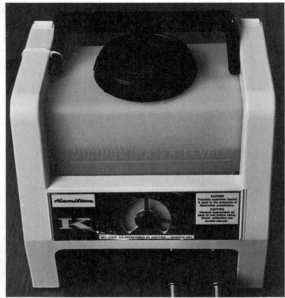

The Aquathermic Pad provides dry heat at a consistent temperature. It is regulated by a set, controlled electrical unit.

### Procedure

1. Fill water bottle two-thirds full, using water temperature of no more than 110° F (43.3° C).
2. Expel air from bottle and secure top.
3. Test bottle for water leak by turning upside down.
4. Cover water bottle with protective covering.
5. Place on skin surface, and remove after a few seconds. **Rationale:** This allows you to check skin for redness or burning. Replace bottle on skin surface.
6. Remove water bottle after one hour. Observe skin for untoward effects.
7. Reposition patient for comfort and return bottle to appropriate storage area.

## APPLYING AN AQUATHERMIC PAD

### Equipment

Aquathermic pad

### Preparation

1. Review physician's order to determine treatment area, type of application, and temperature of treatment.
2. Gather equipment and check it for safety factors, i.e., frayed cords, water leaks, etc.
3. Bring equipment to patient's room.
4. Explain procedure to patient.
5. Check that reservoir container is two-thirds full of distilled water and is free of air bubbles.
6. Place the reservoir container on bedside stand, and plug into electrical outlet. **Rationale:** If reservoir is placed below bed level the water will not circulate through the system.
7. Turn on switch. Allow water to circulate through pad to warm pad. Ensure that temperature does not exceed 105° F (40.5° C).

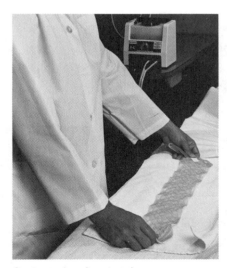

Center pad on face towel.

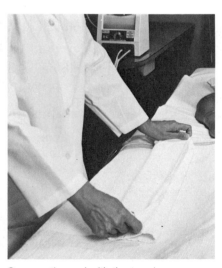

Cover entire pad with the towel.

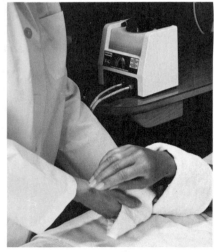

Secure pad with tape or gauze.

## Procedure

1. Cover pad with towel or pillow case and place pad on affected area. If arm or leg is used, pad may be tied around extremity using kerlix or towel and tape. **Rationale:** Pins should not be used to secure pad, as pins may puncture pad and cause a leak.

2. Remove pad after 15 to 20 minutes. Observe area for redness, pain, or any untoward reaction.

3. When pad is used to keep dressings or soaks warm, continue treatment longer than 20 minutes if ordered. Treatment may be continuous when used for patients with back pain.

4. Place pad on bedside stand until next treatment or return pad to proper storage area.

5. Reposition patient for comfort.

## CHARTING  *for Warm Dry Heat*

☐ Appearance of area before and after application

☐ Length of time of application

☐ Type of application used

☐ Patient's response to application

---

## CLINICAL PROBLEM SOLVING

### Potential Problems

Cast does not dry as quickly as expected.

Patient experiences discomfort with heat.

Patient's internal (core) temperature rises above normal or desired value.

Patient turns up equipment control settings on own volition.

Patient is losing too much body fluid from a full body warmer (exposure to heat produces sweating and evaporative heat loss).

### Suggested Solutions

☐ Continue with heat treatment until cast is shiny, indicating that it is dry.

☐ If room is cold and/or humid, increase room temperature to at least 72° F (22.2° C) and use dehumidifiers if possible. Cast drying is delayed under these conditions.

☐ Do not move wet casted area with your fingers as indentations in the cast can lead to decubiti formation.

☐ Elevate casted extremity above level of heart to prevent edema formation.

☐ Reduce the control settings.

☐ Remove heat application.

☐ Examine patient for burns or tissue damage.

☐ Check for malfunctioning equipment.

☐ Remove the heat source.

☐ Avoid chilling the patient.

☐ Take patient's vital signs frequently, including temperature, until returned to normal.

☐ Explain reasons why settings must not be changed, e.g., burns.

☐ Reset and observe settings frequently.

☐ Assess for tissue damage. Report to physician.

☐ Discuss reasons why patient may have not been sensing the true temperature of the equipment (peripheral receptors become depressed after a time and pad may not feel hot).

☐ Give fluids unless contraindicated.

☐ Use fluid retaining material between the patient and ambient air (e.g., saran wrap) to allow heat to come through but retard fluid and heat loss through evaporation.

Patient is burned by presence of creams and/or ointments on the skin.

☐ Remove creams or ointments. Notify physician.
☐ Assess skin carefully for damage.
☐ Obtain order for and apply cooling measures such as ice bag to area.

## UNIT THREE   COLD APPLICATIONS

### NURSING PROCESS DATA

#### ASSESSMENT   *Data Base*

Check the purpose for the cool application, e.g., injury, fever.

Determine patient's ability to tolerate cold application.

Assess baseline vital signs and assess any hazards to patient's vital functions with the application of cold.

Check if antipyretic medications have been administered (identify type, amount, time, and response) in addition to the cool application.

Observe fluid and electrolyte status, especially in patients with elevated temperatures.

Assess condition of skin before and after application to determine if alterations occur.

#### PLANNING   *Objectives*

To promote vasoconstriction.

To decrease edema.

To reduce pain.

To decrease temperature.

To decrease or stop bleeding.

#### IMPLEMENTATION   *Procedures*

Providing a Tepid Bath

Using Ice Application

Using Instant Cold Pack

#### EVALUATION   *Expected Outcomes*

Edema is slowed or reduced locally.

Patient's internal (core) temperature is reduced.

Pain is reduced or alleviated.

Bleeding is reduced or alleviated.

## PROVIDING A TEPID BATH

### Equipment

Water source or source of coolant (e.g., water, ice, or alcohol) for equipment

Basin or tub for sponge bath

Washcloth and towels

Thermometer

Bath blanket

Lightweight linens

### Preparation

1. Review order for type of bath to be given: water, ice, or alcohol.
2. Note temperature of solution ordered and length of time of application.
3. Gather equipment and bring to patient's room. Identify patient.
4. Provide privacy and explain procedure to patient.
5. Wash your hands.

### Procedure

1. Remove clothing from body to allow for cooling and observation. Utilize bath blanket for privacy.
2. Observe skin surface before cold wrap is applied, and take vital signs, especially temperature.
3. Monitor body color and vital signs every 15 to 30 minutes during cooling.
4. Immerse washcloths or material for sponging in ordered solution, generally 70° to 80° F (21° to 27° C). **Rationale:** Alcohol is infrequently used due to its drying effect; however, due to efficiency of action, it should be used when the temperature needs to be decreased quickly.
5. Place cloths on forehead, back of neck, axilla, groin, and wrists. **Rationale:** The reason for this placement is that blood circulation is near the surface.
6. Depending on type of bath, change wraps or soaks every five minutes. **Rationale:** This prevents wraps from holding body heat.
7. Replace warmed cloths and continue procedure for 20 to 30 minutes, then stop, and reassess patient's condition.
8. Do not allow shivering to occur. Stop the treatment or modify it to prevent shivering. **Ration-ale:** If the body senses a loss of heat, it will attempt to produce it by thermogenesis, conserve it, or dissipate it.
9. Cool the air to 68° to 72° F (20.0° to 22.2° C) if possible.
10. Promote movement of air (fanning) if possible.
11. If using alcohol, promote ventilation of the room and observe carefully for patient's response.
12. When temperature has decreased to desirable level, dry skin and replace light covering over patient and reposition patient for comfort.
13. Determine patient's response to cool treatment.
14. Take vital signs every one to two hours until temperature is stabilized.
15. Provide high calorie diet. **Rationale:** Increased temperatures cause an increased metabolic rate. Carbohydrates, proteins, and 2500 to 3000 cc fluid intake is essential for maintaining homeostasis.

## USING ICE APPLICATION

### Equipment

Ice cap, ice bag, ice collar, ice glove, freeze bag

Crushed ice

Plastic drape or absorbent pad

### Preparation

1. Review order for type and length of treatment.
2. Gather equipment for specific applications.
3. Wash your hands.
4. Fill container, if needed, two-thirds full with crushed ice, express air, and secure top shut.
5. Place absorbent covering over ice applicator.
6. Take equipment to patient's room.

### Procedure

1. Identify patient by checking identaband.
2. Explain procedure to patient.
3. Provide privacy as needed.
4. Take baseline vital signs, if needed, and observe the skin surface where ice is to be applied.
5. Remove ice pack after one hour or when absorbent cover becomes wet. Observe skin for any untoward effects such as bluish, purple appearance or a feeling of numbness.

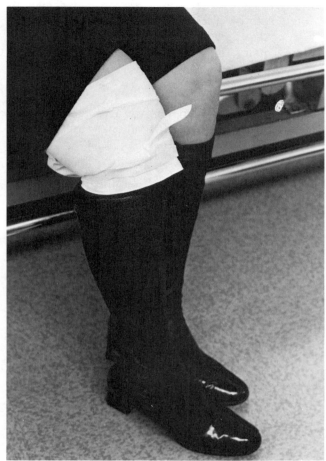

Wrap the cold pack around the injured extremity to decrease edema.

6. Reposition patient for comfort, and provide warmth if needed.
7. Reapply ice pack in one hour if necessary.

## USING INSTANT COLD PACK

### Equipment

Packaged cold pack

### Preparation

1. Review orders and check length of treatment.
2. Gather equipment.
3. Wash your hands.
4. Identify patient by checking identaband.
5. Explain procedure to patient.
6. Provide privacy.

### Procedure

1. Grasp top of cold pack and shake contents to bottom of bag.
2. Hold package in the middle with both hands.
3. Squeeze the package firmly to break the inner pouch.
4. Shake the package gently to mix the chemicals together.
5. Apply directly on the injured area.
6. If package is punctured or opened and the solution touches the skin, flush the area with water. **Rationale:** The chemicals will burn the skin.

### CHARTING  *for Cold Applications*

☐ Specific cold application used to reduce temperature
☐ Effectiveness of treatment
☐ Response of patient to procedure
☐ Vital signs taken during application

---

## CLINICAL PROBLEM SOLVING

**Potential Problems**

Local edema is not reduced.

Bleeding continues even with cold applications.

**Suggested Solutions**

☐ Elevate extremity above level of heart.
☐ Ensure that body surface is sufficiently covered with cold application to cause vasoconstriction.
☐ Apply cold treatment for first 24 hours until edema has dissipated, as ordered.

☐ Reassess area for possible "bleeders," which may require cautery or ligation by the physician.
☐ If bleeding continues for extended time or large

| | |
|---|---|
| | blood loss is observed, notify physician immediately. |
| | ▢ If bleeding occurs in an extremity, elevate the extremity above the level of the heart to decrease blood flow to the area. |
| | ▢ Continue with cold application as cold constricts the arterioles and increases the viscosity of the blood, assisting in the control of bleeding. |
| Patient feels cold. | ▢ Apply warmth to soles of feet. |
| | ▢ Place bath blanket over unaffected area. |
| Internal (core) temperature drops too low. | ▢ Monitor the temperature frequently, every 30 to 60 minutes. |
| | ▢ Warm the patient slowly. |
| | ▢ Take vital signs every 15 to 30 minutes. |
| Skin becomes irritated or macerated from sponging or cooling measures. | ▢ Remove cold application from the area and use alternate surface site. |
| | ▢ Apply petroleum jelly or oil to area when using cold applications. |
| | ▢ Do not massage or rub the area as this action can cause tissue damage. |
| Total numbness occurs at the site of the cold application. | ▢ Warm the area immediately by placing body surface in 110° F (43.3° C) water. Remove extremity from water when red flush appears. |
| | ▢ Apply loose dry dressing if area appears broken down. |
| | ▢ Observe circulation closely for any alterations. |
| | ▢ Observe for signs of frostbite. |
| Pain occurs at the site of cold applications. | ▢ Remove cold application. |
| | ▢ Warm the site a few degrees. |
| | ▢ Inspect for tissue damage. |
| Patient becomes nauseated or disoriented from alcohol fumes. | ▢ Discontinue using alcohol; remove it from area. |
| | ▢ Provide ventilation in room. |
| | ▢ Assess vital signs. |
| Patient becomes very cyanotic and/or mottled. | ▢ Discontinue cooling. |
| | ▢ Assess vital signs. |
| | ▢ Warm the site a few degrees. |
| | ▢ Observe site for signs of frostbite. |

# UNIT FOUR   HYPOTHERMIA BLANKET

## NURSING PROCESS DATA

### ASSESSMENT   *Data Base*

Evaluate if patient's temperature can be reduced by less intensive measures.

Assess skin condition, especially of face, ears, hands, and feet, before, during, and following treatment.

Determine patient's ability to tolerate treatment.

Assess baseline data, i.e., vital signs, neurological signs, mental status, peripheral circulation.

Assess that the cooling blanket and machine are functioning properly.

Evaluate EKG findings throughout treatment.

Assess fluid and electrolyte balance (especially potassium level).

Evaluate fluid intake and output throughout treatment.

Assess for shivering.

### PLANNING    *Objectives*

To protect the skin from injury during use of the cooling blanket.

To prevent shivering during cold applications.

To ensure that the cooling blanket functions properly.

To reduce body's internal (core) temperature.

To provide hypothermia for operative procedures.

To decrease metabolic processes, thereby preventing irreversible states.

### IMPLEMENTATION    *Procedure*

Using a Cooling Blanket

### EVALUATION    *Expected Outcomes*

Skin remains free of injury during use of the cooling blanket.

Cooling blanket functions properly.

Patient's internal temperature is reduced without any untoward effects.

Shivering is avoided during use of the cooling blanket.

## USING A COOLING BLANKET

### Equipment

Cooling blanket, top and/or bottom, machine

Glass thermometer

Sphygmomanometer

Stethoscope

Thermometer probe

### Preparation

1. Check physician's orders and Patient Care Plan.
2. Gather equipment.
3. Check that electrical plugs are grounded.
4. Ensure that amount of coolant is sufficient. If not, add 20 percent isopropyl alcohol solution through the reservoir cap. To mix a 20 percent alcohol solution:
   a. Mix one quart 50 percent alcohol with 1½ quarts distilled water.
   b. Mix one quart 70 percent alcohol with 2½ quarts distilled water.
5. Connect the cooling pad to the machine.
   a. Push back the collar. Insert the male tubing connector of the cooling pad into the inlet opening. Release the collar.
   b. Repeat connection using the outlet opening.
   c. If two pads are being used, connect the second pad in the same manner.
6. Turn the unit on by moving the master temperature control knob to the desired temperature.

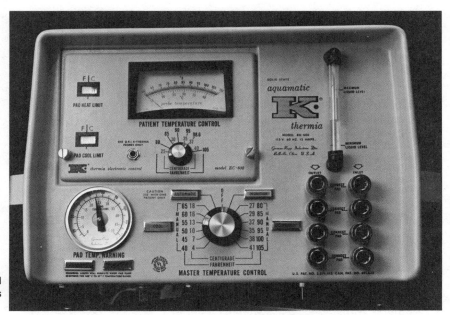

Maintain and monitor temperature control while using a cooling or heating blanket. This prevents complications.

The pads from the machine reservoir fill automatically.

7. Add the alcohol mixture to the reservoir as the pads fill. Observe the reservoir sight gauge to determine the fluid level.

8. Set the master temperature control knob to either automatic or manual operation. **Rationale:** There are two separate temperature control knobs, one for automatic and one for manual operation.

9. When using automatic control, insert the thermister probe plug in the electronic control thermister probe jack.

10. When using manual control, set the master "temperature control knob" to the desired temperature.

11. Bring equipment to patient's room.

12. Identify patient and explain procedure.

13. Provide privacy.

14. Wash your hands.

| Classifications of Hypothermia | |
| --- | --- |
| □ Mild | 32° to 37° C |
| □ Moderate | 28° to 32° C |
| □ Deep | 20° to 28° C |
| □ Profound | 0° to 20° C |

## Procedure

1. Place the cooling blanket on bed and connect it to the machine. Precool blanket to 5° to 10° C.

2. Place a sheet or a thin bath blanket over the cooling blanket.

3. Obtain baseline patient data before starting treatment.

4. Place patient on the cooling blanket. Wrap patient's hands and feet in towels. **Rationale:** This prevents frostbite or skin damage.

   *for automatic control*
   a. Insert the probe into patient's rectum.
   b. Check that patient's temperature control knob is at the desired temperature.
   c. Observe that the automatic mode light is on.
   d. Check that the pad temperature limits are set at desired safety limits.

   *for manual control*
   a. Insert the probe into patient's rectum.
   b. Observe that the cool mode light is on.
   c. Watch that the cool limit warning light does not illuminate. **Rationale:** This light indicates that unit temperature is below 37° C.
   d. Monitor the fluid thermometer, which indicates temperature of pad. **Rationale:** This ensures pad temperature is maintained at desired level.

5. Set the temperature control to 37° C and begin lowering temperature 1° C every 15 minutes until 33° or 34° C is reached.

6. Monitor patient's temperature every 15 minutes.

7. Observe patient for signs predicting onset of shivering: ECG muscle tremor artifact, visible facial muscle twitchings, hyperventilation, and verbalized sensations.

8. If manifestations of shivering occur, obtain order for IV medications, usually chlorpromazine.

9. While patient undergoes hypothermia, monitor vital signs every 30 minutes during reduction of temperature control and then every two hours.

10. Monitor with ECG if the patient has cardiac disease or hypokalemia.

11. Observe obese patients for fluid balance alterations.

12. Remove and clean rectal probe every four hours.

13. Check the automatic temperature control every four hours for accuracy by taking temperature with a glass thermometer. **Rationale:** The type of thermometer, oral, axillary, or rectal, will depend on the condition of the patient. Remember that oral and axillary temperatures tend to be less accurate indicators of the true internal body temperature.

14. Check physician's order for, and apply, thigh-high support stockings. **Rationale:** Stockings prevent venous stasis.

15. Turn, cough, and deep-breathe patient every 30 minutes.

16. Monitor patient's skin condition and massage bony prominences every two hours.

17. When physician orders hypothermia to be discontinued, gradually increase temperature from 30° to 37° C over six hours.

18. Monitor vital signs every 15 minutes.

19. Observe for edema. **Rationale:** This is caused by increased cell permeability, acidotic shock due to shivering, fluid imbalance, and hypothermia.

### CHARTING *for Cooling Blanket*

☐ Patient's temperature and method of taking temperature

☐ Any untoward effects of the treatment, i.e., shivering

☐ Setting of the cooling blanket

☐ Whether the top blanket is used

☐ Skin condition

☐ Skin treatments done prior to use of cooling blanket

☐ Length of cooling blanket treatment

---

## CLINICAL PROBLEM SOLVING

### Potential Problems

Patient's core temperature decreases rapidly and falls below 37° C.

Patient begins to shiver.

The rectal temperature probe does not seem to be accurate.

### Suggested Solutions

☐ Turn off cooling blanket.
☐ Take top blanket off if you are using one.

☐ Stop the procedure and/or warm the solution a few degrees.
☐ Monitor temperature because shivering causes an increase in the metabolic rate leading to an increase in heat production.
☐ Monitor temperature every 15 minutes to detect additional temperature decrease.
☐ If temperature continues to drop, the blanket can be turned on to the warming control and the patient can be warmed.

☐ Assess patient's skin condition for cold, presence of peripheral pulses, and ability to feel pressure.
☐ Take patient's temperature every two hours with glass or electronic thermometer to evaluate the accuracy of the thermister.

Patient's core temperature is not reduced.

□ Calibrate the thermister to ensure that the temperature reading of the thermister is accurate.

□ Check the master temperature control to see what limits are set. May need to decrease lower limit. Do not set below 30° C without checking with physician.

□ Place a top cooling pad on patient to provide a greater body surface area in contact with pads.

□ Place a blanket over the top pad to insulate and provide a more effective and rapid control of temperature.

□ Attach small cooling pads to the extra connections on the machine to provide cold areas to body where the arteries are close to the surface, such as groin, axilla, and neck.

Skin does not remain free of injury during use of the cooling blanket.

□ Make sure patient is turned every 30 minutes.

□ Lubricate skin with petroleum jelly to provide protection.

□ Wrap patient's hands and feet securely to prevent frostbite.

□ Massage bony prominences at least every hour.

□ Ensure that the master control temperature is not set too low.

□ Chart changes in skin condition.

Cooling blanket does not function properly.

□ Check that plug is not disconnected from the outlet.

□ Check that the alcohol level is sufficient and that unit freezing has not occurred.

□ Check that the thermister probe is properly connected.

□ Check that the cool limit on the pad is not set too high.

□ Check that there is no constriction through pads or tubing.

## TERMINOLOGY

**Adipose:** fatty; pertaining to fat.

**Ambient air temperature:** the temperature of the air surrounding a person.

**Antipyretic:** an agent that reduces febrile temperatures.

**Brown adipose tissue:** a special lipid cell that is capable of producing heat through chemical processes; brown fat.

**Circadian biorhythms:** physiologic rhythms that run a full cycle in 24 hours. The high temperature is usually experienced in late afternoon, and the low in the early morning. Temperature can vary up to 2° F.

**Compress:** a pad of cloth applied firmly to a part of the body; compress may be dry or wet, cold or warm.

**Conduction:** transfer of heat by direct contact through fluids or solids or any suitable substance.

**Constriction:** a narrowing or closing in.

**Continuous fever:** consistently elevated fever

**Convection:** transfer of heat by air.

**Crisis:** sudden drop in fever to a normal value.

**Cyanosis:** bluish coloring of the skin and the mucous membrane due to decreased oxygenation.

**Dermatitis:** inflammation of skin evidenced by itching, redness, and skin lesions.

**Diaphoresis:** an excessive amount of perspiration, as when a person's skin is moist and perspiring.

**Erythema:** increased reddish color of the skin due to vasodilatation of capillaries.

**Euthermia:** a normal body temperature.

**Evaporation:** to convert from a liquid or solid state to a gaseous state.

**Fastigium:** the course of a fever, wherein the body attempts to give off heat. The person feels flushed, sweaty, and lethargic.

**Flush:** redness of the skin, as in a blush, usually associated with an elevated temperature. The face and neck are more likely to be affected.

**Hyperemia:** increased blood supply to an area.

**Hyperthermia:** a body temperature much higher than normal.

**Hypothermia:** a body temperature lower than normal.

**Insulator:** substance that is a poor conductor or a nonconductor of heat; a substance that helps prevent the escape or entrance of radiant heat.

**Intermittent fever:** alternates between normal and fever.

**Lysis:** slow or gradual drop to normal temperature.

**Mottling:** blue-gray to purplish blotches seen usually peripherally; it is usually the result of peripheral vasoconstriction.

**Nonshivering thermogenesis:** production of body heat by chemical processes, and not involving the muscle co-contraction (shivering) process.

**Onset:** phase of fever where chills and shivers are experienced.

**Pallor:** loss of reddish hue due to superficial vasoconstriction produced by sympathetic stimulation.

**Palpitation:** rapid, violent, or throbbing pulsation, as of the heart.

**Periphery:** outer part or surface of a body.

**Physiologic:** concerning body function.

**Pyrexia (terminology associated with fever):** a disorder of the thermoregulation where the "set point" is displaced upward and the body actively seeks to raise its temperature; "true fever" temperature.

**Radiation:** transfer of energy (heat) in the form of waves.

**Remittent fever:** alternates between pyrexia and several degrees above normal.

**Resolution:** period when the temperature begins to drop.

**Shivering:** the tremoring of the body usually in response to coolness. It is the result of reflex action coordinated by the hypothalamus.

**Shivering thermogenesis:** production of body heat by shivering or muscle contraction (tremors).

**Sitz bath:** bath to sit in with water above the hips.

**Thermogenesis:** heat production by the body.

**Vaso-constriction:** a narrowing of blood vessels.

**Vasomotor:** pertaining to nerves having muscular control of the blood vessel walls.

*Chapter* **22**

# *Wound Care*

## LEARNING OBJECTIVES

Define the terms second intention and primary healing.

Discuss four factors that affect wound healing.

State two complications associated with wound healing.

Describe the four phases of wound healing.

Write three nursing diagnoses that relate to patients requiring wound care.

Perform the steps of a surgical hand scrub.

Demonstrate proper gloving technique.

Demonstrate removal of sterile supplies from containers.

Prepare a sterile field using sterile technique.

List four objectives for wound care.

Compare and contrast the difference between cleansing a clean and a dirty wound.

Outline the steps in irrigating a wound.

Demonstrate the steps in applying a sterile dressing.

Describe the procedure for cleansing around a drain site.

Outline the steps in irrigating a wound.

State three potential problems in wound care and at least one suggested solution for each problem.

Outline the pertinent data which is included in wound care charting.

Describe the steps in emptying a Hemovac drain.

Outline the procedure for changing wet-to-dry dressings.

Explain the assessment data needed when identifying the presence of a decubitus ulcer.

Describe the four stages of decubitus ulcers.

Compare and contrast the advantage of using Op-Site and Duoderm as a treatment for a decubitus ulcer.

## WOUND HEALING

**Primary Healing** Primary healing, or healing by first intention, is the simplest form of healing. A minimum of tissue damage and tissue reaction occurs when the edges of an incision are brought together to assist in the healing process.

Once the wound closes, a blood clot forms. Then the blood vessels constrict and retract, controlling the bleeding in the smaller vessels. The aggregation of platelets forms clots in the smaller arterioles and capillaries and the release of various enzymes activates several healing cycles of increased permeability; increased number of platelets; increased adhesions; and increased local stasis.

Soon after the formation of the clot, an inflammatory reaction develops at the incision site. Leukocytes enter the clot and begin destroying it by triggering the release of proteolytic enzymes. At the same time, granulation is initiated through the entry of fibroblasts and endothelial cells. Within several days granulated tissue matures and begins to form a scar.

As the scar develops, surface epithelium at the edges of the incision begin to regenerate. The epithelium takes on the appearance of the adjacent skin within a few days and a thin, almost invisible, line results.

**Second Intention** Second intention, or healing by granulation, occurs when wound edges cannot be brought together because of the extent or type of wound. The wound is left open to heal spontaneously. In this process a greater amount of granulation tissue is formed, and a larger scar results because of the necessity for more epithelial regeneration. Healing time is in direct proportion to the extent and depth of the wound. Because of the longer healing time and increased scar formation of healing by second intention, the primary healing method is preferred.

**Healing by Means of Suture Placement**   Sutures are generally placed in surgical wounds to hold the edges of an incision together until epithelial regeneration occurs. Regeneration usually takes seven to ten days. When sutures are removed, only half the sutures (every other suture) should be removed at one time so that the suture line can be observed for any dehiscence which could occur when stress is placed on the surgical site. If the sutures are removed all at once, instruct the patient to splint the wound when coughing or straining for at least two to three days following suture removal. Abdominal binders may be applied after suture removal to prevent complications of wound dehiscence or evisceration.

**Factors Affecting Wound Healing**   Deficient blood supply to the affected area can result in poor wound healing. Nutrition-related conditions, such as anemia, diabetes, or obesity, will also impair wound healing. Lack of vitamin C, low levels of the essential amino acid methionine, and high doses of corticosteroids delay wound healing. Infection, improper alignment of wound edges, rough handling, and unnecessary dressing changes can all retard the healing process.

**Complications Associated with Wound Healing**   One complication that may occur after wound healing has seemed to progress satisfactorily is adhesions. Adhesions frequently form in the peritoneal cavity after abdominal surgery and can either constrict or fold around the intestines.

Frequently patients are admitted to the hospital with incisional strangulated internal hernias that may even be gangrenous. Other complications are surgical or incisional hernias which may occur when the intraperitoneal pressure is such that it pushes against the scar tissue and causes a hernia (or outpouching) through the incision.

Contractures, formed as a result of a shortening of scar tissue, can decrease mobility and joint movement. Contractures caused by incisional scars are far less common than those caused by scar tissue from burns.

Excessive collagen formation results in the formation of a keloid, a complication that does not present a serious problem with body function; however, it generally causes an altered self-image if the keloid is large or in a prominent place on the body.

## WOUND INFECTIONS

The clinical symptoms of wound infections generally begin in 36 to 48 hours postoperatively or following injury. When the patient's temperature and pulse rate increase, an associated tachypnea occurs. As the inflammatory process proceeds, the wound becomes progressively more tender and edematous. Erythema surrounds the edges of the wound unless the infection is in the deeper tissues. An absence of local signs of infection does not necessarily mean that deep wound infections are not present.

Several microorganisms are responsible for the majority of wound infections. *Staphylococcus aureus* is still a major cause of postoperative infection. *Escherichia coli*, *Streptococcus pyogenes*, *Proteus vulgaris*, *Aerobacter aerogenes*, and *Pseudomonas aeruginosa* are also closely associated with wound infection. Antimicrobial agents themselves can promote infection by increasing the susceptibility of patients to colonization with nosocomial microflora, they can also select and concentrate antibiotic-resistant organisms on or in the host.

Maintaining strict asepsis during dressing changes assists in preventing wound infections. Using sterile equipment, including gloves, is the first barrier against infection. A mask should be worn during dressing changes if the patient is at risk for developing an infection. Nurses need to keep hair off their faces and tied back and to avoid coughing or sneezing when caring for a patient with an open wound. In fact, health team members who are not healthy should not be providing direct patient care.

When wounds become grossly infected or are extensive in nature, the physician may order wound irrigations. Irrigating solutions vary from normal saline solution to antibiotic solutions.

Each hospital has its own protocol for wound irrigation and you should become familiar with the procedure. This chapter presents one method of wound irrigation that is helpful in most clinical situations.

**Wound Cultures**   Exudate, or purulent drainage, from infected wounds can contain a variety of aerobic and anaerobic microorganisms. In the majority of wound infections the causative agent is usually found in the upper respiratory tract, gastrointestinal tract, and genitourinary tract. When these organisms invade other body parts, they can cause severe infections and sometimes death.

The best specimen for culture is one from the exudate itself, excised tissue, or from the discharge found on wound dressings. If swabs are used to obtain the culture, they should be serum-coated and sterile. At least three swabs should be used.

**Decubitus Ulcers**   Decubitus ulcers are considered a form of wound infection. Once skin breakdown occurs it is difficult to avoid bacterial invasion and secondary infection. Management of the decubitus ulcer begins on admission with a thorough assessment. Emphasis is placed on observing bony prominences and reddened areas of the skin.

The primary nursing objective is to prevent additional areas of breakdown and/or to heal the already formed ulcer. Patients with diabetes, vascular disease, or who are immobilized, comatose, dehydrated or those with poor nutrition are prone to develop decubitus ulcers.

Preventative steps need to begin on admission. Keeping the bed dry and wrinkle-free, providing adequate fluids and a balanced diet high in protein are essential components of care. In addition, the use of pressure-relieving devices, turning every two hours and thorough assessment of the skin to detect reddened areas or impaired skin integrity must be an integral part of the care for any high risk patient. Immediate institution of decubitus care and follow-up care on all shifts is mandatory if the ulcer is to heal. Decubitus ulcers often look worse when treatment begins due to the debriding and sluffing of tissue in the wound. Healing of a stage three or four decubitus ulcer may take months.

While treatment procedures and products have changed over the years, the need for uniformity and consistency of care has remained the same. The newest treatment for decubitus ulcers centers on creating a moist wound environment that encourages debridement and granulation. These barriers create a membrane that allows for air exchange but maintains body fluid in the wound. They draw the protein and antibodies into the wound and promote granulation. A major advantage in using this treatment is that it is the same regardless of the stage of the ulcer. Several commercial preparations are available including: Op-Site; Ensure; Tegaderm; Duoderm; Vergilon; Barrier film and Bio-occlusive dressings.

The following nursing diagnoses may be appropriate to include in a Patient Care Plan when the components are related to the patient requiring wound care.

## NURSING DIAGNOSES

| Nursing Diagnosis (Potential) | Defining Characteristic; Etiology (Examples) |
|---|---|
| ☐ Comfort, Alteration in: Pain, *related to* | Extreme tissue irritation, e.g., extensive dressing changes (burns). |
| ☐ Self-Concept, Disturbance in: Body Image, *related to* | Perceived change in body appearance, e.g., open lesion, potential scarring. |
| ☐ Skin Integrity, Impairment of, *related to* | Interruption in skin integrity, e.g., surgical incision. |
| | Altered circulation and/or pressure on a bony prominence, e.g., long-term bedrest. |
| | Poor protein intake, e.g., lack of adherence to diet. |
| ☐ Tissue Perfusion, Alteration in, *related to* | Altered blood supply, e.g., constrictive dressings. |

---

## UNIT ONE    PREVENTION OF INFECTION

### NURSING PROCESS DATA

**ASSESSMENT**    *Data Base*

Identify patients at risk for infection.

Identify length of time patient remained in surgery (the more hours in surgery the more patient is at risk for infection).

Identify the components necessary to prevent infection for individual patients.

Assess need for sterile technique compliance in patient care.

> **Clinical Alert**
> Admission histories are an important adjunct in identifying potentially contagious patients as they enter the hospital. Initiation of appropriate isolation techniques needs to begin immediately.

**PLANNING**    *Objectives*

To prevent patients with impaired resistance from becoming infected.

To prevent microorganisms from entering the wound.

To provide a sterile working field for dressing changes.

### IMPLEMENTATION  *Procedures*

Completing a Surgical Hand Scrub

Using Sterile Gloves

Removing Sterile Supplies from Container

Using Sterile Forceps

Pouring from a Sterile Container

Preparing a Sterile Field

### EVALUATION  *Expected Outcomes*

Infection is prevented in patients with impaired resistance.

Sterile technique is maintained throughout wound care.

Sterile field is set up appropriately.

## COMPLETING A SURGICAL HAND SCRUB

### Equipment

Plastic or orangewood stick

Antiseptic solution (hexachlorophene or chlorhexidine)

Sterile towel

### Procedure

1. Turn on water using foot or knee pedal or hand lever.
2. Wet your hands thoroughly.
3. With your arms held up in front of you, begin to scrub by cleaning your fingernails with a plastic or orangewood stick.
4. Next, scrub your hands for four to five minutes with either an iodophor, hexachlorophene, or chlorhexidine antiseptic.
   a. Scrub may be done using brush or friction of hands.
   b. Start at fingertips and with circular motion work around each finger and between each finger.
   c. Move to back of hand and use circular motion with scrub.
   d. Move to palm of hand, wrist and then up arm to elbow continuing with circular scrubbing motion.
   e. Placing arms under water faucet, keep fingertips pointed upward and rinse thoroughly with water flowing down toward elbows. **Rationale:** This method keeps fingers and hands free of contamination.
5. Dry your hands with a sterile towel starting at the fingertips and moving toward the elbows.
6. If hand levers are used to control water flow, turn faucets off with sterile towel used for drying hands. Do not touch faucet or sink with hands. **Rationale:** Contamination of hands occurs if objects are touched after handwashing.

## USING STERILE GLOVES

### Equipment

Packaged sterile gloves

### Procedure

1. Wash and dry your hands.
2. Open glove wrapper, keeping both package and gloves sterile. Open wrapper from the middle of the package outward.
3. With your nondominant hand, remove the first glove by grasping the section that has a folded edge. Lift the glove up and away from the wrap-

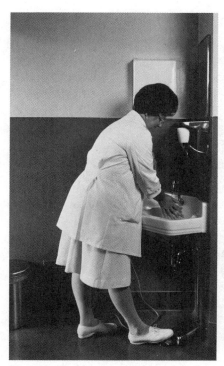

Wash hands using foot pedals and dry thoroughly before putting on sterile gloves.

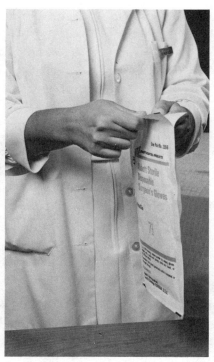

Grasp the two upper edges at the red mark of the package and pull laterally.

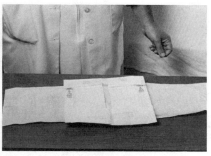

Place the glove package on a clean, flat working area and then open wrapper.

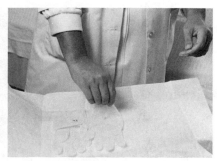

Pick up sterile glove by rolled edge; do not touch outer surface to maintain sterility.

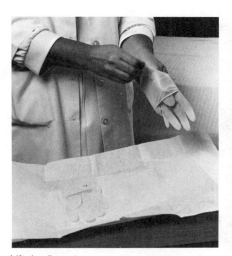

Lift the first glove up and away from sterile package to prevent contamination.

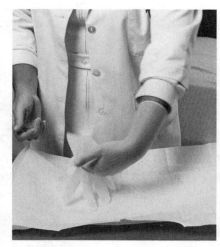

Pick up second glove by placing fingers under cuff and lifting away from wrapper.

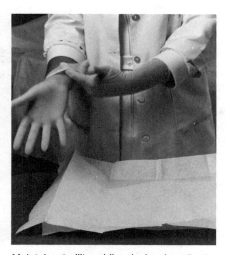

Maintain sterility while gloving by allowing only the sterile surfaces to touch.

per. Be careful not to touch the inside of the package or any part of the glove except the inner surface of the cuff.

4. Slip your dominant hand into the glove opening. Gently pull the glove into place with your nondominant hand, touching only the folded-up cuff. **Rationale:** Don't worry if you have difficulty easing your fingers all the way into the glove. After you have placed both gloves on your hands, you can move your fingers into place.

5. With your dominant, gloved hand, remove the other glove from the package, making sure you touch only the inside of the folded cuff. Lift this glove up and away from the wrapper.

6. Place your ungloved fingers into the new glove opening. Gently pull the glove over your hand as before.

7. Adjust both gloves, remembering to touch sterile surfaces with sterile surfaces.

8. Keep both sterile gloves in front of you above your waist level. **Rationale:** When you can see gloves at all times, you can prevent potential contamination.

## REMOVING STERILE SUPPLIES FROM CONTAINER

### Equipment

Sterile forceps

Sterile container with supplies

### Procedure

1. Gather necessary equipment.

2. Wash your hands.

3. Place closed sterile container on a table at appropriate working height.

4. Open sterile container by removing lid. **Rationale:** The under side of the lid is considered sterile; thus, if you must put lid down, invert it so that outer surface is touching table.

5. Grasp lid on top and, holding it above your waist, face lid downward. Do not move it around or tip upside-down. **Rationale:** This position allows fewer microorganisms to come in contact with the lid.

6. Remove supplies with sterile forceps, without touching the rim of the container. **Rationale:** The rim is considered unsterile when it has come in contact with the air.

7. Once sterile supplies have been removed, replace lid without touching outer surface. **Rationale:** Never return unused supplies to sterile container, as they are now considered to be contaminated.

## USING STERILE FORCEPS

### Equipment

Pickup forceps

Container with disinfectant

### Procedure

1. Wash your hands.

2. Lift forceps by the handles vertically from the container.

3. Do not allow tips to touch the container sides.

4. Keep tips pointed downward. **Rationale:** Solution from the tips could run to the unsterile area, then back to tips, thus contaminating them.

5. Hold tips above waist and table level.

6. Use forceps to transfer or arrange sterile items.

7. Replace forceps in container.

8. If forceps become contaminated, wash in soap and water, rinse and dry. Then follow hospital protocol for sterilization solution and procedure. Place forceps in a labeled container with date and time forceps will again be sterile, or autoclave before replacing in container.

## POURING FROM A STERILE CONTAINER

### Equipment

Sterile container

Nonsterile container

Sterile liquid

### Procedure

1. Wash your hands.

2. Gather equipment.

3. Open sterile container according to procedure.

4. Place container on firm surface.

5. Take cap off the bottle and invert the cap before laying on firm surface. **Rationale:** This will keep the cap sterile.

6. Hold the bottle with the label facing up.

7. Pour a small amount of liquid into a nonsterile container. **Rationale:** This action cleans the lip of the bottle.

8. Pour the liquid into the sterile container while keeping the label facing up and not touching the container with the bottle. Do not reach over a sterile field if the container has been placed on one.

9. Replace the cap if liquid remains in the bottle. If total contents have been used dispose of bottle in trash.

10. Replace partially-filled bottle to storage area if it is to be reused.

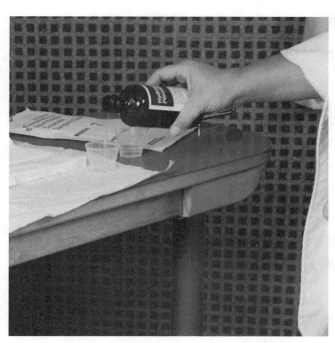

Pour liquids by placing container close to the edge of the working area, and prevent bottle from touching container.

## PREPARING A STERILE FIELD

### Equipment

Commercially prepared sterile tray for dressing change

Antiseptic cleansing solution, as ordered

If commercial tray not available, gather the following equipment:
    Two packages of sterile towels
    Number and type of dressings required for dressing change
    Tape
    Container for antiseptic solution
    Disposable paper bag for soiled dressings
    Transfer forceps if used in facility

---

**Clinical Alert**

The primary purpose for performing interventions associated with infection control is to establish and maintain asepsis so that infection can be prevented.

---

### Preparation

1. Check physician's orders and Patient Care Plan.
2. Gather equipment from supply area.

3. Clean off overbed table.
4. Place commercial package or tray on overbed table or on another surface close to table.

### Procedure

1. Wash your hands, using surgical aseptic techniques.

2. Place sterile towel packages on overbed table or on another surface close to the table. Place packages so that first wrapper edge can be opened away from the sterile area. **Rationale:** This prevents contamination from crossing over a sterile field.

3. Using both hands, pick up the two side edges of the first wrapper and open them away from the middle of the sterile field.

4. Unfold the last edge toward you, without touching the wrapper.

5. Using pickup forceps or gloved hands (or ungloved hands if allowed in the facility), pick up one edge of the sterile towel and move away from the table. Gently shake the towel away from the sterile area.

6. When the towel is open, use your other hand to pick up the two edges that are away from you.

7. Lower the towel onto the tray or bedside stand so the towel is furthest away from you. Then lay the towel down on the tray by bringing it toward you, covering the entire tray.

8. Repeat the same steps with a second sterile towel.

9. If solutions for cleansing the skin are required, place sterile medicine cups on the tray near one side.

10. Take the cap off the antiseptic bottle.

11. Pour a small amount of solution into a container, not on the sterile field, keeping the label in uppermost position. **Rationale:** This action will rinse contaminated particles from the lip of the bottle.

12. Pour the antiseptic solution, from the side of the sterile field, directly into the medicine cup.

13. Open sterile packages of dressings and place on sterile surface.
    *Commercially prepared packages:*
    a. Open package at designated end by pulling edges apart and downward to expose contents.
    b. Grasp the edges of the two sides of the pack-

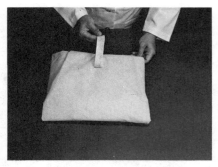

Check sterilization tape to ensure that package has been autoclaved properly.

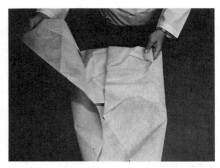

Open sterile package away from sterile field to prevent crossing over the sterile field.

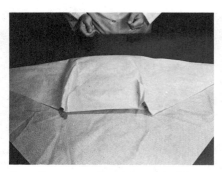

Open the corner closest to you last to prevent reaching over the sterile field.

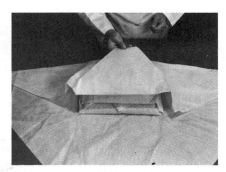

Move away from the sterile field as the package is opened to maintain sterility.

age and invert the package over the edge of the sterile field. Allow the contents to drop onto the sterile field.

c. Repeat procedure for each item to be placed on sterile field.

*Hospital wrapped packages:*

a. Hold package in your hand and securely grasp one edge.

b. Open package wrapper by allowing edges to drop down, away from package.

c. Grasp the edges of the wrapper with your free hand and pull them toward your wrist, thus exposing the sterile contents.

d. Gently drop the contents on the sterile field. **Rationale:** Touching the sterile field with the wrapper will contaminate it.

e. Repeat procedure for each item to be placed on the sterile field.

14. If sterile tray is not to be used immediately, cover with sterile towels.

a. Open sterile towel package by opening wrapper away from you so that you do not cross over a sterile field.

b. Pick up one towel at the edge and open towel by moving yourself away from the sterile field and allowing towel to fall open.

c. Grasp corner of towel opposite to one you are holding. Keep towel from touching contaminated areas.

d. Place towel over sterile field starting at edge nearest you. Lay the towel down without touching the tray with your hand. Move the towel across the tray toward the opposite edge.

e. Repeat procedure with second sterile towel.

---

**Guidelines for Sterile Field**

Never turn your back on a sterile field

Avoid talking, coughing, sneezing, or reaching across a sterile field

Keep sterile objects above waist level

Do not spill solutions on the sterile field

Open all sterile packages away from the sterile field to prevent crossover and contamination

---

**CHARTING** *for Prevention of Infection*

☐ Type and amount of sterile dressings used

☐ Antiseptic solution used

## CLINICAL PROBLEM SOLVING

| Potential Problem | Suggested Solution |
|---|---|
| Hole develops in glove while performing sterile technique. | ☐ Discard gloves and replace with sterile gloves. |
| | ☐ Examine hands for cuts if hole caused by sharp object. |
| | ☐ If hands are cut, scrub hands and replace sterile gloves. |
| Sterile field becomes wet or damp. | ☐ Discard supplies on sterile field. |
| | ☐ Set up new sterile field. |
| Sterile transfer forceps not available. | ☐ Use sterile gloves to transfer articles. |
| | ☐ Open packages and drop contents on sterile field following step 13 in *Preparing A Sterile Field*. |

# UNIT TWO   WOUND CARE

## NURSING PROCESS DATA

### ASSESSMENT   *Data Base*

Identify type of dressing needed, e.g., occlusive, non-occlusive, nonadhering, wet-dry, medicated.

Assess level of pain associated with wound care and dressing change.

Determine if infection is present.

Assess for function of Hemovac suction.

Assess for extent of wound healing.

Assess need for support with scultetus binder.

### PLANNING   *Objectives*

To promote wound granulation and healing.

To prevent microorganisms from entering the wound.

To decrease the presence of purulent wound drainage.

To maintain sterility during a dressing change.

To maintain patency of Hemovac suction.

To absorb fluid and provide a dry environment.

To immobilize and support a wound.

To assist in removal of necrotic tissue.

To apply medication to wound.

### IMPLEMENTATION   *Procedures*

Changing a Sterile Dressing

Caring for a Wound with Drain

Applying a Scultetus Binder

Maintaining Hemovac Suction

Irrigating Wounds

**EVALUATION** *Expected Outcomes*

Granulation takes place and healing occurs.

Sterility is maintained during dressing change.

Drain is advanced appropriately.

Hemovac suction remains patent.

Scultetus binder keeps dressing in place and supports abdomen.

## CHANGING A STERILE DRESSING

### Equipment

Sterile, prepackaged dressing(s) as needed

Tape; micropore, paper, or Montgomery tie tapes

Disposable suture removal kit for disposable scissors and forceps

Sterile gloves

Clean gloves

Cleansing solution as ordered, e.g., Betadine, hydrogen peroxide, normal saline

Plastic bag

### Preparation

1. Check physician's orders and Patient Care Plan.
2. Wash your hands.
3. Gather equipment.
4. Provide privacy.
5. Identify the patient and explain procedure.
6. Clean off overbed table.
7. Place sterile supplies on the overbed table.
8. Raise bed to HIGH position and lower side rails on working side of bed.
9. Place bag for soiled dressings near wound site. Expose wound area.
10. Open sterile packages and place on overbed table. Arrange packages to ensure that you don't cross over the sterile field when using dressings. **Rationale:** Commercially prepared sterile packages can be opened and used for the sterile field; the inside of the package is sterile.

### Procedure

1. Remove tape slowly by pulling tape toward the wound. **Rationale:** Pulling toward the wound decreases the pain of tape removal by not putting pressure on the incision line.
2. Put on clean gloves.
3. Remove soiled dressings and place in bag for disposal. Soaking dressings that are dried to skin or incision with sterile normal saline will prevent tissue damage and pain when dressings are removed.
4. Obtain wound culture if ordered.
5. Remove clean gloves and discard into plastic bag.
6. Bring overbed table close to working area.
7. Open cleansing solution and pour over dressings to be used for cleansing the wound.
8. Cut tape into appropriate length strips and place on edge of overbed table.
9. Put on sterile gloves.
10. Cleanse wound. When cleansing an area, always start at the cleanest area and work away from that area. Never return to an area you have previously cleaned.
11. Use sterile forceps to hold the gauze pads while cleansing the wound. **Rationale:** This action prevents contamination of your hands during cleansing.
12. If a drain is present, cleanse under the drain and around the site with a 4 × 4 gauze pad and cleansing solution.
13. Place several gauze pads under the drain.
14. Place several 4 × 4 gauze pads over the wound. Cover with an ABD pad if necessary, remove

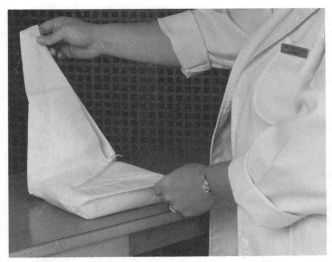

Open the sterile package by not crossing over the sterile field.

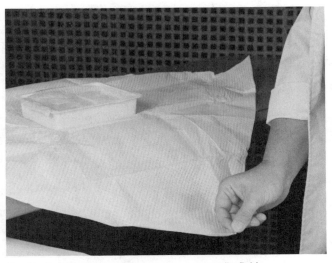

Use the inside of the package cover as a sterile field.

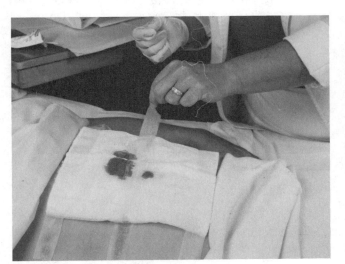

Gently remove tape by pulling toward the wound.

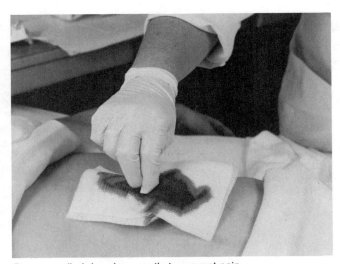

Remove soiled dressings gently to prevent pain.

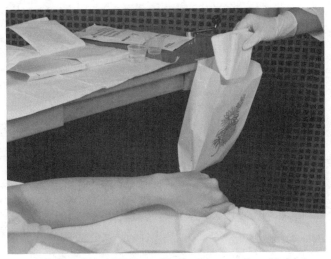

Place soiled dressing in disposable bag to prevent contamination.

*Clean wound:* no purulent drainage
a. Cleanse the wound with a 4 × 4 gauze pad.
b. Start at the incision and work outward in a circular motion.
c. Discard the pad after each stroke.

*Dirty wound:* purulent drainage
a. Cleanse the wound with a 4 × 4 gauze pad.
b. Start at the outer margin and work inward in a circular motion.
c. Place the soiled pad in a plastic bag.

gloves and tape securely. (Montgomery straps may be used if frequent dressing changes are required or the patient has sensitive skin). **Rationale:** Once a dressing has been placed over the

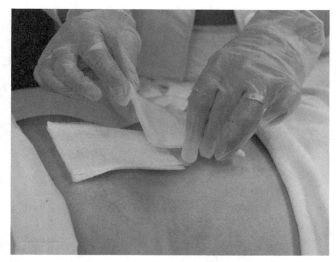

Place several gauze pads over incision, being careful not to readjust them once they have been placed.

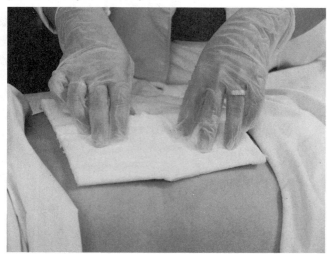

Cover the gauze dressings with ABD pads in sufficient numbers to absorb drainage from the wound.

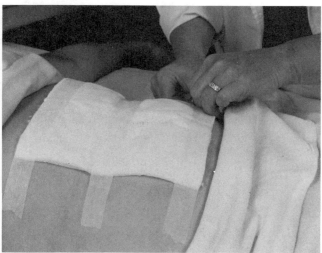

Take off gloves and tape dressings securely with nonallergenic tape to maintain placement of dressings.

wound it is not to be moved and readjusted as microorganisms from the skin could be introduced into the wound.

15. Cover patient.
16. Close the plastic bag and dispose of bag as isolation material.
17. Wash your hands thoroughly.
18. Check with patient to see that he is comfortable before leaving room.
19. Lower the bed and raise the side rail.

---

**Clinical Alert**

☐ Frequent dressing changes are preferable to reinforcing the same dressing.
☐ Avoid pooling of excessive drainage under saturated dressing. Pools of drainage increase the number of organisms that come in contact with the suture line.

---

## CARING FOR A WOUND WITH DRAIN

### Equipment

Same items as for Changing a Sterile Dressing

Sterile cotton applicators

Sterile safety pin

ABD dressings

Sterile scissors

Protective skin covering, e.g., petroleum jelly

### Preparation

1. Check physician's orders and Patient Care Plan.
2. Wash your hands.
3. Gather equipment.
4. Provide privacy.
5. Identify patient and explain procedure.
6. Clean off overbed table.
7. Raise bed to HIGH position and lower side rails on working side of bed.
8. Place plastic bag for soiled dressings on bed near wound site.
9. Open sterile packages and place on overbed table.

### Procedure

1. Remove tape from patient's skin by pulling *toward* the incision.

2. Put on clean gloves.

3. Remove soiled dressing.

4. Discard gloves and dressings into plastic bag.

5. Observe wound closely for signs of infection or healing. Put on sterile gloves.

6. If pin on the Penrose drain is crusted, replace it with a sterile pin. Be careful not to dislodge drain or suction tubing.

7. Using cotton applicators or gauze pads, cleanse drain site with cleansing solution and then saline.

8. Start cleansing at drain site, moving in a circular motion toward the periphery.

9. Discard applicators in plastic bag.

10. Advance drain if ordered:
    a. Using sterile forceps, pull drain out of wound the ordered number of centimeters.
    b. Reposition the safety pin so it is at the level of the skin. **Rationale:** The pin prevents the drain from slipping back into the wound.
    c. Cut off the excess tubing with sterile scissors. Leave at least two inches of tubing on the outside.

11. Apply protective covering, such as petroleum jelly, to the skin. **Rationale:** Drainage from the wound contains enzymes and secretions which cause severe skin breakdown.

12. Place several 4 × 4 dressings around the drain.

13. Apply gauze pad with a precut slit under the drain site.

14. Apply dry, sterile gauze pads over drain.

15. Apply ABD pads over sterile gauze.

16. Remove gloves and dispose of them in refuse bag.

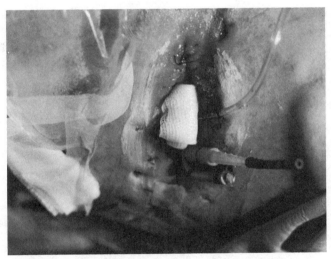

Drains are often inserted in open wounds to prevent the accumulation of secretions and exudate.

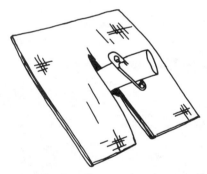

Place a pre-cut sterile 4″ × 4″ gauze dressing around the drain site to prevent skin excoriation.

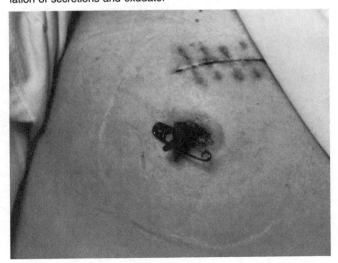

Safety pins are inserted into penrose drains to prevent the drains from slipping back into the wound.

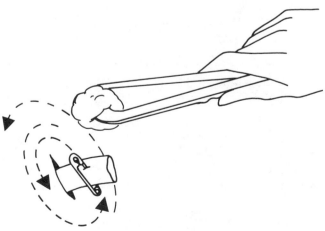

Cleanse the drain site; using a circular motion move from the inside to the periphery of the wound.

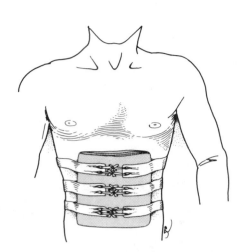

Montgomery straps are used when frequent dressing changes are needed to prevent skin irritation from tape removal.

17. Tape dressing or retie Montgomery straps.

18. Remove bag with soiled dressing from room.

19. Wash your hands thoroughly.

20. Position patient for comfort.

21. Lower bed and raise side rail.

## APPLYING A SCULTETUS BINDER

### Equipment

Scultetus binder

Safety pin

### Procedure

1. Obtain binder from appropriate department. Most facilities now use commercial velcro binders or supports in place of the scultetus binder.

2. Explain use of the binder to the patient.

3. Place the patient on his or her back.

4. Examine the binder to ensure that the tails are pointing toward the top of the abdomen.

5. Ask patient to raise hips, and then slide the binder under patient's hips at about the top of pubic area.

6. Start the binder application by bringing the bottom tails up toward the waist to anchor the binder.

7. For each successive tail, overlap the preceding tail by at least 1 inch, using a spiral effect.

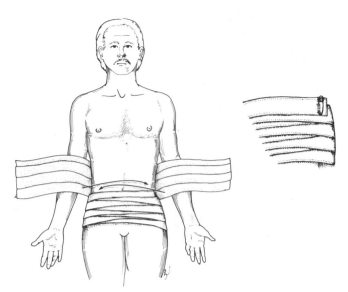

Scultetus binders are frequently used to hold bulky dressings in place or provide abdominal support.

8. Pull each tail tightly to the side and maintain pressure with your hand while you bring the other tail across. Alternate sides of the binder as you move each tail upward toward the patient's waist.

9. Secure the top of the binder with a safety pin.

10. Assess patient's ability to move freely, take in a deep breath, and feel secure pressure over abdominal incision or fundal area.

11. Assess effectiveness of binder every four hours and rewrap every eight hours. Many patients use this binder only when ambulating.

## MAINTAINING HEMOVAC SUCTION

### Equipment

Graduate for measuring drainage

I & O bedside record

Absorbent pad

---

**Clinical Alert**

A Jackson-Pratt catheter or similar drainage system is connected to a drainage system or suction. This prevents the accumulation of secretions on the skin.

---

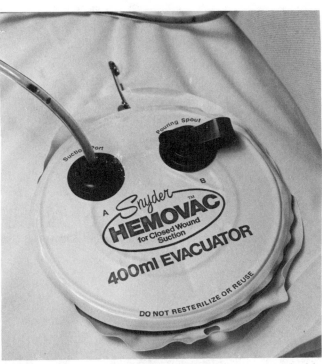

Hemovac suction container should always be kept on the bed in clear view for easy assessment.

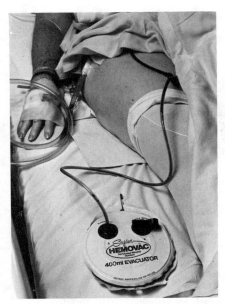

Empty drainage, compress evacuator and replace plug.

## Preparation

1. Check physician's orders and Patient Care Plan.
2. Bring graduate to bedside.
3. Identify patient and explain procedure, giving patient time to ask questions.
4. Provide for comfort and privacy.
5. Wash your hands thoroughly.
6. Elevate bed to workable height.

## Procedure

1. Expose catheter insertion site while keeping patient draped. Place Hemovac on absorbent pad.
2. Examine pump and catheter for patency, seal, and stability. If catheter occluded, notify physician.
3. Remove Hemovac plug, which is labeled "Pouring Spout."
4. Pour drainage into graduate.
5. Compress the Hemovac by pushing the top and bottom together with your hands.
6. Hold pump tightly compressed and reinsert plug to reestablish closed drainage system.

7. Position catheter and evacuator on bed.
8. Measure and record amount of drainage.
9. Examine drainage for color, consistency, and odor.
10. Discard drainage, rinse container, and wash hands.
11. Send culture specimen to laboratory if ordered.
12. Make patient comfortable and lower bed.
13. Compress evacuator at least every four hours to provide suction. Measure drainage at least every 8 hours.

## IRRIGATING WOUNDS

### Equipment

Sterile irrigation solution at 90° to 95° F

Sterile irrigating set
  or
Sterile Robinson catheter

Sterile asepto syringe

Sterile graduate

Sterile basin

Absorbent pad

Sterile gloves

Equipment for dressing change

### Preparation

1. Check physician's orders and Patient Care Plan.
2. Gather irrigation equipment and dressing material.
3. Check patient's identaband.
4. Assemble equipment.
5. Explain procedure to patient and answer any questions.
6. Wash your hands thoroughly.
7. Open sterile packages on the overbed table as with dressing change.
8. Pour sterile irrigating solution into graduate.

### Procedure

1. Place absorbent pads under the patient. Place a bath blanket under absorbent pads when irrigating a large wound. The blanket will absorb any spilled irrigation solution.
2. Position patient so that solution will flow from wound to basin.
3. Put on clean gloves.
4. Remove and discard used dressing.
5. Remove gloves and discard into plastic bag.
6. Place bedside stand near working area with all packages open.
7. Put on sterile gloves following correct procedure.
8. Inspect area surrounding wound for redness, tissue integrity, and signs of granulating tissue.
9. Gently place Robinson catheter into uppermost area of wound to prevent tissue trauma. (For large wounds, position Robinson catheter in several areas of the wound.)
10. Attach barrel of asepto syringe to Robinson catheter.
11. Place sterile basin under wound area.
12. Pour room temperature irrigating solution from sterile graduate into asepto syringe.
13. Allow irrigating solution to flow over wound so that all organisms, tissue debris, and drainage are washed into basin. Cleanse from cleanest to dirtiest area of wound if possible.

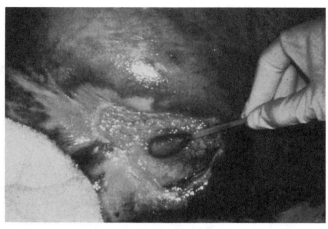

Cleansing of the wound site aids in removing the exudate and thus promotes wound healing.

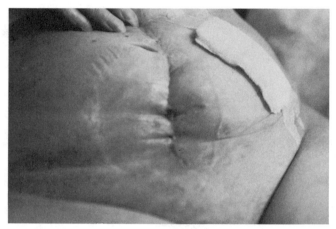

Wound irrigations are frequently used in this type of wound to aid in the removal of excretions.

14. Repeat until all irrigation solution has been used.
15. After the irrigation, cleanse patient's skin and dry the surrounding area.
16. Apply sterile dressing.
17. Dispose of equipment according to isolation protocol, and obtain fresh supplies for next irrigation.
18. Check to see that patient is comfortable before leaving the room.
19. Lower bed and raise side rails.
20. Wash your hands.

### CHARTING *for Wound Care*

☐ Observation of wound site, including amount, color, and odor of drainage, and appearance of suture site

- ☐ Observation of granulating tissue and redness
- ☐ Pertinent observations concerning patient's tolerance of procedure
- ☐ Observation of skin condition around incision site
- ☐ Changes in vital signs that indicate possible infection

- ☐ Type of dressing applied; scultetus binder, if used
- ☐ Observations on wound irrigation
- ☐ Type and amount of irrigation solutions used
- ☐ Unusual tension on sutures if present
- ☐ Amount and color of hemovac drainage

## CLINICAL PROBLEM SOLVING

**Potential Problems**

**Suggested Solutions**

Wound becomes infected with different microorganisms.

- ☐ Notify physician about changes in color and/or odor of drainage.
- ☐ Obtain culture and sensitivity if physician orders one.
- ☐ Wash your hands thoroughly after caring for patient to prevent the spread of infection.
- ☐ Pay strict attention to changing dressings.

Edges of wound split open (wound dehiscence).

- ☐ Place patient in supine position. Apply butterfly tape to wound edges. Cover opening with sterile dressings.
- ☐ Apply binder for abdominal incisions after obtaining order.
- ☐ Notify physician if signs of infection are present.
- ☐ Obtain culture of drainage if physician orders one.
- ☐ Observe patient for signs of shock. If patient in shock, notify physician immediately.
- ☐ Encourage high-protein diet.

Evisceration occurs (protrusion of bowel contents).

- ☐ Institute emergency measures. Place the patient in supine position. Cover bowel with sterile gauze moistened with sterile saline. Have certified IV nurse insert intravenous catheter and infuse normal saline. Reassure patient. Obtain vital signs, and treat for shock if present.
- ☐ After above measures are completed, notify physician and prepare patient for return to surgery.
- ☐ After surgical repair, notify dietician for diet change to increase protein and vitamin C in diet.
- ☐ Apply abdominal binder if ordered.

Wound hemorrhages.

- ☐ Outline area of blood on dressing with a pen and observe outline to see how quickly the bleeding spreads.
- ☐ If bleeding is excessive, notify the physician immediately.
- ☐ Apply pressure dressing to site if there is excessive bleeding.

| | |
|---|---|
| Leakage appears around adhesive-backed drainage bag. | ☐ Clean skin thoroughly with ivory soap and water. Apply stomahesive or hollihesive ⅛ to ¼ inch larger than drainage site. |
| Skin appears red and broken. | ☐ Clean area with ivory soap and water.<br>☐ Cut one sheet stomahesive or hollihesive ⅛ to ¼ inch larger than wound.<br>☐ Remove paper and apply thin ring of karaya or stomahesive paste.<br>☐ Center and apply to wound (the paste may cause mild burning for 5–10 minutes after application).<br>☐ Apply new pouch. |
| Skin is weeping with ulcerated areas. | ☐ Clean area with ivory soap and water. Dry thoroughly.<br>☐ Cut one sheet stomahesive or hollihesive ⅛ to ¼ inch larger than wound.<br>☐ Remove paper and apply thin ring of karaya or stomahesive paste.<br>☐ Apply a base to ulcerated areas.<br>☐ Center and apply stomahesive to wound (the paste may cause mild burning for 5–10 minutes after application).<br>☐ Apply new pouch and reinforce edges with tape and belt. |
| Wound is too extensive for application of a drainage bag or ABD pads cannot contain drainage. | ☐ Obtain stomahesive or hollihesive 8 × 8 sheets and cut on diagonal ⅛ to ¼ inch larger than wound.<br>☐ If larger barrier needed, stomahesive may be pieced together to form larger barrier reinforcing juncture points with karaya paste.<br>☐ A super adhesive pouch may then be applied.<br>☐ If dressings are used, they may be secured with Montgomery straps. |
| Scultetus binder is not effective in supporting incisional area. | ☐ Evaluate the effectiveness of the scultetus binder.<br>☐ Assess if the binder is properly positioned at the hip level and waist level to provide support.<br>☐ Ensure that tails are brought toward the waist in a spiral-like manner.<br>☐ Assess if the binder is too loose for the patient. The binder will loosen if the end of each tail is not tucked in. |
| Patient is too large for the scultetus binder. | ☐ Fold a drawsheet in half lengthwise and place under patient. Position the edges at the waist and pubic area.<br>☐ Pull tightly on the drawsheet and secure the edges with safety pins. |

# UNIT THREE    WET-TO-DRY DRESSINGS

## NURSING PROCESS DATA

### ASSESSMENT    *Data Base*

Assess wound edges for presence of granulation tissue.

Assess for changes in amount of drainage.

Assess if necrotic tissue is decreasing in amount.

Identify if solution is appropriate for wound care.

### PLANNING    *Objectives*

To promote wound healing by secondary intention.

To maintain an environment conducive to wound healing.

To provide the most appropriate solution and type of gauze for wound care.

To treat wound infections effectively.

To maintain sterile technique throughout procedure.

### IMPLEMENTATION    *Procedure*

Applying Wet-to-Dry Dressings

### EVALUATION    *Expected Outcomes*

Wound heals without complications.

Sterile technique is maintained throughout procedure.

## APPLYING WET-TO-DRY DRESSINGS

### Equipment

Sterile 4 × 8 noncotton gauze dressings

Sterile gloves

Nonsterile gloves

Tape

Plastic bag for contaminated dressings

Solution for dressings

Sterile receptacle (round basin or emesis basin)

Montgomery straps, if desired

### Preparation

1. Check physician's orders and Patient Care Plan

2. Wash hands.

3. Gather equipment.

4. Explain procedure to patient.

5. Provide privacy.

6. Raise bed to HIGH position and lower side rail nearest you.

7. Remove tape by pulling it toward the wound. **Rationale:** This action prevents injury to newly formed tissue.

8. Don nonsterile gloves.

9. Remove wound packing. **Rationale:** Touch only the gauze, not the wound itself, to prevent contamination of the wound.

10. Place soiled dressings in disposable bag.

11. Remove gloves and dispose of them in bag.

12. Wash your hands.

**Procedure**

1. Open packages of dressings and the sterile receptacle. Keep the receptacle on the sterile surface of the package.

2. Pour solution in the receptacle. **Rationale:** The type of solution used is determined by the condition of the wound and reason for dressings.

---

**Types of Solutions**

| | |
|---|---|
| Betadine: | Used for draining wounds, especially staphylococcus and aerobic bacteria; usually 10% solution. |
| Acetic acid: | Used for infected wounds with gram positive and gram negative organisms, especially pseudomonas; 0.25% solution. Observe for excoriation of skin surrounding wound. |
| Hydrogen peroxide: | Not as frequently used today; usually 3% solution. Observe for alterations in new tissue formation due to effervescent action. |
| Normal saline: | Used for clean wounds only; has no bactericidal properties. |

---

3. Don sterile gloves.

4. Place dressings into receptacle and thoroughly soak dressings with solution. **Rationale:** Dressings are noncotton material to prevent filaments sticking to the wound, which would encourage bacterial growth.

5. Wring out excessive moisture from dressings. **Rationale:** Dressings should be wet enough to dry in four to six hours.

6. Pack gauze in the wound, covering all exposed surfaces. Press gauze into depressions or cracks. **Rationale:** Necrotic tissue is more prevalent in these areas.

7. Unfold a dry, sterile 4 × 8 dressing into a single layer and place it on top of the wet dressings covering the entire area. **Rationale:** This procedure will absorb excess drainage.

---

**Clinical Alert**

The dressing should be thick and wet enough to dry between dressing changes. The moistened gauze traps necrotic material in the interstices as it dries. A thick, very wet layer of gauze will not dry out enough to trap debris and can lead to tissue breakdown and promote bacterial growth in the wet environment. A dry dressing cannot trap the debris adequately.

---

8. Place a folded 4 × 8 pad over the dressing to hold it in place.

9. Remove gloves and place in plastic bag.

10. Tape only the edges of the dressing. **Rationale:** An occlusive dressing will prevent air circulation and impede drying. Montgomery tapes may be used to prevent excessive skin irritation and damage due to frequent dressing changes.

11. Position patient for comfort. Lower bed and raise side rail to UP position.

12. Discard soiled material in appropriate container.

13. Wash your hands thoroughly.

14. Observe wound for excessive drainage between dressing changes. **Rationale:** Unless excessive drainage occurs, dressings are usually changed every six hours to provide adequate time for the dressing to dry between changes. The drying process promotes the entrapment of debris into the dressing.

15. Provide patient and/or family teaching regarding wound care, if appropriate.

**CHARTING** *for Wet-to-Dry Dressings*

☐ Condition of wound

☐ Solution used

☐ Number of dressings used

☐ Signs and symptoms indicative of wound infection

☐ Color, consistency, presence of odor, amount of drainage on soiled dressings

☐ Condition of skin surrounding wound

☐ Patient's reaction to procedure

## CLINICAL PROBLEM-SOLVING

| **Potential Problems** | **Suggested Solutions** |
|---|---|

Wound drainage increases.

☐ Decrease time between dressing changes. Change every 4 hours.
☐ Obtain order for culture and sensitivity to determine if different microorganisms are present or antibiotic medication is not sensitive to drug.

Dressings do not dry between dressing changes.

☐ Determine if the dressing has been taped to form an occlusive dressing that does not allow air circulation.
☐ Wring out solution from dressings (they are too moist).
☐ Make sure a dry dressing is placed over the wet dressings to absorb excess drainage.
☐ Consider alternating dry gauze dressings with wet dressings to help absorb excess drainage.

# UNIT FOUR   DECUBITUS ULCERS

## NURSING PROCESS DATA

### ASSESSMENT   *Data Base*

Assess stage of ulcer.

Identify if infection is associated with decubitus ulcer.

Evaluate effectiveness of ulcer treatment.

Assess healing process of the ulcer.

Assess other bony prominences for potential formation of decubiti.

Assess for presence of conditions that inhibit wound healing.

### PLANNING   *Objectives*

To identify the stage of the ulcer.

To provide appropriate treatment for specific ulcer stage.

To promote healing of established ulcer.

To prevent new ulcer formation.

To prevent spread of pathogens from ulcerated area.

### IMPLEMENTATION   *Procedures*

Applying Moist Wound Barriers

Using Skin Care Tray

Using Duoderm Dressing

**EVALUATION** *Expected Outcomes*

Stage of decubitus ulcer is accurately assessed.

Decubitus ulcer is treated effectively according to stage of ulcer formation.

---

### Stages of Decubitus Ulcers

Stage 1: Erythematous skin not relieved by stimulation or relief of pressure

Stage 2: Superficial tissue damage; involves excoriation, vesiculation, or skin breakdown

Stage 3: Ulceration involves the dermis (full thickness loss of skin); may or may not include subcutaneous tissue level; produces serosanguineous drainage

Stage 4: Ulceration deep into structures (full thickness loss of skin) with invasion of deep tissue and/or structures such as fascia, connective tissue, muscle or bone

## APPLYING MOIST WOUND BARRIERS

### Equipment

Soap and water

Op-Site kit (or other moist wound barrier kits)

Alcohol soaks

Sterile 4 × 4 gauze pads

Betadine prep pad

Scissors

Paper tape

### Preparation

1. Check physician's orders and Patient Care Plan.

2. Obtain Op-Site kit (all moist wound barriers are applied in the same manner). Op-Site can be used for any stage of ulcer formation. Choose appropriate size of Op-Site. Apply to flat surface for application. Coccyx area cannot be treated with Op-Site.

3. Wash your hands.

4. Explain procedure to patient.

5. Provide privacy.

### Procedure

1. Wash area around decubitus ulcer with soap and water.

2. Wash decubitus ulcer with sterile saline or hydrogen peroxide.

3. Apply Betadine prep pads over decubitus ulcer and surrounding tissue.

4. Rinse decubitus ulcer and surrounding area with sterile saline and dry thoroughly. **Rationale:** To ensure that dressing adheres to skin.

5. Apply plasticizing agent (skin prep, skin gel) over surrounding tissue. **Rationale:** Do not apply on ulcer because the agent contains alcohol, which will burn ulcer area.

6. Raise bed to HIGH position and lower side rail on working side of bed.

7. Loosen Op-Site from one side of backing paper.

8. "Walk on": start at one edge of site and gently lay the Op-Site down, keeping it free of wrinkles. Overlap wound at least 1 inch on all sides.

9. Cut off green tabs from Op-Site after wound is completely covered.

10. Position patient for comfort. Lower bed and raise side rail.

11. Remove and discard equipment.

12. Wash your hands.

---

### Clinical Alert

Observe ulcer area daily to determine if large amount of secretions or serous fluid has accumulated under Op-Site. If fluid has increased, aspirate with a number 26-gauge needle. If you remove Op-Site, "walk-off" Op-Site from one edge to the other.

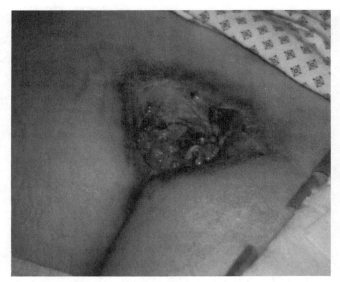

Stage II decubitus ulcer.

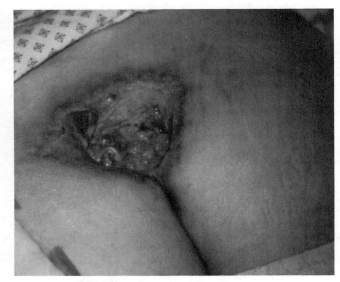

Stage III decubitus ulcer.

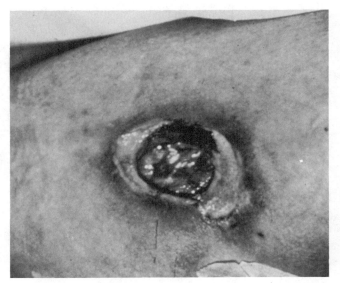

Stage IV decubitus ulcer.

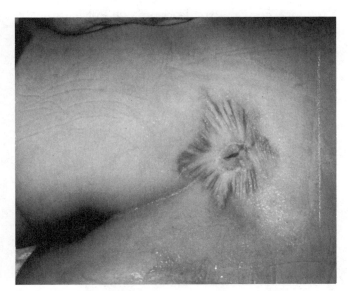

Healing decubitus ulcer.

## USING SKIN CARE TRAY

### Equipment

Soap and water

Appropriate skin care tray for stage of ulcer

### Preparation

1. Check physician's orders and Patient Care Plan.

2. Obtain appropriate tray for stage of ulcer. (Stage 2 kit is explained in this procedure).

3. Wash your hands.

4. Explain procedure to patient.

5. Provide privacy.

6. Place bed in HIGH position and lower side rails on working side of bed.

**Procedure**

1. Wash decubitus ulcer with povidone-iodine for three minutes.

2. Rinse area with water and dry thoroughly. (May use heat lamp for drying.)

3. Apply Maalox and allow to dry. If area is infected, an antibiotic ointment may be used instead of Maalox.

4. Dust Karaya powder over Maalox, removing the excess powder.

5. Apply protective skin prep to area surrounding the ulcer. Allow to dry.

6. Apply Stomahesive. Do not cut Stomahesive, but use entire sheet.

7. Secure edges of Stomahesive with nonallergic plastic tape. (Picture-frame the Stomahesive in a similar manner as with colostomy bag.) Change Stomahesive every 24 hours. Do not tear off the wound.

8. Position patient for comfort. Lower bed and raise side rail.

9. Remove equipment from room.

10. Wash your hands.

## USING DUODERM DRESSING

**Equipment**

Soap and water

Duoderm dressing

Duoderm granules, if needed

Silk or hy-tape

**Procedure**

1. Select dressing size to ensure coverage 1¼–1½″ beyond ulcer margin. (Dressing available in 4 × 4″ and 8 × 8″ size.)

2. Cleanse skin with mild soap, rinse with water and pat dry. If necrotic tissue is present, rinse wound with 3% hydrogen peroxide, rinse with normal saline and pat dry. **Rationale:** Hydrogen peroxide works as a debriding agent and thus will aid in cleansing the area of necrotic tissue.

3. Fill ulcer area with Duoderm granules if ulcer deep or exudate is present. Do not over-fill with granules. Remove excess granules from wound edge. **Rationale:** Granules absorb exudate and

fluid; therefore, they should be removed from healthy tissue.

4. Remove paper backing from dressing.

5. Center dressing over affected area. Mold it gently to skin and hold down with hand approximately one minute.

6. Apply skin prep to area to be covered by tape. Allow to dry. *Do not apply skin prep under Duoderm.*

7. Picture-frame sides of Duoderm with silk or hy-tape.

8. Check dressing daily for leakage.

9. Dressing should not be left on longer than 7 days and should be changed at first sign of leakage.

10. To remove dressing, free one edge from the skin and continue around periphery until all edges released, then lift away carefully.

11. Record stage, size and appearance of ulcer, date and reason for removal of Duoderm, then repeat procedure.

---

**Clinical Alert**

Duoderm should not be used if thick eschar or obvious infection is present.

---

**CHARTING** *for Decubitus Ulcer*

☐ Patient's general skin condition

☐ Assessment of wound, i.e., drainage, evidence of tissue granulation

☐ Type of ulcer care given, i.e., kit used

☐ Stage of ulcer

☐ Decubitus Ulcer Record completed

*ILLUSTRATION:* Mark the exact location of the decubitus

*SIZE:* Indicate size in centimeters

*STAGE:* Write the number of the stage which corresponds to the description of the decubitus ulcer (Stage 1–4)

*TREATMENT:* Chart treatment used, e.g., Duoderm dressing applied; Op-Site applied; etc.

*POSITION:* Indicate position to which patient turned. Use position numbers depicted in drawing, e.g., position 1, patient turned to left side

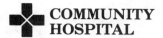 **COMMUNITY HOSPITAL**

## DECUBITUS ULCER RECORD

**STAGES:**

I.   Reddened only

II.  Reddened with skin break vesiculation or excoriation

III. Full thickness loss of skin which may or may not include the subcutaneous tissue and which produces serosanguinous drainage

IV.  Full thickness loss of skin with invasion of deeper tissues

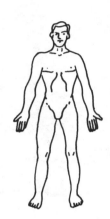 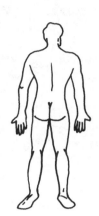

**POSITIONS:**

1. Left side
2. Right side
3. Supine
4. Prone

| DATE | | | | | | | | | | |
|------|---|---|---|---|---|---|---|---|---|---|
| SIZE | | | | | | | | | | |
| STAGE | | | | | | | | | | |
| TREATMENT | | | | | | | | | | |
| SIGNATURE | | | | | | | | | | |

| | | POSITION | INITIAL | POSITION | INITIAL | POSITION | INITIAL | POSITION | INITIAL | POSITION | INITIAL |
|---|---|---|---|---|---|---|---|---|---|---|---|
| **P O S I T I O N  C H A N G E** | 0700 | | | | | | | | | | |
| | 0900 | | | | | | | | | | |
| | 1100 | | | | | | | | | | |
| | 1300 | | | | | | | | | | |
| | 1500 | | | | | | | | | | |
| | 1700 | | | | | | | | | | |
| | 1900 | | | | | | | | | | |
| | 2100 | | | | | | | | | | |
| | 2300 | | | | | | | | | | |
| | 0100 | | | | | | | | | | |
| | 0300 | | | | | | | | | | |
| | 0500 | | | | | | | | | | |

## CLINICAL PROBLEM SOLVING

| Potential Problems | Suggested Solutions |
|---|---|

**Potential Problems**

Patient does not have sufficient exercise and appetite decreases.

Patient's wound does not heal with traditional types of treatments.

**Suggested Solutions**

☐ Encourage small frequent feedings.
☐ Offer high-calorie drinks like eggnog or Isocal.

☐ Discuss with physician the possibility of trying one of the following alternative treatments:
Apply vitamin E to ulcer area—open capsules and place liquid on affected area.
Sprinkle granulated sugar over ulcer.
☐ In patient care conference discuss the following:
Is everyone following same treatment?
Are causative agents preventing healing?
Should treatment be adjusted or changed?
Would use of a flotation or minimal pressure bed be useful?
Is surgical debridement and grafting necessary for healing?

## TERMINOLOGY

**Adhesions:** formation of fibrous scar tissue around the incision as a result of surgical intervention. Adhesions can cause obstruction or malfunction by distorting the organ.

**Aerobe:** a microorganism that lives and grows in the presence of free oxygen.

**Anaerobe:** an organism that lives and grows in the absence of molecular oxygen.

**Antimicrobial:** an agent that prevents the multiplication of microorganisms.

**Asepsis:** prevention of contact with microorganisms.

**Collagen formation:** formation of the protein substance of the white fibers of skin, bone, and cartilage.

**Contracture:** abnormal shortening of muscle tissue making the muscle resistant to stretching.

**Decubitus ulcer:** a break in the skin caused by pressure and restricted blood flow to the area. The ulcer generally occurs over bony prominences of the heels, sacrum, hip, and shoulder.

**Dermis:** synonym for corium; the skin layer beneath the epidermis; contains vascular connective tissue.

**Dehiscence:** a bursting open, as a graafian follicle or wound, especially abdominal wounds.

**Edematous:** the presence of abnormally large amounts of fluid in the intercellular tissue spaces of the body.

**Epidemiology:** division of medical science concerned with defining and explaining the interrelationships of the host, agent, and environment in causing disease.

**Epithelium:** outer covering of the body; top layer of skin.

**Erythema:** redness of the skin due to congestion of capillaries.

**Evisceration:** protrusion of the viscera; removal of the viscera.

**Exudate:** material obtained from a wound as the result of the inflammatory process.

**Gangrene:** death and putrefaction of body tissue precipitated by poor or absent blood supply to the tissue. Occurs as a result of infection, injury, or disease processes.

**Granulation:** formation of granules; fleshy projections formed on the surface of a gaping wound that is not healing by the normal joining together of skin edges.

**Incision:** a cut made with a knife.

**Infection:** morbid state caused by multiplication of pathogenic microorganisms within the body.

**Inflammatory process:** localized response when injury or destruction of tissue has occurred; destroys, wards off, or dilutes the causative agent or the injured tissue.

**Irrigate:** to rinse or wash out with a fluid.

**Isolation:** limitation of movement and social contacts of a patient; especially those having communicable diseases.

**Keloid:** scarlike growth of collagen that results in a rounded, hard, shiny, white benign tumor.

**Microorganism:** minute living body not perceptible to the naked eye.

**Occlusion:** the closure or state of being closed, of a passage.

**Organism:** a living thing, plant or animal.

**Pathogen:** disease producing organism.

**Primary healing:** the first stage in the wound healing process in which the blood clot forms and the inflammatory reaction develops at a wound site.

**Purulent:** containing pus, or caused by pus.

**Pus:** an inflammation containing leukocytes and exudate.

**Second intention healing:** second stage in wound healing in which granulation occurs.

**Wound dehiscence:** the separation of layers of a surgical wound.

**Wound evisceration:** protrusion of the internal viscera or organs through an opened incisional site.

# Chapter 23

# Infection Control

## LEARNING OBJECTIVES

Describe three methods the body uses to resist infection.

Explain what is meant by the body's natural defenses.

List and describe eight conditions which predispose patients to infection.

State the main purpose of handwashing.

Compare and contrast strict isolation with contact isolation.

Demonstrate putting on and removing a gown.

List the equipment usually found in an isolation cart.

Outline the steps in putting on isolation clothing before entering the room.

Outline the steps in taking off isolation clothing before leaving the room.

State the isolation procedure for removing specimens and equipment from an isolation room.

List the steps necessary for implementing protective (reverse) isolation.

Identify two potential problems in maintaining isolation and state a clinical option for each problem.

Define the words barrier nursing and sepsis.

State the pertinent data that should be included in charting.

## BARRIER NURSING

Ten percent of all patients enter the hospital with clinical infections. Another five percent acquire infections during their hospital stay. Patients become colonized by endogenous flora in the hospital after 72 hours. This type of flora tends to be highly resistant to antibiotics. Barrier nursing is concerned with the prevention and reduction of all infections. It should be practiced at all times to protect hospital personnel as well as patients. Barrier nursing is directed at isolating the infective agent, not the patient.

An individual's ability to resist infection is determined by the status of the body's defense mechanisms and by the person's general health. Factors that contribute to susceptibility to infection include altered nutritional status, stress, fatigue, disease, drugs, metabolic functions, and age. Patients with severe underlying diseases are most likely to develop nosocomial infections. The body is protected against infection by immunities, by the inflammatory process, and by anatomical barriers that include the skin and mucous membranes.

## BARRIERS TO INFECTION

When the integrity of the skin is broken, both resident and transient flora or bacteria have a direct route to the internal tissues of the body. To prevent the spread of infection, the body's internal defense mechanisms mobilize and begin clearing and repairing the damaged site. How quickly a wound heals depends on the degree of vascularization in the injured area, the location and cleanliness of the wound, and the degree of tissue damage.

The second way the body resists infections is through immunity, antitoxins and vaccines. Natural immunity is inherited. Acquired immunity occurs after an individual has been exposed to a disease or infection.

The third way the body resists infection is through the inflammatory process. Inflammation involves utilization of metabolic energy, increased blood flow to the inflamed area, and, in many cases, drainage of inflammatory debris to the external environment.

When an area becomes inflamed, cells at the site activate the plasmin system, the clotting system, and the kinin system. The result of the activation of these systems is the release of histamine, which creates increased vascular permeability around the injured site, and the release of chemotaxic agents, which summon phagocytes into the vascular and tissue spaces. Phagocytes are white blood cells that combat and prevent infection by ingesting harmful microorganisms.

**The Body's Natural Defenses**   Any alteration in the body's natural defenses increases the probability that an infection will occur. Given the proper circumstances, almost any organism can be the cause of a significant hospital-related infection. Some of the variables that help determine which organism emerges as the pathogen are the virulence and number of organisms, the exposure and attachment of the organism to a susceptible site, and the duration of the patient's exposure to the infectious challenge. The inherent health and immunologic status of the patient are also major factors in determining whether an infection occurs.

Alterations in the skin barrier include any physiologic break in the integrity of the skin. Intentional breaks are caused by the use of percutaneous catheters and needles and by surgical procedures. Unintentional causes of skin breakdown include the development of decubitus ulcers and traumatic wounds.

## CONDITIONS PREDISPOSING INFECTION

Certain conditions and invasive techniques predispose patients to infection because the integrity of the skin is broken or the illness itself establishes a climate favorable for the infectious process to occur. Among the most common are surgical wounds, changes in the antibacterial immune system, or alterations to the body.

**Surgical Wounds**   From 40 to 65 percent of the patients who enter general hospitals are admitted as surgical patients. Approximately one-half of these patients will have surgery, and out of this population 8 percent will develop a postoperative wound infection. It has been documented that the longer a person is hospitalized prior to the surgical procedure the greater the risk of postsurgical infection. Other factors that influence infection rates are duration of time in the operating room, time surgery is done (between midnight and 8:00 A.M. is period of greatest risk), and whether the patient has postsurgical drains in place. It would be well for the nurse to be aware of those conditions that increase the risk of postsurgical infection so that preventative steps (additional showering with antiseptic solution before surgery, prolonged scrubbing, clipping versus shaving hair at surgical site, etc.) can be taken.

**Antibacterial Immune Mechanisms**   There are three categories of abnormalities in antibacterial immune mechanisms: those affecting inflammatory responses, those affecting phagocytic functions, and those affecting opsonins (humoral immunity).

Anything that interferes with the migration of phagocytic cells to the area of contamination or with the physical contact of phagocytes and bacteria will enhance the development of an infection. Examples of such interferences include deficient blood supplies, the presence of ischemic or dead tissue, sutured material, foreign bodies, and hematomas. Vasopressor agents, radiation injury, uremia, severe nutritional deficiencies, and steroid therapy inhibit the synthesis of antibodies and other essential proteins.

Patients with severe thermal injuries and severe nutritional deficiencies have abnormalities involving the number of neutrophils collected at the site of an inflammatory response and defects of bactericidal chemotaxic capacity. Patients with Hodgkin's disease have a specific defect in cell-mediated immunity.

Genetic inabilities to synthesize complement components or specific antibodies can cause abnormalities in opsonins. Burn patients may have complement inactivated by a circulating substance released by the damaged tissue. Without complement, lysis of cells and destruction of bacteria cannot take place.

**Respiratory Tract**    Common alterations in the respiratory tract that facilitate the development of an infection include endotracheal intubation, tracheostomy, and bronchotracheal suctioning.

The bronchi and trachea are so sensitive to foreign matter that they initiate the cough reflex whenever irritation occurs. Ciliated, mucus-coated epithelium lining the trachea and lungs aids in clearing the respiratory tract of bacteria and mucus by the beating motion of the cilia. Intubation bypasses the cough reflex and compromises the effectiveness of this action. Although the trachea is usually considered sterile, it does not remain sterile after 48 to 72 hours of intubation. Infections associated with endotracheal intubation include pneumonia, tracheitis, and purulent bronchitis.

Catheters placed directly in the trachea can force pathogenic microorganisms into the respiratory system. In addition, catheters can damage the mucous lining of the respiratory tract, further compromising the effectiveness of its clearing mechanisms.

**Genitourinary Tract**    Instrumentation, including catheterization of the bladder, and complicated obstetric delivery after prolonged confinement in bed are two procedures that introduce potentially pathogenic bacteria into the genitourinary tract. Acute urinary tract infection and pyelonephritis often occur after the use of a catheter or cystoscope.

The most common alteration is the placement of an indwelling urinary catheter. Research has demonstrated that significant bacteriuria develop in only 2 percent of the patients who have a single "straight" catheterization (in and out) to empty a distended bladder. Although bacteriuria may be considered benign and will resolve after removal of the catheter (sometimes augmented with antibiotic therapy), bacteriuria following catheterization may result in symptomatic cystitis and, occasionally, in acute pyelonephritis, chronic pyelonephritis and persistent asymptomatic bacteriuria. Lack of adequate emptying of the bladder or highly concentrated urine increases possibility of infection.

**Invasive Devices**    Most nosocomial septicemias occur as a result of significant alterations in normal host defenses. These infections may be primary (caused by direct introduction of microorganisms into the bloodstream) or secondary (arising from an infection at another site, such as the urinary tract).

The use of IV therapy greatly increases the risk of introducing harmful microorganisms. Of the thirty-two million patients admitted to hospitals each year, almost eight million receive some form of IV therapy. The incidence of septicemia in patients receiving IV therapy varies from zero to 8 percent, with an even higher incidence when plastic catheters are used.

Septicemia may also be caused by the introduction of microorganisms from contaminated fluids, infected venipuncture sites, or foci of septic thrombophlebitis as a complication of using an indwelling IV catheter.

Infusion-related sepsis is also associated with contaminated infusion fluid, which may be contaminated either during manufacturing (intrinsic contamination) or during hospital use (extrinsic contamination).

Infusion phlebitis is a common sequela of IV therapy. Although phlebitis does not always represent systemic infection, its presence connotes an eighteen-fold increased risk of related sepsis as compared with an absence of phlebitis. Approximately one-half the patients who have catheter-related sepsis will develop phlebitis.

**Venipuncture Sites**    The wounds made by a percutaneous stick at the venipuncture site may become contaminated and infected, providing a reservoir of bacteria that move along the catheter into the bloodstream.

Organisms that travel down the catheter will ultimately reside in the thrombus, which is almost uniformly present on a catheter tip. Around the thrombus, bacteria are shielded from the immune response and antibiotics, and grow undisturbed. When these microorganisms attain a critical level of colonization, they seed the bloodstream and cause bacteremia.

**Total Parenteral Nutritional Therapy**    Total parenteral nutrition therapy (TPN) is a means of achieving an anabolic state in patients who would otherwise be unable to maintain normal nitrogen balance. Problems with IV-related sepsis in TPN are the same as those seen in conventional IV therapy, only greatly magnified.

Because patients of TPN are critically ill and malnourished, catheters are left in place for long periods of time. The hypertonic solution used with these patients supports the growth of a wide variety of organisms, especially fungus, to a greater extent than conventional IV solutions.

**Implanted Prosthetic Devices**    Commonly used implanted devices include artificial cardiac valves, synthetic vascular grafts, orthopedic prosthetic joints, neurosurgical shunts, cerebrospinal fluid pressure monitoring devices, permanent artificial arteriovenous fistulas for hemodialysis, intraocular lenses, and breast and penile implants. Most infections associated with prosthetic devices do not respond well to antimicrobial therapy. These infections usually require removal and replacement of the prosthesis.

**NURSING DIAGNOSES**

The following nursing diagnoses may be appropriate to include in a Patient Care Plan when the components are related to patients requiring isolation protocol or sterile procedures.

| Nursing Diagnosis (Potential) | Defining Characteristic; Etiology (Examples) |
| --- | --- |
| ☐ Health Maintenance, Alteration in, *related to* | Diminished immune system function, e.g., steroid and antineoplastic drug therapy. |
| ☐ Knowledge Deficit, *related to* | Misunderstanding of information, e.g., inadequate data and/or explanation. |

□ Noncompliance, *related to*     Contamination or transmission of infection, e.g., break in isolation protocol technique.

□ Social Isolation, *related to*     Decreased social interaction, e.g., isolation protocol (restricted visitors).

Restricted resources and stimuli, e.g., isolation protocol and procedures.

## UNIT ONE    ISOLATION

### NURSING PROCESS DATA

**ASSESSMENT** *Data Base*

Identify appropriate times for handwashing.

Identify type of protective clothing required for barrier nursing.

Identify epidemiology of the disease to determine how to prevent infection from spreading.

Identify equipment needed to prevent spread of organisms.

Assess method of terminal cleaning and disposing of equipment.

**PLANNING** *Objectives*

To prevent spreading endogenous and exogenous flora to other patients and personnel.

To reduce potential for transferring organisms from the hospital environment to the patient.

To protect hospital personnel from becoming infected.

**IMPLEMENTATION** *Procedures*

Preparing for Isolation

Washing Your Hands

Using Clean Gloves

Putting on and Removing a Gown

Using a Mask

Assessing Vital Signs

Removing Items from an Isolation Room

Removing a Specimen from an Isolation Room

Transporting an Isolation Patient Outside the Room

Removing Large Equipment Items from an Isolation Room

**EVALUATION** *Expected Outcomes*

Isolation environment is maintained to prevent contamination of surrounding area.

Personnel working with isolation patients remain free of infection.

Patients who are in a medically compromised state remain free of pathogens.

## PREPARING FOR ISOLATION

### Equipment

Soap and running water

Antimicrobial cleansing agent

Isolation cart containing mask, gown, gloves (sterile and/or clean), plastic bags, isolation tape

Linen hamper and trash cans

Sterile brush or sponge

Sterile towel

Paper towels

Cards indicating type of isolation

### Procedure

1. Check physician's order for type of isolation.
2. Obtain isolation cart from central supply.
3. Check that all necessary equipment to carry out appropriate isolation protocol is available on the cart. **Rationale:** Once you are in the patient's room, you cannot leave to obtain an item without repeating all the steps of isolation protocol.
4. Place correct isolation card for type of isolation on patient's door.
5. Ensure that linen hamper and lined waste paper basket are in the room.
6. Explain purpose of isolation to patient and family.
7. Instruct family in procedure required for entrance and exit from isolation room.

## WASHING YOUR HANDS

### Equipment

Germicidal soap

Paper towels

### Procedure

1. Wet your hands.
2. Place small amount of soap on your hands.
3. Rub hands vigorously, keeping fingers pointed down to facilitate mechanical removal of organisms.
4. Wash your hands for 30 seconds.
5. Clean under your fingernails with an orangewood stick.
6. Rinse your hands under running water, keeping your fingers pointed downward.
7. Dry your hands well with a paper towel. **Rationale:** When hands remain moist, they tend to gather and support more organisms from the environment.
8. Turn off water faucets, holding handles with paper towel.

---

### Clinical Alert

Handwashing before and after contact with each patient is the single most important means of preventing the spread of infection. The major source of cross-contamination among patients is direct transmission of microbes by hands.

---

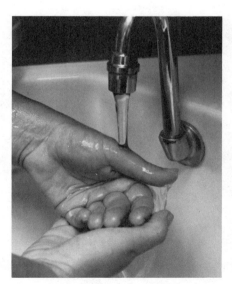

Thoroughly wet hands before applying soap.

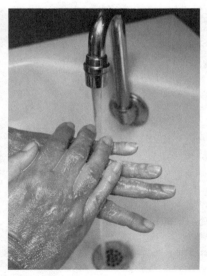

Wash for at least 30 seconds.

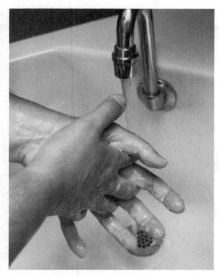

Keep all fingers pointed downward.

**TABLE 1** ISOLATION PRECAUTIONS BY DISEASE CATEGORY

| TYPE OF ISOLATION | DISEASE | TYPE OF ISOLATION | DISEASE |
|---|---|---|---|
| *STRICT*<br>Diseases spread by both air-borne droplets and direct contact | Diphtheria, pharyngeal<br>Chickenpox<br>Smallpox<br>Zoster | *ENTERIC*<br>Diseases spread by direct or indirect contact with feces | Hepatitis A<br>Amoebic dysentery<br>Cholera<br>Coxsackie virus<br>Diarrhea, acute with suspected infectious etiology |
| *CONTACT*<br>Diseases spread by close or direct contact | Acute respiratory infection in infants and young children: Croup<br>    Colds<br>    Bronchitis<br>    Bronchiolitis<br>Influenza, in infants and young children<br>Conjunctivitis, gonococcal, in newborns<br>Endometritis, group A, streptococcus<br>Furunculosis, staphylococcal, in newborn<br>Herpes simplex<br>Pediculosis, scabies<br>Pneumonia, viral in infants and young children, staphylococcus or streptococcus A<br>Wound, skin infections | | Echovirus<br>Encephalitis<br>Enterocolitis:<br>    Clostridium<br>    Staphylococcus aureus<br>Enteroviral<br>Gastroenteritis caused by:<br>    Escherichia coli<br>    Salmonella<br>    Shigella<br>    Virus<br>Meningitis, viral<br>Poliomyelitis<br>Typhoid fever |
| | | *RESPIRATORY*<br>Diseases spread through air-borne droplets, direct or indirect contact | Epiglottitis<br>Measles<br>Meningitis:<br>    Haemophilus<br>    Meningococcal<br>Pneumonia, meningococcal<br>Mumps<br>Pertussis<br>Pneumonia, Haemophilus influenza |
| *DRAINAGE/SECRETIONS*<br>Diseases spread by direct or indirect contact with purulent material or drainage from infected body site | Abscess<br>Burns, infected<br>Conjunctivitis<br>Decubitus ulcers<br>Skin infection<br>Wound infection | *TUBERCULOSIS* (AFB Isolation)<br>Diseases spread by air-borne droplets | Adults with positive sputum smear<br>Chest x-ray suggestive of TBC<br>Laryngeal TB |
| *BLOOD/BODY FLUID*<br>Diseases spread by direct or indirect contact with infective blood or body fluids | AIDS<br>Yellow fever<br>Hepatitis B<br>Hepatitis:<br>    Non-A<br>    Non-B<br>Leptospirosis<br>Malaria<br>Syphilis, primary and secondary with skin or mucous membrane lesions | | |

**TABLE 2** ISOLATION PROTOCOL

| TYPE OF ISOLATION | PRIVATE ROOM | HANDS | GOWNS | MASKS | GLOVES | ARTICLES |
|---|---|---|---|---|---|---|
| Strict Isolation | Closed door | Wash before entering and after leaving room | All persons entering room | All persons entering room | All persons entering room | Discard or bag and send for sterilization |
| Contact Isolation | Desirable, but patients with same organism may share room | Wash before entering and after leaving room | If soiling is likely | While in close contact with patient | When touching infective material | Discard or bag and send for sterilization |
| Drainage/ Secretions Isolation | Not indicated | Wash before entering and after leaving room | For direct contact with infected wound | Not indicated | While in direct contact with infective material | Discard or bag and send for sterilization |
| Blood/Body Fluid Isolation | Necessary if poor hygienic habits. Patients with same organisms may share room | Wash immediately if in contact with blood or body fluid. Wash before entering and after leaving room | If soiling of clothing with blood or body fluids is likely | Not indicated | When touching blood or body | Discard or bag and send for sterilization |
| Enteric Isolation | Necessary for children or if poor hygienic habits | Wash before entering and after leaving room | For direct patient contact | Not necessary | While in contact with articles contaminated with fecal material | Discard or bag and send for sterilization |
| Respiratory Isolation | Closed door | Wash before entering and after leaving room | Not necessary | While in close contact with patient | Not necessary | Discard or bag and send for sterilization |
| Tuberculosis (AFB) Isolation | Closed door, special ventilation. Patients with same organism may share room | Wash before entering and after leaving room | If gross contamination of clothing could occur | If patient coughing and not reliable to cover mouth | Not necessary | Thoroughly clean and disinfect or discard |

Recommended categories for Isolation developed by the Center for Disease Control, Atlanta, Georgia, 1983.

## USING CLEAN GLOVES

### Equipment

Germicidal soap

Paper towel

Box of clean gloves

### Procedure

1. Wash and dry your hands.

2. Take clean glove out of the box.

3. Slip fingers in openings and pull glove up to wrist. Repeat step with second glove.

4. If you are wearing a gown, place gloves so that they cover gown wristlets. If you are not wearing a gown, place gloves so that they cover your wrists.

5. Remove gloves by pulling them over your wrists and fingers until each glove is turned inside out.

## PUTTING ON AND REMOVING A GOWN

### Procedure

1. Take gown from isolation cart. Put on a new gown each time you enter an isolation room.

2. Hold gown so that the opening will be in the back when you are wearing the gown.

3. Put the gown on by placing one arm at a time through the sleeves. Pull the gown up and over your shoulders.

4. Wrap the gown around your back, tying the strings at your neck. (These ties are considered clean.)

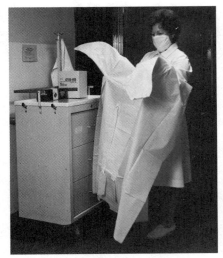

Put mask on first, then don gown.

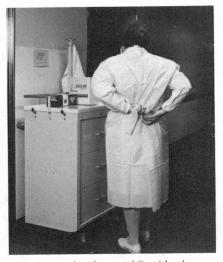

Overlap gown's edges and tie at back.

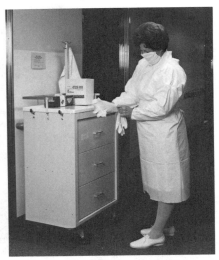

Gloves must completely cover wristlets.

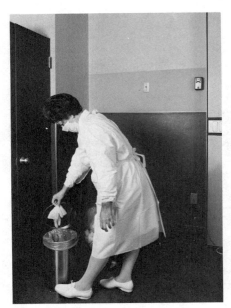

Take off gloves first.

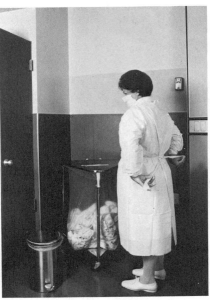

Untie the gown at the waist before the neck.

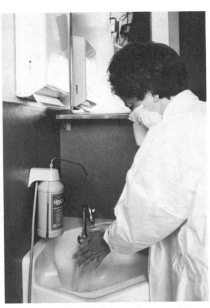

Wash your hands after untying waist ties.

5. Wrap the gown around your waist, making sure your back is completely covered. Tie the strings around your waist. (These strings are considered dirty.)

6. To remove the gown, take gloves off, then untie the waist strings. Wash your hands.

7. Next untie the neck strings, bringing them around your shoulders so that the gown is partially off your shoulders.

8. Using your dominant hand, pull the sleeve wristlet over your nondominant hand. Repeat this procedure, using your nondominant hand to pull the sleeve wristlet over your dominant hand.

9. Grasp the outside of the gown through the sleeves at the shoulders. Pull the gown down over your arms.

10. Hold both gown shoulders in one hand. Carefully draw your other hand out of the gown, turning the arm of the gown inside out. Repeat this procedure with your other arm.

11. Hold the gown away from your body. Fold the gown up inside out.

12. Discard the gown if it is disposable. If the gown is reusable, hang it in the appropriate place.

13. Wash your hands. Use a paper towel to turn off the water.

14. Take off mask and discard.

15. After leaving room, proceed to sink and wash hands thoroughly. **Rationale:** This action is necessary to prevent cross-contamination to other patients.

## USING A MASK

### Equipment

Clean mask

### Procedure

1. Obtain mask from box.

2. Position mask to cover your nose and mouth.

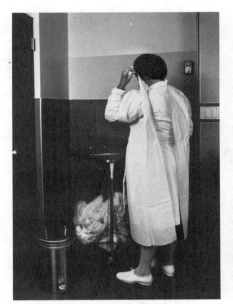
Untie neck string and pull gown off.

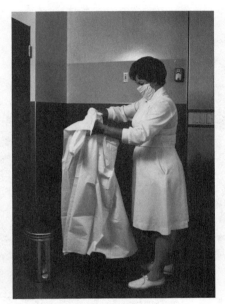
Fold gown inward after removing.

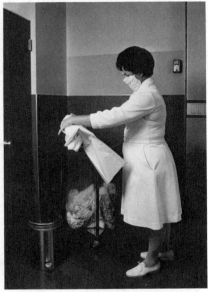
Roll gown away to prevent contamination.

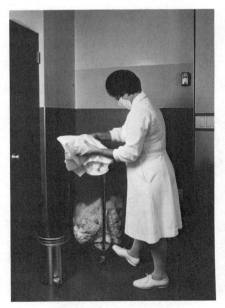
Place rolled-up gown in trash container.

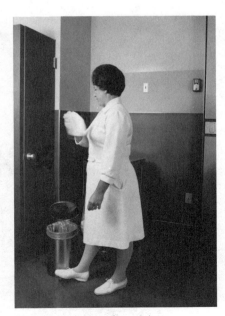
Discard mask in trash container.

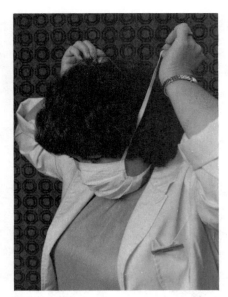

Untie mask at top first.

3. Bend the nose bar so that it conforms over the bridge of your nose.

4. If you are using a mask with string ties, tie the top strings on top of your head to prevent slipping. If you are using a cone-shaped mask, tie the top strings over your ears.

5. Tie the bottom strings around your neck to secure the mask over your mouth. There should be no gaps between the mask and your face.

6. To remove the mask, untie the strings without touching the mask. **Rationale:** Only the strings are considered clean.

7. Discard the mask in a trash container.

8. Wash your hands.

## ASSESSING VITAL SIGNS

### Equipment

Single use thermometer

Disposable stethoscope

Blood pressure cuff and sphygmomanometer

Thermometer stand with disinfectant solution

Paper towel

Disinfectant spray

Watch with sweep second hand

### Preparation

1. Wash your hands.

2. Don isolation clothing as required by type of isolation.

3. Place your watch on a paper towel.

4. Enter patient's room and place the paper towel on the bedside stand in a position where you can visibly see the sweep second hand without touching the watch.

5. Proceed to take vital signs as you would for any patient.

6. If equipment is to be left in room, place in appropriate area.

7. Remove isolation clothing according to protocol.

8. Wash hands before picking up watch. Be careful to not touch the surrounding area.

9. Pick up paper towel by grasping the middle of the towel and placing in the trash.

10. Place watch on the isolation cart outside the room, wash your hands and then replace the watch on your wrist.

11. If watch is accidently contaminated, it can be sprayed with disinfectant spray while inside the room. After spraying, allow to dry before removing from room.

---

**Protocol for Leaving Isolation Room**

Take off gloves
Untie gown at waist
Wash hands
Untie gown at neck
Pull gown off and place in laundry hamper
Wash hands
Take off mask
Leave room and wash hands

---

## REMOVING ITEMS FROM AN ISOLATION ROOM

### Procedure

1. Close the half- to three-fourths-full contaminated bag inside the isolation room.

2. Set up a new bag for continued use inside the room.

3. Have someone outside the room hold a clean bag with the top of the bag cuffed over her hands. If

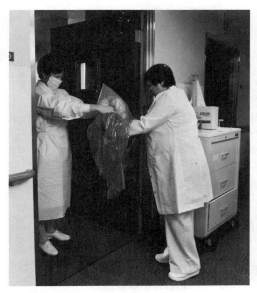

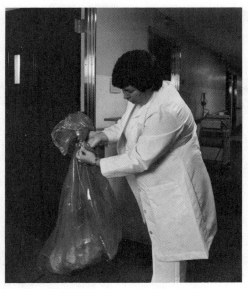

Double-bagging may be required.    Close bag securely and label ISOLATION.

no one is available to help, assemble a clean bag in a hamper stand before you go into the isolation room.

4. Position the hamper stand outside the room for easy access.

5. Place the contaminated bag into the clean bag being held by another person or in the hamper outside the room. Be careful not to contaminate the outside of the clean bag.

6. Close the clean bag and mark it "Isolation." (Many hospitals use color-coded bags to indicate isolation contents.)

7. Double-bag (one bag from inside the room and one bag from outside the room) all items used for the care of a patient in isolation and mark "Isolation" to protect the environment. All items contained in isolation bag to be returned to CSR are listed on tag which is placed on outside of bag. **Rationale:** All items used for the care of a patient in isolation are considered contaminated.

8. Dispose of isolation room equipment using these guidelines:
   a. Disposable glass items are placed in isolation bag separate from burnable trash. Place in appropriate hospital area for disposal.
   b. Metal equipment to be returned to central supply is bagged together and returned to CSR.
   c. Glass equipment to be returned to CSR is bagged together and separately from metal equipment.
   d. Rubber and plastic items for gas sterilization are bagged separately and returned to CSR.
   e. Soiled linen is placed in laundry bag and brought to separate area of laundry room for special care.
   f. Plastic or paper dishes are disposed of in the burnable trash.
   g. Food and liquids are disposed of down the toilet.

---

### Clinical Alert for Disposal Precautions

*Secretion:* Patient should be instructed to expectorate into tissue held close to mouth. Suction catheters and gloves should be disposed of in impervious, sealed bags.

*Excretion:* Strict attention should be paid to careful handwashing; disease can be spread by oral-fecal route.

*Blood:* Needles and syringe should be disposable. Used needles should *not* be recapped. They should be placed in a puncture-resistant container that is prominently labeled "Isolation." Specimens should be labeled "Blood Precaution."

## REMOVING A SPECIMEN FROM AN ISOLATION ROOM

### Procedure

1. Before entering an isolation room, mark a specimen container with the patient's name, the type of specimen, and the word "Isolation."

2. Collect the specimen and place it in a plastic bag, using the same two-person approach as in double-bagging contaminated items. Use clear bags so that laboratory personnel can see the specimen easily.

3. Wash your hands.

4. Label the clean bag with the word "Isolation," and then take the bag to the laboratory with the appropriate lab slip.

## TRANSPORTING AN ISOLATION PATIENT OUTSIDE THE ROOM

### Procedure

1. Explain procedure to patient.

2. If patient is being transported from a respiratory isolation room, tell him to wear a mask for the entire time the patient is out of isolation. **Rationale:** Patients being transported from a strict isolation room should wear a mask and a cap to prevent contamination.

3. If patient is being transported from a wound and skin, gastrointestinal, strict isolation, or protective isolation room, cover the transport vehicle, i.e., wheelchair, guerney, with a clean sheet *before* you enter the room.

4. Help the patient into the transport vehicle. Cover the patient, from shoulders down, with a sheet.

5. Tell the receiving department what type of isolation the patient will need and what precautions hospital personnel should follow with the patient.

6. When the patient returns to the original isolation room, help him or her into bed. Cover the transportation vehicle with a clean sheet and remove it from the room.

7. Instruct all hospital personnel to wash their hands before they leave the area.

8. Clean the transportation vehicle with an antimicrobial agent.

## REMOVING LARGE EQUIPMENT ITEMS FROM AN ISOLATION ROOM

### Procedure

1. Don isolation garb.

2. Wash equipment with an antimicrobial agent. **Rationale:** Washing is preferred to spraying to ensure all surfaces are cleaned.

3. Cover equipment with a plastic bag.

4. Discard linen and wash your hands inside the room.

5. Wash your hands outside the room and take equipment to CSR to the decontamination area.

### CHARTING  *for Isolation Equipment*

☐ Type of barrier nursing being practiced

☐ Patient's reactions to sensory deprivation

☐ Specimens sent to laboratory

---

## CLINICAL PROBLEM SOLVING

### Potential Problems

Outbreak of disease occurs in isolation environment.

Hospital personnel do not follow isolation procedures.

### Suggested Solutions

☐ Identify cause of outbreak and contact the infection control practitioner for consultation.

☐ Examine handwashing and barrier nursing practices among staff.

☐ Attend in-service education program on isolation techniques to increase your awareness of appropriate procedures.

☐ Identify and report personnel who do not follow protocol.

☐ Notify infection control practitioner and have her/him discuss isolation techniques with personnel.

☐ Complete incident report and send to nursing office.

# UNIT TWO   PROTECTIVE ISOLATION (REVERSE)

## NURSING PROCESS DATA

### ASSESSMENT   *Data Base*

Identify patients at risk for nosocomial infections.

Identify extent of protective isolation required.

Assess health status of visitors and nursing staff prior to entering room.

### PLANNING   *Objectives*

To prevent infections in patients with altered immune systems.

To provide health teaching to visitors of patients with altered immune systems.

To provide appropriate equipment for patient care.

### IMPLEMENTATION   *Procedure*

Providing Protective Care

### EVALUATION   *Expected Outcomes*

Patients with altered immune systems remain free of nosocomial infections.

Visitors with infectious processes are identified and prohibited from entering patient's room.

Isolation protocol is maintained throughout hospitalization.

## PROVIDING PROTECTIVE CARE

### Equipment

Isolation cart

Sterile bed linen

Sterile gowns

Shoe covers

Box of caps

Box of masks

Linen hamper

Isolation tape

Sterile gloves

Sterile personal hygiene equipment

Soap

### Preparation

1. Check physician's order for type of isolation.

2. Provide a private room. (Room with laminar flow is ideal.)

3. Order sterile (or disinfected) bed linen and isolation linen from laundry department (or central supply).

4. Have room cleaned thoroughly with disinfectant.

5. Provide clean curtains for room.

6. Provide new or sterilized personal hygiene equipment, e.g., bedpan, washbasin, leaving wrappers outside unit.

7. Check isolation cart each shift and reorder equipment as necessary.

## Procedure

1. Check isolation cart for linen.

2. Put on shoe covers if required.

3. Put on mask and cap.

4. Open sterile glove package and leave on isolation cart in preparation for putting on after gown.

5. Open sterile packages for equipment and supplies that need to be brought into room.

6. Take gown out of sterile package by grasping the gown by the back neck area.

7. Move gown away from isolation cart and gently shake out gown to open it.

8. Grasping gown by the inside only, place both arms in sleeves and work arms down sleeves and out through wristlets.

9. Tie neck ties.

10. Put on sterile gloves, covering the entire wristlet with each glove.

11. Grasp waist ties on gown and pull around to tie in the front. Be careful not to contaminate gloves by touching gown.

12. Enter room by opening door with your foot. **Rationale:** This procedure avoids contamination of hands by touching the door.

13. Bring into the room all equipment necessary for the patient's care.

14. When you are ready to leave isolation room, remove isolation gown outside the patient's room.

15. Discard in the proper receptacle.

## CHARTING   *for Prevention of Infection*

☐  Type of isolation procedure

☐  Isolation protocol maintained

☐  Disposition of equipment

☐  Patient's response to isolation

---

## CLINICAL PROBLEM SOLVING

| Potential Problems | Suggested Solutions |
|---|---|
| Infection occurs in patient. | ☐ Administer antibiotics specific to microorganism as ordered.<br>☐ Review reverse isolation procedures.<br>☐ Attend in-service program on infection control procedures. |
| Wound becomes infected. | ☐ Notify physician of wounds that appear red, warm to touch, and swollen.<br>☐ Obtain culture and sensitivity if ordered.<br>☐ Request that staff evaluate dressing change protocols and procedures necessary to prevent infection.<br>☐ Wash hands thoroughly to prevent spread of infection. |
| Visitor who has infectious process enters room. | ☐ Explain reason for not allowing visitation.<br>☐ Ask visitor to please leave room.<br>☐ Explain to patient reason for not allowing visitation.<br>☐ Ensure that isolation sign is posted on door to prevent this from happening again. |

# TERMINOLOGY

**Antimicrobial:** an agent that prevents the development or pathogenic action of microbes.

**Antiseptics:** agents that are applied to body tissues, such as skin or mucous membrane, to destroy or retard the growth of microorganisms.

**Asepsis:** the absence of disease-producing microorganisms.

**Aseptic technique:** a method to eliminate contamination, germs, or infection.

**Autoinfections:** infections that arise from an individual's own body flora.

**Bacteriostatic:** a substance that prevents the growth or multiplication of bacteria.

**Barrier nursing:** any technique that reduces the risk of cross-contamination.

**Carrier:** a person or animal without signs of illness but who carries pathogens on or within his body that can be transferred to others.

**Cell-mediated immunity:** reactions to antigens by cells rather than antibody molecules present in body fluids.

**Chemotaxis:** attraction and repulsion of living protoplasm to a chemical stimulus.

**Colonization:** organisms present in body tissue, but not multiplying or invading the tissue.

**Contagious disease:** a disease conveyed easily to others.

**Contamination:** introduction of disease, germs or infectious materials into or on normally sterile objects.

**Depilatory:** agent that removes hair from skin surfaces.

**Disinfectants:** chemical agents that are used to destroy or reduce microorganisms on inanimate surfaces and objects.

**Disinfection:** a process that employs physical and chemical means to remove, control, or destroy most of the organisms that may be present on equipment or materials.

**Duration of the infectious challenge:** sustained exposure to even a relatively small number of organisms that poses a significant risk to the patient (e.g., intravenous catheters become colonized with microorganisms).

**Endogenous:** organisms natural to an individual's own body.

**Enteric precautions:** isolation practices designed to prevent transmission of pathogens through contact with fecal matter and vomitus.

**Exogenous:** organisms external to an individual's own body.

**Granulation:** formation of granules (roughened prominences). Each granulation represents an outgrowth of new capillaries and enriched blood supply.

**Host:** an animal or person upon which or within which microorganisms live.

**Humoral immunity:** acquired immunity where the circulating antibody is predominant.

**Hygiene:** study of health and observance of rules pertinent to health.

**Infection:** establishment of a disease process that involves invasion of the body tissue by microorganisms and the reaction of the tissues to their presence and to the toxins generated by them.

**Isolation technique:** practices designed to prevent the transmission of communicable diseases.

**Microorganism:** minute living body, such as a bacterium or protozoan, not perceptible to the naked eye.

**Nosocomial infection:** an infection acquired while in the hospital that was not present or incubating at the time of admission.

**Opsonin:** a substance in blood serum that acts upon microorganisms and other cells and facilitates phagocytosis.

**Outbreak:** a critical incident where infections occur above an established level and are caused by the same etiological agent.

**Protective isolation:** practices designed to protect a highly susceptible person from contagious diseases, reverse isolation.

**Protocol:** description of steps taken in exact order.

**Resident (normal) flora:** organisms natural to an individual's own body. Organisms multiply in the environment, not merely survive there.

**Sepsis:** condition resulting from the presence of pathogenic bacteria and their products.

**Sterile:** free from any living microorganisms.

**Subungual:** an area beneath a fingernail or toenail.

**Surgical asepsis:** practice to keep area free from microorganisms, as by a surgical scrub.

**Susceptible sites:** an area that is sensitive to or can be invaded by a bacterium or other infectious agent.

**Virulence:** recognized pathogenic organisms designated because of their ability to invade and propagate in normal, intact, uncompromised individuals. Some organisms that are avirulent for normal individuals become pathogenic when defense mechanisms are impaired.

Chapter *24*

# Respiratory Care

## LEARNING OBJECTIVES

Outline the four phases of respiration.

Explain at least two alterations that can occur in normal respiration.

Describe the steps for teaching a patient deep breathing and coughing exercises.

Discuss the purpose of using an incentive spirometer.

Differentiate between the positions used for percussion, vibration and drainage of upper, lower, and middle lobes.

Differentiate between the suctioning techniques used for naso-oral and pharyngeal suctioning.

State the pounds of pressure used for suctioning adults and children.

Compare and contrast the $FIO_2$ delivered and specific nursing interventions required by at least four of the common types of oxygen administration sets.

Describe the nursing actions included in performing tracheostomy care.

Explain the procedure for inflating and deflating the tracheostomy cuff.

Identify at least four interventions that promote chest tube drainage.

List the safety measures that are carried out to promote safe, effective care for patients with chest tubes in place.

Describe the difference between two- and three-bottle suction.

Demonstrate the steps of endotracheal intubation.

Discuss the nursing actions necessary for managing patients requiring mechanical ventilation.

Compare and contrast the purpose of administering PEEP, CPAP, and IPPB.

## THE RESPIRATORY SYSTEM

The respiratory system provides for the exchange of gases between the blood and the external environment. The respiratory structures in this system include the lungs, trachea, bronchi, nose, pharynx, larynx, intercostal muscles, ribs, and diaphragm.

The nose, pharynx, and larynx are the structures of the upper respiratory tract. These structures filter particles of dust and bacteria. They also humidify and moisten the air as it passes through the respiratory tree. When the upper respiratory tract is bypassed due to intubation and tracheostomy, an artificial humidification process must be carried out.

The trachea is composed of smooth muscle reinforced with C-shaped rings of cartilage lined with a membranous sheath branching into the right and left main stem bronchi. The right main bronchus extends vertically from the trachea. The left main bronchus extends from the trachea at an angle. Because of this division and the ease with which an endotracheal or tracheostomy tube could slip into the right bronchus, a chest x-ray may be taken to ensure proper placement of the tube.

The bronchi divide into terminal bronchioles and finally into alveolar ducts, sacs, and alveoli. Each alveolus is surrounded by capillaries, which allow the exchange of oxygen and carbon dioxide. Because the alveoli are so important for the exchange of gases, they must be adequately ventilated to prevent respiratory failure.

**The Respiratory Cycle** Respiration occurs when oxygen is transported from the atmosphere to the cells and carbon dioxide is carried from the cells to the atmosphere. Respiration is divided into four phases. The first phase is ventilation, which is the constant replenishment of air in the lungs. The

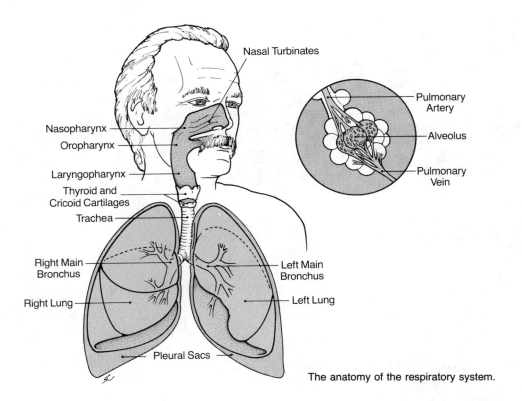

Nasal Turbinates

Pulmonary Artery

Alveolus

Pulmonary Vein

Nasopharynx

Oropharynx

Laryngopharynx

Thyroid and Cricoid Cartilages

Trachea

Right Main Bronchus

Left Main Bronchus

Right Lung

Left Lung

Pleural Sacs

The anatomy of the respiratory system.

alveolar pressures increase as the diaphragm descends, the external costal muscles contract, and the chest expands. This process allows air to flow into the lungs. The second phase is movement of oxygen from the alveolar air to the blood and movement of carbon dioxide in the opposite direction. Next, there is transportation of oxygen and carbon dioxide in the blood to and from the cells; oxygen moves out of the blood and into the cells, and carbon dioxide moves from the cells into the blood. The fourth phase of respiration is the regulation of ventilation.

Respiration involves inspiration, when air flows into the lungs and expiration, when alveolar pressures decrease so that air can flow out of the lungs. This is normally a passive process, whereas inspiration is an active process. In order for adequate respiration to take place, oxygen must be carried to the cells, and carbon dioxide must be carried away from the cells. Without this exchange of gases, survival is not possible.

Alterations in normal respiration can result from biochemical reactions, malfunctions of the circulatory system, obstructions blocking the airways, and inadequate ventilation and gaseous exchange.

## ALTERATIONS IN RESPIRATION

**Biochemical Alterations**   Biochemical alterations are any physiological disturbances in the acid-base balance of the body. Acid-base balance is the ratio of acids and bases in the body necessary in order to maintain a chemical balance conducive to life. Acid-base ratio is 20 base to 1 acid. Acid-base balance is measured by arterial blood samples and recorded as blood pH. Normal range is 7.35 to 7.45. Acids are hydrogen ion donors. They release

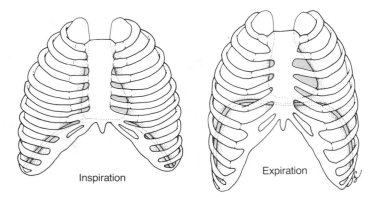

Inspiration

Expiration

Diaphragm movement in the respiratory cycle.

hydrogen ions to neutralize or decrease the strength of the base. Bases are hydrogen ion acceptors. They accept hydrogen ions to convert strong acids to weak acids. The body controls the pH balance by use of buffers. Chemical buffers work fastest. Then lungs, cells, and kidneys act as buffers, giving slower but more reliable protection against acid-base imbalance.

When the pH balance is disturbed, the chemical buffers react in an attempt to keep the pH within normal limits. The three primary buffer systems— bicarbonate, plasma proteins, and hemoglobin—all respond to the imbalance. Next to react are the lungs. They take 10 to 30 minutes to inactivate hydrogen molecules by converting them to water molecules. The carbonic acid that was formed by neutralizing bicarbonate is taken to the lungs. There it is reduced to carbon dioxide and water and exhaled. Therefore, when there is excessive acid in the body, the respiratory rate increases in order to blow off the excessive carbon dioxide and water. When there is too much bicarbonate or base in the body, the respirations become deeper and slower. This process builds up the level of carbonic acid. The result is that the strength of the excessive bicarbonate is neutralized. The lungs can only inactivate the hydrogen ions carried by carbonic acid. The other ions must be excreted by the kidneys.

When carbon dioxide is retained through hypoventilation, the condition of respiratory acidosis occurs. This condition, caused by defective functioning of the lungs, refers to the increased carbonic acid concentration, which is accumulated carbon dioxide combined with water. The basic problem in respiratory acidosis is a change in the lungs, so the kidneys must be the major compensatory mechanism. The kidneys work much slower than do the lungs; it takes from hours to days for the compensation to take place.

Respiratory alkalosis occurs when an excessive amount of carbon dioxide is exhaled, usually caused by hyperventilation. One of the causes of this condition is hypoxia, which stimulates the person to breathe more vigorously. Hyperventilation results in decreased carbon dioxide. The loss of carbon dioxide results in a decrease in the $H^+$ concentration along with a decrease in $pCO_2$ and an increase in the ratio of bicarbonate to carbonic acid. The result is an increase in the pH level. Since the basic problem is related to the respiratory system, the kidneys will compensate by excreting more bicarbonate ions and retaining $H^+$. This process will return the acid-base balance to a normal ratio.

**Circulatory Alterations**   An adequate cardiac output is essential for the exchange of oxygen and carbon dioxide. Sufficient amounts of blood must be delivered to the pulmonary system for gas exchange to occur. The amount of oxygen that is available to the tissues depends on the oxygen content of the blood as well as the cardiac output.

The pulmonary and cardiac systems work together to maintain normal tissue respiration. These two systems are influenced by the heart and buffer mechanisms, which act to maintain normal circulation and blood pressure.

The buffer mechanisms in the body assist in maintaining the exchange of oxygen and carbon dioxide. The capillaries respond to decreased $pO_2$ or increased $pCO_2$ levels by vasodilatation. When vasodilatation occurs, the flow of blood is reduced and the amount of time for gaseous exchange is increased. As the flow of blood decreases, peripheral resistance is lowered and venous return reduced.

Whenever there is a decreased venous return, alterations in cardiac output take place, which result in the accumulation of excessive amounts of fluid in the pulmonary system. This excess fluid reduces the space available for $O_2$-$CO_2$ exchange and can cause vasoconstriction. When this happens, the blood is shunted to capillaries in better ventilated areas of the lungs to allow for better tissue oxygenation.

Another result of decreased venous return is a drop in blood pressure. Aortic and carotid baroreceptors respond to increases or decreases in blood pressure. A decrease in the arterial blood pressure results in a reflex increase in respiratory rate. The baroreflex mechanism restores the blood pressure to normal. If these mechanisms cannot respond adequately, the blood flow to the tissues will be decreased and normal metabolic activities will be altered.

Alterations in intrapulmonic pressure occur when pressures in the lungs and thorax change which alters respiration. Intrapulmonic pressure must be less than atmospheric pressure for air to flow into the lungs. If air enters the intrapleural space, the negative pressure is lost, leading to a collapse of the lung and expansion of the thoracic cage.

**Airway Alterations**   Obstructions which block the airways can cause pathological conditions, such as bronchiectasis, atelectasis, or pneumothorax. Whenever an obstruction occurs in the respiratory tract, regardless of cause, a change in the respiratory status of the patient occurs.

Maintaining a patent airway is essential for respiration to be sustained. Obstruction of the airway can be caused by a mucus plug, particles of food lodged in a small opening, epiglottitis, croup, and laryngeal paralysis.

Pathological changes can affect the mechanics of respiration by interfering with the movement of air into and out of the airways. Tumors can put pressure on the airway and decrease airway space. Edema, accumulated secretions, and spasms of smooth muscle can compromise the bronchioles and increase airway resistance, causing expiratory difficulties. Anatomical alterations such as scoliosis and kyphosis can also restrict the total vital capacity of the lungs.

**Gaseous Exchange Alterations**   Adequate gas exchange within the lung fields depends on the effective ventilation of air and perfusion of blood in both lungs. The thickness and permeability of the alveolar membrane, the amount of surface area available for diffusion, and the pressure gradient are also factors that affect gas exchange.

Ventilation replenishes the supply of oxygen in the alveoli and removes the carbon dioxide released by the capillaries. If ventilation is not uniform throughout all the lung fields (due to a change in perfusion of one area of the lung), then the rate of oxygen replenishment is reduced, which can lead to hypoxemia.

Ventilation-perfusion problems are usually the result of chronic conditions such as heart failure, asthma, and chronic obstructive pulmonary disease (COPD), as well as acute conditions such as pneumonia.

In the normal lung the capacity for diffusion of both oxygen and carbon dioxide is so great and the alveolar capillary membrane so thin that gas exchange occurs long before the blood reaches the end of the pulmonary capillary.

Diseases that cause thickening of the alveolar membrane, such as COPD, will impair this gas exchange and cause hypoxemia and hypercapnia. When the alveolar surface area is decreased in chronic conditions such as COPD, serious problems in gas exchange can occur.

## NURSING INTERVENTIONS

The primary purpose for performing nursing interventions associated with respiratory function is to improve vital capacity and pulmonary ventilation.

Nursing interventions are utilized routinely as preventative measures in most clinical settings. These interventions help prevent respiratory complications for patients on extended periods of bed rest, for patients who are prone to respiratory complications, or for surgical patients who have undergone general anesthesia.

To maintain maximum vital capacity with minimal effort, assist the respiratory patient to Fowler's position. It is also beneficial that the patient remain in a forward-leaning position on an over-bed table for a period of time. In addition to positioning, the removal of secretions from the tracheobronchial tree requires that humidity be consistently administered. This liquefies the secretions and enables the patient to expectorate the mucus or the nurse to suction more effectively. Turning, coughing and deep-breathing exercises also assist in removing secretions as well as increasing oxygen-carbon dioxide exchange. Additional therapy with the IPPB or medication may be necessary for the severely compromised patient.

The most common clinical manifestations which indicate hypoxia are:

Tachycardia
Gasping and/or irregular respirations (dyspnea)
Restlessness
Flaring nostrils
Cyanosis
Substernal or intercostal retractions
Increased blood pressure followed by decreased blood pressure

Hypoxia is a common condition associated with respiratory disorders. The early detection of hypoxia will assist in preventing respiratory complications.

## NURSING DIAGNOSES

The following nursing diagnoses may be appropriate to include in a Patient Care Plan when the components are related to respiratory conditions.

| Nursing Diagnosis (Potential) | Defining Characteristic; Etiology (Examples) |
|---|---|
| ☐ Activity Intolerance, *related to* | Dyspnea, fatigue, e.g., physiological impairment of respiratory system, decreased respiratory reserve. |
| ☐ Airway Clearance, Ineffective, *related to* | Inability to clear secretions, obstructed respiratory tract, e.g., chest trauma, surgical interventions, pain. |
| ☐ Anxiety, *related to* | Ineffective breathing patterns, e.g., chronic respiratory disorders (COPD). |
| ☐ Breathing Pattern, Ineffective, *related to* | Inability to maintain sufficient oxygen supply to cells, e.g., neuromuscular impairment, chronic respiratory disease states. |
| ☐ Comfort, Alteration in: Pain, *related to* | Inflammatory process, e.g., acute respiratory states (pleurisy, pneumonia), terminal states (cancer). |
| ☐ Nutrition, Alteration in: Less Than Body Requirements, *related to* | Excessive expectoration, intubation, fatigue, prolonged coughing, e.g., chronic respiratory states, chest trauma. |
| ☐ Oral Mucous Membrane, Alteration in, *related to* | Prolonged mouth breathing, bypassed airway, e.g., disease state, intubation, comatose state. |
| ☐ Self-Care Deficit: Total, *related to* | Fatigue, ineffective breathing, hypoxic states (confusion), e.g., chronic respiratory disorders, impaired gas exchange. |

# UNIT ONE   DEEP BREATHING EXERCISES

## NURSING PROCESS DATA

### ASSESSMENT   *Data Base*

Observe patient's physical ability to perform exercise (e.g., to assume Fowler's position, the degree of pain experienced, and the amount of medication needed to control pain).

Auscultate breath sounds.

Observe rhythm, rate, and depth of respiration.

Note presence of cough reflex.

Note placement of incision in relation to diaphragmatic muscles necessary for breathing. The incision may interfere with lung expansion.

### PLANNING   *Objectives*

To improve vital capacity and pulmonary ventilation.

To conserve energy.

To loosen secretions and promote full lung expansion.

To assist abdominal breathing to become more automatic and respirations more efficient and relaxed.

To counteract effects of hypoventilation and effects of anesthetic agents.

**IMPLEMENTATION**   *Procedures*

Instructing Patients to Deep Breathe

Instructing Patients to Cough

Teaching Diaphragmatic Breathing

Using Flow Incentive Spirometers

Using Volume Spirometers (Triflo or Respirex)

**EVALUATION**   *Expected Outcomes*

Vital capacity and pulmonary ventilation are improved.

Patient reaches predetermined tidal volume level when using incentive spirometer.

Patient's energy is conserved.

Secretions are loosened and lungs fully expanded.

Abdominal breathing is more automatic and respirations more efficient and relaxed.

## INSTRUCTING PATIENTS TO DEEP BREATHE

### Equipment

Hospital bed in upright position or a straight chair
Pillows for positioning and abdominal support

### Preparation

1. Wash your hands.
2. Provide privacy.
3. Explain the rationale for the procedure.
4. Prior to exercise, instruct the patient to clear respiratory tract by coughing.
5. Position patient to sit up in bed as straight as possible, with head and shoulders supported by a firm surface. **Rationale:** This position maintains maximum vital capacity.

### Procedure

1. Demonstrate the deep breathing steps, allowing time for patient to practice each step.
2. Place your hands palm down around the sides of patient's lower ribs. **Rationale:** This action sup-

ports deep breathing and assists you to evaluate depth of inspiration.
3. Tell patient to breathe in slowly through nose until chest is expanded and abdominal muscles rise visibly.
4. Watch for contraction of intercostal muscles and diaphragm. Tell patient to exhale.
5. Check patient's response to determine how often exercise should be performed—varies according to the patient's condition.
   a. After abdominal or chest surgery, patient should practice this exercise every four hours daily, with five to ten breaths during each exercise.
   b. Patients with pulmonary problems such as COPD, cystic fibrosis, or high abdominal surgery should practice this exercise every hour, with a minimum of five deep breaths during each practice.

## INSTRUCTING PATIENTS TO COUGH

### Equipment

Hospital bed in upright position or a straight chair
Pillows for positioning and abdominal support

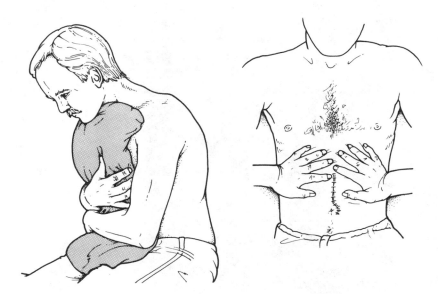

Instruct the patient in deep breathing and coughing exercises preoperatively to enhance their lung expansion postoperatively.

### Preparation

1. Wash your hands.
2. Provide privacy.

### Procedure

1. Place patient in a sitting position to initiate coughing.
2. Instruct patient to inhale deeply and to cough, using abdominal and other respiratory muscles.
3. Support any abdominal incision with the palms of your hands on either side of the patient's incision. You may also place a rolled pillow firmly against the incision. **Rationale:** This will prevent incisional pain and encourage patient to cough more effectively.
4. Encourage patient to cough frequently. Explain why coughing will be beneficial. **Rationale:** Accumulated secretions in the lungs can compromise the bronchioles.

## TEACHING DIAPHRAGMATIC BREATHING

### Equipment

Hospital bed in flat position

### Preparation

1. Check physician's orders and Patient Care Plan.
2. Wash your hands.
3. Provide privacy.

4. Inform patient that the purpose of this exercise is to learn how to breathe by using abdominal muscles.

### Procedure

1. Place patient in a supine position. (After learning the exercise, patient may assume other positions.)
2. Tell patient to breathe in deeply through nose.
3. Tell patient to purse lips and to forcibly exhale air through the mouth to make a slow "whoosh" sound. **Rationale:** Pursing the lips creates a resistance against air flowing out of lungs by increasing pressure within the bronchus.
4. Instruct patient to contract (tighten) abdominal muscles while exhaling. The patient's chest should move as little as possible. **Rationale:** This will assist the patient to forcefully exhale.
5. Tell patient to relax and stretch after completing the exercise.
6. Continue accelerating this exercise, gradually increasing patient's diaphragmatic breathing for five to ten minutes, four times a day.

## USING FLOW SPIROMETERS

### Equipment

Hospital bed in upright position or straight chair

Pillows for positioning

Flow incentive spirometer

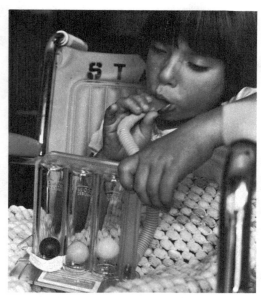

The TRIFLO II facilitates deep inspiration when the patient inhales. Inhaling deeply lifts the Triflo balls to the top of the chambers.

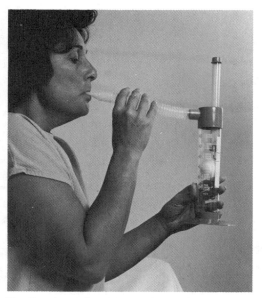

The Respirex spirometer reaches optimal levels of 2700 cc/sec when inspired breath is maintained for 1 second and up to 5400 cc/sec for 3 seconds.

### Preparation

1. Check physician's order and Patient Care Plan.
2. Gather equipment.
3. Wash your hands.
4. Explain purpose and procedure to patient.

### Procedure

1. Have patient hold incentive spirometer upright. **Rationale:** When spirometer tilts less effort is needed to raise ball.
2. Instruct patient to take in a deep breath through the mouth after lips have formed a tight seal around mouthpiece of spirometer. Flow rates range from 100 to 2710 cc/second.
3. Encourage patient to keep the ball elevated for three seconds. **Rationale:** To provide for alveolar inflation.
4. Repeat the procedure hourly. This procedure maintains alveolar inflation.
5. Cleanse the mouthpiece and filter, if spirometer has a filter, with cold water first, then warm water and shake dry. **Rationale:** To prevent the harboring of microorganisms.
6. Store in patient's bedside unit.

## USING VOLUME SPIROMETERS

### Equipment

Hospital bed in upright position or straight chair
Pillows for positioning
Volume incentive spirometer e.g. Triflo or Respirex

### Preparation

1. Check physician's orders and Patient Care Plan.
2. Gather equipment.
3. Wash your hands.
4. Explain purpose and procedure to patient.
5. Set the predetermined volume. Volume ranges are 0 to 5000 cc, depending on type of spirometer.
6. Check that spirometer is functioning before patient begins procedure. **Rationale:** Most spirometers function on batteries.
7. Place spirometer on bedside table.

### Procedure

1. Place patient's mouthpiece on spirometer.
2. Instruct patient to inhale through mouthpiece. As patient inhales, air is drawn into system, causing

piston to rise to preset level. Lights may be illuminated identifying volume obtained or word HOLD may light up when volume is reached.

3. Instruct patient to hold breath for 2½ to 3 seconds. Repeat procedure according to physician's orders.

4. Following breathing exercises remove mouthpiece, cleanse with warm water, and store in bedside unit. **Rationale:** Volume incentive spirometers may be used for many patients, only mouth pieces are individualized.

**CHARTING** *for Deep Breathing and Coughing*

☐ Number and times of breathing exercises

☐ Whether cough is productive or not

☐ Amount and quality of secretions expectorated

☐ Changes in pulse rate, depth of respirations, and color of patient following exercise

☐ Patient's acceptance of, participation in, and feelings about procedure

☐ Number of times and response to flow or volume spirometers

## CLINICAL PROBLEM SOLVING

**Potential Problems**

Patient is unwilling to complete exercise because of fear of pain or dehiscence.

**Suggested Solutions**

☐ Instruct again on rationale and necessity for procedure.

☐ Demonstrate cough exercise after teaching the patient deep breathing.

☐ Support the incision area more fully, using the palms of your hands or a firmly rolled pillow to allay fears of dehiscence.

☐ Medicate 30 to 60 minutes before using spirometer or participating in breathing exercises.

Nasal congestion inhibits patient's breathing capability.

☐ Ask patient to blow nose prior to the breathing exercise.

☐ Check with physician so he may prescribe medications that will open nasal passages.

Patient is unable to master use of incentive devices.

☐ Encourage patient to start slowly and increase volume over several exercise sessions.

☐ Position patient in Fowler's position to assist with lung expansion.

☐ Provide positive reinforcement with increments in volume.

# UNIT TWO   PERCUSSION, VIBRATION, AND DRAINAGE (PVD)

## NURSING PROCESS DATA

### ASSESSMENT   *Data Base*

Listen to breath sounds. Check for adventitious sounds, ventilation, and air exchange.

Determine rhythm, rate and depth of respirations.

Note time elapsed since eating (at least one hour to prevent patient discomfort or regurgitation).

Observe quality of secretions. Thick, tenacious secretions will require manual chest percussion and vibration as well as drainage.

Note any complicating conditions: hypertension, CHF, cerebral edema, abdominal distention, arrhythmias.

### PLANNING  *Objectives*

To facilitate expectoration of retained secretions.

To decrease rales and/or rhonchi.

To reduce shortness of breath.

To assist coughing to be more productive/effective.

To decrease respiratory rate and increase ventilation and air exchange.

To minimize potential complications.

### IMPLEMENTATION  *Procedures*

Preparing Patient for PVD

Performing Percussion

Performing Vibration

Performing Postural Drainage

### EVALUATION  *Expected Outcomes*

Lungs cleared of retained secretions.

Breath sounds clearer to auscultation.

Rales and/or rhonchi decreased.

Shortness of breath reduced.

Coughing is more productive/effective.

Potential complications minimized.

## PREPARING PATIENT FOR PVD

### Procedure

1. Establish the location of each lung segment. If the entire lung field is to undergo chest physiotherapy, the most affected lobe or segment should be drained first. **Rationale:** Usually the lower or middle lobes are the most affected.

2. Protect patient from falling by keeping siderails up when possible.

3. If possible, arrange for privacy during procedure. (Patient may be embarrassed and/or uncomfortable.)

4. Remain with patient during initial procedure.

5. Administer treatment every two to four hours as ordered.

6. Prepare patient by discussing aeration exercises.

7. Explain importance of practicing PVD exercises after an operation to counteract effects of hypoventilation and to prevent complications.

8. Demonstrate steps, allowing time for patient to practice. Place towel over skin to prevent reddened areas when performing PVD.

9. Instruct patient, especially those with COPD, to perform diaphragmatic breathing with daily ac-

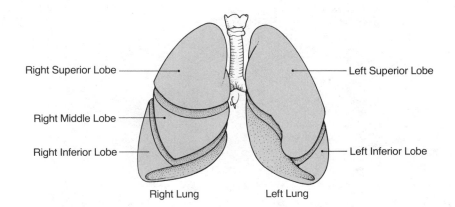

The lobes of the lungs.

tivities (sitting, walking) and to practice graded exercises to improve general physical fitness.

10. Auscultate all lobes for adventitious sounds prior to initiating PVD.

## PERFORMING PERCUSSION

### Equipment

Pillows for positioning

Hospital bed that can be placed in Trendelenburg (optional)

Container for sputum

Towel

### Preparation

Same as *Preparing Patient for PVD*

### Procedure

1. Cover area to be percussed with gown or towel to prevent skin trauma.

2. Cup your hands and clap rhythmically, alternating hands over area to be drained. Each percussion should sound hollow and not cause redness of skin.

3. Relax wrist and elbows when percussing.

4. Percuss for three to five minutes over each segment.

5. Encourage patient to cough between each segment percussion.

6. Auscultate all lobes for changes in breath sounds.

## PERFORMING VIBRATION

### Equipment

Pillows for positioning

Hospital bed that can be placed in Trendelenburg position

Container for sputum

### Preparation

Same as *Preparing Patient for PVD*

### Procedure

1. Instruct patient to breathe deeply through nose and exhale slowly through mouth.

2. Place your hands flat over area to be drained, keeping your arms and shoulders straight.

3. As patient exhales, vibrate by quickly contracting and relaxing your arms and shoulders for ten seconds.

4. Vibrate for several minutes, depending on viscosity of secretions and patient's tolerance.

5. Encourage coughing between vibrations of each segment.

6. Auscultate all lobes for changes in breath sounds.

## PERFORMING POSTURAL DRAINAGE

### Equipment

Hospital bed that can be placed in Trendelenburg position

Container for sputum

Mouthwash and emesis basin

### Preparation

Same as for *Preparing for PVD*

### Procedure

1. Loosen any binders or tight clothing.

2. Lower head of bed so that patient's head is po-

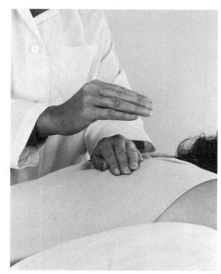

Cup your hands and use a rhythmic motion when performing percussion.

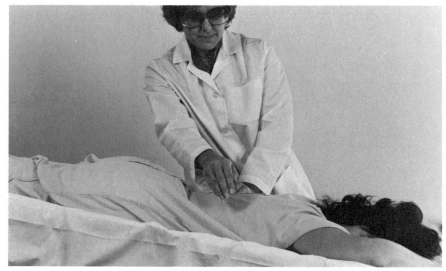

Position the patient so the "most affected" lobe is drained first, or place the patient in Trendelenburg's position to drain lower lobes first.

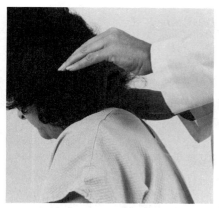

An upright, slightly forward position allows secretions to drain from the upper lobes.

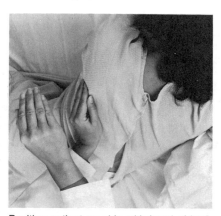

Position patient on side with head of bed raised slightly to facilitate drainage.

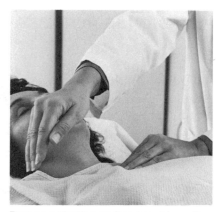

Percuss patient's anterior upper lobes after lower lobes to facilitate drainage.

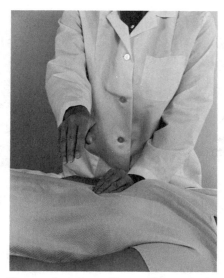

Place patient in positions which assist in draining affected lobes.

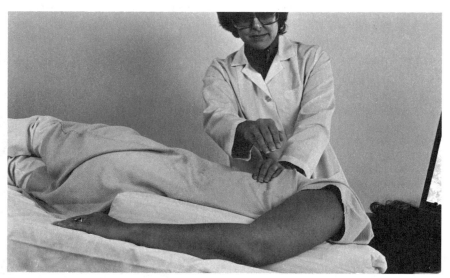

To drain the anterior base of the lobes, place patient in side-lying position with foot of bed elevated slightly. Observe for respiratory distress.

sitioned in a 30-degree downward angle if not contraindicated. (Head is lower than chest.)

3. Place sputum container and tissues within patient's reach.

4. Tell patient to remain in position from 5 to 15 minutes to allow secretions to drain. (Amount of time will vary, depending on patient's need and tolerance.)

5. Instruct patient to make short, rapid-fire coughs to expectorate secretions.

6. Ask patient to maintain deep abdominal breathing. **Rationale:** Assists with ventilating the lungs. (Patient should deep breathe and cough between each position change.)

7. Assist patient to slowly return to normal sitting position.

8. Offer oral hygiene with mouthwash.

9. Discard container and/or send sputum specimens to lab, if ordered.

10. Remain with patient for 5 to 10 minutes and observe patient's condition.

11. Auscultate lobes for breath sounds.

### CHARTING  *for PVD*

☐ Quantity and character of sputum

☐ Rate, depth of respiration, and pulse

☐ Any unusual symptoms following procedure, e.g., vertigo

☐ Patient's physical tolerance, including strength and stamina to complete procedure

☐ Patient's acceptance of and willingness to participate in procedure

☐ Lung sounds before and after PVD

---

## CLINICAL PROBLEM SOLVING

| **Potential Problems** | **Suggested Solutions** |
|---|---|
| Patient experiences vertigo or syncope during postural drainage. | ☐ Change position so that patient's head is not as low, especially if patient is elderly or very weak. <br> ☐ Report to physician so that mechanical means, such as suctioning, may be used to remove secretions. |
| Patient is unable to assume extreme head-down position for postural drainage. | ☐ Use all positions but modify degree of Trendelenburg's position so that the patient's head is slightly lower than chest. <br> ☐ Turn patient on side with pillow support to facilitate bronchial drainage. |
| Patient coughs and vomits with PVD treatment. | ☐ Give treatments immediately before the meal. <br> ☐ Report to physician so that an order for antiemetic before every treatment may be obtained. <br> ☐ Encourage use of other treatment modalities until sputum is more readily expectorated without vomiting. |

---

# UNIT THREE  SUCTIONING

## NURSING PROCESS DATA

### ASSESSMENT  *Data Base*

Assess patient's need for suctioning.

Observe vital signs for increases in pulse and respiration and for changes in skin color.

Auscultate for adventitious sounds to evaluate lung field.

Observe respiratory status for tachypnea, shortness of breath, noisy respirations, and restlessness.

Observe level of consciousness to assess hypoxia.

### PLANNING *Objectives*

To provide patent airway.

To remove secretions.

To increase respiratory ventilation.

To decrease respiratory rate.

To increase tissue oxygenation.

### IMPLEMENTATION *Procedures*

Suctioning Using Separate Catheter and Glove

Suctioning Using Catheter and Sleeve

Suctioning Infants with Bulb Syringe

### EVALUATION *Expected Outcomes*

Secretions removed without complications.

Increased respiratory ventilation with increased tissue oxygenation.

Breath sounds clear; no adventitious sounds auscultated.

## SUCTIONING USING SEPARATE CATHETER AND GLOVE

### Equipment

Portable suction machine or wall suction with Y connector or release port

Disposable suction catheter (size 5 for infants, size 8–10 for children, and to size 18 for adults)

Sterile or clean (check policy) gloves

Container for sterile saline

Sterile saline, labeled with date and time opened (opened bottles should be discarded after 24 hours)

Receptacle for used equipment

### Preparation

1. Check physician's orders and Patient Care Plan.

2. Select a catheter that is one-half the diameter of the patient's nares.

3. Wash your hands before starting procedure.

4. Assess lung sounds.

5. Open catheter package, leaving protective covering over catheter.

6. Attach catheter to tubing on suction machine.

### Procedure

1. Explain procedure and rationale to patient regardless of level of consciousness. Allocate time for patient to express fears and concerns or clarify steps of procedure if alert.

2. Place patient in semi-Fowler's position. (Or use dorsal recumbent position, with patient's head turned toward you.)

3. Put clean glove on the hand that will hold the sterile catheter unless otherwise dictated by hospital policy.

4. Turn on suction machine with ungloved hand. Set pressure of wall suction.

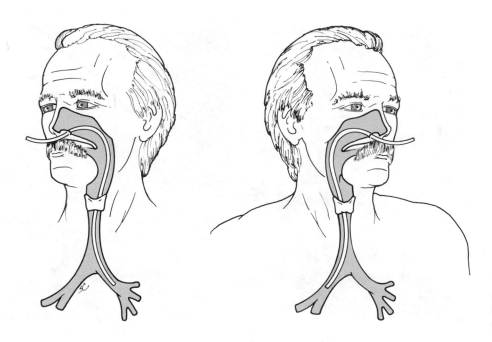

Suction the right and left main bronchus by turning the patient's head in the opposite direction of the bronchus being suctioned.

---

**Indications for Suctioning**
Decreased or absent cough reflex.
Semi-comatose or comatose patient.
Thick, tenacious mucus.
Debilitated, weak patient.
Impaired pulmonary function.

---

**Clinical Alert:**
When performing naso-oral suctioning the same procedure is used, but the catheter is inserted only 2 to 4 inches into the nares or within the oral cavity. The catheter does not extend down to the pharynx or trachea.

---

5. Pour sterile saline into container and lubricate catheter with sterile normal saline.

6. Instruct patient to cough to mobilize secretions into pharynx, or if patient is unable to cough, tickle back of throat with catheter. **Rationale:** Prevents irritation to respiratory tract.

7. Insert catheter 6 to 8 inches into nares. *Do not apply suction.* To introduce catheter into right and left main bronchi, turn patient's head away from the bronchus to be suctioned. **Rationale:** The sternocleidomastoid muscle assists in guiding the catheter into the left bronchus. The right bronchus, because of the angle of the trachea, easily allows the entrance of the catheter into the right side.

8. Advance catheter as far as possible. **Rationale:** To reach area where most mucus is sequestered.

9. Begin suctioning by using a rotating motion as the catheter is withdrawn.

a. To provide suction, place your thumb over valve or Y connector on catheter.
b. To release pressure, remove your thumb from valve or Y connector.

10. If cough reflex is stimulated, withdraw catheter slightly to prevent excessive reflex stimulation.

11. Prevent removal of excessive oxygen by limiting suction to no more than 10 or 15 seconds at one time.

12. Rinse catheter in sterile saline, and repeat suctioning procedure in opposite nares. **Rationale:** To clear tubing of mucus and increase suction in system.

13. Repeat procedure as necessary. If larger amounts of secretions are present, allow at least three minutes between suctionings. **Rationale:** To prevent loss of oxygen.

14. When procedure is completed, turn off suction machine.

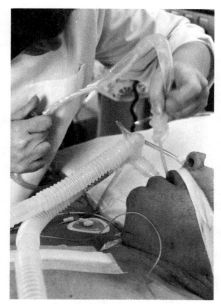

Suction patient's nose and mouth before performing tracheal or endotracheal suction.

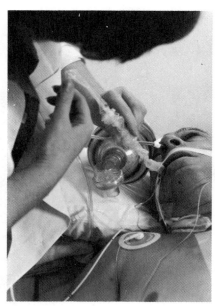

Slide plastic protector back over catheter as it is inserted through endotracheal tube.

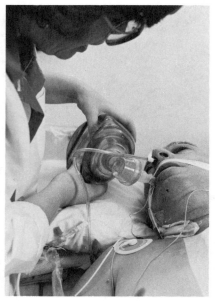

Hyperoxygenate patient with a manual resuscitator bag following suctioning.

15. Dispose of glove.

16. Dispose of catheter, or if catheter is to be reused, rinse it thoroughly in sterile saline and place it in receptacle as outlined in hospital policy. Replace catheter every eight hours or as directed by hospital policy.

17. Offer oral hygiene.

18. Place patient in comfortable position.

19. Assess lung sounds for changes.

20. Wash your hands.

21. Empty suction bottle at the end of every shift. **Rationale:** To prevent harboring of microorganisms in bottle.

## SUCTIONING USING CATHETER AND SLEEVE

### Equipment

Portable suction machine or wall suction with Y connector or release valve

Disposable suction catheter (size 5 for infants, size 8–10 for children, and to size 18 for adults)

Container for sterile saline

Bottle of sterile saline, labeled with date and time opened (opened bottles should be discarded after 24 hours)

---

**Suction Catheters**

Disposable plastic or rubber French catheters.

| | |
|---|---|
| Adults: | 12 – 18 French |
| Children: | 8 – 10 French |
| Infants: | 5 – 8 French |

**Suction Machines**

Wall Unit

| | |
|---|---|
| Adults: | 120 – 150 mm Hg |
| Children: | 80 – 120 mm Hg |
| Infants: | 60 – 100 mm Hg |

Portable Unit

| | |
|---|---|
| Adults: | 5 – 10 cm Hg |
| Children: | 0 – 5 cm Hg |

Portable units may be calibrated in inches or pounds of pressure.

---

Receptacle for used equipment

### Preparation

1. Check physician's order and Patient Care Plan.

2. Gather equipment.

3. Select a catheter that is one-half the diameter of the patient's nares.

4. Wash your hands before starting procedure.

5. Open catheter package, leaving protective covering over catheter.

---

**Clinical Alert:**
Do not suction patients who exhibit signs of laryngo or bronchospasm, as this could lead to occlusion of airway.

---

6. Attach catheter to tubing on suction machine.

7. Explain procedure and rationale to patient.

8. Place patient in semi-Fowler's position. (Or place in dorsal recumbent position, with patient's head turned toward you.)

9. Auscultate lung sounds.

## Procedure

1. Take container for normal saline out of package.

2. Pour 30 to 50 cc sterile saline in receptacle. Slide back protective covering over catheter.

3. Turn on suctioning machine. Set pressure of wall unit according to chart.

4. Lubricate catheter tip with saline.

5. Continue to slide back protective covering over catheter as you insert catheter in nose or mouth.

6. Insert catheter 6 to 8 inches for nasotracheal suctioning. *Do not apply suction.* **Rationale:** To prevent trauma to mucous membranes.

7. Advance catheter as far as possible.

8. Begin suctioning by using a rotating motion as the catheter is withdrawn.
   a. To provide suction, place your thumb over valve or Y connector on catheter.
   b. To release pressure, remove your thumb from valve or Y connector.

9. Withdraw catheter slightly if patient begins to cough.

10. Limit suction to 10 or 15 seconds at one time. **Rationale:** To prevent removal of excessive oxygen.

11. Rinse catheter in sterile saline, and repeat suctioning procedure in opposite nares.

12. Repeat procedure as necessary. If large amounts of secretions are present, allow at least three minutes between suctionings. **Rationale:** This prevents oxygen depletion.

13. When procedure is completed, turn off suction machine.

14. Dispose of catheter after each use.

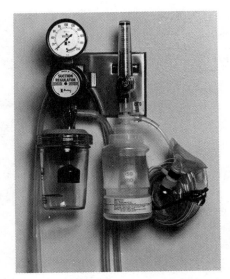

Turn on wall-mounted suction machine to appropriate setting.

15. Offer oral hygiene.

16. Place patient in comfortable position.

17. Assess lung sounds for changes.

18. Wash your hands.

19. Empty suction bottle at the end of every shift.

## SUCTIONING INFANTS WITH BULB SYRINGE

### Equipment

Bulb syringe for newborn

### Procedure

1. Identify infant by checking arm band.

2. Place infant in supine position.

3. Squeeze air from bulb of syringe.

4. Insert tip of syringe into infant's mouth and release finger pressure from bulb, then insert into external nares and repeat. **Rationale:** It is important to suction mouth first, as delicate receptors in nose may be stimulated and cause infant to inhale mucus from the mouth.

5. Release bulb and remove from mouth or nares.

6. Squeeze bulb to expel secretions into basin or gauze.

7. Repeat steps 3 to 6 until mouth and nares are clear of secretions.

8. Rinse the syringe by immersing tip in water, expanding bulb, and squeezing bulb to expel water.

9. Reposition infant on side or on abdomen with head turned to one side. **Rationale:** This promotes drainage of secretions.

## CHARTING  *for Suctioning*

☐  Amount, color, and consistency of secretions

☐  Changes in breath sounds

☐  Respiratory rate

☐  Unanticipated problems and patient's response

☐  Patient's tolerance to procedure

☐  Number of times patient was suctioned

☐  Fluid intake

☐  Hyperinflation of oxygen with ambu or Laerdahl bag

---

## CLINICAL PROBLEM SOLVING

**Potential Problems**

Obstruction in nares.

Irritation from frequent nasopharyngeal suctioning.

Hypoxia may occur if incorrect techniques are used for suctioning.

Excessive secretions that require frequent suctioning are present.

Bleeding from nose or mouth.

**Suggested Solutions**

☐  Remove catheter from the nares, and insert into the other nares. (Deviated septum is more frequently found on left side of nose.)

☐  If ordered, a nasal airway can be inserted and used to suction through.

☐  If both nares are obstructed, suction through mouth.

☐  Report to physician and obtain order and insert decongestive nose drops to decrease irritation.

☐  Provide frequent care of nares.

☐  Observe for signs of increased restlessness, shortness of breath, yawning and/or cyanosis while suctioning.

☐  Limit suctioning time to no more than 15 seconds.

☐  Ensure that catheter is half the diameter of the tube or nares.

☐  Suction once, then reapply oxygen for a couple of minutes before continuing suctioning.

☐  If ordered, hyperinflate lungs with oxygen, using ambu or Laerdahl bag and 100% oxygen.

☐  Administer oxygen as ordered.

☐  After suctioning, attach new suction catheter to tubing on suction machine so that you have a catheter available in case of an emergency.

☐  Suction more frequently but use ambu or Laerdahl bag to administer 100% oxygen before and after suctioning.

☐  Use smaller size catheter to prevent irritation.

☐  Place patient in semi-Fowler's position to prevent aspiration of blood.

☐  Prevent irritation to mucous membrane by applying suction after inserting catheter and by keeping suction pressure low.

| | |
|---|---|
| | ☐ Administer oral hygiene and/or care of nares to prevent infection of mucous membranes. |
| | ☐ Suction in different area of mouth or nose if area is excoriated. |
| Wheezing sounds occur following suctioning due to laryngospasm. | ☐ Do not repeat suctioning. |
| | ☐ Administer oxygen with mist if ordered. |
| | ☐ Place patient in semi-Fowler's position to assist in lung expansion. |
| | ☐ Encourage to take slow, deep breaths. |
| Suctioning equipment is nonfunctioning. | ☐ Examine suction equipment to determine if it is securely attached to wall outlet or plugged into electrical outlet. |
| | ☐ Check that suction equipment is turned ON. |
| | ☐ If "hissing" sound is present, check that seal is around the top of the bottle. |
| | ☐ Observe that connections between catheter and suction equipment are secure and tight without evidence of catheter or tube kinking. |

# UNIT FOUR OXYGEN THERAPY

## NURSING PROCESS DATA

### ASSESSMENT  *Data Base*

Check if patient has a patent airway.

Assess patient's vital signs.

Observe patient for signs of hypoxia.

Assess skin under oxygen mask for irritation.

Assess for signs of carbon dioxide narcosis.

### PLANNING  *Objectives*

To return arterial $pO_2$ to normal range.

To correct hypoxic condition so that patient is adequately oxygenated.

To assist respiration to return to normal rate.

To increase comfort and breathing efficiency for patients with chronic lung disease.

### IMPLEMENTATION  *Procedures*

Monitoring Patients with Oxygen

Using an Oxygen Cylinder

Using an Oxygen Analyzer

Using a Nasal Cannula

Using a Nasal Catheter

Using an Oxygen Face Mask

Using a Pediatric Oxygen Mask

Using an Oxygen Tent

Using a Pediatric Oxygen Tent

Using a Croupette

Using an Oxygen Hood

**EVALUATION** *Expected Outcomes*

Arterial $pO_2$ returns to normal range.

Correction of hypoxic condition results.

Increased comfort and breathing efficiency for patients with chronic lung disease.

## MONITORING PATIENTS WITH OXYGEN

### Equipment

Oxygen administration set

Oxygen flowmeter

Bed in high-Fowler's position

### Procedure

1. Check physician's order in chart for type of oxygen therapy, administration set and desired oxygen liter flow.

2. Place patient in semi- or high-Fowler's position to ensure adequate lung expansion.

3. Turn and reposition patient frequently to prevent skin decubiti.

4. Encourage deep breathing and coughing exercises unless directed otherwise.

5. Ensure adequate hydration, especially if secretions are thick and tenacious.

6. Check equipment frequently to ensure functioning of oxygen flow, humidifier, and temperature.

7. Assess patient's progress by frequently checking vital signs, color, and level of consciousness.

8. Assess patients with chronic obstructive lung disease frequently for signs of carbon dioxide narcosis:
   a. Bounding peripheral pulses
   b. High blood pressure
   c. Increased pulse pressure

> **Clinical Alert**
> Oxygen is used very conservatively on anyone with chronic lung disease because high levels of oxygen will disrupt carbon dioxide center and lead to respiratory arrest.

   d. Warm, clammy skin
   e. Cerebral edema

9. Remain with patients who are frightened or anxious until they feel secure.

## USING AN OXYGEN CYLINDER

### Equipment

Source of oxygen supply: steel cylinder (oxygen tank) or wall oxygen outlet

Regulator: flowmeter

Humidifier

Sterile distilled water

### Procedure

1. Place oxygen cylinder in secure, upright position.

2. Check tag to determine amount of oxygen in the tank. Tag should say "Full."

3. Slowly turn hand knob on cylinder clockwise to crack tank open for a brief second to clear opening of tank; then close.

**TABLE 1** SPECIAL OXYGEN EQUIPMENT

*Nasal Cannula and Prongs*

This equipment is easily tolerated by most patients. It is also simpler than a mask, but provides less humidification. The $FIO_2$ will vary depending on the flow.

| | | | |
|---|---|---|---|
| $FIO_2$: | 24–38% | Flow: | 1–2 liters |
| $FIO_2$: | 30–35% | Flow: | 3–4 liters |
| $FIO_2$: | 38–44% | Flow: | 5–6 liters |

*Nasal Catheter*

This catheter is less comfortable than a cannula and is used infrequently.

| | | | |
|---|---|---|---|
| $FIO_2$: | 30% | Flow: | 4–8 liters |

Size: No. 8–10 F for children, No. 10–12 F for women, and No. 12–14F for men.

*Face Mask without Reservoir Bag*

This equipment requires fairly high flows to prevent rebreathing of carbon dioxide. Accurate $FIO_2$ is difficult to estimate.

| | | | |
|---|---|---|---|
| $FIO_2$: | 35–45% | Flow: | 8–12 liters |
| $FIO_2$: | 45–55% | Flow: | 8–12 liters |
| $FIO_2$: | 55–65% | Flow: | 8–12 liters |

*Mask with Reservoir Bag*

The reservoir allows higher $FIO_2$ to be delivered. At flows of less than 6 l/min, the risk of rebreathing carbon dioxide increases.

| | | | |
|---|---|---|---|
| $FIO_2$: | 50–60% | Flow: | 6 liters |
| $FIO_2$: | 60–70% | Flow: | 7 liters |
| $FIO_2$: | 70–100% | Flow: | 8–10 liters |

Two types are available:

*Partial rebreathing mask:* No inspiratory valve so that the beginning portion of exhaled air returns to the bag and mixes with the inspired air. Ports are present so that expired air escapes.

*Nonrebreather:* Valve is present which closes during expiration so that any exhaled air is forced through the expiratory valve on the face piece.

*Venturi Mask*

This mask allows a fixed or predicted $FIO_2$ to be delivered. It is utilized effectively on patients with COPD when accurate $FIO_2$ is necessary for proper treatment. Carbon dioxide buildup is kept at a minimum.

| | | | |
|---|---|---|---|
| $FIO_2$: | 24% | Flow: | 2–4 liters |
| $FIO_2$: | 28% | Flow: | 4–6 liters |
| $FIO_2$: | 35% | Flow: | 6–8 liters |

*Face Tent*

This tent is well tolerated by patients but is sometimes difficult to keep in place. It is convenient for providing humidification and compressed air in conjunction with nasal prongs.

| | | | |
|---|---|---|---|
| $FIO_2$: | 35–50% | Flow: | 8–10 liters |

*Oxygen Tent*

An oxygen tent is useful for high concentration of oxygen (50–60%) and for circulation of moist air around the patient. It will provide low-to-moderate concentration of oxygen in a temperature-controlled environment.

An oxygen tent is also useful for patients who fear suffocation or experience claustrophobia. It allows the patients to move freely but may produce feelings of isolation.

| | | | |
|---|---|---|---|
| $FIO_2$: | 50–60% | Flow: | 10+ liters |

*Oxygen Hood*

This is a hood that fits over a child's head to provide warm humidified oxygen at high concentrations. It is useful because it includes an oxygen limiter to prevent oxygen concentration from exceeding 40%, thus reducing the hazard of retrolental fibroplasia.

| | | | |
|---|---|---|---|
| $FIO_2$: | 28–40% | Flow: | 5–8 liters |
| $FIO_2$: | 40–85% | Flow: | 8–12 liters |

*Less than 5 liters flow may lead to carbon dioxide narcosis.*

*Croupette*

A croupette is used with premature infants to provide oxygen and to maintain temperature. It is also useful for a child who requires oxygen and/or high humidification. The unit prevents chilling in an atmosphere of aerated mist.

| | | | |
|---|---|---|---|
| $FIO_2$: | 28–40% | Flow: | 10 liters |
| $FIO_2$: | 40–50% | Flow: | 10–15 liters |

## Conditions Requiring Oxygen Therapy

Atmospheric hypoxia: oxygen therapy will correct depressed level of oxygen.

Hypoventilation hypoxia: 100% oxygen will yield five times more oxygen into the alveoli than normal air.

## Conditions Where Oxygen Therapy Is Not Corrective

Hypoxia caused by anemia, carbon monoxide poisoning, or abnormality of hemoglobin transport.

Inadequate tissue use of oxygen (cyanide poisoning).

Chronic obstructive lung disease requires that oxygen be used with caution since oxygen could suppress respiratory drive and result in respiratory arrest.

## Symptoms of Hypoxia

*Early symptoms*

Restlessness
Headache
Visual disturbances
Slight confusion
Hyperventilation
Tachycardia
Hypertension
Dyspnea

*Advanced symptoms*

Hypotension
Bradycardia
Metabolic acidosis (production of lactic acid)
Cyanosis

*Chronic hypoxia*

Polycythemia
Clubbing of fingers and toes
Thrombosis

## Safety Precautions

☐ Set up "No Smoking" and "Oxygen in Use" signs at the site of administration and at the door.
☐ Remove matches and lighters from bedside.
☐ Disconnect grounded electrical equipment.
☐ Remove all volatile materials except solutions and equipment to be used during intervention.
☐ Make sure that all electrical monitoring equipment is properly grounded.
☐ Locate fire extinguishers.

4. Attach regulator to valve outlet. **Rationale:** Regulates gas flow in liters/minute.

5. Fill humidifier with sterile distilled water to indicated level on bottle. Prefilled/disposable humidifier bottles are now available. **Rationale:** Humidity prevents mucous membranes from drying out.

6. Attach top of humidifier to oxygen flowmeter. Turn oxygen cylinder hand knob to open flow.

7. Slowly open handwheel and adjust flowmeter to prescribed liters/minute.

8. Change sign on oxygen cylinder to read "In Use."

## USING AN OXYGEN ANALYZER

### Equipment

Analyzer

### Procedure

1. Calibrate analyzer with room atmosphere prior to each reading.

2. Open tubing to the air, and compress two full times to fill analyzer.

3. Depress button. Analyzer should read 20% for room air. Adjust dial as necessary to obtain this reading.

4. Place tubing close to patient's nose.

5. Compress bulb 3 to 6 times, depress button, and read findings.

6. Based on reading, adjust oxygen flow.

7. Check analyzer with 100% oxygen at least one time per day.

## USING A NASAL CANNULA

### Equipment

O$_2$ supply

Regulator

Humidifier

Nasal cannula

### Preparation

1. Check physician's orders for oxygen.

2. Gather equipment.

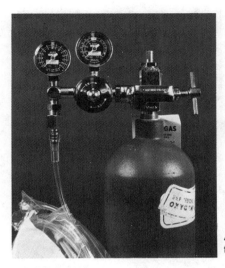

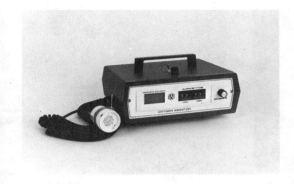

An oxygen analyzer used for in-line respirator oxygen checks.

After regulator and flow meter have been attached, crack the cylinder to clear dust.

## Procedure

1. Explain the purpose and procedures of oxygen therapy to patient.

2. Place tips of cannula no more than one-half inch into patient's nares.

3. Fasten tubing to pillow and bed sheets if bed rest is maintained.

4. Adjust flow of oxygen. Should be limited to 6 liters/minute for nasal prongs. **Rationale:** There is variable oxygen concentration since atmospheric air mixes with prescribed oxygen concentration.

   The $FIO_2$ will vary depending on the flow.

   | | | | | |
   |---|---|---|---|---|
   | $FIO_2$: | 24–38% | Flow: | 1–2 liters |
   | $FIO_2$: | 30–35% | Flow: | 3–4 liters |
   | $FIO_2$: | 38–44% | Flow: | 5–6 liters |

5. Monitor vital signs and check patient's condition frequently.

6. Provide nose care every four hours.

7. Change equipment (tubing, catheter, cannula) daily.

## USING A NASAL CATHETER

### Equipment

Nasal catheter:
   No. 8–10F for children
   No. 10–12F for women
   No. 12–14F for men

Water-soluble lubricating jelly

Adhesive tape

Flashlight and tongue depressor

Oxygen supply

Regulator

Humidifier

### Preparation

1. Check physician's order for oxygen.

2. Gather equipment for insertion of catheter.

3. Wash your hands.

### Procedure

1. Explain procedure to patient.

2. Attach catheter to connecting tubing. Attach humidifier to flowmeter, then to wall outlet or oxygen tank after cracking tank.

3. Turn on oxygen to 3 liters/minute, and test oxygen flow by placing over your hand to feel for flow.

4. Lubricate tip of catheter with water-soluble lubricant.

5. Position patient with neck hyperextended.

6. Ensure flow of oxygen.

7. Slowly insert catheter no more than 5 inches into nares.

8. Examine placement (entrance to oropharynx) by depressing patient's tongue with tongue blade and observing throat with the aid of a flashlight.

9. Adjust flow rate to the liters ordered. (Flow

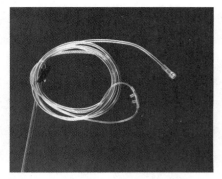

Nasal prongs, the most frequently used method, delivers up to 44% oxygen.

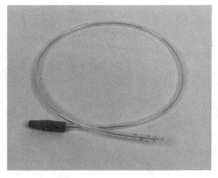

Nasal catheters are used less frequently and can deliver no more than 45% oxygen.

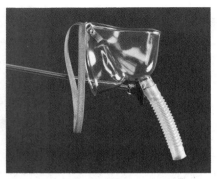

The oxygen face tent delivers an unpredictable oxygen flow, but provides high humidity.

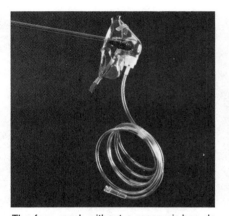

The face mask without a reservoir bag delivers a high oxygen concentrate.

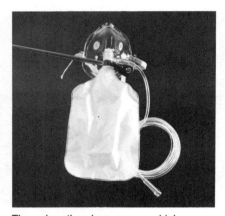

The rebreather bag ensures high oxygen concentration when inflated on inspiration.

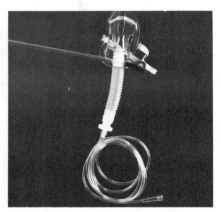

The Venturi mask is used when an exact amount of oxygen must be delivered.

should be limited to 5 liters/minute.) **Rationale:** Provides $FIO_2$ of 30%.

10. Secure catheter to bridge of patient's nose with tape.

11. Attach connecting tube to bed with enough slack for free movement.

12. Observe for gastric distention by palpating epigastrium.

13. Remain with patient until he feels secure and is not coughing or gagging.

14. Remove catheter and insert a new catheter in the opposite nare every eight hours.

## USING AN OXYGEN FACE MASK

### Equipment

Oxygen mask

Oxygen source

Flowmeter

Humidifier

### Preparation

1. Check physician's orders for oxygen.

2. Gather equipment.

3. Wash your hands.

### Procedure

1. Explain procedure and rationale for administration of oxygen to patient.

2. Check size of face mask to make sure it fits patient.

3. Turn on oxygen flow to number of liters prescribed. If reservoir bag is attached, partially inflate it with oxygen.

4. Place patient in semi- or high-Fowler's position.

5. Fit mask to patient's face from nose downward

during expiration. If reservoir bag is attached, oxygen flow must be at a level to prevent bag from collapsing. **Rationale:** A tight fit prevents oxygen from escaping around eyes or nose.

6. Place elastic band around patient's head.

7. Attach tubing to pillows and bedclothes, keeping tubing free of kinks.

8. Stay with patient until patient feels at ease with mask. **Rationale:** Some patients may be afraid of suffocating.

9. Assess patient's condition by checking vital signs and respiratory process.

10. Change mask and tubing daily, and provide skin care to face.

11. Observe for any change in patient's condition.

12. Check equipment frequently. If humidifier is attached, check water level.

13. Check with physician to order a nasal cannula during meals.

## USING A PEDIATRIC OXYGEN MASK

### Equipment

Pedi mask

Oxygen source

Flowmeter

Humidifier

### Procedure

1. Choose a mask that will fit the child. **Rationale:** The mask should cover child's mouth and nose, but not eyes.

2. Place mask so that it fits tightly.

3. Secure mask with elastic strap.

4. Adjust oxygen concentration as ordered.

5. Remove mask at frequent intervals for skin care if the child's condition is stable and provided no

ABGs are scheduled within one hour. **Rationale:** Taking mask off would distort ABG findings.

6. Observe child frequently for complications.

7. Spend extra time with the child as an oxygen mask may be frightening.

## USING AN OXYGEN TENT

### Equipment

Oxygen tent

Oxygen machine

Non-electric call bell

Plasticized mattress or cover

Draw sheet

Oxygen analyzer

### Preparation

1. Check physician's orders for oxygen.

2. Gather equipment.

3. Explain purpose and reason for tent to patient.

### Procedure

1. Secure tent and place machine at head of bed with control knobs on opposite side where working area is required.

2. Connect regulator into oxygen source.

3. Plug in machine.

4. Set up humidifier and check to make sure that water level (tray at back of machine) is adequate.

5. Adjust temperature control to 19° to 22° C (68° to 70° F).

6. Set circulation dial between high and low.

7. Turn on oxygen flow, and flush with high liter rate, or press flush button for one minute until desired concentration is reached.

8. Position canopy one-half to one-third over length of bed.

9. Flush oxygen tent with 15 liters/minute flow rate for 1 to 2 minutes.

10. Tuck all sides of canopy into mattress, and use draw sheet to secure seal over thighs.

11. Regulate flowmeter to 12 to 15 (minimum of 10) liters/minute. **Rationale:** Carbon dioxide is removed with oxygen flow.

12. Give patient a special call button that can be at-

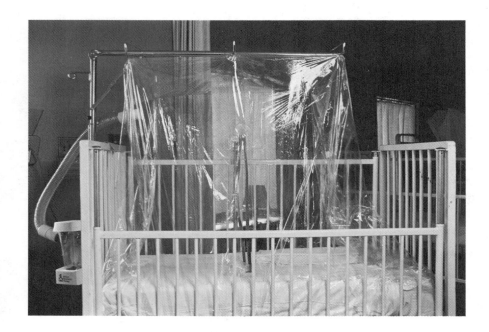

Turn on oxygen supply or compressed air and mist before placing child in oxygen tent.

tached to bed. **Rationale:** Electrical call bells can be an electrical hazard.

13. Test oxygen concentration with oxygen analyzer every four hours.

14. During use, open tent as infrequently as possible.

15. Flood tent with oxygen after tent has been opened.

16. If patient complains of coldness, furnish additional clothing, wrap patient's head and shoulders, or adjust the temperature of the tent.

17. Check equipment every four hours for liter flow, temperature, amount of water in humidifier, and oxygen in tank. Oxygen vent should remain unobstructed.

18. Observe patient's progress by making a general status check every hour and by assessing vital signs every four hours.

## USING A PEDIATRIC OXYGEN TENT

### Equipment

Oxygen tent

Oxygen machine

Oxygen analyzer

Bath blankets (2)

### Preparation

1. Check physician's orders.

2. Gather equipment.

3. Select a tent that will deliver the desired concentration of oxygen to the child.

4. Explain purpose of tent to child and/or parents.

### Procedure

1. Secure tent and place machine at head of bed with control knobs on opposite side where working area is required.

2. Connect regulator into oxygen source.

3. Plug in machine.

4. Set up humidifier and check to make sure that water level (tray at back of machine) is adequate.

5. Pad the frame that supports the canopy.

6. Turn on the oxygen to desired concentration (30 to 50%), and maintain temperature at 17.8° to 21.2° C (64° to 70° F).

7. Secure the canopy by tucking in all sides and maintaining closure whenever possible. **Rationale:** To prevent oxygen leak.

8. Analyze and record tent atmosphere, and check child's vital signs every two hours.

9. Leave crib sides up for safety.

10. Select toys that are washable, do not produce static electricity, and are appropriate to the child's age.

11. Assist in placing on cardiac or apnea monitor.

12. Keep the child warm and check dampness of clothes.

13. Change bed linen and child's clothing as necessary.

## USING A CROUPETTE

**Equipment**

Croupette

Oxygen source or compressed air

Ice

Warm clothing

**Procedure**

1. Connect croupette to wall oxygen.

2. Secure oxygen tent and regulate oxygen flow according to prescribed orders (10-15 liters). The croupettte may be operated with compressed air when only high humidity is required.

3. Fill the receptacle in back of the croupette with ice if cool mist is ordered.

4. Check child frequently for signs of chilling or need for suctioning. Keep crib rails up.

5. Complete postural drainage if secretions need to be drained.

6. Supply additional clothing or change clothing during the procedure if child is receiving high humidity.

## USING AN OXYGEN HOOD

**Equipment**

Oxygen hood

Oxygen source

Oxygen analyzer

Flexible oxygen tubing

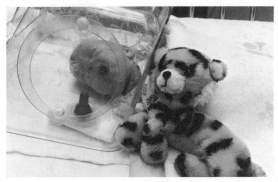

The oxygen hood is opened to provide care. The lid can be opened without disturbing oxygen concentration.

**Procedure**

1. Place hood around child's head and attach tubing to oxygen supply. (Hood may be used alone or with isolette.)

2. Infants are cared for through portholes or lid. **Rationale:** This avoids decreasing oxygen level.

3. Maintain oxygen levels at 40% to 50% and check the amount of moisture that can accumulate inside hood.

4. Measure oxygen concentration as you would in isolette.

5. Observe usual oxygen administration precautions.

**CHARTING** *for Oxygen Therapy*

☐ Ordered oxygen given

☐ Arterial $pO_2$

☐ Vital signs

☐ Type of equipment used for oxygen administration percentage of $FIO_2$ and liter flow

☐ Data from oxygen analyzer

☐ Patient's status every hour

---

## CLINICAL PROBLEM SOLVING

**Potential Problems**

Difficulty breathing.

**Suggested Solutions**

☐ If conscious, the patient can usually tell you what he is experiencing and cough up mucus. Encourage coughing; suction if necessary.

☐ If patient is unconscious, be alert for wet, gur-

Abnormal signs and symptoms: changes in blood pressure, tachycardia, increased respirations, cloudy consciousness, and abnormal color.

□ gling respirations, which indicate need for suctioning. Suction frequently.
□ Utilize Sims's position so that secretions can run out of patient's mouth.

□ Determine if acute acidosis and/or carbon dioxide narcosis is present and report. These conditions can occur if hypoxic drive is removed by the administration of high oxygen concentration.
   a. Check oxygen equipment and use oxygen analyzer to measure oxygen concentration.
   b. Reduce oxygen concentration as ordered.
□ Carbon dioxide retainers may require controlled low oxygen concentration method. Change oxygen therapy from cannula/catheter to Venturi mask as ordered.

Atelectasis.

□ Lower the oxygen concentration as ordered.
□ Encourage deep breathing, coughing, frequent position changes, and ambulation if possible. Avoid constrictive dressings and use sedatives carefully.
□ IPPB, postural drainage, and suctioning may be ordered.
□ Check breath sounds. (They are decreased with this condition.)

Tachypnea.

□ Report symptoms and check oxygen concentration immediately, since inadequate flow rates may be causing the problem.
□ Increase flow rate as ordered and monitor with oxygen analyzer.
□ Monitor vital signs and patient's discomfort, as pulmonary embolus may be the cause.
□ Check patient's breathing pattern and breath sounds as mucus plug may be the cause.

Retrolental fibroplasia.

□ Make sure the premature infant receives no more than 40% oxygen unless infant suffers from sustained tachypnea or respiratory distress syndrome.
□ If higher concentrations of oxygen are ordered, maintain and monitor the oxygen so that the range is 50 to 70 mm Hg in radial artery.

Infection.

□ Change humidifier every 24 hours.
□ Keep water at appropriate level in humidifier.

Oxygen toxicity occurs.

□ Toxicity occurs 24 hours after initiation of oxygen therapy.
□ Monitor closely for signs of nausea, restlessness, pallor.
□ Maintain 40% oxygen concentration unless frequent arterial blood gas monitoring occurs.

# UNIT FIVE   INTERMITTENT POSITIVE PRESSURE BREATHING (IPPB)

## NURSING PROCESS DATA

### ASSESSMENT   *Data Base*

Evaluate patient's need for IPPB.

Evaluate arterial blood gases, sputum cultures, and chest x-rays.

Review the physician's IPPB order for settings, length of treatment, and medications to be used.

Assess patient's lung sounds before and after each treatment.

Observe consistency, amount and color of expectorated sputum.

Assess need for additional physiotherapy to improve respiratory function.

Assess pulse and respiratory rate to establish baseline data.

### PLANNING   *Objectives*

To deliver aerosol medications.

To decrease the work of breathing.

To promote a better ventilation/perfusion ratio by increasing bronchodilatation and alveolar ventilation.

To prevent or treat atelectasis.

To loosen secretions.

To decrease pulmonary edema.

### IMPLEMENTATION   *Procedures*

Setting up the Puritan-Bennett PR 2

Setting up the Bird Mark 7

Administering a Nebulized Treatment

### EVALUATION   *Expected Outcomes*

Increased expectoration of secretions occurs.

Patient experiences less labored breathing.

Improved blood gas values are documented.

Lung sounds are improved.

Aerosol medications administered into deep air passages and ventilation improves.

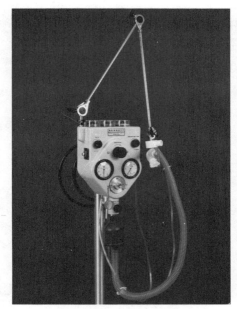

The Bennett PR-2 respirator is the one most commonly used for IPPB treatments.

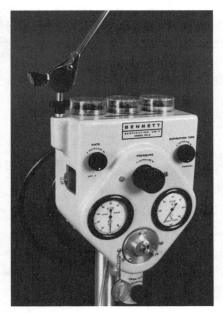

Check all of the settings on the Bennett respirator before each IPPB treatment.

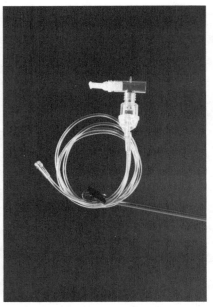

The misty nebulizer with tee adapter is a type of nebulizer for IPPB treatments.

## SETTING UP THE PURITAN-BENNETT PR 2

### Equipment

IPPB machine (Bennett) or pressure-preset ventilator

Ventilator tubing

Nebulizer and manifold

Mouthpiece

Nose piece or clip (optional)

Power source (oxygen, compressed air, or electricity, depending on the machine)

Tidal volume spirometer

### Preparation

1. Check physician's orders and Patient Care Plan.
2. Notify respiratory therapy department regarding the order for IPPB therapy.
3. Gather equipment if nursing performs this activity in your facility. The PR 2 can be used as an IPPB machine or a pressure-preset ventilator.
4. Identify patient via identaband.
5. Explain procedure to patient.
6. Wash your hands.

### Procedure

1. Connect pressure hose to wall oxygen outlet or compressed air.
2. Attach tubing to the machine.
3. Unscrew the nebulizer cup.
4. Place medication or distilled water in the cup and replace it.
5. Adjust the air mix knob: pull it out to give 100 percent oxygen and push it in to administer an air mix.
6. Set the pressure: turn the pressure control knob (in the middle front of the machine) clockwise until the right-hand pressure control gauge reads the ordered pressure.
7. Check that the peak flow knob is completely open (at the maximal counterclockwise position). Do not adjust peak flow without checking with a therapist or physician.
8. Turn the ventilation rate off. **Rationale:** This dial is turned on only for use of the PR 2 in controlled ventilation.
9. Remove the nebulizer from the manifold. Remove the dust cap and lift the drum pin.
10. Adjust the inspiration nebulization knob until a fine mist appears.

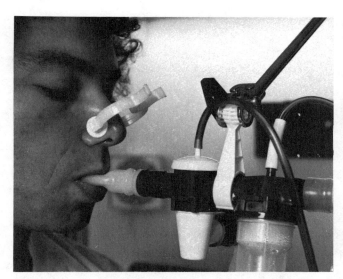

Place nose clip on patient and instruct patient to inhale through mouthpiece. Observe that nebulizer emits a fine mist.

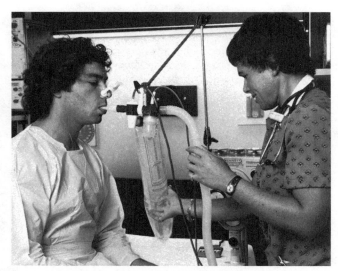

Ensure that patient is receiving an adequate tidal volume. The tidal volume can be measured while giving the IPPB treatment.

11. Lower the drum pin and replace the dust cap.

12. Replace the nebulizer in the manifold.

13. Set the sensitivity control to off by turning the knob clockwise.

## SETTING UP THE BIRD MARK 7

### Equipment

IPPB machine (Bird) or pressure-preset ventilator

Ventilator tubing

Nebulizer and manifold

Mouthpiece

Nose piece or clip (optional)

Power source (oxygen, compressed air, or electricity, depending on the machine)

Tidal volume spirometer

### Preparation

Same as for *Setting up Puritan-Bennett*.

### Procedure

1. Attach tubing to the machine.

2. Hold the nebulizer unit with the cap uppermost. Remove the cap, instill the medication or distilled water, and replace the cap.

3. Adjust the air mix. Push the knob in for 100 percent oxygen and pull it out for an air mix. (The positioning of this knob for 100 percent oxygen is the exact opposite of that for the Bennett PR 2.)

4. Connect the pressure hose to the oxygen outlet.

5. Set the pressure, using the pressure control on the right side of the machine. The usual initial setting is 15 cm.

6. Turn off the dial marked "expiratory time for apnea."

7. Set the sensitivity to 15. The sensitivity control is on the left side of the machine.

8. Set the flow rate dial (on the right side of the machine) to 15 cm. This turns the machine on.

## ADMINISTERING A NEBULIZED TREATMENT

### Equipment

Puritan-Bennett with all appropriate equipment
　　or

Bird Mark 7 with all appropriate equipment

Medication or distilled water

### Preparation

1. Gather equipment.

2. Identify patient.

**Clinical Alert**

IPPB is contraindicated in any condition predisposing to pneumothorax (such as bullous emphysema), in some cardiovascular disorders, and for patients unable to cooperate.

**Clinical Alert**

The higher pressure automatically increases sensitivity, so you may need to lower sensitivity by pulling the control level toward the front of the unit (higher number equals less sensitivity). You must also increase flow rate whenever you increase pressure; turn the flow rate dial to a higher number (higher number equals shorter inspiration and increased flow).

3. Explain the rationale for the treatment in understandable terms.

4. Assess best position for treatment.

5. Place patient on side of bed in sitting position with feet on floor, or have patient sit in chair.

6. Instruct patient on the following:
   a. Keep lips closed tightly around the mouthpiece.
   b. Breathe only through mouth.
   c. Breathe slowly.
   d. To trigger the machine, breathe in slightly. Then relax and let the machine complete the breath while patient expands lower chest and abdomen.
   e. Hold breath briefly at the end of each inspiration.
   f. Exhale normally, around the mouthpiece.

7. Wash your hands.

**Procedure**

1. Complete patient teaching.

2. Administer pain medication about 30 minutes before treatment if patient has postsurgical chest or abdominal pain. **Rationale:** If patient is in pain, he will be reluctant to utilize this treatment to facilitate breathing.

3. Post a "No Smoking" sign and alert visitors and other patients in the room not to smoke.

4. Check patient's pulse and respiratory rate before, during, and after treatment.

5. Begin treatment by placing nose clip on patient and having patient inhale through the machine.

6. Provide instruction until patient has mastered the correct technique.

7. Gradually increase pressure until patient is receiving the ordered pressure.
   a. On the Puritan-Bennett PR 2, turn the pressure control knob until the left-hand delivered pressure gauge reads the ordered pressure.
   b. On the Puritan-Bennett AP 5, turn the pressure control knob until the pressure gauge shows the ordered pressure at the end of inspiration.
   c. On the Bird, turn the pressure control until the gauge on the front of the machine shows the ordered pressure.

8. Observe the chest for full expansion.

9. Encourage periodic coughing to remove secretions.

10. Tap the nebulizer cup periodically. **Rationale:** This action moves moisture to the bottom.

11. Continue treatment until the nebulizer is empty, usually about 20 minutes. If the nebulizer becomes empty before the end of the prescribed treatment period, add distilled water.

12. Check pulse, blood pressure, and respiratory rate at the end of treatment.

13. Assist patient to a comfortable position. Remind patient of the value of the treatment and give positive reinforcement for cooperation.

14. Wash your hands.

**CHARTING** *for IPPB*

☐ Medication and dosage

☐ Type of machine used for IPPB

☐ Settings used on IPPB machine

☐ Duration of treatment

☐ Amount, consistency, and color of secretions obtained

☐ Patient's tolerance for treatment

☐ Vital signs before and after treatment

## CLINICAL PROBLEM SOLVING

**Potential Problems**

**Suggested Solutions**

There is no increase in the expectoration of secretions.

☐ Check that the nebulizer is expelling a fine mist.
☐ Notify physician for medication order change to a drug that lowers surface tension of sputum, thereby facilitating expectoration.
☐ Encourage deep breathing and coughing between IPPB treatments.
☐ Obtain order for PVD.

Breathing continues to be labored.

☐ Ensure that patient is positioned in Fowler's or at least semi-Fowler's position to facilitate breathing.
☐ Have patient expectorate mucus. If unable to cough productively, suction patient.
☐ Evaluate need for additional treatments or potential need for assisted mechanical ventilation.
☐ Use relaxation techniques if patient is anxious.

Lung sounds do not improve.

☐ Monitor lung sounds before and after each treatment.
☐ Identify area of lung that contains adventitious sounds, and administer PVD to the specific area.
☐ Obtain order to change medications or increase number of treatments.

Inability to trigger the machine at the usual sensitivity setting.

☐ On the PR 2, increase sensitivity by turning the sensitivity knob to the left. On the Bird, increase sensitivity by pushing the sensitivity control level toward the back of the machine (toward a lower number).

Pressure setting reached too quickly.

☐ Check tubing for kinks.
☐ Encourage patient to cough.
☐ Suction patient if patient is unable to expectorate secretions.
☐ Instruct patient not to resist the airflow or blow back into the machine.
☐ Decrease the flow rate (and the pressure) in the Bird.

Machine will not cycle off.

☐ Check for leak in tubing.
☐ Check for leak around mask, mouthpiece, or tracheostomy tube.
☐ Increase the flow rate (and the pressure) in the Bird.

# UNIT SIX    TRACHEOSTOMY CARE

## NURSING PROCESS DATA

### ASSESSMENT  *Data Base*

Note if there are dried or moist secretions surrounding cannula or on tracheal dressing.

Note excessive expectoration of secretions.

Assess if routine tracheal care is adequate for this patient.

Observe patient's ability to sustain respiratory function by ability to breathe through normal airway.

Assess respiratory status: breath sounds, respiratory rate, use of accessory muscles for breathing while tracheal tube is plugged.

Observe for labored breathing, flaring of nares, retractions, and color of nail beds.

Observe vital signs for increases in pulse or respirations and for changes in skin color.

Auscultate for adventitious sounds to evaluate lung field.

Listen for audible hissing sounds indicating an air leak.

Check if pilot balloon is deflated or inflated.

### PLANNING  *Objectives*

To prevent airway obstruction by liquefying and mobilizing secretions.

To prevent infections of tracheal site.

To improve respiratory function so patient can breathe normally, without artificial support.

To suction secretions more easily.

To deflate tracheostomy cuff to facilitate suctioning.

To prevent aspiration while feeding.

To prevent tracheal damage.

### IMPLEMENTATION  *Procedures*

Cleaning the Inner Cannula

Changing Trach Ties

Performing Tracheostomy Suctioning

Using a Manual Resuscitator

Instilling Normal Saline

Plugging a Tracheostomy

Deflating a Tracheal Cuff

Inflating a Tracheal Cuff

## EVALUATION  *Expected Outcomes*

Patient adequately ventilated with absence of respiratory distress.

Secretions easily liquefied and mobilized with saline instillations.

Secretions easily suctioned.

Tracheostomy site remains free of infection.

Patient able to eat without aspirating food.

Tracheal necrosis is prevented.

## CLEANING THE INNER CANNULA

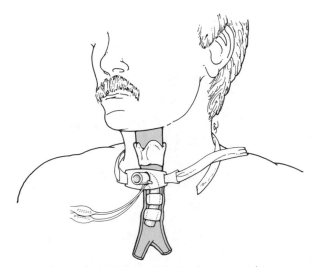

Anatomical placement of a tracheostomy tube.

### Equipment

Tracheal cleaning tray (includes 2 sterile basins, pipe cleaners, brush, 4 × 4 gauze pad)

Sterile gloves

Suction equipment

Complete tracheal tube set for emergency use

Interchangeable inner cannula of same size if available or tracheostomy tube and obturator

Hydrogen peroxide, one-half strength

Sterile normal saline

Sterile nonraveling pre-cut dressings

Clean tracheal ties

### Preparation

1. Check physician's orders and Patient Care Plan.
2. Assemble equipment.
3. Make sure suction equipment and additional tracheal tubes are available.
4. Wash your hands.

### Procedure

1. Explain procedure and rationale to patient.
2. Put on gloves.
3. Suction before cleaning tracheal tube.
4. Unlock the inner cannula by turning the lock to the left about 90°. Secure the outer cannula of the neck plate with your left index finger and thumb.
5. Gently pull the inner cannula slightly upward and out toward you. Place in sterile container with hydrogen peroxide.
6. Soak the cannula in a hydrogen peroxide-filled sterile bowl to remove dried secretions.

7. Cleanse the lumen and outer surface of the cannula with pipe cleaners or brush moistened with hydrogen proxide. (Some hospitals use sterile normal saline.) **Rationale:** To remove dried-on secretions.
8. Rinse cannula thoroughly with sterile water or saline.
9. Place clean tube on sterile 4 × 4 gauze pad and dry tube thoroughly.
10. Replace the inner cannula carefully by grasping the outer flange of the cannula with your other hand as you insert the cannula.
11. Lock the inner cannula by turning the lock to the right so that it is in an upright position.
12. Cleanse around the incision site with applicator sticks soaked in normal saline and/or hydrogen peroxide.
13. Apply antibiotic ointment around the incision site if ordered.

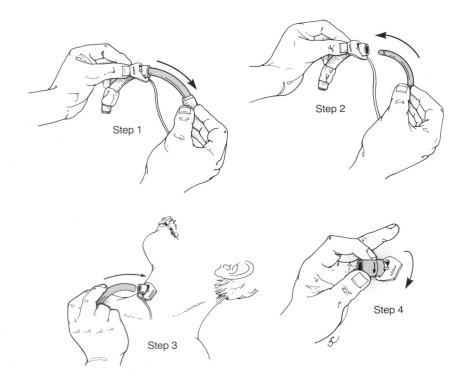

Step 1

Step 2

Step 3

Step 4

Drawing depicts how the inner cannula is removed and then replaced for cleaning. Outer cannula is not removed when cleaning.

---

**Clinical Alert**

A packaged sterile trach tube is kept at the bedside for emergency use. If the trach tube becomes dislodged, the new tube can be immediately inserted.

---

14. Apply pre-cut, nonraveling trach dressing around insertion site, and change tracheal ties if needed. **Rationale:** Nonraveling dressing will prevent lint from entering trach tube.

15. If tracheal ties are to be changed, ask another person to hold the tracheal tube in place while you change the ties. **Rationale:** This procedure prevents accidental extubation if patient coughs.

16. Make patient comfortable.

17. Discard soiled dressings, tapes, and cleaning equipment.

18. Wash your hands.

## CHANGING TRACH TIES

### Equipment

Sterile scissor

Kelly forceps

Twill tape or commercial trach ties

Packaged sterile trach tube set-up

### Preparation

1. Seek assistance from another person. **Rationale:** It is safer to have someone hold the trach tube in place when changing ties. The patient isn't as likely to cough the tube out.

2. Explain procedure to patient.

3. Wash your hands.

4. Gather equipment.

5. Place patient in semi- to high-Fowler's position as condition warrants.

### Procedure

1. Cut trach ties length you desire, if not pre-cut.

2. Fold ends of the trach ties over 1½″ and cut a slit in the piece starting at the folded edge.

3. If assistance is available, have the person hold the trach tube in place. Cut the old trach ties and remove and discard.

4. Pass the slit end of the ties through the flange loop of the trach tube about 2 to 3 inches. **Rationale:** Leave the old trach tie in place if you are changing the ties without assistance. This will prevent accidental dislodging of the trach tube.

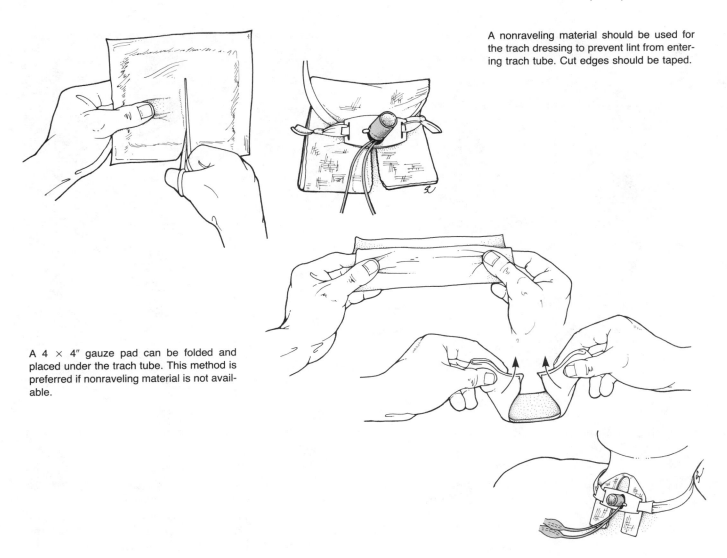

A nonraveling material should be used for the trach dressing to prevent lint from entering trach tube. Cut edges should be taped.

A 4 × 4″ gauze pad can be folded and placed under the trach tube. This method is preferred if nonraveling material is not available.

5. Thread the other end of the tie all the way through the slit. Pull it firmly in place. **Rationale:** This action will anchor the tie around the flange loop.

6. Repeat steps 4 and 5 on other flange loop.

7. Bring ties around patient's neck and tie in a square knot to one side of neck leaving one fingerbreadth under tie. **Rationale:** This is more comfortable for the patient and prevents pressure necrosis on the neck and jugular vein.

8. Cut off soiled trach ties if not already done, and discard in soiled trash.

9. Position patient for comfort.

10. Wash your hands.

## PERFORMING TRACHEOSTOMY SUCTIONING

### Equipment

Syringe with sterile saline

Suction catheter

Sterile gloves

Portable suction machine or wall suction with Y connector or release valve

Receptacle for used equipment

Container for sterile saline

Ambu or Laerdahl bag

Oxygen source

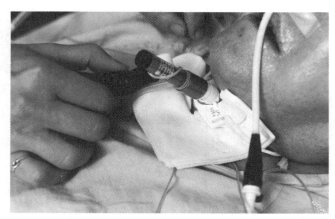

Place 4 × 4″ pad under trach tie to prevent tie from cutting into skin.

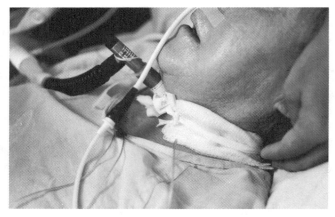

Tie trach ties at the side of patient's neck for comfort and safety.

## Preparation

1. Check physician's orders and Patient Care Plan.
2. Gather equipment.
3. Explain procedure to patient.
4. Wash your hands.
5. Assess lung sounds.
6. Complete nasopharyngeal or oropharyngeal suctioning.
7. Prepare sterile syringe with 2 to 10 cc sterile normal saline for tracheal lavage when applicable. (Amount is determined by hospital protocol.)

## Procedure

1. Change catheter and glove or obtain new catheter and sleeve package after nasopharyngeal or oropharyngeal suctioning.

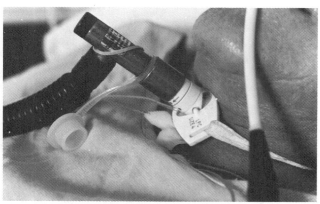

When respirator is disconnected from trach, place cap over adapter.

2. Suction patient no more than 10 seconds at a time, using sterile technique with tracheal cuff inflated.
3. Hyperinflate lungs on adult with ambu or Laerdahl bag at 100% oxygen. **Rationale:** This prevents oxygen loss.
4. Rinse catheter and deflate cuff. If using separate catheter and glove for suctioning, use ungloved hand to deflate cuff.
5. Instill prescribed amount of sterile normal saline slowly into tracheal tube. If feasible, ask patient to take a deep breath while instilling saline. Allow solution to remain in bronchus for several seconds if possible; then complete suctioning procedure. **Rationale:** The cough reflex will be stimulated when the bronchus is reached with the catheter.
6. Inflate tracheal cuff again and hyperinflate lungs with ambu or Laerdahl bag and 100% oxygen.
7. Position patient for comfort.
8. Assess breath sounds.
9. Wash your hands.
10. Empty suction bottle at the end of every shift.

## USING A MANUAL RESUSCITATOR

### Equipment

Laerdahl or ambu bag

Oxygen source and tubing

Trach adapter or face mask

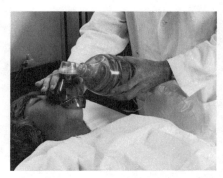

Form a tight seal by placing the apex of the mask over nose and base over mouth.

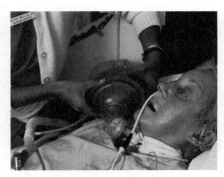

Use the manual resuscitator bag with patients who have trach tubes in place.

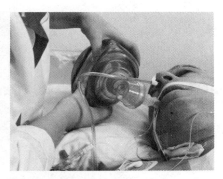

Compress the manual resuscitator bag every five seconds for an adult patient.

## Preparation

1. Check physician's orders and Patient Care Plan.
2. Gather equipment.
3. Connect mask or trach adapter, oxygen tubing, and oxygen flowmeter (reservoir) to bag.
4. Wash your hands.

## Procedure

1. Turn on oxygen flowmeter to 15 l/minute as ordered.
2. When using a mask, hyperextend patient's neck and place the apex of the mask over the nose. Place the base of the mask between the lower lip and chin. You may have to open patient's mouth by pressing down on the chin. **Rationale:** This ensures a tight seal.
3. When using a trach adapter, attach the universal adapter to the bag. Attach the adapter to the patient's endotracheal or tracheostomy tube.
4. Compress the ambu or Laerdahl bag every five seconds for an apneic adult and every three seconds for an apneic infant.
5. If patient is able to breathe spontaneously, give the breaths in synchrony with his breaths.
6. When using the bag to hyperinflate the lungs following suctioning, compress the bag three to five times each time you suction.
7. To keep the airway open when using a mask, seal mask tightly by pressing down on the mask with thumb and index finger of one hand and lifting up patient's mandible with your remaining fingers.
8. Observe the patient's chest rise and fall with each compression. **Rationale:** This ensures adequate ventilation.

9. Observe for possible gastric distention with continued use of the bag.
10. If gastric distention persists, notify physician for nasogastric tube insertion orders.

## INSTILLING NORMAL SALINE

### Equipment

Sterile normal saline (not bacteriostatic) bottle or disposable one-time-only packages

Sterile 10-cc syringe with needle

Sterile suction catheter and glove

Suction machine

Resuscitation bag

Tracheostomy plug

### Preparation

1. Check physician's order and Patient Care Plan.
2. Wash hands.
3. Gather equipment.
4. Explain procedure to patient.

### Procedure

1. Attach sterile catheter to suction machine tubing.
2. Draw up prescribed amount of normal saline (usually 3 to 5 cc) in syringe. Open top of disposable package if using.
3. Remove needle from syringe.
4. Turn on oxygen supply to resuscitation bag.
5. Turn on suction equipment.
6. Pull sterile glove on dominant hand.
7. Instill prescribed amount of normal saline into

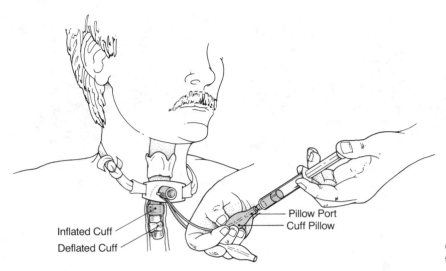

Inflated Cuff
Deflated Cuff
Pillow Port
Cuff Pillow

Check pillow port for pressure level and tautness to determine if balloon is inflated.

tracheostomy or endotracheal tube with un-gloved hand.

8. Give patient 3 to 5 breaths with resuscitation bag if patient can tolerate this procedure.

9. Begin deep suctioning. Patient may be hyperventilated with resuscitator bag after suctioning.

10. Turn off oxygen for resuscitator bag.

11. Discard used equipment.

12. Make patient comfortable.

## PLUGGING A TRACHEOSTOMY

### Equipment

Trach plug

Suction machine

Sterile suction catheters and glove

10cc syringe

### Preparation

1. Check physician's order and Patient Care Plan to determine length of time it should remain plugged.

2. Wash hands.

3. Gather equipment.

4. Explain procedure to patient and reassure that he won't suffocate.

5. Place patient in semi- to high-Fowler's position. **Rationale:** This assists with lung expansion and will decrease fear of not being able to breathe.

### Procedure

1. Suction nasopharynx.

2. Change suction catheters, and suction trachea.

3. Deflate tracheal cuff; suction again if necessary.

4. Place tracheal plug in either the inner cannula or outer cannula with inner cannula removed. Clean inner cannula while plug is in place.

5. Observe patient for respiratory distress.

6. Stay with patient until he is comfortable and exhibits no difficulty in breathing.

7. Remove plug when time elapsed. Cleanse plug and return to clean area for reuse or discard according to hospital policy.

8. Suction patient and replace inner cannula if removed.

9. Position for comfort.

10. Change trach dressings if necessary.

11. Dispose of used equipment.

12. Wash your hands.

## DEFLATING A TRACHEAL CUFF

### Equipment

10 cc syringe

Suction equipment

### Preparation

1. Check physician's orders and Patient Care Plan.

2. Gather equipment.

3. Wash your hands.

4. Prepare patient by explaining procedure.

5. Provide patient privacy.

**Procedure**

1. Suction nose and/or mouth and tracheostomy before deflating cuff.

2. Attach 10-cc syringe to distal end of inflatable cuff, making sure seal is tight.

3. Slowly withdraw 5 cc of air. **Rationale:** Amount of air withdrawn is determined by type of cuff used and whether minimal air leak is utilized.

4. Keep syringe attached to end of cuff.

5. Suction if cough reflex stimulated.

6. Keep cuff deflated for five minutes if patient can tolerate.

## INFLATING A TRACHEAL CUFF

### Equipment

10-cc syringe

Hemostat with padded rubber tubing on ends for some tracheal tubes

Suction equipment

### Procedure

1. Suction tracheostomy before inflating cuff.

2. If syringe is not already attached, attach 10-cc syringe to distal end of inflatable cuff, making sure seal is tight.

3. Inflate prescribed amount of air to create leak-free system. Cuff is inflated correctly when you cannot hear the patient's voice or any air movements from nose or mouth. **Rationale:** Some authorities believe a minimal air leak is best. A minimal leak can be detected by listening for a hissing sound with a stethoscope held over the trachea.

4. Remove syringe and apply rubber-tipped forceps to maintain air in cuff, depending on the type of tube used. **Rationale:** Some cuffs have a one-way valve which prevents air leaks.

5. If cuff has two balloons, alternately inflate them every hour.

6. If high volume/low pressure cuff is used, cuff is not routinely deflated.

**CHARTING** *for Tracheostomy Care*

☐ Location of plug: outer or inner cannula

☐ Baseline vital signs before procedure

☐ Respiratory status during procedure

☐ Vital signs, any indications of cyanosis or respiratory distress after procedure

☐ Amount of normal saline instilled into tracheal tube

☐ Trach care completed

☐ Appearance of trach site

☐ Characteristics of secretions

☐ Trach ties changed

☐ Patient's tolerance of procedures

*for Tracheostomy Suctioning*

☐ Amount, color and consistency of secretions

☐ Changes in breath sounds

☐ Respiratory rate changes

☐ Patient's tolerance to procedure

☐ Unanticipated problems and patient's response

☐ Number of times patient suctioned

☐ Use of ambu or Laerdahl bag for hyperinflation of lungs

*for Tracheal Cuff Care*

☐ Tracheal cuff release time

☐ Amount of air used for cuff inflation

☐ Changes in respiratory status during deflation/inflation

☐ Amount, color, and consistency of secretions

## CLINICAL PROBLEM SOLVING

**Potential Problems**
*for Tracheostomy Tube Cleaning*

Accidental extubation.

**Suggested Solutions**

☐ Have second tracheal set available.

|  |  |
|---|---|
|  | ☐ Keep airway open by inserting obturator or sterile forceps through trach opening. |
|  | ☐ Insert new trach tube or notify physician as hospital policy dictates. |
| Excessive secretions and coughing while inner cannula is cleansed. | ☐ Perform oral suctioning before removing inner cannula. |
|  | ☐ Suction lumen if necessary, while soaking inner cannula. |
|  | ☐ Place another interchangeable cannula in trach tube and continue to soak cannula. |
| Inner cannula is dislodged. | ☐ Insert extra cannula from emergency set if cannulas are interchangeable. If not, insert new tracheal set. |
|  | ☐ If cannula is metal, send it to CSR for autoclaving. If cannula is disposable, discard in trash. If plastic, soak in hydrogen peroxide for one hour, then rinse in sterile saline. |
| Patient unable to be off ventilator long enough for cleansing of inner cannula. | ☐ Insert new inner cannula (interchangeable) and place patient back on ventilator. |
|  | ☐ Proceed to clean inner cannula and keep it clean for next change. |
| Coughing and/or shortness of breath occurs when plug inserted. | ☐ Remove plug. |
|  | ☐ Suction if necessary. |
|  | ☐ Reassure patient that he can breathe, even with the plug in place. |
|  | ☐ Reinsert plug and instruct patient to take slow, deep breaths. |
|  | ☐ If unable to keep plug in place, notify physician. |

### for Tracheostomy Suctioning

|  |  |
|---|---|
| Hypoxia may occur if incorrect techniques are used for suctioning. | ☐ Observe for signs of increased restlessness, shortness of breath, yawning, and/or cyanosis while suctioning. |
|  | ☐ Limit suctioning time to no more than 15 seconds. |
|  | ☐ Ensure that suction catheter is half the diameter of the tube. |
|  | ☐ Hyperinflate lungs with 100% oxygen using ambu or Laerdahl bag before and after suctioning. |
| Excessive secretions that require frequent suctioning are present. | ☐ Replace suction catheter with new one immediately after suctioning in order to have it ready for next time |
|  | ☐ With frequent suctioning, hyperinflate lungs with 100% oxygen using an ambu or Laerdahl bag. |
| After suctioning intubated patient he still sounds congested. | ☐ Allow rest period before suctioning again. |
|  | ☐ Instill normal saline (2 to 5 cc) through endotracheal or tracheostomy tube if ordered. |

☐ Hyperinflate lungs with 100% oxygen using an ambu or Laerdahl bag if ordered.
☐ Encourage deep breathing and coughing exercises.
☐ Notify physician for bronchodilator drugs.

### for Tracheal Cuff Care

Balloon ruptures and herniates over the end of the tube.

☐ Replace tube immediately and report to physician.
☐ Assess patient for respiratory dysfunction. A portion of the cuff may have been aspirated.

Patient is unable to tolerate cuff deflating for prescribed five minutes.

☐ Release cuff for as long a time as patient can tolerate.
☐ May hyperinflate lungs with manual resuscitator while cuff deflated.

Accidental extubation occurs when the tube is deflated.

☐ Place patient flat on his back and insert an oropharyngeal airway until reintubation can be accomplished if endotracheal tube in place.
☐ Insert forceps into tracheostomy stoma until intubation can be accomplished.

## UNIT SEVEN   WATER-SEAL DRAINAGE SYSTEMS

### NURSING PROCESS DATA

#### ASSESSMENT   *Data Base*

Assess patient's respiratory status while tubes inserted.

Check to see that all connections between the water-seal system and the patient are securely taped.

Check patency of chest tubes.

Assess if mediastinal shift present.

Auscultate breath sounds.

Observe for bilateral chest expansion.

Note chest drainage.

#### PLANNING   *Objectives*

To evacuate air or a combination of air and serosanguineous fluid from the intrapleural space.

To reestablish negative pressure after an intrathoracic procedure.

To provide continued suction that functions as a safeguard against pneumothorax.

To facilitate drainage of accumulated fluid within the thoracic cavity after open heart surgery.

**IMPLEMENTATION** *Procedures*

Establishing a Closed Drainage System

Setting up Disposable Water-Seal Suction

Maintaining a Closed Drainage System

**EVALUATION** *Expected Outcomes*

Closed water-seal drainage system maintained until patient's lung is reexpanded and air or serosanguineous fluid is removed from pleural space.

Normal respiratory function restored.

Chest tubes remain patent.

Water-seal system remains intact.

## ESTABLISHING A CLOSED DRAINAGE SYSTEM

### Equipment

Chest-tube insertion tray with appropriate chest-tube size

Tape or wire for connectors

Water-seal drainage system as ordered

Rubber-tipped hemostats (carmalts) for clamping tube to prevent air leak

Tape for drainage bottle markings

### Preparation

1. Check physician's orders and Patient Care Plan.
2. Assemble chest-tube insertion tray, sterile gloves, chest tubes, and water-seal drainage equipment.
3. Explain procedure to patient to decrease anxiety.
4. Plug water-seal drainage equipment into the suction source.
5. Place patient in a semirecumbent position. **Rationale:** This allows air to rise to the apex of the pleural space.
6. Open equipment tray and prepare tray as needed.

### Procedure

1. Following chest-tube insertion, connect chest tube to water-seal drainage equipment.
2. Turn suction control to low suction.

---

**Check Points for Chest Tube Air Leaks**

*Check Insertion Site:* Pinch chest tube at insertion site. Bubbling will stop in the water-seal chamber if there is an air leak at insertion site.

*Check Tubing:* Pinch between chest tube and rubber connecting tubing. Bubbling will stop if there is a leak at connector site.

*Check Water-Seal Drainage System:* Pinch between chest tube and rubber connecting tubing. Bubbling will continue if there is a leak in water-seal drainage system.

---

3. Secure connection sites with wire or tape.
4. Make sure that all stoppers in bottles fit tightly if bottle suction is used.
5. Check tubing to make sure fluid does not collect. **Rationale:** This prevents suction from being exerted.
6. Provide a straight line of tubing from bed to collection system. **Rationale:** Straight-line tubing will prevent pooling of fluid.
7. Keep collection system below level of chest-tube insertion site. **Rationale:** This will enable fluid to flow by gravity.
8. Make sure that tubing is free and not coiled. Do not use pins or restrain tubing. **Rationale:** Pins could puncture tubing causing an air leak.
9. Observe for possible air leaks or excessive suction in the system.

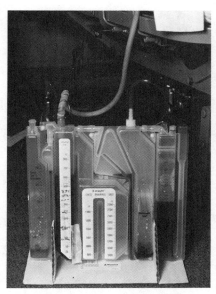

Mark drainage on the collection chamber at least every 8 hours. Only change system when chamber is full.

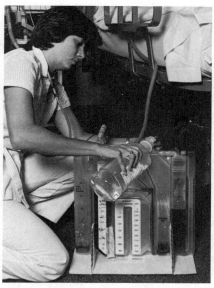

Refill chambers of the water-seal container when the fluid level is low. This maintains negative pressure.

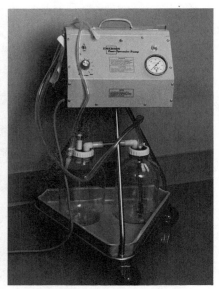

Chest tubes may be attached to the Emerson suction machine when wall suction is not available.

## SETTING UP DISPOSABLE WATER-SEAL SUCTION

### Equipment

Disposable water-seal suction, e.g., Pleur-evac, Argyle

Stand

60 cc asepto sterile syringe

Sterile water in pouring bottle

Tape or wire

Suction source

### Procedure

1. Gather equipment.

2. Unwrap the Pleur-evac.

3. Place the Pleur-evac on its disposable floor stand.

4. Remove the plastic connector on the short tube that is attached to the water-seal chamber.

5. Remove the plunger from the large 50- to 60-cc Asepto syringe. Attach the barrel of the syringe to the short rubber tube.

6. Pour sterile water into the barrel of the syringe, if not using a pouring bottle of sterile water.

7. Fill the water-seal chamber to the 2-cm level. **Ra-**

**tionale:** This level provides sufficient fluid to create a one way valve.

8. Remove the plastic plug from the vent to the suction control chamber.

9. Attach the syringe barrel to the vent. Pour sterile water into the chamber. (The tip of the syringe fits into the top of the chamber vent. There is no rubber tubing attached.)

10. Fill the suction control chamber to the 20-cm level. **Rationale:** This level is equal to the osmotic pressure of blood.

11. Insert the plastic plug into the vent.

12. After the physician has inserted chest tubes, remove the long tube adapter from the collection chamber and attach it to the chest tubes.

13. Tape or wire the connector sites.

14. Attach short rubber tube on the water-seal suction to the suction machine (wall or portable), using an adapter connection piece.

15. Turn suction device on slowly until bubbling occurs in the suction control chamber. **Rationale:** Excessive bubbling reduces drainage.

16. Monitor water levels daily in both the water-seal chamber and the suction control chamber. Refill to level with sterile water as needed.

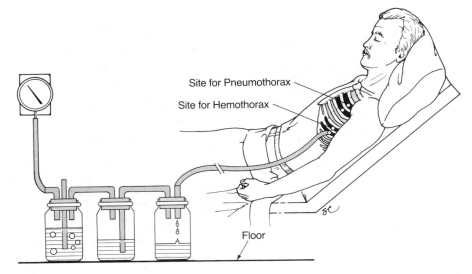

Keep collection system below level of chest tube insertion site.

## MAINTAINING A CLOSED DRAINAGE SYSTEM

### Equipment

Lundy roller

Alcohol wipes

Lotion

Rubber-tipped hemostats

### Procedure

1. Monitor safety.
   a. Monitor tubes for air leaks, which may cause the patient's lung to collapse.
   b. If air leaks occur, clamp off tube momentarily (if you have orders to do so) and inform physician immediately.
   c. Keep rubber-tipped hemostats at the patient's bedside. Place clamps facing in opposite directions. **Rationale:** If ordered, the tube can be clamped off nearest to chest insertion site.
   d. Obtain a chest x-ray to identify the correct placement of chest tubes if ordered.

2. Maintain pressure.
   a. Keep suction bottles or Pleur-evac system below level of bed.
   b. Keep suction control pressure where ordered. (Make sure that bubbling is not excessive in the control bottle.)
   c. Maintain water level in water-seal bottle.

3. Maintain chest-tube patency.
   a. Milk chest tubes every 30 to 60 minutes when constituents are blood. Milk every 4 to 8 hours when constituents are serous.

> **Clinical Alert**
> Do not pinch tubing for longer than *one* minute, as a pneumothorax could occur.

   b. Milk away from patient toward the drainage receptacle (Pleur-evac or bottles). **Rationale:** Force clot away from patient and into receptacle.
   c. Pinch tubing close to the chest with one hand as you milk the tube with your other hand. Continue going down tube in this method until you come to the drainage receptacle. (You may use a Lundy roller for this procedure. If you do, use the roller with caution.)
   d. Use lotion or alcohol wipes to make stripping easier. **Rationale:** These substances decrease friction on tubing.

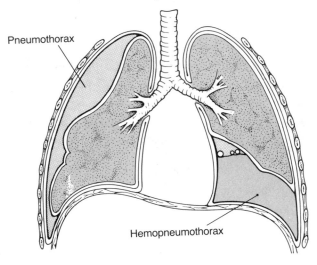

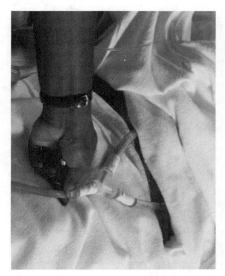

Seal all tube connections to prevent accidental interruption of the water-seal system.

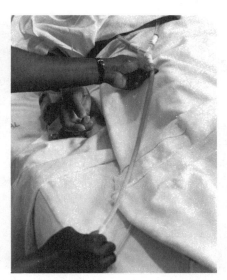

Maintain chest tube patency by milking tubes every 30 to 60 minutes.

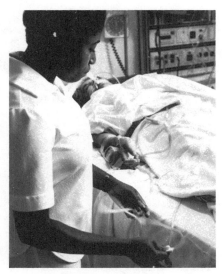

Start milking from the chest tube connection site until you reach the collection system.

4. Record intake and output.
   a. With Pleur-evac suction equipment, visually measure and mark level of chest drainage as ordered. (System holds up to 2800 to 3000 cc drainage.) Change equipment only when the drainage chamber is full.
   b. With two- or three-bottle suction, estimate drainage and mark bottle. Change drainage bottle only when full.
5. Assess patient's status.
   a. Instruct patient to deep breathe and cough at frequent intervals. **Rationale:** Frequent deep breathing helps to expand lungs.

b. Tell the patient to change positions frequently.
c. Observe and report any unusual respiratory signs/symptoms: rapid, shallow breathing, cyanosis, pressure in chest, or hemorrhage.

### CHARTING *for Chest Tubes*

☐ Size of chest tubes inserted and pressure levels

☐ Amount, color and characteristics of drainage

☐ Patient's tolerance of procedure

☐ Vital signs

☐ Breath sounds and chest expansion

## CLINICAL PROBLEM SOLVING

**Potential Problems**

Air leaks occur at the insertion site and/or in tubing.

Chest tube becomes dislodged.

**Suggested Solutions**

☐ Apply Vaseline gauze around opening at insertion site.
☐ Secure all connections with tape.
☐ Clamp tubing (if not tension pneumothorax); turn suction motor off; report to physician for orders.

☐ Apply pressure over insertion site with the palm of your hand or any available material, e.g., sheet, dressings. Notify physician.
☐ When sterile pressure dressing is obtained, instruct the patient to exhale. Then compress the opening and provide tight seal with dressing.

Chest tube comes apart from rubber tubing and becomes contaminated.

□ Observe for signs of respiratory distress: symmetry of chest, respiratory rate, changes in color, or level of consciousness.
□ Observe for mediastinal shift to unaffected side from tension buildup.
□ Submerge chest tube in sterile container filled with water.
□ Replace tubing with sterile tubing.
□ Observe for signs of tension pneumothorax while chest tubes are being replaced.
□ Wire or tape all the connections.

---

## UNIT EIGHT   WATER-SEAL MONITORING

### NURSING PROCESS DATA

#### ASSESSMENT   *Data Base*

Assess patient's respiratory rate, rhythm, and breath sounds for signs of respiratory distress.

Check to make sure all connections on tubing are airtight and the suction control is connected.

Examine system to see if it is set up and functioning properly.

Identify any malfunctions in system, i.e., air leaks, negative pressure, or obstructions.

#### PLANNING   *Objectives*

To remove air and fluid from pleural space so that reexpansion of lung may occur.

To maintain closed system.

To assist in the evacuation of drainage.

To reestablish negative pressure and reexpand lung.

#### IMPLEMENTATION   *Procedures*

Monitoring a Three Bottle System
Monitoring Disposable Water-Seal System
Obtaining Chest Drainage Specimen

#### EVALUATION   *Expected Outcomes*

Closed chest drainage maintained, drainage evacuated, and lung reexpanded.

Negative pressure reestablished and lung reexpanded.

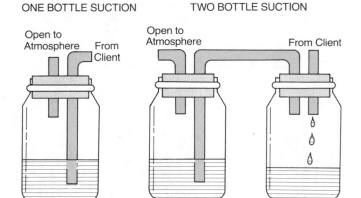

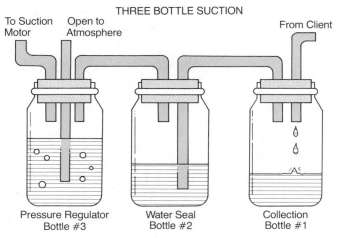

ONE BOTTLE SUCTION

Open to Atmosphere   From Client

Water Seal and Collection Bottle

TWO BOTTLE SUCTION

Open to Atmosphere   From Client

Water Seal Bottle #2

Collection Bottle #1

THREE BOTTLE SUCTION

To Suction Motor   Open to Atmosphere   From Client

Pressure Regulator Bottle #3

Water Seal Bottle #2

Collection Bottle #1

## MONITORING A THREE BOTTLE SYSTEM

### Equipment

Appropriate water-seal bottles and stand

Suction source

Tape and plastic cables or wires for connectors

Two hemostats

### Procedure

1. Examine the control bottle (bottle #3) to check if 10 to 20 cm negative water pressure is maintained. The depth is determined by how deep the longest tube is submerged in the water. This depth determines the pressure in the drainage system.

2. Regulate the wall suction to maintain continuous suctioning. **Rationale:** Constant bubbling in the control bottle indicates the desired pressure level has been reached.
   a. To increase pressure, increase the depth to which the longest tube in the control bottle is submerged.
   b. To decrease negative pressure, decrease the depth to which the longest tube is submerged.

3. Examine the water-seal bottle (bottle #2).
   a. Make sure the longer tube is covered with water to maintain the water-seal. **Rationale:** This prevents air from getting into tubing and pleural space which prevents pneumothorax.

---

### Bottle Systems

One Bottle: One bottle functions as a collection bottle as well as pressure regulator. Used mainly to reinflate lung from pneumothorax.

Two Bottle: Drainage bottle and collection bottle are separate. System not usually connected to suction source. Used following thoracic and/or cardiac surgery.

Three Bottle: Third bottle is connected to an external suction source. The other two bottles are the same as for two bottle system. Used following thoracic and/or cardiac surgery.

---

   b. Check the water level in this bottle to prevent changes in the amount of negative pressure the patient receives.
   c. Tape all connections between the water seal and the patient to prevent air leaks. You may also band taped connections with wire or plastic cable as an extra precaution against air leaks.

4. Monitor the water-seal bottle for air leaks in the system. **Rationale:** These leaks can be identified by constant bubbling in the water-seal bottle.

5. If air leaks occur, clamp tubing close to patient's chest (if you have standing orders to do so) and notify the physician immediately.

6. Examine the collection bottle (bottle #1) to make sure it is not constantly bubbling, indicating an air leak.

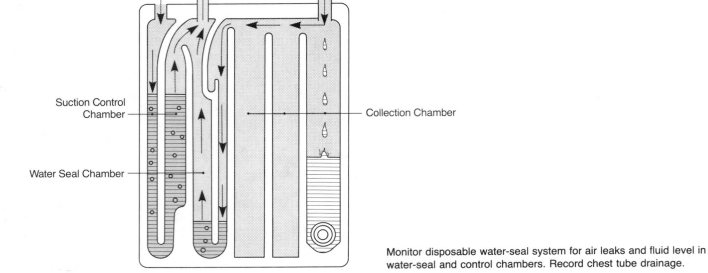

Monitor disposable water-seal system for air leaks and fluid level in water-seal and control chambers. Record chest tube drainage.

7. Observe and record the drainage level on the collection bottle as ordered:
   a. Every hour immediately after surgery, or if there is a large amount of drainage.
   b. At least every eight hours while chest tube is inserted; mark the time on the drainage bottle every shift.

8. Whenever the suction motor is off, keep the drainage system open to the atmosphere by detaching the tubing from the motor to provide a vent.

## MONITORING DISPOSABLE WATER-SEAL SYSTEM

### Equipment

Black marking pen

Tape

### Procedure

1. Monitor the collection chamber for chest drainage every 15 minutes immediately after surgery and every hour for first 24 hours and then as ordered by the physician. Record the results.

2. Mark the drainage on the collection chamber every shift. Place a line at the top level of fluid and place the time on the chamber next to the line.

---

**Principles of the Water-Seal System**

☐ The water-seal mechanism operates on the principle of negative pressure. (The pressure in the chest cavity is lower than the pressure of atmosphere, which causes air to rush into the chest cavity when an injury, such as a stab wound, occurs.)

☐ When the chest has been opened, a vacuum must be applied to chest to reestablish negative pressure.

☐ Water acts as a seal and keeps the air from being drawn back into the pleural space.

☐ An open-drainage system would allow air to be sucked back into the chest cavity and collapse the lungs.

---

3. Observe the suction control chamber for excessive bubbling in the chamber. (Suction control set on low suction.) **Rationale:** This bubbling has no relationship with the amount of pressure exerted on the pleural space. Excessive bubbling just evaporates the water. The control bottle regulates vacuum in the system.

4. Observe the water-seal chamber; there should be no air bubbles present if chest tubes are inserted for drainage. **Rationale:** Bubbles will be present if the lung is being reinflated. When the lung is inflated, the bubbles will cease.

5. Check tube in water seal chamber. It should be under the water. **Rationale:** If it isn't submerged, air can escape into pleural space.

6. Check that all connections are secured with wire or tape.

7. Check that there are no kinks or dependent loops in the extension tubing. **Rationale:** Kinks can create positive pressure on pleural space.

8. Observe and strip chest tubes for drainage and possible clots at least every 15 minutes immediately after surgery and every hour until discontinued.

## OBTAINING CHEST DRAINAGE SPECIMEN

### Equipment

10 cc syringe

18–20 gauge needle

Requisition form

Betadine swab

### Procedure

1. Obtain 18- or 20-gauge needle with 10-cc syringe.

2. Swab self-sealing diaphragm on back of the collection chamber with Betadine swab.

3. Insert needle into diaphragm.

4. Withdraw specified amount of drainage.

5. Place needle protector on needle, label specimen with name, hospital number, and source from where specimen was collected.

6. Fill out requisition form and send to the lab with the specimen.

### CHARTING *for Water-Seal Chest Drainage*

☐ Drainage—amount, color, presence of clots

☐ Any abnormalities in the system and treatment of abnormalities

☐ Respiratory status, including rate, rhythm, and breath sounds

☐ Frequency of chest-tube milking

---

## CLINICAL PROBLEM SOLVING

### Potential Problems

Air leak indicated by bubbling in water-seal bottle.

### Suggested Solutions

☐ Check for specific leak area by clamping chest tube (if physician's orders allow) between water-seal bottle and patient.
  a. If water-seal bottle continues to bubble, the leak is in the tubing.
  b. If water-seal bottle stops bubbling, the leak is in the patient's chest tube at the site of the insertion.

☐ Secure all connections with tape or wire.

☐ Change tubing if necessary (after obtaining physician's order).

☐ Apply sterile Vaseline gauze and pressure dressing around chest-tube insertion site if air leak is at insertion site.

Control bottle not bubbling.

☐ Pressure is too low. Check gauge to wall suction for proper amount.

Chest tube becomes disconnected from water-seal drainage system at any one of the connection sites.

☐ Clamp chest tube near catheter insertion site while replacing extension tubes to prevent pneumothorax from atmospheric air entering intrapleural space during inspiration.

☐ Replace the extension tubing leading from the

chest tube with sterile tubing as infection can occur from contamination of the lumen.

☐ Turn suction source down before clamping chest tube to prevent rapid increase in intrapleural pressure when clamps removed.

☐ Unclamp chest tube as soon as extension tubing replaced to prevent tension pneumothorax.

☐ Reset suction pressure. Observe force of bubbles in suction control compartment to prevent suction from being too great.

☐ Tape or wire new extension connection sites to prevent disconnection.

☐ Observe for signs of respiratory distress due to potential pneumothorax and report.

Chest tubes become obstructed by a clot, kink in the chest tube, or pressure on the chest tube.

☐ Observe for respiratory distress especially if suction is being used to reexpand the lungs and report immediately.

☐ Observe entire system for kinks in tubing. Loop the tubing on bed. Do not secure with tape. Loop rubber band around the chest tube and put safety pin through rubber band and then pin to linen. Allow sufficient slack.

☐ Observe tubing for signs of clot, decreased flow of fluid through tube, visualization of clotted material in tube.

☐ Milk chest tubes several times to force clot out into drainage bottle.

Suction source for water-seal drainage malfunctions due to defect in suction pump, wall plug outlet, or disconnection of suction tube.

☐ Open up the distal end of the chest tube by disconnecting the suction tube to prevent back pressure. Plug system into outlet or replace suction pump.

☐ Observe for decreased flow of fluid through chest tube.

☐ Monitor respiratory rate, rhythm, and chest excursion for signs of respiratory distress and report.

Loose connection on rubber stopper caps (bottle suction) or suction tubes.

☐ Check each suction tube connection site for looseness and tighten each site.

☐ Push rubber stopper caps down into bottles.

☐ Push rubber tubing down securely on stopper caps.

☐ Tape rubber stoppers to bottles.

# UNIT NINE   INTUBATION

## NURSING PROCESS DATA

### ASSESSMENT   *Data Base*

Assess patient's level of consciousness.

Observe for shortness of breath, severe dyspnea, tachypnea, or tachycardia.

Note quality and quantity of secretions.

Check if all lung lobes are ventilated adequately.

Note presence of rhonchi, rales, or wheezes.

Determine if gag and swallowing reflex are present.

Assess patient's use of accessory muscles for breathing.

Observe patient's ability to control tongue.

Listen to cough for signs of weakness.

Listen to chest for signs of right ventricular failure.

Assess patient's ability to understand and cooperate with procedure.

## PLANNING  *Objectives*

*Oropharyngeal or Nasopharyngeal Intubation*

To provide patent airway in an emergency situation.

To provide patent airway when physician is not available.

*Endotracheal Intubation*

To provide patent airway for surgical interventions.

To provide route for short-term mechanical ventilation.

To facilitate removal of pulmonary secretions.

To provide cardiopulmonary rest after cardiovascular surgery.

To relieve carbon dioxide retention in clients with chronic pulmonary disease.

To treat acute respiratory failure.

To prevent aspiration.

## IMPLEMENTATION  *Procedures*

Inserting an Oropharyngeal Airway

Inserting a Nasopharyngeal Airway

Assisting with Endotracheal Intubation

Providing Endotracheal Care

## EVALUATION  *Expected Outcomes*

Patent airway maintained in emergency situation.

Route established for mechanical ventilation in either short-term or long-term therapy.

Secretions easily suctioned so that pulmonary complications can be treated or prevented.

Lungs aerated more easily.

Artificial airway provided when upper airway is obstructed.

## INSERTING AN OROPHARYNGEAL AIRWAY

### Equipment

Oropharyngeal tube

Tongue depressor

### Procedure

1. Select appropriate size airway.

2. Wash your hands.

3. Open patient's mouth with tongue depressor. You may need to hyperextend patient's neck to insert tube.

4. Turn airway sideways and slide it along buccal mucosa until the flange on the end touches the lips.

5. Turn airway so that the curve fits over the tongue. It will extend from the lips to the pharynx, displacing the tongue anteriorly. **Rationale:** Proper positioning will help to prevent injury to lips, teeth, tongue, and posterior pharynx.

6. Tape airway in position. **Rationale:** Stabilization of the tube will prevent injuries.

7. For an uncooperative patient, turn airway upside down and, once the flange on the end touches the lips, turn the airway as described.

---

Oral or nasal endotracheal tube (size of tube determined by patient's needs, physician's orders, and type of intervention) may be rubber or plastic with cuff or no cuff. Use smallest cuff-diameter tube that will accomplish goal of ventilation to prevent damage to upper airway.

---

## INSERTING A NASOPHARYNGEAL AIRWAY

### Equipment

Nasopharnygeal tube

Water-soluble lubricant

### Procedure

1. Select appropriate size tube.

2. Wash your hands.

3. Lubricate entire length of tube.

4. Insert tube gently through one nares. If obstructed, try other nares.

5. Tape tube in position if necessary.

## ASSISTING WITH ENDOTRACHEAL INTUBATION*

---

**\*Only nurses with special preparation or those who are ACLS certified will actually perform endotracheal intubation.**

---

### Equipment

Topical and local anesthetic agents: usually 4% xylocaine spray for tongue, gums, and pharynx; 10% cocaine hydrochloride for nares

Laryngoscope with several blade sizes

Water-soluble lubricant

McGill forceps

2.5-cm micropore tape

Disposable plastic syringes (5–10 cc) for cuff inflation

Stylet to guide endotracheal tube, if needed

### Preparation

1. Explain procedure and rationale to patient or to family.

2. Assemble all equipment.

3. Wash your hands.

4. Remove dentures or bridgework.

5. Check laryngoscope light. (Extra batteries and bulbs should be available.)

6. Inspect tracheal cuff for intactness by inflating cuff.

7. Lubricate tube.

8. Make sure that all necessary mechanical devices are plugged in and operational.

### Procedure

1. Place patient in supine position with head and neck hyperextended and a pillow under shoulders. **Rationale:** Proper positioning will prevent complications such as erosion and necrosis of the nasal septum and turbinates.

2. Restrain patient's hands if necessary. Verbally explain why you are using restraints.

3. Suction and oxygenate patient before procedure begins.

4. Explain procedure as you proceed, to reduce patient's anxiety.

5. Mark tube at level of patient's mouth, and tape securely with micropore tape. **Rationale:** Secure taping prevents tube from slipping.

6. Insert oral airway or bite block when tube is positioned orally. (Benzoin may be applied before taping to secure tube.)

7. After intubation is completed, inflate cuff and place patient on ventilator or administer humidity and/or oxygen with T-piece.

8. Auscultate lung fields for ventilation and aeration. **Rationale:** This action helps to determine that the tube is in position and not in the right mainstem bronchus.

9. Prepare patient for chest x-ray. **Rationale:** X-ray is important to determine the exact placement of the tube.

10. Place patient in semi-Fowler's or Fowler's position to increase ventilation.

11. Place call bell within patient's reach.

12. Discard disposable equipment.

13. Clean and return nondisposable equipment to designated place.

## PROVIDING ENDOTRACHEAL CARE

### Procedure

1. Monitor breath sounds every 4 hours.

2. Check marked points on tube at insertion point to determine if tube has moved.

3. Inspect positioning and stabilization of tube to avoid erosion and necrosis of tissues.

4. Inspect mouth and nose for evidence of pressure areas or ulceration.

5. Provide frequent mouth care.

6. Support patient's head and tube when turning. **Rationale:** This prevents severe head motion and helps to prevent complications.

7. Provide alternate means of communication when cuffed tube is in place. **Rationale:** No air passes over larynx, so patient will not be able to talk.

8. Support patient during this time by spending extra time, using touch and anticipating patient's needs.

### CHARTING *for Intubation*

☐ Clinical manifestations indicating need for intubation

☐ Specific reason for intubation

☐ Size and type of inserted endotracheal, nasopharyngeal, or oropharyngeal tube

☐ Preoxygenation if completed

☐ Type and quantity of secretions

☐ Patient's tolerance of procedure

☐ Type of ventilator connected to tube

---

## CLINICAL PROBLEM SOLVING

### Potential Problems

Pharyngeal airway cannot be inserted.

Laryngospasm occurs when endotracheal tube is inserted.

### Suggested Solutions

☐ Change size of tube.
☐ Relubricate nasopharyngeal airway and attempt to reinsert.
☐ Hyperextend patient's neck.
☐ Insert tube at different angle.

☐ Provide humidity to prevent edema.
☐ If not severe, remove tube and wait a few minutes.
☐ If severe, give patient a muscle relaxant such as succinylcholine chloride. You also may need to perform an emergency cricothyrotomy. Physician's orders are required for this action.
☐ If severe and causing respiratory distress, you may need to prepare for a tracheostomy.

Endotracheal tube is inaccurately placed into right main bronchus.

- ☐ Obtain order for chest x-ray to ascertain exact placement of tube.
- ☐ Pull back slightly on tube, and assess for ventilation of left lung field.

Prolonged endotracheal intubation causes laryngeal damage.

- ☐ Decompress cuff five minutes every hour unless contraindicated. (There is controversy that this procedure is effective.)
- ☐ Listen to trachea. Inflate cuff until there is a slight hissing sound at the peak of inspiration. You may also inflate cuff and remove ½–1 cc of air when you do not hear any leak. Cuff pressure should not exceed 20 mm Hg.
- ☐ Tell the physician how long the patient has been intubated, and discuss the possible need for a tracheostomy.

Accidental extubation occurs.

- ☐ Call physician immediately. Obtain laryngoscope, blades, and extra endotracheal tubes.
- ☐ Observe the marking on the tube every 2–4 hours to ensure tube placement and to prevent accidental extubation.
- ☐ Consider use of soft wrist restraints to prevent extubation if patient if not fully conscious.

Patient is unable to eat with tube inserted.

- ☐ Reassess dietary needs for increased calories.
- ☐ Weigh daily.
- ☐ Consider instituting total parenteral nutrition.

---

## UNIT TEN   Tracheostomy Intubation

### NURSING PROCESS DATA

#### ASSESSMENT   *Data Base*

Assess severity of respiratory distress.

Determine need for tracheostomy as compared to less intrusive methods of providing patent airway.

Assess patient's level of consciousness to determine patient's ability to understand explanation and instructions.

Observe patient's respiratory status: shortness of breath, severe dyspnea, tachypnea, or tachycardia.

Note presence of rhonchi, rales, or wheezes.

#### PLANNING   *Objectives*

To provide patent airway.

To provide route for long term mechanical ventilation (as necessary with pulmonary edema or lung surgery).

To facilitate removal of pulmonary secretions.

To increase respirations if patient is unconscious or has respiratory paresis.

**IMPLEMENTATION** *Procedure*

Assisting with Tracheostomy Intubation

**EVALUATION** *Expected Outcomes*

Artificial airway provided when upper airway is obstructed.

Anatomic dead space decreased in patients with chronic obstructive disease.

Route established for long-term ventilatory assistance.

Secretions easily suctioned.

Pulmonary toilet with hyperinflation of lungs accomplished, and effective treatment for atelectasis or other pulmonary complications.

## ASSISTING WITH TRACHEOSTOMY INTUBATION

### Equipment

Sterile tracheostomy tray

Betadine solution for cleansing skin

Xylocaine for local anesthesia

Sterile tracheal tube with obturator, sized

Sterile gloves

Suction equipment

Manual resuscitator bag

Mechanical ventilator

T-piece, mask, oxygen equipment if needed

Humidifier

Antibiotic ointment

Applicator sticks

Hydrogen peroxide

Sterile dressing

### Preparation

1. Assemble all necessary equipment.
2. Wash your hands.
3. Explain procedure and rationale to patient and/ or relatives.
4. If not an emergency situation, obtain permit from patient or other legally responsible individual prior to tracheostomy.
5. Set up tracheostomy tray where sterile field may be maintained; open tray when physician is ready.

### Procedure

1. Open sterile gloves.
2. Assist physician by pouring Betadine solution into sterile containers on tray. To maintain sterile technique, Xylocaine is usually held by the nurse while the physician draws it out of vial.
3. Restrain patient, if necessary, with soft hand restraints.
4. If patient is alert, explain procedure as it is being done.
5. Have suction equipment ready when tracheal tube is inserted. **Rationale:** Secretions will have accumulated and patient may panic if he feels he is choking.
6. Suction when tube is inserted. If necessary, suction when tube is in place.
7. Secure tracheal ties using two people. **Rationale:** Two people are required to hold tracheostomy tube and to secure ties.
   a. Turn end of twill tape back on itself 5 cm.
   b. Make 2.5-cm cut horizontally in tape.
   c. Thread one end of tape through flange of tracheal tube.
   d. Pull other end of tape over flange and through slot in the tape.
   e. Repeat for other side of flange.
   f. Tie two ends of tape to side of patient's neck to secure tracheal tube in place.
   g. For children, pull tape through each side, doubling it, and tie all pieces in the back of the neck.
   h. To ensure ties are not too tight, insert one finger between neck and tape before securing and knotting ties.

---

**Prevent infections during intubation:**

Maintain sterile technique during intubation and suctioning.

Maintain good handwashing technique.

Administer good oral care every four hours.

If patient is on ventilator, do not drain condensed water from tubing into lungs.

Change ventilatory equipment every 24 hours.

Change sterile water in humidifier every eight hours.

---

8. Attach tracheal tube with an adapter to mechanical ventilator or to humidification system.

9. Cleanse tracheal opening with applicator sticks and hydrogen peroxide and/or normal saline to remove blood from site. (This is a clean procedure; gloves may or may not be worn, depending on hospital policy.)

10. Apply antibiotic ointment if hospital policy allows.

11. Apply sterile tracheal dressing around tracheal opening under tube.

12. Reposition patient for comfort. If not contraindicated, place in semi-Fowler's position. **Rationale:** This position makes breathing easier for patient.

13. Place call bell where patient can reach it.

### CHARTING *for Tracheostomy Intubation*

☐ Clinical manifestations and need for intubation

☐ Size and type of tracheal tube inserted

☐ Name of physician performing procedure

☐ Patient's tolerance of procedure

☐ Amount, color, and consistency of secretions

☐ Respiratory status before and after procedure

☐ Any equipment attached to tracheal tube, type of ventilator, and percent oxygen

---

## CLINICAL PROBLEM SOLVING

### Potential Problems

Artificial airway cannot be inserted due to upper airway obstruction.

### Suggested Solutions

☐ Obtain smaller size tracheostomy tube or change type of tubes (i.e., use rubber instead of plastic).

☐ Hyperextend neck more.

☐ Have CPR cart available for immediate use.

☐ Auscultate all lung fields to assess degree of ventilation.

Secretions cannot be easily suctioned.

☐ Change suction catheter size.

☐ Provide warm, humidified air through ventilator, tracheostomy mask, or T-piece.

☐ Before suctioning, instill 5–10 cc sterile normal saline (not bacteriostatic water) into tracheal tube to liquefy and mobilize secretions. Allow saline to remain in tube for a few seconds, or ventilate 5–6 times with ambu bag before suctioning again.

Patient begins choking while tracheal tube is inserted.

☐ Suction through tracheal opening or through nose.

☐ If possible, prevent choking by premedicating patient with muscle relaxant.

☐ Tube is inaccurately placed in prebronchial tissue.

☐ Auscultate all lung fields at least every four hours to ensure ventilation.

☐ Observe for signs of surgical emphysema or cardiopulmonary collapse.

|  |  |
|---|---|
|  | ☐ Obtain physician's order for x-ray to verify tube placement. |
|  | ☐ Replace tube with different size. |
| Accidental extubation occur. (Usually occurs within first five days or during suctioning when cuff is deflated.) | ☐ Have emergency equipment at bedside.<br>    Sterile tracheal set of same size and style<br>    Ties and syringes for inflating cuff<br>    Tracheal dilator, scissors, and hemostats<br>    Sterile gloves and dressings |
|  | ☐ Insert old tube if new one not available to preserve patent airway. |
|  | ☐ Immediately insert tracheal dilator into stoma to preserve airway. |
|  | ☐ Suction stoma, if there is time. Then reinsert new tracheal tube, secure with tapes, and establish ventilation. Oxygenating with ambu bag is desirable, especially if any signs of respiratory distress are present. |
| Sudden overventilation occurs resulting in rapid reduction of $pCO_2$. May occur if patient is on mechanical ventilator. | ☐ Ventilate patient adequately prior to intubation to prevent build-up of carbon dioxide. |
| Hemorrhage from tracheostomy site is noted. | ☐ Apply pressure if hemorrhage site accessible. |
|  | ☐ Have physician cauterize bleeding vessels. |
|  | ☐ Take patient to operating room for exploration of site and ligation of bleeding vessel if physician orders surgery. |
| Tracheostomy is obstructed. | ☐ If no physician available, follow these procedures:<br>    Deflate cuff.<br>    Cut tracheostomy ties.<br>    Remove tube.<br>    Insert tracheal dilator (if at bedside).<br>    Establish airway. (You may need to suction through tracheal stoma although this is contraindicated if tracheostomy is new.)<br>    Insert new tube and reestablish ventilation. |

# UNIT ELEVEN   MECHANICAL VENTILATION

## NURSING PROCESS DATA

### ASSESSMENT   *Data Base*

Assess patient for presence of risk factors for acute respiratory distress syndrome: massive trauma, massive fat embolism, aspiration pneumonia, and other disorders characterized by abnormal gas distribution (due to airway or alveolar closure) and pulmonary interstitial edema.

Auscultate heart and lung sounds for baseline data.

Assess vital signs and measure arterial blood gases and hemodynamic pressures if CVP and Swan-Ganz lines are in place.

Identify if need for mechanical ventilation is present. Criteria for non-COPD patients:
- Vital capacity is less than 15 ml/kg of body weight.
- Inspiratory pressure is less than $-25$ cm $H_2O$.
- $PaCO_2$ is below 30 mm Hg or above 50 mm Hg.
- Alveolar-arterial oxygen difference (A-a $\Delta$ $pO_2$) is greater than 350 mm Hg on 100 percent oxygen.
- Pulmonary shunt is greater than 30 percent.
- Deadspace-tidal volume ($V_D$-$V_T$) ratio is greater than 60 percent.
- $PaO_2$ is less than 60 mm Hg on an $FIO_2$ of 1.0.

Observe for trend of respiratory values (trend is more important than isolated measurements).

Assess patient for indications for PEEP:
- Inability to maintain arterial $pO_2$ of at least 70 mm Hg on 50 percent oxygen during continuous mechanical ventilation.
- Failure of other methods to reduce pulmonary shunt, e.g., treatment of cardiac failure or pneumonia.
- Normovolemia. (Normal state of blood volume.)

Check physician's orders regarding amount and duration of PEEP. (Usual range is 5 to 15 cm $H_2O$ although 20 to 35 cm $H_2O$ have been used.)

Review physician's order for amount and duration of CPAP.


## PLANNING  *Objectives*

To maintain physiological functioning in: respiratory center failure (brainstem injury or narcotic overdose), neuromuscular diseases (myasthenia gravis), musculoskeletal disorders (flail chest), and pulmonary disorders (adult respiratory distress syndrome).

To maintain cardiopulmonary functioning in cardiopulmonary arrest.

To maintain acid-base balance of the body.


*For PEEP*

To assist in keeping the alveoli open on expiration, thereby reducing shunt, increasing functional residual capacity (FRC), and improving compliance.

To assist in surfactant regeneration.

To improve oxygenation without prolonged use of high oxygenation concentrations.

To maintain respiratory function in adult respiratory distress syndrome (ARDS).

To increase functional residual capacity.


*For CPAP*

To improve oxygenation for patients who are able to spontaneously ventilate without the use of mechanical ventilation.

To establish a resistance to expiration to maintain the airway under constant positive pressure.

To enable patients to avoid mechanical ventilation when pulmonary dysfunction is acute and reversible.

## IMPLEMENTATION *Procedures*

Managing Patients on Ventilators

Providing Positive End Expiratory Pressure (PEEP)

Providing Continuous Positive Airway Pressure (CPAP)

## EVALUATION *Expected Outcomes*

Adequate respiratory function is maintained for patients with altered respirations.

Acid-base balance is improved in altered respiratory states.

Oxygenation of tissue is improved and $pO_2$ is maintained at 80 to 100 mm Hg on low oxygen concentration with PEEP or CPAP.

Pulmonary pathology is reduced with PEEP or CPAP.

Functional residual capacity and compliance are increased with PEEP.

---

### Airway Pressure Therapies

Intermittent positive-pressure breathing (IPPB)—inspiration by positive airway pressure; expiration is passive.

Intermittent mandatory ventilation (IMV)—spontaneous ventilation intermittently interspersed with positive-pressure ventilation.

Positive end-expiratory pressure (PEEP)—an expiratory airway pressure modality in which the airway pressure is maintained above atmospheric at the end of expiration.

Continuous positive airway pressure (CPAP)—spontaneous ventilation and PEEP. Inspiratory airway pressures are maintained above atmospheric.

## MANAGING PATIENTS ON VENTILATORS

### Equipment

Specific ventilator ordered, i.e. Bennett MA-1, Bennett PR 2, etc.

Handheld resuscitator connected to oxygen flowmeter (ambu or Laerdahl bag)

Sterile suction supplies

Ventilator flowsheet

### Preparation

1. Double check the ventilator settings against those ordered by the physician.

2. Plug the machine in and turn it on.

3. Familiarize yourself with location of alarm systems on the ventilator and turn on all alarm systems.

4. Connect the ventilator tubing to patient's endotracheal tube or tracheostomy tube.

### Procedure

1. Monitor patient's pulse and blood pressure every five minutes until stable.

2. Obtain arterial blood gases 15 minutes after ventilation is established.

3. Monitor ventilator settings and delivered values every hour: tidal volume, inspiratory pressure, peak pressure, rate, $FIO_2$, I:E ratio, in addition to PEEP or IMV when ordered.

---

### Initial Ventilator Settings

☐ Tidal volume of 10 ml/kg (High tidal volumes help prevent atelectasis.)

☐ Respiratory rate of 10 to 15 per minute

☐ Inspiratory pressure of 25 cm $H_2O$

☐ Inspiratory-expiratory (I:E) rate 1:2 (I:E ratio should be set at less than 1:1 to prevent air trapping in the lungs.)

☐ Pressure pop-off setting of 50 cm $H_2O$

☐ $FIO_2$ of 0.4 to 1.0

---

4. Check thermometer every hour in inspiratory

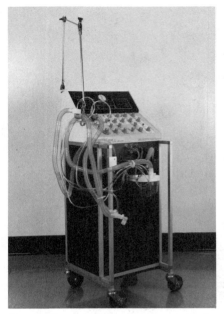

Commonly used adult volume respirator for patients requiring respiratory maintenance.

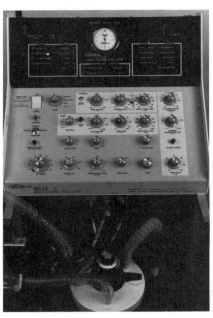

Check all ventilator settings with physician's orders before placing patient on ventilator.

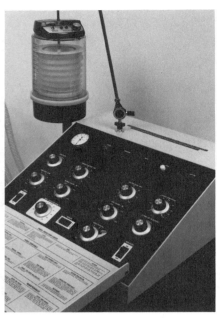

Identify location of alarm systems and what these alarms mean when triggered.

tubing line. Maintain temperature of inspired air between 32°C and 35°C.

5. Check humidifier fluid level every eight hours and refill as necessary.

6. Record intake, output, and daily weights. Positive pressure ventilation may cause a positive water balance due to humidification of inspired air.

7. Suspend ventilator tubing from an IV hook or support it on a pillow to reduce traction on the endotracheal or tracheostomy tube.

8. Change ventilator tubing every 24 hours.

9. Check vital signs every hour and auscultate lungs. **Rationale:** Positive pressure ventilation may decrease venous return and cardiac output.

10. Observe and listen for possible cuff leaks around tracheostomy or endotracheal tubes.

11. Empty accumulated water in the ventilator tubing as needed. Disconnect the tubing, stretch it to release water trapped in the corrugated areas, and drain the water into a basin or trap in tubing. Do not drain water back into the humidifier. **Rationale:** This action increases the risk of infection.

12. Provide patient with a method of communication, such as a "magic slate."

13. Test the nasogastric drainage pH every hour and administer antacids to maintain the pH above 5. Stress ulcers are frequently associated with mechanical ventilation.

---

Compliance is determined by $\dfrac{TV}{PIP}$

where TV = tidal volume
PIP = peak inspiratory pressure

---

14. Test the nasogastric drainage and fecal matter daily for occult blood.

15. Assess lung compliance frequently. **Rationale:** Lung compliance falls before changes are evident in blood gas analysis or clinical manifestations.

16. Implement methods of stress reduction, such as careful explanation of procedures even if patient appears comatose.

17. Keep ventilator alarms *ON*.

18. "Sigh" the patient six to eight times an hour. Use the sigh button if the ventilator has one, or ventilate the patient manually, using a volume larger than the ventilator set tidal volume. **Rationale:** To prevent atelectasis.

## PROVIDING POSITIVE END EXPIRATORY PRESSURE (PEEP)

### Equipment

Mechanical ventilator with built-in PEEP device or

Mechanical ventilator without PEEP

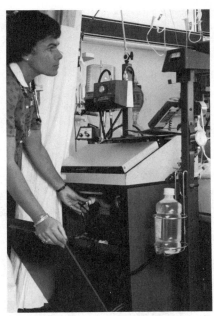

PEEP and CPAP settings are checked hourly to ensure accuracy of treatment.

Connecting tubing attached to ventilator expiratory port

Cylinder containing water, under which the end of the connecting tubing is submerged

### Procedure

1. Notify respiratory therapist of order for PEEP.

2. Briefly explain procedure to patient.

3. Gradually increase PEEP to specified level while monitoring respiratory and cardiovascular status.

4. Monitor vital signs every 15 minutes × 4 and then hourly. Transient hypotension is common with PEEP.

5. Check blood gases 15 to 30 minutes after stabilization and adjust PEEP accordingly.

6. Check inspiratory pressure and PEEP setting dial hourly on ventilators with built-in PEEP. On other setups, check inspiratory pressure and level of water column hourly.

7. Check exhalation port tubing hourly for kinks or other obstructions.

8. Monitor blood gasses every two to four hours.

9. Inspect, palpate, and auscultate chest hourly to detect subcutaneous emphysema, or pneumothorax development.

10. Monitor cardiac outputs hourly if Swan-Ganz catheter is in place and PEEP is more than 5 cm $H_2O$. **Rationale:** May see fall in cardiac output.

11. As condition improves, lower PEEP pressure.

## PROVIDING CONTINUOUS POSITIVE AIRWAY PRESSURE (CPAP)

### Equipment

Clear face mask with straps

Inspiratory and expiratory tubing with one-way valves

Oxygen source

Oxygen-air mixer

Reservoir bag

Humidification warming device

CPAP device with safety pop-off (PEEP valve, cylinder containing water)

Pressure gauge

### Preparation

1. Notify respiratory therapist of physician's order.

2. Briefly explain procedure to patient and family.

3. Start flow of warm, humidified oxygen through CPAP system.

4. Strap facemask on patient to form tight seal.

5. Connect CPAP device to expiratory tubing.

### Procedure

1. Slowly increase expiratory resistance to level specified by physician. CPAP is usually not delivered at more than 10 cm of $H_2O$.

2. Reassure patient especially if dyspneic, that CPAP will help to ease her underlying condition.

3. Instruct patient to breathe slowly and deeply. **Rationale:** Patients may panic due to mask over nose and mouth. In addition, there is the increased work of breathing caused by CPAP.

4. Monitor vital signs, blood gases, respiratory and cardiovascular status hourly. **Rationale:** CPAP may precipitate acute respiratory failure, due to $CO_2$ retention from fatigue, or cardiac failure due to increased intrathoracic pressure.

5. Observe frequently for air leaks in system, especially around mask.

6. Check pressure gauge frequently.

7. Observe for abdominal distention. **Rationale:** This can be caused from air swallowing.

8. Interrupt CPAP every 2 hours and provide warm, humidified oxygen via face tent for ten minutes.
   a. During this time, check respiratory and car-

diovascular status to aid in determining resolution of pulmonary disorder.

  b. Clean and dry face. Lotion may be applied to reddened areas.

  c. Provide time to eat and talk in addition to relieving pressure on face.

9. Reapply CPAP.

10. Change the tubing every 48 hours. **Rationale:** This will minimize infection.

11. Provide communication method such as a "magic slate" for patient while mask is in place.

## CHARTING  *for Mechanical Ventilation*

☐ Type of ventilator used

☐ Ventilator settings

☐ Time mechanical ventilation started

☐ Any problems with ventilator and actions taken

☐ Results of suctioning, i.e., amount of secretions obtained and color and odor of secretions

☐ Tidal volume obtained, sighing volume if indicated

## CHARTING  *for PEEP*

☐ Pre-PEEP assessment including presence of risk factors

☐ Time of trials on PEEP and levels of PEEP used, with patient's responses

☐ Volume of PEEP on which patient is stabilized

☐ Arterial blood gas values

☐ CVP and/or PAWP readings

☐ Results of lung and cardiac auscultation

## CHARTING  *For CPAP*

☐ Pressure volume of CPAP utilized

☐ Patient's ability to tolerate CPAP

☐ Findings of cardiac and respiratory assessment

☐ Vital signs

☐ Complications that occurred and specific treatment

☐ Blood gas values and pulmonary artery wedge pressures

---

# CLINICAL PROBLEM SOLVING

| **Potential Problems** | **Suggested Solutions** |
|---|---|
| Adequate respiratory function is not maintained. | ☐ Auscultate lungs to determine if air flow through the lungs is adequate.<br>☐ Auscultate lungs to identify presence of adventitious lung sounds.<br>☐ Suction lungs frequently to increase pulmonary ventilation.<br>☐ Assess that the ventilator is set at the proper settings and that the system is functioning properly.<br>☐ Observe for possible leak in cuff if pressure settings are not maintained. |
| Arterial blood gas values are not improved. | ☐ Auscultate lungs for adventitious lung sounds and suction as needed.<br>☐ Obtain order to "sigh" patient, if not already doing so.<br>☐ Assess if patient is ventilated adequately via the respirator. |
| Patient breathes out of synchronization with the ventilator. | ☐ Check arterial blood gases; as anxiety increases, struggling occurs, which is a common sign of hypoxemia.<br>☐ Remove patient from the ventilator, and hand ventilate at a rate faster than the machine (to |

| | |
|---|---|
| | blow off carbon dioxide and diminish patient's ventilatory drive). Slowly decrease rate until it is the same as the ventilator setting. Place patient back on the ventilator, while reassuring and coaching patient to breathe in synchronization with ventilator. |
| | ☐ If problem persists and arterial blood gas values and ventilator settings are adequate, consult with physician about the use of sedation or neuromuscular blocking agents to paralyze patient. |
| | ☐ Remove patient from the ventilator, and hand ventilate with ambu or Laerdahl bag connected to 100 percent oxygen. |
| | ☐ Request therapist or physician to recheck accuracy of settings. |
| Sudden respiratory distress, cyanosis, distended neck veins, or a possible tracheal shift occurs. | ☐ Immediately remove patient from ventilator and hand ventilate. |
| | ☐ Immediately notify physician as these are signs of a tension pneumothroax. |
| | ☐ If physician is not immediately available and you are trained in performing emergency chest decompression, insert a large bore (15 gauge) needle in the second intercostal space. |
| | ☐ Prepare equipment and patient for chest tube insertion. |
| | ☐ Assist the physician with chest tube insertion. |
| Patient experiences decreased compliance, and diminished breath sounds. | ☐ Suction patient more frequently as these are signs of atelectasis. |
| | ☐ Implement program of chest physical therapy. Provide percussion, vibration, drainage, deep breathing/sighing, and suctioning at least every two hours. |
| | ☐ Turn patient frequently. |
| | ☐ "Yawn" patient several times an hour to reopen atelectatic alveoli, hyperinflate lungs with a brief pause at the end of inspiration mimicking a normal yawn. |
| Patient experiences symptoms of dyspnea, burning chest pain on inspiration, decreasing $PaO_2$, and dry cough, indicating oxygen toxicity. | ☐ Prevent oxygen toxicity by returning $FIO_2$ to specified setting after increasing it to 1.0 for oxygenation pre- and post-suctioning or for determination of A-a $\Delta pO_2$ difference. |
| | ☐ Obtain physician's order to reduce the $FIO_2$ as quickly as possible. (The danger of oxygen toxicity is increased with prolonged use of $FIO_2$ over 0.5.) |
| | ☐ Check $FIO_2$ settings hourly. |
| Rales, edema, weight gain, and pulmonary edema, indicating fluid imbalance occurs. | ☐ Notify physician for orders to slow IV rates. |
| | ☐ Administer diuretics. |
| | ☐ Apply rotating tourniquets. |
| Pressure alarm is activated. | ☐ Check for kinks or obstructions in tubing and take corrective measures. |

Volume alarm is activated.

□ Suction patient for possible mucus obstruction.
□ Obtain order for and administer bronchodilators.
□ Assess for pneumothorax.
□ If unable to find cause for alarm, remove patient from the ventilator and hand ventilate while respirator is checked for malfunction.

□ Check if inspiratory phase is shortened due to pressure being reached earlier than normal. Tidal volume is decreased when this occurs.
□ Check for disconnected tubing.
□ Check for loose connections and tighten them if present.
□ Check whether the plug has been pulled out of the wall socket.
□ Check the volume indicator stick on the ventilator bellows. In some models, the arm that supports the ventilator tubing may become jostled and obstruct the movement of the stick. If so, readjust the arm so the bellows can move freely.
□ Deflate and reinflate the airway cuff to detect a cuff leak.
□ If unable to identify and relieve the cause immediately, disconnect the ventilator tubing, hand ventilate the patient and summon help.

Patient has fever, elevated white blood cell count, or changed odor or color of respiratory secretions.

□ Send sputum specimen for culture and sensitivity.
□ Administer antibiotics as ordered.
□ Examine suctioning technique for breaks in aseptic technique.

Subcutaneous or mediastinal emphysema occurs, as manifested by puffy tissues that crackle on palpation, or a crunching sound with each heartbeat when the heart is auscultated.

□ Notify physician.
□ If ordered, assist with chest tube insertion.
□ If chest tube already in place, switch to a drainage system with an air leak indicator.
□ If ordered, assist physician with expelling air from tissues by placing needles or drains in tissues and "milking" the tissues toward you.
□ Observe patient closely for development of respiratory distress due to tracheal compression.

*For PEEP*

Mechanical ventilator fails or patient needs to be transported.

□ Start oxygen flow through handheld ventilating device.
□ Attach expiratory resistance, for example PEEP valve.
□ Disconnect ventilator tubing from airway at end of inspiration.
□ Attach handheld ventilator to airway during expiration.
□ Watch chest and provide breaths in synchrony with patient's inspirations (if any) or at rate of 10 to 12/minute.
□ Notify respiratory therapist to check machine.

Oxygenation of tissues is not improved and $pO_2$ is not maintained at 80 to 100 mm Hg.

- ☐ Continue delivery of PEEP at ordered prescribed volume. If this is not effective, obtain an order for increased volume.
- ☐ Do not attempt to wean patient off PEEP until parameters are maintained or improved.

Pulmonary pathology is not reduced.

- ☐ Continue with PEEP.
- ☐ Evaluate other treatment modalities for effectiveness.
- ☐ Monitor drug therapy, such as antibiotic or diuretic and cardiotonic for effectiveness.
- ☐ Evaluate the results of respiratory toilet and monitor amount, type, and consistency of secretions.

Significant decrease in cardiac output.

- ☐ Anticipate that patients with decreased sympathetic reserve may have difficulty adjusting to increased intrathoracic pressure. Examples are patients who are elderly, hypovolemic, or on sympatholytic medications.
- ☐ If cardiac output falls abruptly, or severely decreases, terminate PEEP trial and notify physician.

Pneumothorax occurs.

- ☐ Discontinue PEEP and take patient off ventilator; hand ventilate with ambu or Laerdahl bag and 100 percent oxygen.
- ☐ Notify physician and prepare to assist with chest tube insertion.
- ☐ If tension pneumothorax occurs, assist with emergency chest decompression with large-bore needle, three-way stopcock, and large syringe.

### For CPAP

Oxygenation is not improved to the tissues.

- ☐ Monitor blood gases and pulmonary artery wedge pressures. If they remain abnormal even with treatment, notify physician for possible orders for mechanical ventilation and PEEP.
- ☐ Continue to use CPAP and instruct patient to breathe slowly and deeply. Anxiety decreases the patient's ability to utilize oxygen.

Pulmonary pathology is not decreased.

- ☐ Ensure adequate pulmonary toilet is being done in addition to CPAP with patients who have increased secretions.
- ☐ Monitor effects of drug therapy for cardiac or pulmonary disorders.
- ☐ Assess patient's need for mechanical ventilation with PEEP.

Patient complains of nausea.

- ☐ Immediately remove mask and supply oxygen via face tent while assessing cause of nausea.
- ☐ Insert nasogastric tube to remove air and fluid from stomach.
- ☐ If impending vomiting, place patient in supine position with head turned to side or place patient on side to minimize risk of aspiration.

Patient complains of fatigue; increasing dyspnea, coma, or apnea occurs.

- ☐ Assist physician with intubation and mechanical ventilation.
- ☐ Discontinue CPAP and bag the patient with an ambu or Laerdahl bag if necessary. Use 100 percent oxygen with bagging.

Pneumothorax occurs.

- ☐ Notify physician and prepare to assist with chest tube insertion.
- ☐ If tension pneumothorax occurs, assist with emergency chest decompression.

---

## UNIT TWELVE   VENTILATOR WEANING PROCESS

### NURSING PROCESS DATA

#### ASSESSMENT   *Data Base*

Measure vital signs, inspiratory pressure, vital capacity, and arterial blood gases.

Evaluate patient parameters indicating readiness for weaning.

$PaO_2$ of 70 mm Hg or better on an $FIO_2$ of 0.5 or less.

PEEP 5 cm or less, if used.

Vital capacity of 15 ml/kg or better.

Inspiratory pressure of $-25$ cm $H_2O$ or better.

A-a $\Delta pO_2$ difference less than 350 mm Hg on 100 percent oxygen.

Shunt less than 30 percent.

Respiratory rate between 12 to 20 breaths per minute.

Blood pressure and pulse stable.

Note current ECG pattern as a baseline.

Review the physician's order regarding details of weaning.

#### PLANNING   *Objectives*

To identify patients who are capable of maintaining respirations without the use of mechanical ventilators

To reestablish normal breathing patterns for patients on mechanical ventilators

#### IMPLEMENTATION   *Procedure*

Taking Patient Off Ventilator

#### EVALUATION   *Expected Outcomes*

Laboratory parameters indicate patient is ready for weaning.

Patient is able to maintain respiratory status without mechanical ventilation.

Arterial blood gases maintained within normal range for patient.

## TAKING PATIENT OFF VENTILATOR

### Equipment

Heated humidified oxygen source with wide bore tubing

T-piece adaptor

Suctioning supplies

Arterial blood gas sampling supplies

### Procedure

1. Explain the discontinuation process to patient. Reassure patient that you will watch closely and, if necessary, discontinue weaning and attempt later.

2. Suction patient. Hyperinflate patient's lungs with 100 percent oxygen before and after suctioning.

3. Maintain inflated endotracheal or tracheostomy cuff during weaning.

4. If physician orders cuff deflated during weaning, suction secretions that have accumulated above the cuff as follows:
   a. Provide positive pressure to end of tube with a hand-held resuscitation bag and 100 percent oxygen.
   b. Place tip of suction catheter in the posterior pharynx.
   c. Deflate cuff and apply suction to catheter. **Rationale:** Positive pressure will blow the secretions into the pharynx, where they can be suctioned out.
   d. Hyperinflate lungs with 100 percent oxygen for 3 to 5 breaths.

5. Elevate head of the bed to facilitate diaphragmatic excursion.

6. Connect T-piece to wide bore oxygen tubing leading to the source of warm, humidified oxygen.

7. Set oxygen concentration as ordered by physician, usually 0.10 higher than the ventilator $FIO_2$ the patient has been receiving.

8. Remove ventilator tubing from airway and connect airway to the T-piece.

9. Cover end of ventilator tubing with sterile gauze.

10. Monitor vital signs every 5 minutes until stable.

11. Observe for vital sign changes, apprehension, diaphoresis, and dysrhythmias. (A mild increase in blood pressure, pulse, and respiratory rate is normal. Mild-to-moderate anxiety is also normal.)

12. Measure arterial blood gases fifteen minutes after initiating weaning.

13. Proceed with weaning procedure. Length of the weaning is ordered by physician.
    *With patient on ventilator a short time*
    a. Continuous weaning may be ordered.
    b. Leave patient on the T-piece.
    c. Obtain vital signs hourly.
    d. Monitor arterial blood gases every four hours.
    e. If patient tolerates weaning well for two to six hours, weaning may be discontinued and the artificial airway may be removed.
    *With patient on prolonged ventilation*
    a. Gradual weaning may be ordered.
    b. Following intermittent weaning time period, remove T-piece and place patient back on ventilator.
    c. Obtain vital signs hourly.
    d. Monitor arterial blood gases every four hours.
    e. Extend weaning periods 15 to 30 minutes each time until patient is able to tolerate several hours on the T-piece.
    f. Remove the artificial airway.

14. Following weaning, measure vital signs, vital capacity, inspiratory pressure, and blood gases.

---

### IMV (INTERMITTENT MANDATORY VENTILATION)

Provides continuous ventilation and weaning for patients on ventilators.

Primary mode of ventilatory support.

Allows smooth transition from controlled to spontaneous ventilation by gradually decreasing IMV or ventilator rate.

Patient breathes at own tidal volume and rate for majority of time.

Ventilator breaths are not synchronized to patient's own respiratory pattern.

Machine breath can be given during the patient's exhalation or peak inhalation.

Weaning with IMV may take a longer time.

---

### Charting *for Ventilator Weaning*

☐ Preweaning vital signs, vital capacity, inspiratory pressure, and blood gas values

☐ Method of weaning

☐ $FIO_2$

☐ Time weaning started and terminated

☐ Vital signs, blood gases, and physical signs and symptoms during weaning period

# CLINICAL PROBLEM SOLVING

| **Potential Problems** | **Suggested Solutions** |
|---|---|
| Laboratory parameters indicate patient is not ready for weaning. | ☐ Continue mechanical ventilation as ordered.<br>☐ If ventilation settings do not improve patient's respiratory status, notify physician for change in orders.<br>☐ Attempt to use T-piece and 40 percent oxygen for longer time periods each hour until laboratory parameters are reached.<br>☐ Assess patient for possible respiratory complications that may be interfering with the weaning process. |
| Patient is not able to maintain respiratory status without mechanical ventilation. | ☐ Continue use of ventilator.<br>☐ If patient has been extubated, prepare equipment and patient for intubation and placement on a ventilator.<br>☐ If respiratory distress occurs with unintubated patient, ventilate with ambu or Laerdahl bag, using a face mask. |
| Arterial blood gases (ABGs) are not maintained within normal range. | ☐ Notify physician of abnormal ABGs and obtain order for alteration in ventilation, i.e., increased percent of oxygen, added dead space, etc.<br>☐ Maintain mechanical ventilation. Do not attempt to wean or extubate patient.<br>☐ Suction patient frequently if secretions are thick and/or copious in amount.<br>☐ If severe acidosis occurs, obtain order for increasing the respiratory rate to blow off carbon dioxide, or administer sodium bicarbonate to buffer acidotic state. |
| Decreased level of consciousness, dyspnea, severe anxiety, or severe fatigue occurs. | ☐ Obtain arterial blood gases.<br>☐ Place patient back on ventilator. |
| Patient has unstable vital signs, development of premature beats on EKG, or ST segment depression. | ☐ Place patient back on ventilator.<br>☐ Monitor vital signs every 15 minutes and obtain blood gases to determine oxygen concentration. |
| Patient is unable to be weaned because of emotionally-induced anxiety. | ☐ Reassess that anxiety is emotionally based by measuring physical parameters. Anxiety is a common early sign of hypoxia.<br>☐ Provide increased reassurance to patient.<br>☐ Consult with physician about weaning with intermittent mandatory ventilation (IMV). The IMV allows brief rest periods, decreases fatigue, and facilitates psychological adaptation. Since patient is usually unaware of exact rate adjustments, weaning with IMV is less emotionally traumatic than weaning with a T-piece. |

# TERMINOLOGY

**Acidosis:** accumulation of acids in the body disturbing the acid-base balance.

**Adventitious:** arising sporadically; pertaining to adventitia, or the outermost covering of an organ.

**Alkalosis:** condition in which the alkalinity of the body tends to increase beyond normal.

**Antiemetic:** an agent that will prevent or arrest vomiting.

**Apnea:** cessation of breathing, usually of a temporary nature.

**Atelectasis:** condition that may be caused by a mucus plug closing a bronchus; can also occur when nitrogen is washed out of the lungs because a high FIO has been delivered to the patient. Symptoms include dyspnea, chest pain, cyanosis, and sweating.

**Auscultation:** process of listening for sounds produced in some of the body cavities.

**Bradycardia:** slow heart action, below 60 beats/minute.

**Bronchiectasis:** dilatation of a bronchus or bronchi, usually secreting large amounts of offensive pus.

**Chylothorax:** milky chyle that has entered pleural space from the thoracic duct.

**Cyanosis:** slightly bluish, grayish, slatelike, or dark purple discoloration of the skin resulting from reduced hemoglobin or oxygen in the blood.

**Diaphoresis:** profuse sweating

**Dyspnea:** air hunger resulting in labored or difficult breathing.

**Expectorant:** an agent that facilitates the removal of the secretions of the bronchopulmonary mucous membrane.

**Hemothorax:** blood in pleural space as a result of severed blood vessels.

**Hypoventilation:** reduced rate and depth of breathing.

**Hypoxemia:** insufficient oxygenation of the blood.

**Hypoxia:** lack of adequate amount of oxygen transported to the tissues.

**Intercostal:** outer layer of muscles, between the ribs.

**Intrapulmonic:** within the lung.

**Intubation:** to insert a tube into a body opening, as into the trachea.

**Lung volumes:**
   *Expiratory reserve volume* (ERV)—volume of air that can be expelled following a resting expiration.
   *Inspiratory capacity* (IC)—volume of air with maximum inspiration; comprises tidal volume and inspiratory reserve volume.
   *Inspiratory reserve volume* (IRV)—volume of air that can be inspired above the tidal volume.
   *Reserve volume* (RV)—volume of air remaining in the lungs at the end of maximum expiration.
   *Tidal volume* (TV)—amount of air normally inspired.
   *Vital capacity* (VC)—volume of air that is able to be expelled following a maximum inspiration.

**Narcosis:** unconscious state due to narcotics.

**Nares:** the nostrils.

**Nebulizer:** a device for breaking a drug into small particles to produce mist or fog for inhalation

**Percussion:** tapping the body lightly but sharply to determine position, size, and consistency of an underlying structure and the presence of fluid or pus in a cavity.

**Pneumothorax:** presence of air or gas in the intrathoracic space; results in lung collapse.

**Polycythemia:** excess of red blood cells.

**Postural drainage:** the utilization of gravity to drain secretions from the lungs.

**Pyothorax:** exudate in pleural space.

**Rales:** the intermittent sounds heard as air passes through moisture in the trachea, bronchi, or alveoli.

**Respiratory pressures:**
   □ At inspiration the intraalveolar pressure is more negative than the atmospheric pressure.
   □ At expiration the intraalveolar is more positive, thereby pressing the air out of the lungs.
   □ A negative pressure exists in the intrapleural space and aids in keeping the visceral pleura of the lungs against the parietal pleura of the chest wall. Lung space enlarges as the chest wall expands.
   □ Recoil tendency of the lungs is due to the elastic fibers in the lungs and the surfactant.

**Retrolental fibroplasia:** condition marked by the presence of opaque tissue behind the lens, which can lead to blindness. Condition is usually caused by elevated arterial levels of oxygen in premature infants.

**Rhonchi:** synonym for wheezes; continuous sounds produced by air passing through respiratory passages narrowed by secretions.

**Spirometer:** device used for measuring inhalation and exhalation volumes and in alveolar expansion.

**Spontaneous pneumothorax:** a condition developing from air leaks in pulmonary alveoli or from erosion by a disease process through the pulmonary pleura.

**Sputum:** substance expelled by coughing or clearing the throat.

**Subcutaneous:** third layer of tissue; method of administering medications beneath the skin.

**Tachypnea:** abnormal rapidity of respiration, over 40 breaths per minute.

**Tension pneumothorax:** massive lung collapse and shift of the mediastinum resulting from extensive accumulation of air in the intrapleural space.

**Tracheostomy:** operation of cutting into the trachea usually for insertion of a tube to overcome tracheal obstruction.

**Ventilation:** the exchange of gases—oxygen and carbon dioxide—across the alveolar membrane.

**Vibration:** therapeutic shaking of the body; a form of massage using a to-and-fro motion.

# Chapter 25

# Circulatory Maintenance

## LEARNING OBJECTIVES

Identify three properties of the cardiac muscle and define cardiac output.

Define the words inotropic and chronotropic.

State the reason it is important to minimize the patient's stress when hemorrhage occurs.

Outline the assessment actions for a patient who is hemorrhaging.

Identify two interventions for treating pump failure.

Define the term ischemia.

List the nine pressure points in the body which can be used to control bleeding if hemorrhage occurs.

Identify two potential problems which could occur in patients who are bleeding and state one suggested solution for each problem.

Describe how to measure appropriately for elastic hosiery.

Explain when the precordial thump is used with CPR.

List at least four potential problems for patients requiring CPR and two suggested solutions for each problem.

Outline the steps in administering CPR with one rescuer and with two rescuers.

Compare and contrast the differences in administering CPR to an infant or small child.

Demonstrate the steps in performing the Heimlich maneuver.

State two nursing diagnoses relevant to patients with circulatory dysfunction.

Identify three safety measures utilized when administering rotating tourniquets.

Demonstrate proper placement of defibrillator paddles.

Differentiate between a normal and abnormal EKG pattern.

Complete an assessment for a patient with a pacemaker.

## THE CIRCULATORY SYSTEM

The heart is a three-layered, four-chambered vessel, approximately the size of an adult fist. It weighs close to 600 grams in the normal adult. A thick, fibrous sheath, called the pericardium, surrounds about two-thirds of the heart's surface. Most of the mass lies in the heart's middle layer—the myocardium, or cardiac muscle. The endocardium, a thin, inner layer, lines the four chambers.

In considering the heart's chambers, imagine two major pump systems. The right and left atria contract in one phase, and the right and left ventricles contract in the successive phase. The tricuspid, pulmonary, mitral, and aortic valves are the four flow regulators for the chambers.

Three properties of cardiac muscle best illustrate the heart's specialization. Automaticity physiologically differentiates heart muscle from all other muscle tissue. The other two properties—conductivity and contractility—characterize all muscle; however, a cardiac contraction is normally all or none, as opposed to partial contractions in other muscles.

The heart serves as a pump to maintain blood flow and blood pressure. Adequate blood flow perfuses the lungs for oxygenation. Blood pressure is a driving force for that flow and is normally highest during ventricular contractions. The heart pumps 4 to 7 liters of blood per minute. This constitutes a normal cardiac output, formulated by multiplying contraction volume times ventricular rate.

When the heart maintains a safe blood pressure and blood flow, it is in a state of compensation, regardless of cardiac output. If the heart cannot maintain a safe blood pressure and blood flow, it is in a state of decompensation. Three cardiac reserves allow for compensation: inotropic reserve, increased venous filling pressure, and chronotropic reserve.

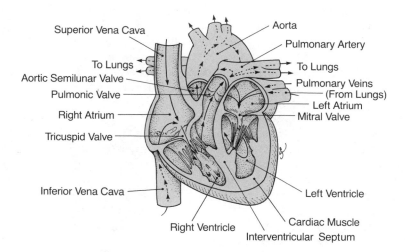

Blood flow pattern through the right and left side of the heart.

Inotropic reserve is under the control of sympathetic nerve stimulation. Adrenergic drugs, as well as some others, exert an inotropic effect by increasing the force of the cardiac contraction and therefore stroke volume. Cardiac output will also increase with additional filling pressure in the atria. Starling's Law of the Heart summarizes the relationship by stating that an increased filling pressure causes an increased force of contraction within the elastic limits of the heart. Finally, chronotropic reserve refers to increased cardiac output. Atropine-like drugs exert a chronotropic effect by increasing the heart rate.

Blood vessels, together with the heart, form a closed circulatory system unless there is damage or abnormalities that result in leakage. When the ventricles contract, blood leaves the right ventricle through the pulmonic valve into the pulmonary artery. Blood is now in the pulmonary circulation for oxygenation of the red blood cells, or erythrocytes. After gas exchange occurs at the cellular level, the blood is returned to the left atrium through four pulmonary veins. This is normally the most oxygenated blood in the human body.

On the left side of the heart during a ventricular contraction, blood travels through the aortic valve out of the left ventricle into the ascending aorta. Five percent, or 200 to 350 ml, of this blood enters coronary circulation for oxygenation and waste removal from the cardiac tissue. Fifteen percent, or 600 to 1050 ml, travels to the brain and twenty-five percent, or 1000 to 1750 ml, goes to the kidneys, and the same amount to other viscera. The extremities and skin normally receive thirty percent of the circulating volume.

Arteries carry blood from the heart throughout the body unless obstructed or severed. The largest subdivision is the aorta and the smallest subdivision is the arteriole. Similar to the heart, arteries have three layers: endothelium, involuntary muscle, and connective tissue. Capillaries join the arterial system to the venous system and are a single cell layer in thickness. The single layer allows gas, nutrients, and waste exchanges to occur throughout the body. Blood enters the venous system from the capillary beds for eventual return to the right side of the heart via the superior and inferior vena cava.

**PATHOLOGY**   There are many ways to categorize disorders of the heart, arteries, and veins. Endocarditis, myocarditis, and pericarditis classify cardiac problems according to inflammation of a particular heart layer. Another classification is congenital heart disease, such as tetralogy of Fallot and transposition of the great vessels. For the purpose of this chapter alterations of circulation are divided into hemorrhage, shock, pump failure, ischemia, thrombosis, and embolism.

**Hemorrhage**   Hemorrhage results when trauma or disease causes leakage in the closed circulatory system. Damage to the heart or arteries usually constitutes the greatest danger because of the high pressure and large volumes. Normally, when a blood vessel is ruptured or severed, compensatory mechanisms protect the body from significant blood loss. The wall of the injured vessel contracts immediately. A platelet plug forms at the site, and blood clotting occurs. New connective tissue penetrates the clot for permanent closure. Interventions for patients who are hemorrhaging are based on one of these compensatory mechanisms.

To prevent, correct, or compensate for hemorrhage, the nurse must assess the patient. She identifies the nature of the bleeding as external and/or internal and establishes baseline data, which includes blood pressure and vital signs. An assessment is made of the body's response, adaptive, excessive, or deficient, and the nurse assists in formulating and planning appropriate interventions. The first concern is to minimize the patient's stress, since sympathetic stimulation of the heart increases heart rate (chronotropic effect) and force of contraction (inotropic effect). Interventions for hemorrhage involve restricting activity, elevating involved body areas above the heart if possible, applying direct pressure, and replacing lost fluid volume. A tourniquet is generally used as a last resort. It is placed proximal to the site of the hemorrhage with the knowledge that the extremity may be sacrificed.

**Shock**   Unchecked hemorrhage eventually leads to hypovolemic or hemorrhagic shock, a serious state with a poor prognosis. Peripheral resistance is of great significance. In hemorrhagic shock, high peripheral resistance is secondary to pronounced peripheral vasoconstriction in the initial stage. Due to the loss of blood volume it becomes very difficult to start an intravenous line in a superficial vein. Vasoconstrictors, such as Levophed, are undesirable since they cause a further decline in tissue perfusion. Successful recognition and early treatment of hemorrhagic shock depends heavily upon sophisticated monitoring devices, the nature of the fluid for volume replacement, and the use of blood components instead of whole blood. Intervention centers on establishing one or more intravenous lines for fluid replacement, drug administration, and blood component therapy. Careful monitoring of peripheral pulses, blood pressure, central venous pressure, and even more sophisticated hemodynamic parameters, such as pulmonary arterial wedge pressures, is desirable.

The use of pressure devices, such as the antigravity suit (G-suit), the Jobst extremity pump, and inflatable splints, are helpful adjuncts in treating patients in hemorrhagic shock. These devices provide pneumatic compression for immobilizing the patient, controlling bleeding, and counteracting hypotension by maintaining venous pressure.

**Pump Failure**   Heart failure results from any condition that reduces the ability of the heart to pump blood. The heart is no longer in a state of compensation, and cardiac output will fall. Cardiac arrhythmias and congestion are the most common types of pump failure.

Effective cardiac contraction depends upon correctly timed depolarization of cardiac cells, which is achieved in normal sinus rhythm. When a dysrhythmia (abnormal rhythm) occurs, the ideal timing of depolarization is disrupted, and pump failure can occur, particularly when the dysrhythmia interferes with proper filling and emptying of the ventricles. This problem occurs when the patient experiences ventricular fibrillation or tachycardia.

Heart failure has three successive phases of variable duration. The first phase is pathologic cardiac overloading due to excessive pressures, too much fluid, and/or myocardial tissue loss. The second phase of failure is cardiovascular compensatory response, such as dilatation and reflex responses. Finally, the heart fails to compensate, producing a wide variety of signs (objective data base) and symptoms (subjective data base).

Heart failure should not be confused with circulatory overload, a condition in which cardiac output is adequate but blood volume and/or venous return is excessive. Excessive infusion of IV fluids in too short a period of time results in circulatory overload.

Pulmonary edema, the most common result of pump failure, is a life-threatening condition. Pulmonary edema is a disorder in which alveoli fill with fluid. It produces severe abnormalities in gas exchange and can lead to death if not treated immediately. There are several disorders that can cause pulmonary edema, all of which produce a high hydrostatic pressure in the pulmonary capillaries. Right ventricular output into the pulmonary capillaries depends in part on the volume of venous return to the heart.

Interventions for treating pump failure and pulmonary edema focus on correcting the arrhythmias and removing excess body fluid. One way to restore ideal timing is to terminate the dysrhythmia by delivering an electrical countershock. This countershock causes simultaneous depolarization of the entire myocardium. It thus interrupts the dysrhythmia, allowing the sinoatrial node to resume control of the sequence and coordination of depolarization. Two types of electrical countershock are used—defibrillation, and cardioversion. Both of these interventions are specialized therapies carried out by trained personnel.

Interventions to reduce congestion include drug therapy and the temporary use of rotating tourniquets. Drug therapy is long-term therapy for treating and preventing pump failure as a result of fluid overload. Drugs most often used are digitalis p.o. or IV, Lasix IV, and potassium chloride IV.

Application of tourniquets to extremities carried out by a registered nurse retards venous flow, thereby decreasing right ventricular output into the pulmonary vascular tree. The use of rotating tourniquets causes a temporary reduction in circulating blood volume, "buying time" while morphine, digitalis, and diuretics take effect to lower pulmonary vascular pressure.

**Ischemia**    Ischemia is a circulatory condition in which blood supply to a body part or region is reduced to a critical level. Relative ischemia occurs with hypotension or the inability to meet increased metabolic demands. Absolute ischemia is usually a sudden, complete occlusion of a blood vessel, resulting in tissue necrosis. Leaving a tourniquet on an extremity for more than 15 minutes may cause tissue necrosis. Other causes of ischemia include Raynaud's disease, Buerger's disease, thromboembolism, mechanical obstruction, arteriosclerosis, and atherosclerosis. Atherosclerosis is currently under study in relation to hypertension, cigarette smoking, genetic factors, obesity, physical activity, hypercholesterolemia, and emotional stress. The actual cause of coronary atherosclerotic disease (CAD) remains a mystery, and the incidence in the United States continues to increase.

**Thrombosis and Embolism**  Blood clot formation within the circulatory system causes thrombi. Endothelial injury, decreased blood flow, and changes in blood constituency lead to blood clot formation and therefore thrombosis. If veins are inflamed, the condition is termed thrombophlebitis. This phlebitis is usually of bacterial origin, with the thrombi firmly attached in the lower extremities. Thrombophlebitis should be differentiated from phlebothrombosis or thrombus in a vein.

A dislodged, or migrating, thrombus becomes an embolus. Embolism is the process of impaction somewhere within the circulatory system and may be solid, liquid, or air. Liquid emboli are usually injected intravenously by accident such as during a hyperalimentation procedure (TPN). Similarly, air emboli occur when air is not removed from intravenous or arterial lines before infusion of solutions.

Elastic hosiery (TED, Jobst, and others) is used to prevent venous stasis and avoid thrombus formation and subsequent emboli. The hosiery produces compression of peripheral leg veins. This pressure forces the venous blood into deeper, larger leg veins for a more rapid return to the heart.

## PACEMAKER

A pacemaker is a device that provides electrical stimulation to the heart muscle in order to maintain an effective rhythm. It takes over the initiating and the maintaining function of the heart rate when the natural pacemaker fails.

Pacemakers have two primary parts—the pulse generator and the electrodes. When temporary pacing is desired, the pulse generator is external. When permanent pacing is desired, the pulse generator is placed internally. Conditions such as heart block and persistent bradycardia usually require permanent placement. Since the monitoring function is not utilized under these conditions, this text will focus primarily on the temporary pacemakers.

The temporary pacemaker is inserted in severe bradycardia or sinus arrest situations. Temporary conditions such as toxic drug reaction or inferior wall myocardial infarction also may require a temporary pacemaker. The temporary pacemaker is a device that provides a low-voltage electrical stimulus to the endocardial surface of the right atrium or ventricle (transvenous method) or into the ventricle itself (transthoracic or epicardial method).

All methods of temporary pacing utilize a pulse generator with rechargeable or replaceable batteries. This battery is the source of the low-voltage output. In addition, all methods use some type of electrode or impulse conductor. These electrodes may be either unipolar or bipolar and differ in sensitivity. Unipolar (single-pole) catheter electrodes have a single cathode tip and are more sensitive to the patient's generated impulses. The catheter electrode wire fits into the negative output terminal on the generator. The bipolar (two-pole) catheter electrodes have both an anode and cathode at the tip and fit into both positive and negative output terminals on the generator. The pace rate determines the rate of beats per minute (BPM) provided by the generator.

Pulse generators have certain abilities that distinguish them from one another: synchronization with patient's own spontaneous heart beats, chamber to be paced, and chamber to be sensed. The chamber to be paced refers to the atrium, ventricle, or both, with several available possibilities: VVI— ventricular inhibited (demand); VDD—atrial triggered; DVI—AV sequential; and DDD—universal.

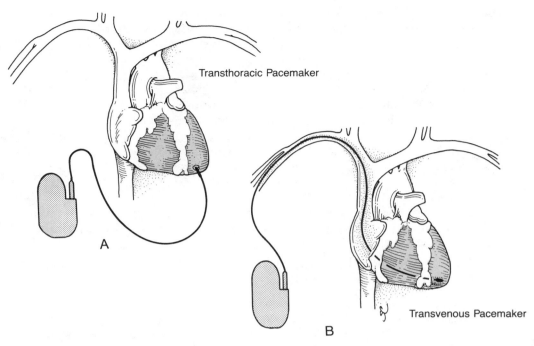

Transthoracic Pacemaker

A

Transvenous Pacemaker

B

Temporary pacemakers have two parts, the pulse generator and the electrodes. The pulse generator is external.

There are three modes of temporary pacemaker therapy. Pacing differs according to the presence and/or function of a sensing mechanism. The first mode is a fixed or continuous rate (asynchronous). This type of pacemaker delivers an uninhibited impulse at a continuous set rate regardless of the patient's underlying rhythm, so it does not have a sensing mechanism. The intervals between stimuli are unchanged even if ectopic or natural beats occur. This type is the simplest; however, its major drawbacks are its competition with the patient's own heart rate and the fact that in competition, the stimulus occurs during repolarization, thus pacing during the heart's vulnerable period.

Demand (synchronous) is the most frequently used. This type fires or stimulates the heart only when the heart's natural pacemaker does not function at predetermined rates. The atrial synchronous pacemaker senses the atrial impulse following a normal P-R interval. If the P wave fails to arrive at a set time, the pacemaker takes over. The ventricular inhibited pacemaker senses QRS waves and immediately discharges an impulse if the patient's ventricular rate falls below the preset rate. This method is noncompetitive and is the most common; however, electromagnetic interference suppresses pacemaker function.

A third mode is AV sequential. Catheter electrode wires are placed in the atria and ventricles. The wires sense in both places and fire in both places. It is a complex mechanism and not as reliable as the other pacer modes.

Initiation of temporary pacing by attaching electrode wires to an external generator source may be accomplished by the following routes:

*Transvenous:* pacemaker wires are threaded percutaneously through the subclavian or femoral vein or through a cutdown venotomy in the brachial or external jugular vein. With either method, the wire is advanced through the vena cava, right atrium, and tricuspid valve and positioned at the apex of the right ventricle on the endocardial surface. The wire is then attached to the generator.

*Transthoracic:* a needle is advanced through the chest wall into the right ventricle. The catheter wire is then threaded through the needle, the needle is removed, and the proximal end of the catheter wire is attached to the generator. Pacemaker wires are frequently inserted in this manner during cardiac surgery. The catheter electrodes are directly attached to the epicardial surface. Instead of being connected to the generator, the proximal ends of the wires are brought out through the chest wall, covered, and are then available for use if necessary.

In terms of pacemaker effectiveness, the nurse should be familiar with EKG monitoring and interpretation. Pacemaker spikes should be seen in relation to their appropriate EKG waveform. In addition, providing an electrically safe environment is essential.

## ALTERED CIRCULATION

**Assessment**    Alterations in circulation are indicated by a variety of signs and symptoms. The nurse should not overlook the behavioral manifestations or the more physical signs and symptoms. Systematic patient evaluation considers whether or not there is a significant blood loss. If bleeding exists, external and/or internal sites must be identified. Special attention is given to the family history for disease conditions of the heart, vessels, liver, spleen, kidneys, brain, lungs, and coagulation mechanisms. Baseline data is gathered for vital signs and arterial blood pressures. The color, temperature, and condition of the skin are closely noted. Cyanosis is differentiated as peripheral versus central. Weakness and fatigue is significant, as well as physical discomforts such as pain, pressure, or numbness. Abnormalities of superficial veins often indicate obstruction and/or pooling. Impaired renal function, especially related to output, is closely considered. Edema is differentiated as dependent versus generalized. Special observations include such findings as clubbing of the fingers, petechiae, and calf tenderness with dorsiflexion of the foot (positive Homan's sign). Information obtained from the drug history and present medications the patient is taking may affect the diagnosis and therefore the nursing intervention. Trauma victims require especially close inspection since more overt signs and symptoms may not appear until days later. Table 1 illustrates an assessment of a hemorrhaging patient.

**Planning and Intervention**    Once an initial assessment of a patient for alterations in circulation has been made, the nurse develops a prioritized problem list for planning and intervention. Nurses monitor circulatory status with a variety of sophisticated tools. Again, however, the most valuable approach is direct observation of the patient. Blood pressure measurements are usually noninvasive, taken with a blood pressure cuff, stethoscope, and sphygmomanometer. The central venous line and the Swan-Ganz catheter for pulmonary arterial pressures (PAP and PAWP) are invasive methods used under certain conditions and by specially trained personnel.

Interventions for circulatory problems cover numerous therapeutic modalities but usually fall into three broad categories: inputs, outputs, and pressure/

**TABLE 1**
ASSESSMENT GUIDE FOR HEMORRHAGING

1. Observable bleeding from skin, mucous membranes. Check under the person, clothing, dressings, casts.
2. Observable bleeding into the skin, mucous membranes. Check for petechiae, ecchymosis, hematomas, purpura.
3. Observable bleeding from body orifice. Check for epistaxis, hematemesis, hemoptysis.
4. Observable bleeding from tubes. Check T-tubes, endotracheal tubes, suction drainage, urinary catheters.
5. Generalized signs and symptoms of bleeding.
   a. Low blood pressure (systolic below 90 mm Hg and diastolic below 50 mm Hg).
   b. Progressive drop in blood pressure.
   c. Rapid, weak pulses or absence of pulses.
   d. Clammy skin and central cyanosis.
   e. Deep, rapid respirations (above 24/minute).
   f. Low body temperature (one or more degrees below 98.6°F, or 37°C, for oral temperature).
   g. Reduced urine output (less than 30 ml per hour).
   h. Behavioral changes.
   i. Syncope and visual disturbance.
   j. Loss of consciousness.
6. Localized signs and symptoms of bleeding.
   a. Painful, swollen, tender, or hot joints.
   b. Soft, spongy uterus high in abdominal cavity during postpartum period.
   c. Pupillary and visual changes, behavioral shifts, tinnitus, vertigo, breathing pattern shifts, loss of consciousness following head injury.

supports. Inputs include arterial lines, venous lines, drug regimens, transfusions, blood component therapies, etc. Outputs include suctioning with specialized equipment like hemovacs and procedures like thoracentesis. Pressure/supports include dressings, bandages, digital compression, tourniquets, and cardiopulmonary resuscitation. This chapter outlines some of the most common skills the nurse will be required to do in the management of circulatory problems.

In coping with alterations in circulation, care should be directed toward promoting, maintaining, or regaining the best possible cardiopulmonary function. The design for nursing action is to assess the situation and patient for stressors. The patient should be interviewed if possible, observed, and examined to identify actual and/or potential circulatory problems. The patient's responses will be appropriate, deficient, or excessive, and interventions should be planned accordingly. The nurse attempts to reduce patient stress, supports adaptive behaviors, replaces deficiencies, modifies or removes excessive responses, and prevents injury and complications. The nurse should always assist in the evaluation of planned actions, report patient responses, and assist in modifying the interventions as indicated.

The following nursing diagnoses are appropriate to utilize on Patient Care Plans when the components are related to circulation.

**NURSING DIAGNOSES**

| Nursing Diagnosis<br>(Potential) | Defining Characteristic; Etiology<br>(Examples) |
|---|---|
| ☐ Cardiac Output, Alteration in: Decreased, *related to* | Cardiac arrhythmias, e.g., cardiac disease states (myocardial infarction). |
| ☐ Fluid Volume, Alteration in: Excess, *related to* | Decompensated cardiovascular system, e.g., disease states (pulmonary edema, congestive heart failure). |
| ☐ Tissue Perfusion, Alteration in, *related to* | Altered blood supply, e.g., tight elastic hosiery, rotating tourniquets. |

# UNIT ONE   CONTROL OF BLEEDING

## NURSING PROCESS DATA

### ASSESSMENT   *Data Base*

Observe the amount of bleeding.

Check for the source of bleeding.

Observe the extent of the wound.

Identify familial history of bleeding disorders.

Assess baseline vital signs and arterial blood pressure readings.

Observe color, temperature, and condition of the skin.

Ask about medications taken routinely by patient.

### PLANNING   *Objectives*

To detect source of bleeding.

To stop or control bleeding or hemorrhage before large blood loss occurs.

To provide pressure as an assist (adjunct) to stop bleeding.

To minimize capillary seepage, hematoma, and serum accumulation.

### IMPLEMENTATION   *Procedures*

Using Digital Pressure to Control Bleeding

Using Pressure Dressing to Control Bleeding

### EVALUATION   *Expected Outcomes*

Early detection of bleeding occurs and loss of blood minimized.

Pressure dressing is applied and bleeding controlled.

Collateral circulation is minimally inhibited.

## USING DIGITAL PRESSURE

### Equipment

Towels or gauze dressing if available

### Procedure

1. Identify the closest artery proximal to the bleeding site. **Rationale:** The rapid loss of more than 25 to 30 percent of the total blood volume leads to death.

2. Apply direct pressure to artery, using your finger.

3. Raise the affected limb above the level of the heart about 30 degrees. **Rationale:** Decreases arterial blood flow to area and promotes venous return.

4. Maintain direct pressure for at least five minutes.

5. Do not remove pressure before five minutes. **Rationale:** Clot formation has not had an opportunity to stabilize.

6. If towels or 4 × 4 gauze pads are available, apply direct pressure to site if wound does not contain glass particles. **Rationale:** If pressure is placed on wound when glass is present, additional tissue damage can occur.

7. When bleeding has subsided, proceed to clean and dress the wound.

8. To control nose bleeds, place patient in sitting position, with head tilted forward. Pinch nose for five minutes. If ordered, apply ice pack to assist in vasoconstriction.

## USING PRESSURE DRESSING

### Equipment

Towel

4 × 4 gauze pad

Sterile dressings—number and size depends on wound

Sterile gloves

Cleansing solution

Tape

### Preparation

1. Check physician's order.

2. Assemble necessary supplies according to extent of wound.

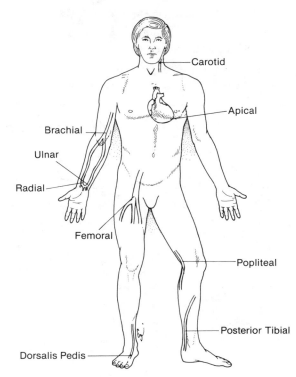

Pulse sites which may be used to control bleeding.

3. If time permits, explain procedure to patient and provide light and privacy.

4. Wash your hands thoroughly if time permits.

5. Set up sterile field and prepare cleansing solution if time permits.

### Procedure

1. Put on sterile gloves.

2. Cleanse wound and apply dressing.

3. To provide an occlusive dressing, place tape over entire dressing. Do not completely circle an extremity or the body. **Rationale:** To ensure that collateral blood flow is maintained.

4. Place all soiled materials in red plastic bag.

5. Wash your hands thoroughly.

6. Monitor vital signs and observe for signs of shock.

7. Position patient for comfort.

8. Elevate extremity to prevent bleeding.

9. Monitor frequently for signs of bleeding and hematoma. Hematomas feel spongy even under bandages.

**CHARTING** *for Control of Bleeding*

☐ Size, location, condition of wound

☐ Color, odor, amount of drainage

☐ Type and number of dressings used

☐ Approximate amount of blood loss

☐ Condition of dressing when changed, e.g., soaked with drainage, etc.

---

## CLINICAL PROBLEM SOLVING

**Potential Problems**

Even with direct pressure and application of pressure dressing, bleeding continues.

**Suggested Solutions**

☐ Monitor IV flow closely.
☐ Notify physician and be prepared to send patient to surgery for wound closure.
☐ Monitor closely for signs of shock.
☐ Aid with placing tourniquets proximal to the site of the hemorrhage to control bleeding.

Wound edges do not approximate.

☐ Notify physician.
☐ Be prepared to assist with wound closure or to send patient to surgery.

Glass particles are evident in wound.

☐ Irrigate wound profusely with sterile saline solution as ordered.
☐ If large amount of glass or if glass is difficult to extract, notify physician and be prepared to send patient to surgery for wound cleansing and debridement.
☐ Do not apply direct pressure or pressure dressing to wound containing glass.
☐ Apply pressure to vessel above wound or, as a last resort, apply a tourniquet.

---

# UNIT TWO   CIRCULATORY MAINTENANCE

## NURSING PROCESS DATA

### ASSESSMENT   *Data Base*

Evaluate patient's overall physical condition, particularly patient's cardiovascular status.

Observe baseline vital signs before procedures are initiated.

Determine if patient is at risk for pooling of blood in extremities. Conditions that require use of elastic stockings are leg varicosities, thrombophlebitis, lymphedema, orthostatic hypotension, immediate postcast removal, postoperative venous ligation or stripping, and venous insufficiencies due to muscular inactivity.

Check lungs for signs of pulmonary edema—rales or rhonchi.

Assess for peripheral edema by palpating pulses and observing color and temperature as well as fluid accumulation.

**PLANNING** *Objectives*

To prevent venous stasis.

To prevent thrombus formation and subsequent emboli.

To temporarily reduce venous return to the heart through use of rotating tourniquets.

To improve oxygenation in pulmonary edema.

To utilize elastic hose to prevent venous stasis.

**IMPLEMENTATION** *Procedures*

Applying Elastic Hosiery

Applying Automatic Rotating Tourniquets

Applying Manual Rotating Tourniquets

**EVALUATION** *Expected Outcomes*

Elastic stockings remain wrinkle-free and pressure is evenly distributed.

Pulmonary edema is relieved following use of rotating tourniquets.

Peripheral pulses are present throughout use of rotating tourniquets.

## APPLYING ELASTIC HOSIERY

### Equipment

Tape measure

Specific type of hosiery, e.g., below-the-knee or above-the-knee

Talcum powder

### Procedure

1. Check orders for specific reason patient is in need of elastic stockings.

2. Check physician's order for type and specifications. Below-the-knee type is the most common.

3. Gather supplies, identify patient, and explain procedure.

4. Wash your hands, and provide for patient's privacy and comfort.

5. Apply drape as top linens are removed. Bathe, dry, and powder patient's legs.

6. Position patient in dorsal recumbent position, and elevate bed to working height.

7. Measure patient for size.
   a. For below-the-knee stockings, measure from the Achilles tendon to the popliteal fold, and measure the midcalf circumference.
   b. For high stockings, measure midcalf and mid-thigh circumference to determine size. Length is determined by measuring the distance from gluteal furrow to bottom of the heel.

8. Compare your measurements to manufacturer's chart to obtain correct hose size.

9. Powder patient's heel and foot.

10. Invert foot of stocking back to heel area.

11. Holding both sides of hose at inverted foot area, pull hose over toes and ease gently toward top of foot.

12. Gather top of hose down to heel area, and with curving motion, cover heel and then pull hose up the leg.

13. Reposition patient and wash your hands.

14. Observe extremities for edema above level of hose.

15. Remove hose two to three times daily for 30 minutes.

16. Wash in mild detergent and warm water as needed.

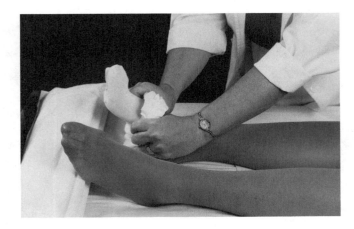

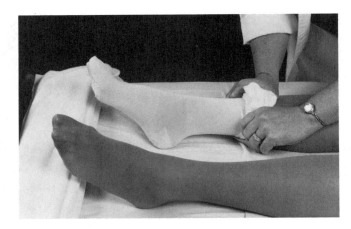

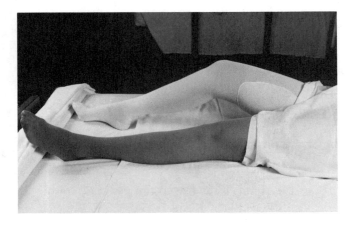

Start applying elastic hose by first inverting the foot of the stocking and pulling the hose over the toes. Ease the stockings over the heel area and work it up the leg to the thigh. Ensure stockings are wrinkle-free.

**TABLE 2** MEASURING FOR ELASTIC HOSIERY

| **Thigh-Hi Measuring** | *Circumference* Measure calf at largest circumference | *Length* Measure leg from bottom of heel to fold of buttocks |
| --- | --- | --- |
| **Knee-Hi Measuring** | *Circumference* Measure calf at largest circumference | *Length* Measure leg from bottom of heel to bend of knee |

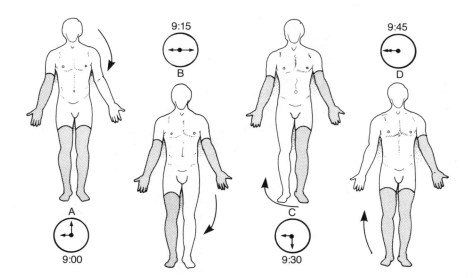

Tourniquets are applied to three limbs at one time and rotated every fifteen minutes in a clockwise direction.

## APPLYING AUTOMATIC ROTATING TOURNIQUETS

### Equipment

Automatic rotating tourniquet machine: four separate blood pressure cuffs

Diagram and chart for tourniquet rotation pattern

Sphygmomanometer

Stethoscope

### Procedure

1. Check the physician's order.

2. Explain the procedure to patient. Alert patient that extremities may be temporarily swollen and discolored during treatment.

3. Place patient in high-Fowler's position. **Rationale:** This position assists patient to breathe.

4. Obtain baseline blood pressure.

5. Assess quality of peripheral pulses and color and temperature of each limb.

6. Mark pulse locations with a pen for future reference.

7. Note extremities in which IV lines are present.

8. Apply the cuffs as proximal or close to the trunk as possible.

9. Connect the air tubes of the cuffs to the valves on the machine.

10. Adjust the cuff release timer to cycle length ordered by physician.

11. Set cuff pressure by using the pressure control valve. Select a cuff pressure 10 mm above the patient's diastolic pressure. **Rationale:** This allows arterial blood flow but decreases venous return to the heart.

12. Activate the alarm system which indicates air leak or failure of rotation.

13. Open cuff valves one at a time while observing patient for shock.

14. Check that the cuffs are inflating and deflating properly. The machine will cycle the cuff inflations automatically.

15. Check blood pressure and pulse every 15 to 30 minutes. To check blood pressure, close valve when cuff is deflated. Disconnect cuff from machine and attach it to a sphygmomanometer. After you have measured the blood pressure, reconnect the cuff to the machine and open the valve.

16. When physician orders procedure terminated, deflate each cuff in sequence.

---

### Clinical Alert

Do not deflate all the cuffs at once, since the sudden return of fluid to the circulation is likely to precipitate another episode of pulmonary edema.

---

17. Leave deflated cuffs in place for a few minutes in case it is necessary to reinstitute the rotating tourniquets.

18. Monitor vital signs, lung sounds, and heart sounds immediately after tourniquets are discontinued and then as ordered.

## APPLYING MANUAL ROTATING TOURNIQUETS

### Equipment

Four soft rubber, 2-inch-wide tourniquets
  or
Four blood pressure cuffs

Sphygmomanometer

Stethoscope

### Procedure

1. Review physician's order.
2. Explain procedure and position patient in high-Fowler's position.
3. Apply blood pressure cuffs or wide rubber tourniquets over pads to three limbs as close to the trunk as possible. **Rationale:** The patient will be more comfortable if the rubber tourniquets are placed over soft pads.
4. If using cuffs, inflate them to a pressure just 10 mm above the diastolic pressure.
5. Palpate peripheral pulses. Lower cuff pressure or loosen the rubber tourniquets if pulses are not palpable.
6. Remove one tourniquet and apply another one on the previously unoccluded limb every 15 min-

utes. **Rationale:** Never occlude all four extremities at once.

7. Measure blood pressure every 15 to 30 minutes.
8. Check pulses, color, and temperature of the extremities every hour.
9. Chart the sequence of cuff or tourniquet rotation meticulously.
10. Assist in removing the tourniquets. Remove one tourniquet every 15 minutes, following the rotation sequence.

### CHARTING  *for Elastic Hose*

- ☐ Size and type of elastic hose applied
- ☐ Condition of skin
- ☐ Presence of pulses
- ☐ Edema formation below or above hose
- ☐ Time and length of time hose removed

### *for Rotating Tourniquets*

- ☐ Time rotating tourniquets applied
- ☐ Presence of peripheral pulses
- ☐ Color and condition of extremities
- ☐ Rotation pattern
- ☐ Patient's response to procedure
- ☐ Time procedure discontinued and patient's response

---

## CLINICAL PROBLEM SOLVING

### Potential Problems

*for Elastic Hosiery*
Elastic hosiery is not available.

Below-the-knee stockings do not fold over at top.

### Suggested Solutions

- ☐ If ordered, use elastic (Ace) bandages. Anchor bandages on top of the foot and in front of the leg, using metal clips or tape. Overlap should be one-third of bandage width; for a 4 inch width each turn overlaps by 1½ inches.
- ☐ Assess that elastic bandages are tight enough for support but do not obstruct arterial flow.
- ☐ While making each turn, place a finger between the bandage and skin to prevent bandage from becoming too tight.
- ☐ Remeasure patient's leg from heel to popliteal fold.

*for Rotating Tourniquets*
On initial assessment, limb is ischemic, infected, or being used for IV infusion.

Shock develops with rotating tourniquet therapy.

Patient is moved before therapy is terminated.

□ If hosiery is not available in proper size, apply Ace bandages or contact charge nurse for thigh-high hosiery order.

□ Do not apply tourniquet on that limb.
□ Rotate tourniquet application among remaining limbs.

□ Notify physician and remove tourniquets as per prescribed procedure.

□ Close all four valves, keeping three cuffs inflated; or, if manual tourniquets are used, leave three tourniquets in place. Transfer patient to stretcher and reopen valves if automatic unit is being used. Continue rotation pattern.

# UNIT THREE   EMERGENCY LIFE SUPPORT MEASURES

## NURSING PROCESS DATA

### ASSESSMENT   *Data Base*

Assess patient for signs of cardiac or respiratory arrest.

Know your own responsibilities for an arrest situation.

Identify location of resuscitation equipment.

Identify the location of the emergency cart, nearest defibrillator/monitor (if none on cart), and 12-lead EKG machine.

Identify procedure for activation of cardiac arrest team.

### PLANNING   *Objectives*

To provide adequate oxygenation of lungs through mechanical support.

To provide oxygenated blood to vital organs.

To support the patient via mechanical intervention or mouth-to-mouth ventilation until other equipment is available.

### IMPLEMENTATION   *Procedures*

Maintaining the Emergency Cart

Using the Emergency Cart

Administering Cardiopulmonary Resuscitation (CPR)

Administering CPR to a Child

Administering the Heimlich Maneuver

Providing Care Following Code

### EVALUATION   *Expected Outcomes*

Basic life support measures established within three minutes after arrest.

Emergency measures performed according to established protocol.

Patient is adequately oxygenated by use of mechanical adjuncts.

No permanent neurological damage is sustained.

## MAINTAINING THE EMERGENCY CART

### Equipment

Cardiac board (head board or foot board of most hospital beds can be removed and used as a cardiac board)

Crash cart with equipment

### Procedure

1. Gather emergency equipment in advance.
2. Place equipment in a logical order on the emergency cart.
3. Familiarize yourself with cart layout so equipment can be retrieved promptly.
4. Time ability to locate items against predetermined standards.
5. Check the completeness of the cart at least once a shift as assigned or as determined by hospital policy.
6. Keep cart in an open area; determine that access to the cart is unimpeded.

## USING THE EMERGENCY CART

### Equipment

Emergency cart

### Procedure

1. Assess and evaluate condition of contents of cart.
2. Observe the expiration date on drugs.
3. Practice retrieving and setting up items from the cart (in anticipation of resuscitation measures) in mock situations.
   a. Airway equipment.
   b. Ventilation equipment.
   c. Circulatory equipment:
      Monitor and defibrillator.
      IV lines.
      Emergency drugs.
4. If assigned, restock the cart promptly and return

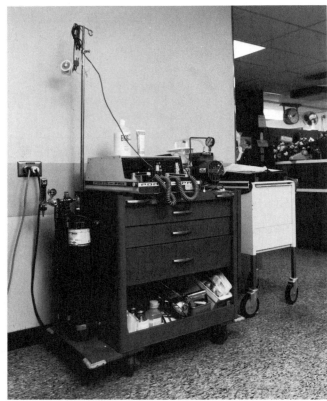

Self-contained emergency cart with defibrillator unit placed on top for easy access. Some carts include an EKG monitor and readout.

it to its usual location following an emergency, or obtain a fully stocked cart from central supply.

5. Fill out charge slips for items used from the cart.

## ADMINISTERING CARDIOPULMONARY RESUSCITATION (CPR)

### Equipment

Cardiac board

### Procedure

*for Unresponsiveness*

1. CPR should be instituted within three minutes.

**Rationale:** Cardiopulmonary resuscitation is usually not effective in preventing brain damage unless initiated within four minutes of an arrest.

2. Call out for help.

3. Quickly approach patient.

4. Check responsiveness. Shake shoulders. Shout, "Are you OK?" **Rationale:** To ensure that patient has not fainted.

5. Obtain proper position. Place victim flat on firm surface and position yourself next to victim at approximately the same level. **Rationale:** CPR is ineffective if the head is above the level of the heart.

*for Airway*

1. Take the following measures if you suspect airway obstruction from food or some other foreign body.
   a. Tilt head: hyperextend neck with chin forward. **Rationale:** Tongue may have occluded the airway.
   b. Remember that one attempt to ventilate will not be successful if airway is obstructed.
   c. If not successful, reposition head and attempt to ventilate.
   d. Deliver four back blows.
   e. Deliver four abdominal thrusts.
   f. Finger probe for obstruction.
   g. Repeat steps until foreign body is removed.

2. Ensure open airway in adult patient:
   a. Use head-tilt method.
   b. Use jaw-thrust or chin-lift method if neck injury is even remotely possible.

*for Breathing*

1. Evaluate respiratory function:
   a. Put your ear down near patient's mouth.

---

**Clinical Alert**
**CPR Protocol**

1. Shake and shout.
2. Open airway.
3. Look, listen, and feel for breathing.
4. Call code.
5. Ventilate patient with four quick breaths.
6. Check carotid pulse for 5 to 10 seconds.
7. Initiate CPR at 15 cardiac compressions to two ventilations.
8. Check for carotid pulse after one minute. If absent, continue CPR.

---

   b. Look for chest movement. **Rationale:** If chest movement occurs but you cannot feel or hear air, the airway is obstructed.
   c. Feel for air flow against your cheek.
   d. Listen for exhalation of breath.

2. Prepare to ventilate if no respirations are present.
   a. Replace victim's dentures. **Rationale:** Necessary to form tight seal.
   b. Pinch off nostrils.
   c. Fit mouth-to-mouth seal.

3. Administer four quick, full breaths. **Rationale:** This action increases oxygenation.
   a. Give breaths as fast as you can.
   b. Between breaths, release seal for exhalation.
   c. Take fresh breath; do not allow complete deflation of lungs (stairstep volume).
   d. Maintain position next to patient.
   e. Provide 800 cc minimum tidal volume per breath.

*for Circulation*

1. Feel for carotid or femoral pulse and palpate one side with two fingers for five seconds.

2. If pulse is absent, begin CPR.
   a. Position hands midline, lower half of sternum, two fingers above xiphoid.
   b. Place heel of one hand on sternum and other hand superimposed on top of first hand.
   c. Interlace fingers and extend fingers off rib cage.
   d. Administer compressions at a rate of 60 to 80 per minute. Compress chest 1½ to 2 inches.
   e. Count compressions: one-and-two-and, etc.
   f. Release pressure between compressions for cardiac refilling but do not take heel of hand off chest. **Rationale:** Leaving the hand on the chest prevents malposition of hands between compressions which could result in injury to the patient.

3. Continue CPR at the following rate:
   a. Lone rescuer: 15:2 for adults.
   b. Two rescuers: 5:1 for adults.

4. If help arrives, follow this protocol for changing roles.
   a. Second rescuer identifies self and states, "Stop compression"; then check pulse for 5 seconds.
   b. If no pulse is found, two rescuer CPR is started by stating "No pulse—begin compression."

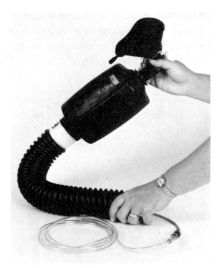

Hope resuscitator bag, used for ventilation; it is often found on emergency carts.

c. Compressor sets pace (one, one thousand, two, one thousand, three, one thousand, four, one thousand, breath).
d. Compressor observes for need and institutes change.
e. Compressor states, "Change 1000, two 1000, three 1000, four 1000, five 1000."
f. Rescuer giving breaths: gets into position to give compression after giving the breath.
g. Rescuer giving compressions: moves to victim's head after fifth compression and counts pulse for five seconds.
h. If no pulse, rescuer checking pulse states, "No pulse, start CPR," and gives a breath, and CPR is begun again.

*for Continuing CPR*

1. Check major pulse after one minute of CPR.
   a. Equal to 4 sets of 15:2 by one rescuer.
   b. Equal to 12 sets of 5:1 by two rescuers.

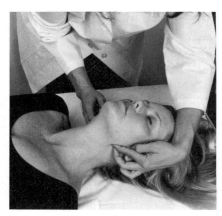

Hyperextend the neck keeping the chin forward to open patient's airway.

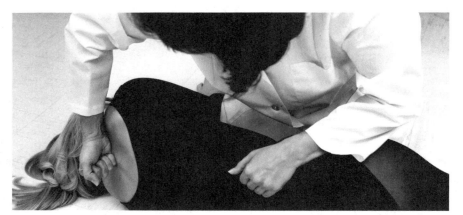

If attempt to ventilate patient is unsuccessful, suspect airway obstruction. Expel foreign objects from airway and deliver four back blows with patient placed on side.

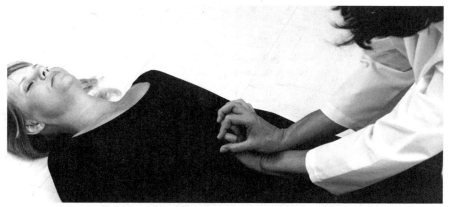

Quickly deliver four abdominal thrusts following the back blows. Finger probe the mouth to determine presence of foreign object. Initiate CPR if needed.

2. Check major pulse every four to five minutes thereafter.

3. Check pupils every four to five minutes (optional if a third trained person is present)—not always a conclusive indicator.

4. Observe for abdominal distention (all age groups).
   a. If evident, reposition airway and reduce force of ventilation.
   b. Maintain a volume sufficient to elevate ribs.

5. Ventilator: check carotid pulse frequently between breaths to evaluate perfusion.

6. Ventilator: observe each breath for effectiveness.

7. If respiratory arrest only, check major pulse after each minute (12 breaths) to ensure continuation of cardiac function.

8. Terminate CPR under the following conditions:
   a. The resuscitation is successful.

b. Spontaneous return of vital functions.
c. Assisted life-support measures are initiated.
d. Patient is transferred to emergency vehicle or code team arrives.
e. Patient is pronounced dead by physician.
f. Rescuer is exhausted and cannot continue.

## ADMINISTERING CPR TO A CHILD

### Procedure

1. If you suspect cardiac or respiratory arrest, follow these steps:
   a. Call for help.
   b. Check responsiveness by shaking child, slapping bottom of feet, or rubbing chest to elicit a cry.
   c. Place child on your lap, over your arm, or on a firm surface.

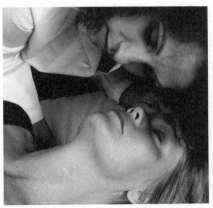

Begin CPR by looking, listening, and feeling for patient's breath.

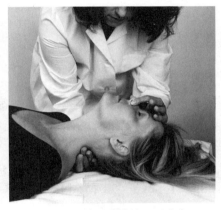

Hyperextend neck and pinch nostrils in preparation for artificial ventilation.

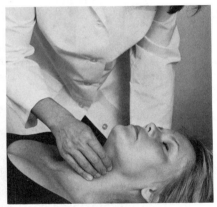

Feel for presence of carotid pulse after giving four quick breaths.

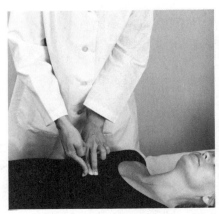

Place heel of hand 2 fingerbreadths above xiphoid for compressions.

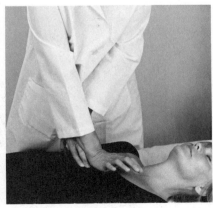

Keep fingers in position when placing heel of hand down on sternum.

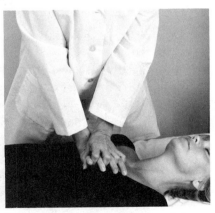

Do not take hands off chest surface between compressions to prevent chest injuries.

2. If foreign body aspiration is suspected, follow steps for CPR.

3. Clear airway by lowering child's head, turning to side, and sweeping mouth with your little finger.

4. If unable to clear airway with sweeping motion, place child in airway position (chin forward with neck slightly extended). This position usually pulls the tongue from the back of the throat and opens the airway.

5. Place rolled towel under shoulders to maintain chin in a jutting-out position, without causing hyperextension of the neck.

6. Evaluate respiratory function by following these steps:
   a. Place cheek next to child's mouth and nose.
   b. Observe for chest movement.
   c. Feel for air flow against cheek.
   d. Listen for exhalation.

7. For absent respirations, begin artificial ventilation.
   a. Maintain open airway. Tip head back. **Rationale:** Trachea can collapse if neck is hyperextended.
   b. Form tight seal by encircling nose and mouth of child. **Rationale:** Infant face is too small for nose-pinch/mouth-seal maneuver.
   c. Maintain tight seal.

8. Administer four quick breaths.
   a. Give breaths as fast as you can.
   b. Fill cheeks with air and use short puffing breaths. Do not use full breaths for children. **Rationale:** Short breaths prevent overinflation of the lungs and gastric distension.
   c. Between breaths, release seal for exhalation, and turn your head to side.
   d. Take fresh breath; do not allow complete deflation of lungs (stairstep volume).
   e. Maintain position.

9. Do not release the child when giving ventilations; just turn your head to side.

10. Administer ventilations at 20 per minute for children under one year of age, and at 15 per minute for children over one year of age.

11. Continue ventilations until child is intubated or ambu bag is available.

12. For cardiopulmonary arrest, follow these steps:
    a. Follow procedure for initiating artificial ventilation.
    b. After administering four quick breaths, check for presence of pulse by placing two fingers over brachial pulse. Palpate for 5–10 seconds.
    c. Begin cardiac compression.

13. For infants to one year of age:
    a. Place two fingers at midsternum or midline of chest.
    b. Alternate method: grasp both hands behind the infant's back for support and overlap your thumbs at midsternum.

14. For children one to four years of age, use the heel of one hand at the junction of the middle and lower third of the sternum.

15. For children over four years of age, use two hands over the lower third of the sternum.

16. Remember that compression depth for children is half that of the adult victim.

17. Do not take fingers or heel off skin between compressions.

18. Perform cardiac compression and ventilate at the rate of one breath to five compressions.
    a. For infants under twelve months, administer compression 100 times per minute to depth of ½ to 1 inch.
    b. For infants over twelve months and up to eight years, administer compression 80 times per minute to depth of 1 to 1½ inch.

19. Follow usual steps in CPR for single rescuer.

20. Continue CPR until code team arrives or you are instructed to stop by a physician.

## ADMINISTERING THE HEIMLICH MANEUVER

### Procedure

1. Assess choking patient for pale color progressing to cyanosis.

2. Be familiar with choking signs.
   a. Ask patient if he can speak.
   b. Ask patient to hold hand on neck if choking.

3. With heel of your hand, rapidly deliver four sharp blows between the shoulder blades. If airway remains obstructed, continue maneuver.

4. Stand behind patient. Place your arms around the patient's waist.

5. Make a fist with one hand. Place other hand over the fist.

6. Position hands halfway between xiphoid process

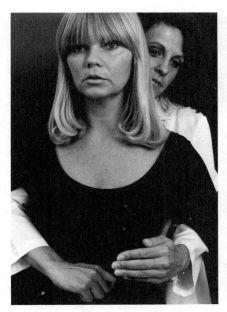

Stand behind patient, make a fist and place it between the xiphoid and umbilicus.

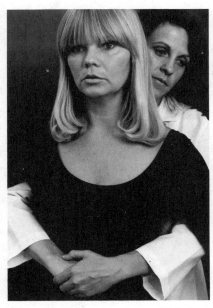

Position second hand over the fist for leverage and a more secure grasp.

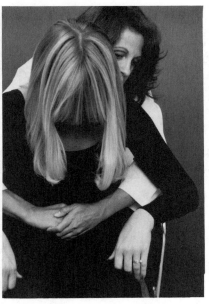

Quickly thrust your hands backwards and up toward you to expel the foreign object.

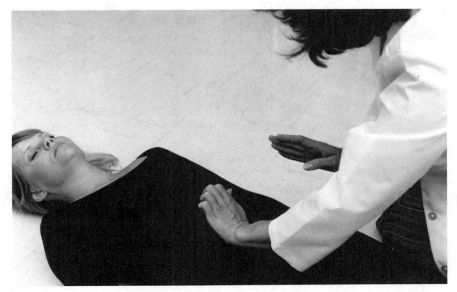

If you find the patient on the floor, kneel over patient and deliver four quick abdominal thrusts to force foreign object out of the airway.

and umbilicus. (Patient will probably fall over your arms.)

7. Press your fist into patient's abdomen.

8. Using a rotating motion of the hands, forcefully thrust your hands in an upward direction to assist in expelling the foreign body.

9. Repeat measures until foreign body is expelled.

### Heimlich Maneuver
The Heimlich maneuver is used when the patient has a foreign body occlusion. The maneuver uses residual air in the lungs to push the foreign body out. This is an alternative intervention for airway obstruction.

## PROVIDING CARE FOLLOWING CODE

### Procedure

1. Remind physician he needs to talk with family.
2. Wash patient's face and hands and provide clean top sheet.
3. Escort family in to see patient.
4. Assist in transfering patient to intensive care unit or morgue, if necessary.
5. Provide one-to-one nursing care for patient until ICU transfer is accomplished.
6. Update charting.
7. If assigned, restock emergency cart or obtain replacement cart.
8. Return all equipment to original location. Remember to recharge defibrillator.
9. Clean room.
10. Allow other patients to return to room.
11. Participate in staff critique of resuscitation management.

### CHARTING  *for CPR*

☐  Time of arrest

☐  Type of arrest

☐  Initial resuscitation efforts before arrival of team

☐  Resuscitation efforts after arrival of team

☐  Time of cessation of resuscitation efforts

☐  Outcome of resuscitation efforts

☐  Outcome of Heimlich maneuver

---

## CLINICAL PROBLEM SOLVING

| Potential Problems | Suggested Solutions |
|---|---|
| Equipment is missing from cart. | ☐ Immediately notify charge nurse. If item is minor, ask if substitute can be used. If item is major, immediately obtain replacement from floor stock or nearby unit.<br>☐ After emergency is over, notify charge nurse of possible breakdown in cart-checking procedure or pilferage.<br>☐ Obtain missing item and place on cart. If any delay in obtaining item, tape warning notice to cart that item is missing. |
| Additional useful equipment is not included on cart. | ☐ When emergency is over, check with charge nurse and ask her to obtain necessary approval to add item to cart on a trial basis. |
| Equipment cannot be located promptly on cart. | ☐ During resuscitation, look for item in other drawers, or ask someone for assistance.<br>☐ After resuscitation, suggest to charge nurse a more logical placement of item.<br>☐ After resuscitation, practice quick retrieval of items. |
| Equipment is inaccessible or malfunctions. | ☐ Notify charge nurse to replace malfunctioning equipment immediately. Obtain additional cart from the nearest unit. |
| Choking patient is found on floor. Heimlich maneuver cannot be performed in usual manner. | ☐ Perform alternate procedure:<br>Lay patient flat on back.<br>Kneel over patient with your head facing patient's head and your legs on each side of the patient's hips. |

Make a fist with one hand. Place second hand over fist.

Place hands between patient's xiphoid and umbilicus.

Make a forceful upward thrust with the heel of the fisted hand.

Team demonstrates poor coordination efforts.

☐ Attend practice CPR drills.
☐ Evaluate own performance after every drill.

Patient is revived but maintained on life-support system.

☐ Continually reassess CPR protocol.
☐ Assist in preparing patient for serial ECGs if brain hypoxia is suspected.
☐ Reassess for developmental level.
☐ Give custodial care if required.

# UNIT FOUR    EKG MONITORING

## NURSING PROCESS DATA

### ASSESSMENT   *Data Base*

Assess chest pain and its relationship to EKG changes.

Assess for signs and symptoms of electrolyte imbalance, particularly calcium and potassium.

Identify patient's previous cardiac history.

Assess patient's level of fear and anxiety related to procedure.

Assess previous EKG strips for any abnormalities.

### PLANNING   *Objectives*

To determine electrocardiographic changes.

To identify EKG abnormalities reflecting electrolyte imbalances.

To determine cardiac irregularities.

To determine if a relationship exists between chest pain and EKG changes.

### INTERVENTION   *Procedures*

Using EKG Monitors

Interpreting an EKG Strip

### EVALUATION   *Expected Outcomes*

EKG leads applied without difficulty.

Abnormal EKG interpreted appropriately.

Heart rate calculated correctly.

EKG pattern clearly displayed on oscilloscope.

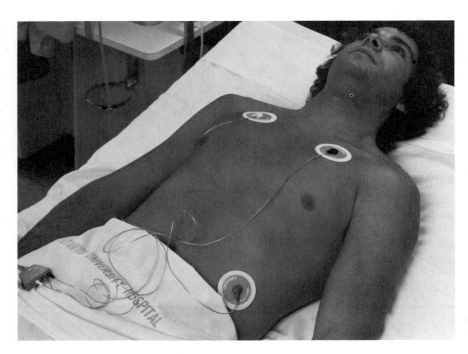

Common sites for EKG lead placement when using three bipolar leads on a patient.

## USING EKG MONITORS

### Equipment

Electrodes

Electrode jelly (if not prejelled)

Cardiac monitor and cable

Alcohol wipes or acetone pledgets

Razor

Wash cloth or 4 × 4s, soap, and towel

### Preparation

1. Gather equipment.
2. Wash your hands.
3. Explain procedure to patient.
4. Wash skin areas on patient where electrodes will be attached with soap and water. Allow to dry or wipe with a 4 × 4 pad. **Rationale:** Washing removes oily substances for better adherence of electrodes.
5. Shave areas which are excessively hairy. **Rationale:** Shaving provides better contact between skin and electrode.
6. Check that EKG monitor is plugged in and turned ON.
7. Attach cable to monitor.

### Procedure

1. Apply electrodes.
   a. Peel off paper backing on electrode. Check that sponge pad in center of electrode is moist with conductive jelly. Place electrode on skin with adhesive side down.
   b. Apply electrodes in areas where there will not be excessive movement.
   c. Place near but not directly on bone surfaces; however, if patient is overly obese, electrodes may have to be placed on the bones, since a large amount of adipose tissue results in a poor image on the oscilloscope.
2. Determine the lead placement which will give the best EKG pattern.

**Lead II:**
*Positive (+) lead*—left side of chest, lowest palpable rib, midclavicular.
*Negative (−) lead*—right shoulder region, below clavicular hollow.
*Ground (G) lead*—left shoulder, below clavicular hollow—opposite negative lead.

**Lead MCL₁ (Modified Chest Lead):**
*Positive (+) lead*—right sternal border, lowest palpable rib.
*Negative (−) lead*—left shoulder, below clavicular hollow.
*Ground (G) lead*—right shoulder, below clavicular hollow—opposite negative lead.

Lead II

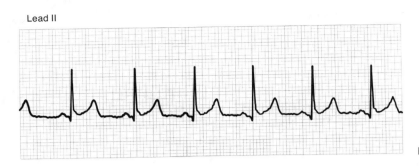

EKG pattern from Lead II placement.

MCL$_1$

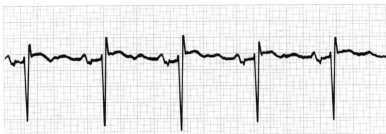

EKG pattern from MCL$_1$ placement.

Lead I

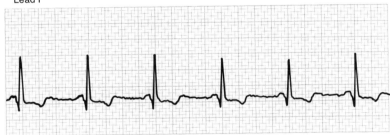

EKG pattern from Lead 1 placement.

Artifact

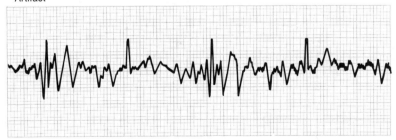

EKG pattern showing artifact.

Other leads such as Lead I and MCL$_6$ can also be useful in specific situations.

3. Attach the chest electrodes to the monitor cable using the appropriate colored lead wires. **Rationale:** The patient end of the cable is coded to facilitate connection with the electrodes.

4. Set High and Low alarm limits on the monitor.

Common codes are − (neg), + (pos) and G (ground) or RA, LA, and LL or color codes. Be sure that the positive lead wire is connected to the electrode in the positive position, the negative lead wire to the electrode in the negative position, and the ground lead wire to the electrode in the ground position.

5. Turn alarm buttons to ON.

6. Observe pattern to determine clarity of image on oscilloscope.

7. Run EKG strip and place in nurses' notes. **Rationale:** This provides a baseline record of the EKG pattern at the beginning of monitoring. To run the strip, turn the switch on the monitor to RUN. A strip of EKG paper will appear with the wave form printed out.

## INTERPRETING AN EKG STRIP

### Equipment

Calipers

### Procedure

1. Determine heart rate by calculating atrial rate (P-P interval) and ventrical rate (R-R interval). Normal pulse is 60 to 100.
   **Heart Rate is calculated by:**
   a. Counting the number of cardiac cycles (QRS complexes) in a six-second strip and multiplying that number by ten to obtain the pulse.
   b. Counting the number of small boxes between R waves, and dividing that number into 1500. The quotient is the ventricular rate.
   c. Counting the number of small boxes between P waves, and dividing that number into 1500. The quotient is the atrial rate.

2. Determine regularity of rhythm (atrial and ventricular). Check if complexes look alike and are equally spaced. Use calipers to check this.

3. Measure P-R interval to determine conduction time in atria and AV junction (0.16 to 0.20 seconds).

4. Measure QRS duration to determine ventricular

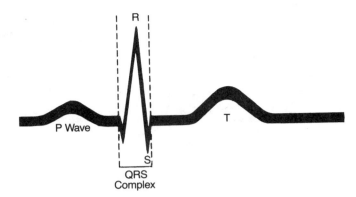

It is important to determine the configuration and location of the wave pattern to interpret an EKG accurately.

conduction (0.04 to 0.12 sec.). There are six complexes.

5. Measure Q-T interval (rate of 70 in one minute occurring 0.36 seconds apart).

6. Check configuration and placement of P waves, QRS complex, ST segment, and T wave.

7. Summarize findings to obtain interpretation.

8. Document interpretation of findings and place EKG strip in patient's chart.

### CHARTING   *for EKG Monitoring*

☐ Findings based on the interpretation of the EKG strip

☐ Nursing interventions carried out, based on the EKG findings

☐ Lead placement used in EKG monitoring

☐ When electrodes were replaced

---

## CLINICAL PROBLEM SOLVING

### Potential Problems

Electrodes do not adhere to skin and interference appears on oscilloscope.

Alarms ring without change in pattern.

### Suggested Solutions

☐ Change placement of electrodes to another area of the body.
☐ Put tincture of Benzoin on the skin before placing electrodes.
☐ Cleanse skin thoroughly with alcohol swab.

☐ Check High and Low parameters, they may need to be changed.
☐ Check GAIN, it may be too low to be sensing pattern.

EKG pattern abnormal.

☐ Recheck each configuration.
☐ Check if pattern is a death producing arrhythmia (PVCs, ventricular tachycardia, ventricular fibrillation); if so, notify physician immediately.

## UNIT FIVE   PACEMAKER MANAGEMENT

### NURSING PROCESS DATA

#### ASSESSMENT   *Data Base*

Assess pre-existing cardiovascular disease.

Identify patient's and/or family's knowledge of and cooperation with procedure.

Assess 12 lead EKG findings.

Assess heart sounds.

Observe patient's general appearance for pallor, cyanosis, and edema.

Assess for hemodynamic abnormalities related to low cardiac output syndrome, including dizziness, weakness, altered level of consciousness, low blood pressure, and decreased cardiac index.

Ensure placement of large gauge intravenous route for administration of fluids and drugs during an emergency.

#### PLANNING   *Objectives*

To provide temporary cardiac electrical stimulation for conditions resulting in alterations of heart rate or function.

To prevent bradycardia.

To improve cardiac function, thereby, improving cardiac output.

To provide a treatment modality for those cardiac dysfunctions impervious to drug therapy.

To assist in the treatment of existing or impending cardiac arrest situations.

#### INTERVENTIONS   *Procedures*

Assisting with Pacemaker Insertion

Maintaining Pacemaker Function

Performing Defibrillation

Providing Patient Teaching

#### EVALUATION   *Expected Outcomes*

Patient's cardiac rate and rhythm are maintained through use of a pacemaker.

Patient is prepared psychologically and physically for insertion of the pacemaker.

Pacemaker is inserted without complications.

Dysrhythmias subside and cardiac output improves.

Defibrillation is effective.

## ASSISTING WITH PACEMAKER INSERTION

### Equipment

Emergency cart with defibrillator

A bolus each of lidocaine, atropine, and isoproterenol

External pacemaker pulse generator

Pacing catheter electrodes

EKG monitor

Patient cable

Rubber glove

Skin antiseptic solution (povidone-iodine)

Sterile gloves and gown, mask and cap

Sterile towels

Lidocaine, 1-2%

Alcohol wipes

Syringe

18– and 25–gauge needle

Suture with attached needle

Sterile 4" x 4" gauze pads

Sterile skin antiseptic ointment

Tape

Cutdown tray

### Preparation

1. Wash hands.
2. Describe the procedure to the patient and/or family and answer any questions.
3. Provide sedation as necessary. (Valium is frequently used.)
4. Connect patient to a continuous EKG monitor.
5. Place the patient in a supine position with head of bed flat. If patient is hypovolemic, the bed may need to be in Trendelenburg's position.
6. If either the subclavian or external jugular vein is to be used, place a towel roll under the patient's shoulders to provide better exposure of the insertion site.

### Procedure

1. Open the sterile gloves.
2. Assist physician as needed.
   a. Physician dons mask, cap, sterile gown, and gloves.

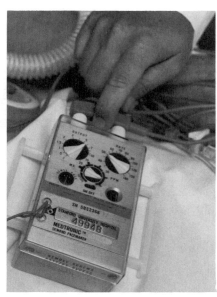
External temporary demand pacemaker.

   b. Insertion site is cleansed with sterile antiseptic solution.
   c. Area is draped with sterile towels.
   d. Top of lidocaine is cleansed with alcohol wipe.
   e. Lidocaine is aspirated with 18–gauge needle, and skin is injected with 25–gauge needle.
   f. Insertion is accomplished (transvenous method via cutdown or percutaneously, or transthoracic method). Catheter electrode wires are positioned, and skin sutures are applied.

3. Continuously observe the EKG during the insertion. (Observe for PVCs—assess number per minute.)

4. Connect the pacing electrode to the appropriate outlet terminal (unipolar to negative and bipolar to both the positive and negative terminals).

5. Turn on power switch on external pacemaker.

6. Set rate according to physician's orders.

7. Set milliamperes (MA) by determining threshold. To do this, observe the EKG while slowly increasing the MA from its lowest setting to a point where a QRS complex is detected following each stimulus.

8. Multiply the threshold level according to hospital policy (usually two to four times) to adjust the MA setting.

9. Set sensitivity mode according to physician's order.

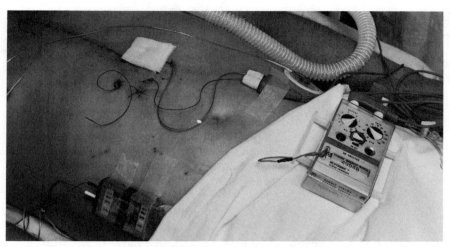

Electrode wires connected to the pacemaker using both a positive and negative terminal.

10. Secure all connections. Put plastic cover back over pacemaker.

11. Place external pacemaker and exposed wires in a rubber glove to ensure insulation if required by hospital policy.

12. Apply sterile antibiotic ointment and sterile dressings to insertion site and tape securely.

13. Order chest x–ray following insertion.

14. Obtain 12–lead EKG.

## MAINTAINING PACEMAKER FUNCTION

### Equipment

4″ x 4″ gauze pads

Povidone-iodine prep swab

Rubber glove

Tape

### Procedure

1. Observe for failure to sense.
   a. Observe the oscilloscope for presence of pacemaker artifact (spikes). Artifact before QRS complex in ventricular paced or preceding the P waves and QRS waves in AV sequential pacing.
   b. Check connections for secure, tight fit.
   c. Observe that pace/sense needle deflects to right, indicating pacing is occurring.
   d. Check sensitivity dial to determine if sensitivity threshold is set correctly.

2. Observe for failure to pace.
   a. Check that external generator is ON.
   b. Check battery to ensure it is functioning.
   c. Check lead connector sites.
   d. Check pace/sense indicator. (Absence of or slight deflection of the pace/sense indicator reveals battery failure.)

3. Observe for failure to capture.
   a. Observe for pacing artifact followed by QRS complex. **Rationale:** This sequence indicates a failure of the stimulus to trigger a ventricular response.
   b. Check the setting of the MA, or output dial, to determine if setting should be increased. **Rationale:** The myocardial threshold may be altered as a result of disuse or drugs.
   c. Check all connector sites for secure, tight fit.

4. Observe that sutures are intact.

5. Check for exposed electrode wire, and insulate, if necessary, by placing in rubber glove.

6. Cleanse insertion site with povidone-iodine prep swabs.

7. Apply sterile dressing and tape securely. Date and label dressing, "Pacer Wire."

8. Assess urine output. **Rationale:** Decreased urine output indicates poor cardiac output.

9. Observe for signs of shortness of breath, rales, or rhonchi.

10. Monitor temperature every four hours.

11. Observe patient for signs of anxiety or fear. Complete pacemaker teaching as necessary.

## PERFORMING DEFIBRILLATION

### Equipment

EKG monitor

Defibrillator with external paddles

Saline gauze pads

Airway

Resuscitator bag

Emergency cart

Oxygen equipment

### Preparation

1. Verify EKG reading of ventricular fibrillation. **Rationale:** Artifact can mimic ventricular fibrillation.

2. Gather equipment.

3. Plug defibrillator and/or emergency cart into electrical outlet.

4. Turn defibrillator power ON and allow to warm up.

5. Place saline soaked pads on patient's chest. One pad is placed below the right clavicle at the sternoclavicular joint and the second pad is placed to the left of the cardiac apex (below and to the left of the left nipple) in the anterior axillary line. **Rationale:** Saline soaked pads reduce electrical resistance to ensure delivery of electrical energy.

6. Set defibrillator in nonsynchronized mode. **Rationale:** The machine will not function in the synchronized mode as there is an absence of R waves in ventricular fibrillation. The synchronized mode is used for cardioversion.

7. Dial the defibrillator to charge at 350 to 400 watt-seconds. **Rationale:** High level current is needed for conversion of ventricular fibrillation.

### Procedure

1. Place paddles on saline pads. Ensure that defibrillator is charged to 350 to 400 watt-seconds.

2. Instruct all persons to move away from the bed area.

3. Stand away from the bed area yourself.

4. Depress discharge buttons on defibrillator simultaneously to ensure appropriate energy discharge.

5. Check EKG pattern to determine effects of defibrillation. Reinstitute CPR and administer sodium bicarbonate or other appropriate medications if ventricular fibrillation continues.

6. Prepare defibrillator equipment for second attempt.

7. Instruct all persons to move away from bed area.

8. Repeat defibrillation procedure.

9. Monitor patient every 15 minutes past defibrillation until stable:
   a. Level of consciousness.
   b. Vital signs.
   c. Presence of peripheral pulses.
   d. Heart and lung sounds.

10. Continue oxygen administration.

11. Continue IV medication administration, e.g., antiarrhythmics, vasopressors, etc.

12. Monitor EKG strip continuously until stable.

13. Observe for EKG signs of pacemaker malfunction:
    a. Absence of pacemaker artifact.
    b. Absence of pacemaker capture.
    c. Competition rhythm.

14. Maintain patient on bedrest.

## PROVIDING PATIENT TEACHING

### Equipment

Audiovisual aids

Written material

### Procedure

1. Ascertain what patient already knows and understands.

2. Determine patient's ability and level of interest in learning about pacemaker.

3. Recognize patient's fears and provide opportunity to talk about them.

4. Review facts: heart anatomy and physiology and pacemaker information. Use illustrations and audiovisual aids.

5. Clarify misconceptions and allay fears.

---

**Clinical Alert**

Observe for pacemaker failure:
   Decreased urine output
   EKG pattern change
   Decreased blood pressure
   Cyanosis
   Shortness of breath

6. Describe insertion procedure.

7. Answer questions and provide additional opportunities to discuss impending procedure.

## CHARTING *for Patient with a Pacemaker*

☐ Date and time of insertion

☐ Model and type of pacemaker used

☐ Type of catheter electrode wires

☐ Method of insertion

☐ Mode of pacing

☐ Pacemaker settings

☐ Patient's tolerance of and response to treatment

☐ Vital signs

☐ Rhythm following pacemaker insertion

☐ Rhythm and strips of pacing obtained during insertion

## CHARTING *for Defibrillation*

☐ Rhythm identified

☐ Number of times defibrillated

☐ Watt-seconds used for defibrillations

☐ Associated treatment, e.g., medications, oxygen, respiratory assistance

☐ Results of defibrillation

## CLINICAL PROBLEM SOLVING

**Potential Problems**

Patient's cardiac rhythm is not stabilized.

**Suggested Solutions**

☐ Check sensitivity setting. (If too high, P or T wave may be sensed; if too low, fixed rate pacing will occur.)

☐ Check MA setting (may be too high).

☐ Check pace indicator for movement.

☐ Check rate setting.

☐ Check all connections.

☐ Check catheter insertion site.

☐ Check for battery depletion and change if necessary.

☐ Check for electrical artifact.

☐ Insulate generator in rubber glove.

☐ Obtain 12-lead EKG.

☐ Anticipate replacement of pulse generator.

Pacemaker is inserted with complications.

☐ Check MA setting (may be too high).

☐ Check sensitivity setting (may be too low).

☐ Assess for signs of bleeding or shock due to trauma of insertion.

☐ Observe for dysrhythmias due to irritability of conduction system upon insertion.

☐ Anticipate cardiac emergency.

☐ Obtain 12-lead EKG for diagnosis.

Patient is unprepared for pacemaker insertion.

☐ If patient is frightened, reassure patient that a pacemaker is not dangerous.

☐ If patient does not understand explanation of how the pacemaker or the heart functions, reexplain the procedure, using illustrated learning aids.

☐ Demonstrate the pacemaker and electrode and allow time for questions and further explanations.

Electrical interference occurs.

□ Describe specifically the insertion procedure, allowing time for questions.

□ Orient your teaching to the patient's intellectual and interest level.

□ Check electrical equipment for proper grounding.

□ Remove microwave ovens, TVs, electric razors, or other electrical equipment from vicinity of patient.

□ Insulate generator, especially output terminals and exposed electrodes, in a rubber glove.

Infection or inflammation at insertion site is observed.

□ Provide daily site care using strict aseptic technique.

□ Keep dressings dry at all times.

□ Monitor vital signs, especially temperature.

□ Instruct patient to decrease extremity movement.

Diaphragmatic pacing occurs.

□ Observe for hiccoughs or muscle twitching.

□ Change position of body.

□ Decrease MA.

Cardiac arrest occurs.

□ Provide CPR and defibrillation, establish IV route, and administer drugs as required.

Failure to capture is suspected.

□ Check patient's heart rate. If heart rate less than the rate set on generator, and if pace indicator shows firing, suspect failure to capture.

□ Check all connections.

□ Anticipate that pacer wires are dislodged.

□ Check battery.

□ Change position of extremity.

□ Turn patient on left side; catheter may float back to epicardial wall.

□ Increase MA after checking threshold.

□ Obtain chest x–ray and 12-lead EKG.

□ Anticipate change of batteries, electrode terminals, or generator.

Battery depletion occurs.

□ Have atropine and isoproterenol on stand-by.

□ Anticipate possible CPR.

□ Turn on power switch, and observe pace indicator. If there is little or no movement, replace battery immediately.

□ Record clock hours of battery usage. (Record should be taped to back of generator.)

□ Determine rate fluctuations.

□ Label each pacemaker with the date battery is inserted.

□ Store extra batteries in refrigerator, and put new battery in pacemaker before use.

□ Disconnect catheter from pacemaker before replacing battery. Contact with battery terminal may be dangerous to the patient.

Pericardial inflammation is observed.

□ Auscultate for a pericardial friction rub.

□ Place in semi-Fowler's position to decrease pain.

| | |
|---|---|
| Pneumothorax occurs. | ☐ Auscultate lung sounds to make sure breath sounds are present in all fields.<br>☐ Notify physician immediately.<br>☐ Have chest tube and equipment ready for insertion.<br>☐ Monitor vital signs. |
| Defibrillation is ineffective. | ☐ Check that defibrillator is charged to 350 to 400 watt-seconds.<br>☐ Check defibrillator paddle placement.<br>☐ Administer sodium bicarbonate IV to reverse lactic acidosis, and defibrillate again.<br>☐ Administer oxygen, and support patient with CPR until defibrillation is effective or treatment is terminated by physician. |
| EKG is not clearly displayed on the oscilloscope. | ☐ Ensure that electrodes are applied in correct position and are securely attached.<br>☐ Observe for electrical interference resulting in a 60-cycle interference on oscilloscope.<br>☐ Observe for excessive patient activity resulting in artifact display on oscilloscope. |
| Electrodes do not adhere to skin and interference appears on oscilloscope. | ☐ Change placement of electrodes to another area of the body.<br>☐ Put tincture of Benzoin on the skin before placing electrodes.<br>☐ Cleanse skin thoroughly with alcohol swab. |
| Alarms ring without change in pattern. | ☐ Check High and Low parameters. They may need to be changed.<br>☐ Check GAIN. It may be too low to be sensing pattern. |
| EKG pattern is abnormal. | ☐ Recheck each configuration.<br>☐ Check if pattern is a death producing arrhythmia (PVC's, ventricular tachycardia, ventricular fibrillation); if so, notify physician immediately. |
| Electrical interference continues after lead wires and cable connections are secured. | ☐ Check all other electrical equipment in the immediate environment.<br>☐ If excessive electrical equipment is used, the electrical bed may need to be changed to a non-electrical bed.<br>☐ Check for proper grounding of monitor.<br>☐ Check all connections. Ensure that cable that goes to patient is pinned to client's gown to prevent disturbance of electrodes.<br>☐ Change electrodes and cable; sometimes poor conduction results in 60-cycle interference.<br>☐ Check that monitor is calibrated. |
| Skin irritation occurs with use of electrodes. | ☐ Remove electrodes, cleanse site, and reapply electrodes on new site. |
| Chaotic rhythm appears on oscilloscope. | ☐ Check patient's other assessment parameters to determine if clinical changes have occurred. |

High or low alarms on monitor continue to sound.

□ Check electrode contact on skin, and ensure that wires are in contact with cable.
□ Determine activity level of patient.
□ Check for loose electrodes.
□ Observe activity level of patient.
□ Check that alarm parameters on monitor are not set too close to patient's pulse.
□ Check position of patient.
□ Reposition electrodes, avoiding large muscle masses or bone.

Patient demonstrates increasing anxiety regarding diagnosis, alarms, or arrhythmias.

□ Elaborate on rationale and necessity for procedure. Answer patient's questions accurately and promptly.
□ Reassure patient by frequently checking to determine that electrodes have not become loose.
□ Demonstrate competence and confidence while caring for the patient.
□ Check monitor immediately when alarm goes off.

Electrodes conduct poorly on diaphoretic patient.

□ Clean skin sites as usual, apply benzoin to the skin, and let dry and apply electrodes.
□ Clean skin sites as usual, apply spray deodorant to the skin, allow skin to dry, and apply electrodes.

Wires do not stay attached to electrodes because patient is restless.

□ Place paper tape over wires and electrodes.

Asystole occurs.

□ Before beginning CPR, check patient's LOC and electrodes, wires, and cables.
□ If the patient has an arterial line, check for an arterial waveform in the absence of an EKG waveform.

---

## APPENDIX

### CONTENTS OF TYPICAL EMERGENCY CART

*Top of cart*
  EKG monitor with readout
  EKG electrodes and extra roll of recording paper
  Defibrillator
  Defibrillator paddles and conductive medium

*First drawer*
  Emergency medications
  IV additive labels

*Second drawer*
  Venipuncture supplies: steel needles, over-the-needle catheters, inside-the-needle catheters, short intracatheters, macrodrop administration sets, microdrop administration sets, extension tubing, stopcocks, syringes, tape, alcohol swabs, tourniquets, tincture of benzoin, gauze pads.
  Blood sampling supplies: venous blood tubes, arterial blood gas kits or glass syringes
  Spinal needles for intracardiac injections
  Scalpels with blades attached
  Alligator clips

*Third drawer*
  Oral airways
  Endotracheal tubes
  Laryngoscope handle, curved blades, straight blades, extra batteries, extra bulbs, stylet

McGill forceps
Tonsil suction
Surgical lubricant
Hand-held self-inflating resuscitation bag
Oxygen masks, connecting tubing, flowmeter
Suction catheters
Nasogastric tubes

*Bottom shelf*
 Tracheostomy tray
 Cutdown tray and sutures

IV solutions, armboards
Portable suction device
Pacemaker and electrodes

*Back of cart*
 Cardiac arrest board

*Side of cart*
 CVP catheters or long intracaths
 Emergency cart checklist
 Cardiac resuscitation recording sheet and clipboard

## TERMINOLOGY

**Antiembolic:** a preventative measure used to help prevent the formation of an embolism, such as elastic hosiery.

**Atherosclerosis:** a form of arteriosclerosis in which there are localized accumulations of lipid-containing material within the surfaces of the blood vessels.

**Cardio:** pertaining to the heart.

**Cardiovascular:** pertaining to the heart and blood vessels.

**Chronotropic:** modification of a repetitive event such as the heartbeat through external causes.

**Conductivity:** the specific electric conducting capability of a substance.

**Congestion:** the presence of an excessive amount of blood or fluid in an organ or tissue.

**Contractility:** having the ability to contract or shorten.

**Cyanosis:** slightly bluish, grayish, slatelike, or dark-purple discoloration of the skin resulting from reduced hemoglobin or oxygen in the blood.

**Dilatation:** expansion of an organ or vessel.

**Dorsiflexion:** movement of a part at a joint so as to bend the part toward the dorsum or posterior aspect of the body.

**Ecchymosis:** a form of macula appearing in large irregularly-formed hemorrhagic areas of the skin; color is blue-black changing to greenish-brown or yellow.

**Edema:** a condition in which the body tissues contain an excessive amount of fluid.

**Embolism:** obstruction of a blood vessel by foreign substances or a blood clot.

**Endocardial:** within the heart or arising from the endocardium.

**Endocardium:** serous lining membrane of the inner surface and cavities of the heart.

**Endotracheal:** within the trachea.

**Epistaxis:** hemorrhage from the nose.

**Hematemesis:** vomiting of blood.

**Hematoma:** a swelling or mass of blood, usually clotted, confined to a specific space and caused by a break in a blood vessel.

**Heme:** prefix meaning blood.

**Hemodynamic:** the study of the circulation of the blood.

**Hemoptysis:** expectoration of blood arising from hemorrhage of the larynx, trachea, bronchi, or lungs.

**Hemorrhage:** abnormal internal or external discharge of blood.

**Homan's sign:** pain in the calf when the toe is dorsiflexed. An early sign of deep vein thrombosis in the calf.

**Hydrostatic:** pertaining to the pressure of liquids in equilibrium and that exerted on liquids.

**Hypotension:** low blood pressure; a deficiency of tone.

**Immobilize:** the making of a part or limb immoveable.

**Inotropic:** influencing the contractibility of muscle tissue.

**Ischemia:** local and temporary anemia due to the obstruction of the circulation to a part.

**Perfusion:** passing of fluid through spaces.

**Petechiae:** small, purplish, hemorrhagic spots on the skin, which appear in certain severe fevers.

**Phlebitis:** inflammation of a vein.

**Precordial:** pertaining to the precordium or epigastrium.

**Purpura:** hemorrhage into the skin, mucous membranes, internal organs, and other tissues.

**Resuscitation:** act of bringing one back to full consciousness.

**Sclerosis:** hardening or induration of an organ or tissue due to excessive growth of fibrous tissue.

**Shock:** term used to designate a clinical syndrome with varying degrees of disturbances of oxygen supply to the tissues and return to the heart.

**Stasis:** standing still; stagnation of normal flow of fluids.

**Syncope:** fainting; transient loss of consciousness due to inadequate blood flow to the brain.

**Thoracentesis:** surgical entry into the thoracic cavity in order to remove fluid.

**Thrombosis:** formation of a blood clot.

**Tinnitus:** subjective ringing in the ear.

**Vertigo:** sensation of moving or having objects around you move when they are actually still, due to a disturbance of balance.

# Chapter *26*

# *Intravenous Therapy*

## LEARNING OBJECTIVES

Describe the role the kidneys play in maintaining fluid and electrolyte balance.

Discuss the two regulatory systems that influence urinary excretion through the kidneys.

State the major cations and anions in the body.

Identify the assessment modalities used to determine the patient's fluid balance.

Compare and contrast the clinical manifestations associated with overhydration and dehydration.

Outline the steps in preparing the IV bottle for administration.

Describe the steps in the procedure for performing a venipuncture using a winged-tipped needle.

Calculate an IV flow rate using a standard formula.

State at least two potential problems that can occur with IV insertion and one suggested solution for each problem.

Describe the reason for hanging the partial fill bottle higher than the primary IV bottle.

Outline the nurse's responsibility for assisting the physician with a CVP insertion.

Explain the protocol for maintaining sterility during a CVP dressing change.

Describe the safety checks utilized to ensure proper blood is administered to the patient.

Differentiate between the signs and symptoms associated with bacterial, allergic, and hemolytic blood transfusion reactions.

## FLUID AND ELECTROLYTES

Fluid and electrolytes do not exist independently. They exist in a state of dynamic equilibrium which demands a stable composition of the various elements that are essential to life. The primary elements that control this state of equilibrium are fluids, or body water, and electrolytes, most of which are minerals.

**Fluids**  Body fluid is primarily water. Depending on the amount of body fat, a person's total body weight is usually made up of between 50 and 70 percent water. Since fat is essentially water-free, an obese adult's body weight will be 50 percent water. In a leaner individual the percentage of body weight due to body water is closer to 70 percent.

Body water is divided into three compartments: intracellular fluids, extracellular fluids, and intravascular fluids. The majority of the body water is located inside the cell. Most extracellular fluid is found in the interstitial spaces surrounding body cells. Only a small percentage of the body's total water is located in the intravascular fluid compartment, or the body's plasma.

Communication between these fluid compartments varies. Intracellular body water does not move out of the cell readily. In contrast, body water in the intravascular and interstitial spaces can diffuse easily and is similar in electrolyte composition. The diffusion of fluid from the vascular compartment to the interstitial spaces back to the blood is controlled by a variety of factors such as hydrostatic pressure, osmotic pressures, and the diameter of the vessels.

The overall maintenance of body water is the result of adjustments made between the gains and losses of water that occur on a daily basis. The major sources of water coming into the body are fluids or solid foods. A small amount of water is also produced as a by-product of cellular metabolism. Most fluid leaves the body through urinary excretion. Water is also lost by fecal elimination, sweating, and diffusion and evaporation through the skin and the lungs.

The major organ of excretion is the kidney. Because the kidney handles the end-products of cellular metabolism, as well as the intake of fluids, it must excrete a minimum of 500 to 600 cc of urine every 24 hours. Depending on the amount of fluid intake, the amount usually excreted on a daily basis varies from 600 to 1600 cc.

The regulation of the volume and concentration of body fluids is handled by two mechanisms: thirst and urinary excretion. Thirst is stimulated by receptors in the central nervous system. Under normal circumstances, an individual will ingest fluids when these receptors are activated. During an illness or an altered level of consciousness, the thirst response may change, causing such conditions as hypovolemia and increased tonicity or concentration of the extracellular fluids.

Urinary excretion through the kidney is directed or influenced by two regulatory systems. The first regulatory system involves the antidiuretic hormone (ADH). By increasing and decreasing ADH, this system helps to regulate the balance of fluids in the body.

When extracellular body fluids become concentrated, osmoreceptors located in the hypothalamus stimulate the release of ADH from its storage place. ADH then acts on the kidney, causing it to retain more water.

As this retained water circulates through the extracellular fluid compartment, the concentration of body fluid is reduced. The osmoreceptors, sensing this change, slow the secretion of ADH, which then acts on the kidney, causing it to excrete more water.

Other conditions that can stimulate the secretion of ADH and lead to increased water retention by the kidney include hemorrhage, decreased cardiac output, trauma, pain, fear, surgery, and dehydration. Drugs such as morphine, barbiturates, and nicotine and some anesthetics and tranquilizers will also increase the secretion of ADH. The secretion of ADH can be inhibited by alcohol, decreased concentration of body fluids, and hypervolemic states.

The second system that regulates urinary excretion involves the hormone aldosterone. Like ADH, aldosterone is secreted by the adrenal cortex and regulates the levels of sodium in the body. Because sodium is exchanged for either potassium or hydrogen, aldosterone indirectly affects the levels of potassium and hydrogen. Secretion of aldosterone is increased in response to several stimuli which include decreased sodium and increased extracellular potassium, hypovolemia, and physical or emotional stress.

When the level of sodium is lowered, or when hypovolemia occurs, the receptor-like area in the glomerulus of the nephron releases an enzyme substance called renin. As renin circulates in the body, it converts a plasma protein in the liver into a vasoconstrictor substance called angiotensin I. When this substance enters the lungs it is converted into angiotensin II. Angiotensin II acts directly on the adrenal cortex and increases the level of aldosterone secretion. Aldosterone then stimulates the kidney's tubule cells to retain sodium and to secrete either hydrogen or potassium. The sodium that is retained in the body increases the overall concentration of extracellular fluids, which stimulates the osmoreceptors in the hypothalamus to increase the secretion of the hormone ADH. The hypersecretion of ADH, in turn, causes the kidney to retain more water.

**TABLE 1** FLUID GAINS AND LOSSES

| INTAKE | OUTPUT | |
|---|---|---|
| Oral intake 1,500 – 3,000 | Urine | 600 – 1,600 |
| Cellular catabolism | Skin | 300 – 600 (insensible loss) |
| of PRO, CHO | Lung | 350 (insensible loss) |
| AND FAT | Feces | 200 |
| | Sweat | 100 – 300 |

**TABLE 2** MAJOR ELECTROLYTES

| CATIONS⁺ | | ANIONS⁻ | |
|---|---|---|---|
| $Na^+$ | Sodium | $Cl^-$ | Chloride |
| $K^+$ | Potassium | $HCO_3^-$ | Bicarbonate |
| $Ca^{++}$ | Calcium | $HPO_4^{--}$ | Phosphate |
| $Mg^{++}$ | Magnesium | | |

**Electrolytes** In partnership with body fluids are substances called electrolytes. These substances, mostly minerals, contribute to body function in many ways and are essential to life.

Electrolytes are distributed throughout the body, both intracellularly and extracellularly. In the extracellular compartment, the main electrolytes are sodium, chloride, and bicarbonate. Intracellular electrolytes are potassium, magnesium, phosphate, and sulfate.

Electrolytes, in body fluids, possess an electrical charge when placed in water. Electrolytes with a positive charge are called cations. Negatively charged electrolytes are called anions. Positive cations and negative anions are attracted to each other because of their opposite electrical charges. When they combine with each other, they form neutral compounds that either remain in body fluids or dissociate and regain their electrical charges. When they do dissociate or ionize, they are referred to as ions.

**Alterations** Alterations in fluid and electrolytes may occur as a primary event or as secondary responses to a preexisting disease state or to a sudden, unexpected traumatic episode. When alterations among the fluid and electrolytes exceed the narrow limits consistent with health, the body needs to adjust quickly.

Changes in the composition of body fluid and electrolytes may be relative or absolute. Relative losses or gains can occur when fluids or electrolytes shift from one body space to another. Absolute losses or gains can occur when electrolytes and fluids are lost outside the body or added to the overall body stores by IV fluid and blood replacement because of injury or medical/surgical procedures. Because body elements are in a state of continual change, minor alterations in one element can affect all the other elements within the body's matrix. Excess or deficit fluid and electrolytes may be due to loss of function of the regulatory mechanisms. The kidney is an electrolyte computer. If it is functioning correctly, it will supply the body with optimum intravascular volume so that many mild to moderate imbalances will correct themselves.

The kidney has an obligatory urine output and the body has an insensible water loss which must be replaced daily. A daily minimum fluid intake of 1500 cc is essential to maintain this fluid balance. A loss of body water greater than fluid intake results in weight loss. A gain of body water greater than output results in weight gain. One kg of body weight gain or loss is equal to 1000 cc or one liter of fluid.

In addition to obtaining assessment data, the chapter will discuss methods of providing fluid and electrolytes to patients who have experienced alterations in their homeostasis.

The primary purpose for performing these interventions associated with alterations in either fluids or electrolytes is to maintain homeostasis and regulate and maintain essential fluids and nutrients.

Patients undergoing major surgery or trauma may be subjected to blood loss necessitating replacement therapy. Administration of blood and blood products will be discussed. Patients requiring intravenous therapy frequently have associated nutritional needs that are not always met. The nutritional needs of patients cannot be met by intravenous fluids alone. If the patient will need to remain on parenteral therapy, other means of nutritional support must be considered.

This chapter will present the methods of supplying fluid and electrolytes through IV medications, blood and blood components, and intravenous therapy. These interventions provide baseline data as well as sequential measurements in the assessment of fluid and electrolyte gains or losses.

The following nursing diagnoses may be appropriate to include in a Patient Care Plan when the components are related to intravenous therapy.

**NURSING DIAGNOSES**

| Nursing Diagnosis (Potential) | Defining Characteristic; Etiology (Examples) |
|---|---|
| ☐ Fluid Volume, Alteration in: Excess, *related to* | Excessive fluid intake, e.g., inaccurate IV drip. |
| | Ineffective fluid output, e.g., fluid retention. |
| ☐ Fluid Volume Deficit, *related to* | Restricted fluid intake, excess fluid loss, e.g., nausea and vomiting. |
| ☐ Noncompliance, *related to* | Inaccurate I & O records, e.g., not using bedpan/urinal for voiding. |
| ☐ Self-Care Deficit: Bathing/Hygiene, Dressing/Grooming, *related to* | Inability to perform ADL's, e.g., immobilized arm. |
| ☐ Skin Integrity, Impairment of, *related to* | Alterations in skin turgor, tissue damage, e.g., IV infiltration. |

## UNIT ONE   INTRAVENOUS THERAPY

### NURSING PROCESS DATA

**ASSESSMENT**   *Data Base*

Determine physician's order for IV therapy.

Determine patient's need for psychological support.

Assess need for patient explanation about IV therapy.

Identify appropriate site for venipuncture. Vein should be superficial, large enough for the needle to be inserted smoothly, rapidly palpated, and easily followed.

Evaluate patient for proper placement of needle.
    Placement is based on patient convenience and functional use (left vs. right hand).

If possible, the needle is not placed in joints that bend, e.g., antecubital space, wrist. When a needle must be placed in a joint, a splint must be used to immobilize the joint.

Assess type and size of needle necessary.

**PLANNING** *Objectives*

To maintain fluid and electrolyte balance.

To identify the appropriate method for IV infusion.

To administer medications through the most therapeutic intravenous route.

To provide a ready access for emergency medications, particularly in critically ill patients.

To provide the appropriate means for administering blood and blood products.

**IMPLEMENTATION** *Procedures*

Preparing IV System

Preparing IV Site

Using a Winged-Tip Needle

Using an Over-the-Needle Catheter

**EVALUATION** *Expected Outcomes*

Appropriate IV equipment is identified.

IV site is prepared appropriately.

IV therapy is initiated without difficulty.

---

## PREPARING IV SYSTEM

### Equipment

IV solution in either bottle or bag, as ordered by the physician

Administration set: drip system, which includes drip chamber and IV tubing with clamp or adjuster

Extension tubing to lengthen the original tubing or to provide extra ports for the administration of additional medication

IV pole: free-standing, bed-attached, or ceiling-affixed

### Procedure

1. Wash your hands before preparing IV equipment.

2. Compare the type and amount of solution with physician's orders and Patient Care Plan.

3. Check IV solution container for expiration date and for signs of contamination or deterioration.

4. Hold in both a dark and bright light to examine for discoloration, cloudiness, or particulate matter, which indicates contamination.

5. Examine glass bottles for cracks or leaks; examine bags for tears.

6. Select IV tubing according to hospital policy.

7. Prepare the IV solution for infusion:
   *For using a glass container*
   a. Remove metal cap, metal disc, and rubber diaphragm from IV bottle. If pharmacy has added medications, remove protective additive cap.
   b. Listen for the escape of air when rubber diaphragm is removed.
   c. Close control clamp on IV tubing administration set.
   d. With the container placed on a firm surface,

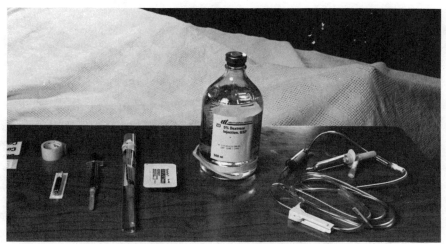

Prepare necessary equipment before beginning venipuncture procedure. This ensures a smooth process when starting the IV.

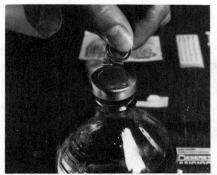

Remove metal cap from IV bottle. Listen for escape of air when cap lifted.

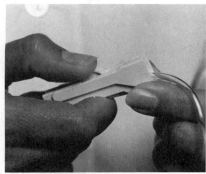

Close clamp on IV tubing before inserting into bottle to prevent air in tubing.

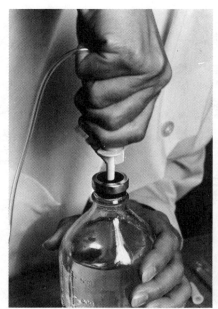

Squeezing the drip chamber, insert spike through the rubber stopper of the IV bottle.

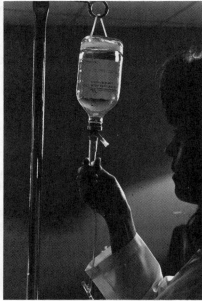

Invert IV bottle and place on IV pole. Ensure that bottle is securely placed on pole.

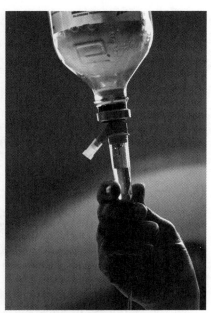

Squeeze the drip chamber to fill it at least one-third full of IV solution.

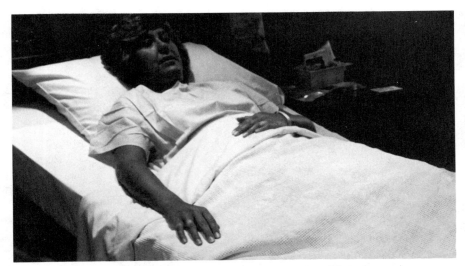

Position patient and adjust lighting to assist in identifying the best IV site.

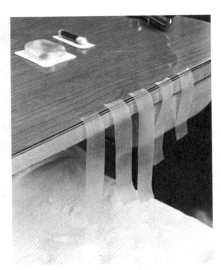

Cut tape in appropriate length strips.

squeeze the IV drip chamber and insert the spike through the appropriate area on the bottle cap.

e. Invert IV bottle and place it on the IV pole. Release drip chamber until it is one-third to one-half full of fluid.

f. Open tubing control clamp and clear the tubing of air over a receptacle such as an emesis basin or a sink. (It may be necessary to remove the adaptor cap at the end of the tubing so that fluid can flow through tubing.) Reclamp tubing.

g. Readjust the adaptor cap or place covered needle over the tubing insertion site to maintain sterility before infusion is established.

*For using a plastic container*

a. Remove outer wrap surrounding IV container.

b. Remove plastic protector from the administration set. **Rationale:** Since there is no vacuum in the plastic container, you should not hear any escaping air.

c. Close control clamp on IV tubing administration set and squeeze the IV drip chamber.

d. Insert the spike into the port, holding the neck of the port tightly to prevent slipping and possible contamination of the setup.

e. Invert the IV container and release pressure on the drip chamber.

f. Hang the IV container on the IV pole.

g. Open the IV tubing control clamp and clear the tubing of air; then reclamp.

h. Readjust the adaptor cap or place covered needle over tubing insertion site. **Rationale:** This action maintains sterility before infusion is established.

8. Before taking IV equipment to patient's room, tell the patient what you will be doing and what type of equipment you will be using.

## PREPARING IV SITE

### Equipment

Prepared IV system

Tourniquet or blood pressure cuff

Antimicrobial wipe (povidone-iodine or iodophors are preferred; alcohol is acceptable if patient is allergic to iodine)

Sterile winged-tip needle:
 Adults use size 16- to 19-gauge for viscous solutions and 20- to 25-gauge for less viscous solutions
 Neonates use a 25- to 27-gauge needle
 Older children use a 21- to 25-gauge needle

Tape (check patient for adhesive allergy)

Sterile two- by two-inch strips or bandaids

Antimicrobial ointment

### Procedure

1. Assemble equipment and take to bedside.

2. Check patient's ID band.

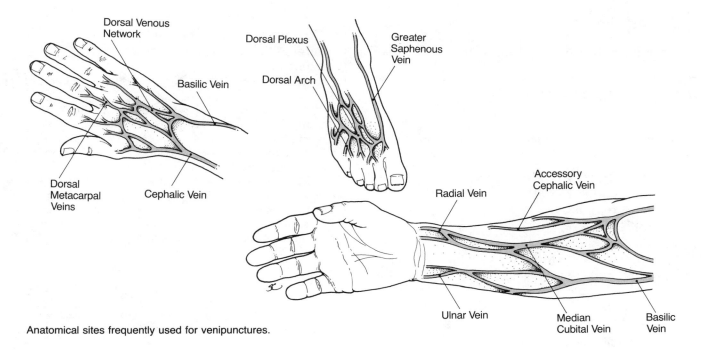

Anatomical sites frequently used for venipunctures.

3. Hang bottle and place covered end of administration set within easy reach.

4. Position patient and adjust lighting as necessary.

5. Cut pieces of tape. Open two-inch by two-inch strips or bandaids and squeeze a dollop of antimicrobial ointment on the sterile surface.

6. Wash your hands again. **Rationale:** Handwashing decreases the numbers of both endogenous and exogenous microorganisms, reducing the risk of cross-contamination of the catheter.

7. Select a vein. Inspect both of the patient's arms, palpating and visualizing the exact course of the veins. If the patient's skin is thick or darkly colored, you may not be able to visualize the veins easily. Instead, palpate them until you find a vein that feels full and superficial.
   a. Veins should be superficial, easily palpated and followed, and large enough for a needle to be smoothly inserted.
   b. Veins should be free of sclerosis, hematomas, and pain.
   c. Veins should be selected according to the IV solution that will be infused. Larger veins are preferable for caustic solutions, blood, and viscous fluid.
   d. Distal end of veins should be punctured first. Proximal ends should be preserved for further IV therapy.

> **Clinical Alert:**
> Do not shave the venipuncture site. Shaving can facilitate the development of infection through the multiplication of organisms in microabrasions that occur. Hairy sites can be clipped with scissors.

   e. Needle should be placed in the arm that is not used for writing.
   f. Needle should not be placed near joints, which require immobilization.

8. Prepare the site with povidone-iodine or a 70% ethyl-alcohol solution if the patient is allergic to iodine. **Rationale:** A vigorous skin prep will decrease endogenous and exogenous organisms at the venipuncture site.

9. Let the iodine or alcohol solution dry on the patient's skin before continuing with the intervention.

10. Dilate the patient's vein by using one of these methods:
   a. Ask the patient to open and close his fist several times. You may also slap the vein lightly.
   b. Place the patient in a low or semi-Fowler's position with patient's arm over the edge of the mattress for one or two minutes.
   c. If the vein is difficult to dilate, apply warm, moist compresses for 10 to 15 minutes.

11. Distend the vein by applying a tourniquet or blood pressure cuff. If using a cuff, pump it to a pressure between the patient's systolic and diastolic pressures.

## USING A WINGED-TIP NEEDLE

### Equipment

Prepared IV system

Tourniquet or blood pressure cuff

Antimicrobial wipe (povidone-iodine or iodophors are preferred; alcohol is acceptable if patient is allergic to iodine)

Sterile winged-tip needle:
> Adults use size 16- to 19-gauge for viscous solutions and 20- to 25-gauge for less viscous solutions
> Neonates use a 25- to 27-gauge needle
> Older children use a 21- to 25-gauge needle

Tape (check patient for adhesive allergy)

Sterile two- by two-inch strips or bandaids

Antimicrobial ointment

### Procedure

1. Select a winged-tip needle. (A 20- to 22-gauge needle is adequate for an adult.) **Rationale:** Winged-tip needles are used in short-term therapy with adults and in normal therapy with children, infants, and elderly patients who have small or fragile veins.

2. Carefully affix the end of the IV administration tubing to the end of the winged-tip needle. Remove sterile cover from needle. Run fluid through the needle.

3. Hold needle by its wings.

4. Anchor vein by placing your thumb below the patient's vein and gently stretching the skin by pulling down distally.

5. With bevel of the needle up, enter the patient's skin at a 45-degree angle. You may use either of these methods:
   a. Enter skin at a 45-degree angle next to the vein. Flatten the angle once the needle is under the skin and enter vein from the side.
   b. Enter skin and vein in one smooth motion from above. You will feel a gentle "pop" or release as the needle enters the vein. Observe for flashback of blood in needle tubing. **Rationale:** This method requires experience and

**Each time the closed body system is entered the potential for contamination exists.**

☐ Strict attention should be directed to maintaining the infusion system aseptically.

☐ Once the needle has been inserted, it should be anchored with tape to prevent a rocking motion, which may irritate the vein or push bacteria into the bloodstream from the skin.

☐ The sterile dressing should be applied in such a way that daily dressing changes and venipuncture site inspection can occur without undue problems.

☐ The IV administration set should be changed every 24 to 48 hours to decrease levels of microbial contaminants in the infusion solution.

judgment, since it is easy to put the needle through the vein.

6. Advance needle carefully up the course of the vein.

7. Release tourniquet or blood pressure cuff.

8. Open clamp on IV tubing and observe drip chamber. **Rationale:** Fluid should flow easily, and there should be no sudden swelling around the IV site.

9. Reduce flow rate to keep open until you have taped the needle and the tubing in place.

10. Apply antimicrobial ointment to needle site and cover with sterile two- by two-inch strips or bandaids.

11. Tape winged-tip needle and tubing to patient's skin.

12. Using a watch, set drip rate according to physician's orders.

13. Label IV site with pertinent information, according to hospital policy.

## USING AN OVER-THE-NEEDLE CATHETER

### Equipment

Tourniquet or blood pressure cuff

Antimicrobial wipe (povidone-iodine or iodophors are preferred; alcohol is acceptable if patient is allergic to iodine)

Sterile over-the-needle catheter
> sizes 12-gauge to 22-gauge, 1¼" to 5½" long

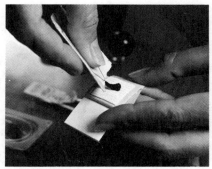

Place antimicrobial ointment on gauze pad before performing a venipuncture.

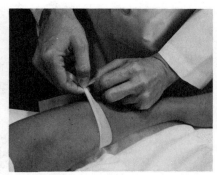

Tie tourniquet tightly in a method for easy removal once the needle is in the vein.

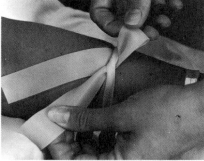

Apply tourniquet proximal to IV puncture site in order to dilate the veins.

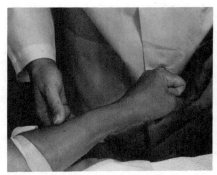

Instruct the patient to open and close fist several times to dilate the vein.

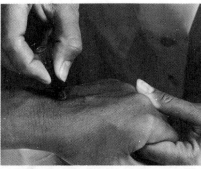

Apply povidone-iodine to puncture site and allow area to dry thoroughly.

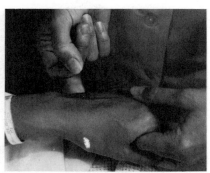

Start venipuncture at the distal end of vein to preserve future IV sites.

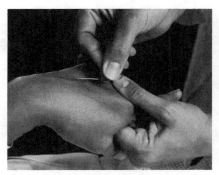

Keep winged-tip needle bevel up and insert needle at 45-degree angle to the skin.

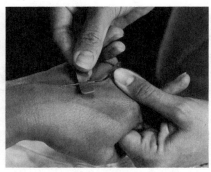

Observe IV tubing for blood backflow indicating that the needle is in the vein.

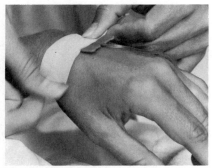

Place tape directly over the needle insertion site to secure it to the skin.

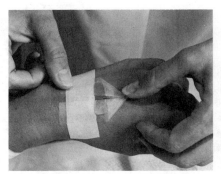

Tape down wings of needle securely to prevent accidental dislodging.

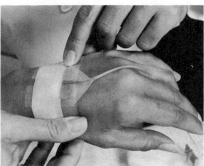

Secure IV site with additional tape; position tubing to prevent pulling.

IV solution in either bottle or bag, as ordered by physician

Administration set: drip system, which includes drip chamber and IV tubing

Extension tubing, if necessary

IV pole

Tape (Check patient for adhesive allergy.)

Sterile two-by two-inch strips or bandaids

Antimicrobial ointment

Filter (used whenever the IV system is entered to administer drugs)

IV controller or pump, if required

## Procedure

1. Prepare IV equipment following steps in preparation.

2. Select appropriate sized over-the-needle catheter.

3. Prepare IV site following steps 1–11 in procedure Preparing IV Site.

4. Just prior to insertion, carefully remove needle cover. Inspect both needle and catheter. **Rationale:** Barbs or rough edges can occur even with new needle bevels.

5. With bevel of needle up, insert needle and catheter together, as one unit into the patient's skin. **Rationale:** Bevel needle in the "up" position assists with needle insertion.

6. Insert the cannula into the vein.

7. Advance catheter and needle gently as one unit into the lumen, making sure that both are inside the vein. Observe for backflow of blood in plastic hub of needle.

8. Place small, sterile gauze sponge under the hub of the over-the-needle unit.

9. As soon as the catheter and needle are fully in place, release the tourniquet.

10. Gently withdraw the needle from inside the catheter with one hand, placing your fingertip firmly above the catheter tip to occlude the vein and prevent sudden bleeding.

11. Connect hub to IV administration set.

12. Open clamp on set briefly and observe drip chamber. Fluid should flow rapidly without obstruction, and there should not be any sudden swelling at IV site.

13. Reduce flow and proceed with taping, using chevron method.

14. Apply antimicrobial ointment to needle site and cover with sterile two-by two-inch strips or bandaids.

15. Tape tubing to the patient, using two strips of tape.

16. Using a watch, set drip rate according to physician's orders.

17. Label IV site with pertinent information, according to hospital policy.

## CHARTING  *for Preparing IV System*

☐  Location of insertion site

☐  Gauge of needle inserted

☐  Time of insertion

☐  Type of solution infusing

☐  Rate of infusion

☐  Condition of IV site

---

## CLINICAL PROBLEM SOLVING

### Potential Problems

Venipuncture attempt does not result in insertion into vein.

### Suggested Solutions

☐  Remove needle. Apply dressing.

☐  Move to other side of body for vein assessment. If necessary, move up proximally on the same vein. Select new site and use fresh needle.

☐  After two attempts, ask more experienced personnel to perform venipuncture.

☐  Ensure that the needle enters the skin at 45 degree angle and to one side of the vein.

Veins roll and are difficult to enter.

☐  Use firmer pressure to anchor skin and vein.

Veins are fragile and appear to "balloon" around the needle once the vein has been entered.

During insertion, the needle enters an artery. This may result in a rapid, backward movement of the syringe plunger and the appearance of bright red blood.

☐ Loosen tourniquet to reduce pressure in the vein. If possible, use a smaller gauged winged-tip needle.

☐ Completely remove the syringe and needle. Apply pressure to the puncture site *if possible* for a minimum of ten minutes.

## UNIT TWO  IV MANAGEMENT

### NURSING PROCESS DATA

#### ASSESSMENT  *Data Base*

Assess flow rate for accuracy.

Determine if pump or controller cassette or modular unit needs to be changed.

Assess venipuncture site for edema, erythema, and infiltration.

Assess IV solution for correct solution, amount, and timing.

Assess need to discontinue IV needle or catheter.

Assess need to change patient gown while IV infusing.

#### PLANNING  *Objectives*

To maintain the IV site free from redness, edema, and purulent drainage.

To calculate and monitor the IV infusion rate accurately and to reassess throughout the therapy.

To remove IV equipment without complications.

To change a gown while maintaining the IV site.

#### IMPLEMENTATION  *Procedures*

Regulating IV Flow Rate

Using a Controller and Pump

Using a Syringe Pump (Harvard)

Managing IV Site

Changing Gown for Patient with IV

Removing IV Equipment

#### EVALUATION  *Expected Outcomes*

Fluids, additives, and medications are administered without adverse effects on the patient.

IV site remains free from redness, edema, and purulent drainage.

IV infusion rate is accurately calculated and reassessed throughout the therapy.

Patient gown is changed while maintaining IV placement.

IV therapy is discontinued without complications.

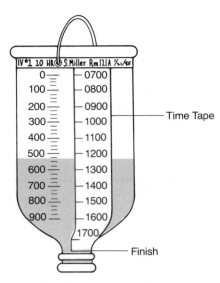

Time Tape

Finish

Before hanging time-tape the bottle.

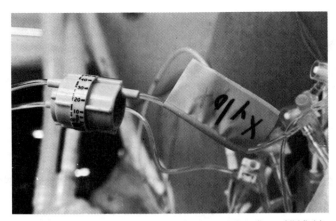

The Dial-A-Flo in-line device is a method to regulate flow of IV fluids.

## REGULATING IV FLOW RATE

### Procedure

1. Check manufacturer's drip rate calibration on administration set package. Macrodrip sets vary from 10 gtts to 20 gtts to equal 1 ml.

2. Check physician's order for amount of fluids to be delivered per unit of time. Some physicians state one liter to be given over eight hours; others specify hourly flow rate, such as 60 ml per hour.

3. Calculate flow rate. There are several formulas which may be useful. Here is one two-step method.
   a. To find ml to be given per hour:
   $$\frac{\text{Total solution}}{\text{No. of hours to run}} = \text{ml per hour}$$
   b. To find drops per minute:
   $$\frac{\text{ml/hr} \times \text{drop factor}}{60 \text{ minutes}} = \text{gtts/minute}$$

---

**IV Calorie Calculation**
- ☐ 1000 cc $D_5W$ provides 50 g of dextrose.
- ☐ 50 g of dextrose provides four calories per gram (actually 3.4 calories); therefore, multiply 50 gms × 4 calories.
- ☐ 1000 cc $D_5W$ provides 200 calories.
- ☐ Usual IV total/day is 3000 cc (600 calories/day).

---

4. Stand near the drip chamber and count the drops for one minute, using a watch with a sweep hand.

5. Adjust clamp until the chamber drips the desired number of drops.

6. Affix tape to bottle and mark the hourly flow rate.

## USING A CONTROLLER AND PUMP

### Equipment

Controller or pump

Compatible IV tubing

Cassette or modular unit if required

### Preparation

1. Identify if type of medication or amount of medication requires use of the controller or pump.

2. Bring equipment to patient's room and explain use of the machine.

3. Plug the machine into the electrical outlet.

### Procedure

1. Place IV solution container and tubing on the IV pole.

2. Fill the drip chamber of the IV tubing at least one-third full.

3. Flush the tubing to expel all air bubbles. Some types of controllers or pumps have modular units attached that need to be changed every 24 hours.

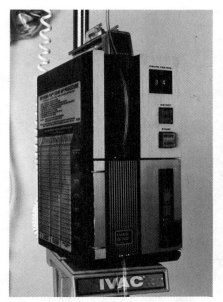

The IVAC 530 pump infuses IV fluids up to 99 drops per minute.

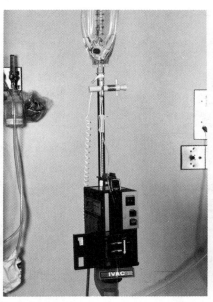

The electronic drop sensor monitors the drops per minute set on the IVAC.

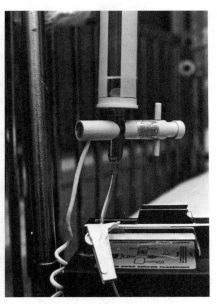

Place the electronic drop sensor below the needle and above fluid level.

The IV extension tubing and regular IV tubing are attached directly to the modular unit.

4. Raise the IV pole to ensure that the drip chamber is at least 30 inches above the infusion site.

5. Attach the drip sensor device to the IV drip chamber.

6. Lift the door handle and open the door of the controller or pump.

7. Place the IV tubing through the tubing guides on the machine.

8. Close the door and push the handle down.

9. Open the IV control clamp completely.

10. Select the appropriate drops per minute on the dial. Check the side of the machine for conversion table.

11. Connect the IV tubing to the venipuncture site.

12. Press the power button to the ON position.

13. Press the start button.

14. Count the drops for one full minute. **Rationale:** Counting verifies that the drop rate is correct as set.

15. Assess the drops being delivered, the condition of the tubing in the guide, and the fluid level in the drip chamber at least every four hours.

---

**If alarm sounds, check the following:**

☐ Ensure that drip chamber is only one-third full.

☐ Assess that height of the IV container is at least 30 inches above the venipuncture site.

☐ Examine the IV tubing in the guides to ensure it is not pinched down.

☐ Assess that drop sensor is placed properly to sense the drops.

☐ Evaluate the position of the needle and tubing to prevent kinking.

---

16. Change the site of the tubing in the guide at least every eight hours.

17. Listen for the alarm and respond immediately to determine the problem.

## USING A SYRINGE PUMP (HARVARD)

### Equipment

Infusion pump

Syringes 20cc, 35cc, 50cc (disposable or glass)

IV extension tubing

IV solution

Medication

Diluent for medication (if required)

Syringe 5cc or 10cc

### Procedure

1. Check physician's order for drug, dosage, and amount of fluid to be delivered over specified time. Check patient's ID band.

2. Identify the amount of medication and/or fluid to be delivered per minute.

3. Check the chart on the syringe pump to identify proper syringe size and machine setting according to amount of drug to be delivered.

4. Set dial on side of pump.

5. Assemble equipment, i.e., syringes, extension tubing, and pump.

6. Draw up medication in syringe. Predilute the medication in another syringe or bottle before withdrawing into large syringe.

7. Place extension tubing on the syringe and flush the tubing to expel all air bubbles.

8. Place syringe in holder clamp on pump.

9. Position carriage carefully over plunger of syringe. **Rationale:** Glass syringes can easily break when machine is turned on if not positioned carefully.

10. Plug machine into electrical outlet at the bedside.

11. Make sure the switch of the pump is set on the infusion site and not on the withdrawal site.

12. Connect the extension tubing to the IV site by either piggy-backing the tubing into the existing IV line or inserting the tubing directly into an IV site.

13. Double check the dials and recalculate the rate of infusion.

14. Turn syringe pump on.

15. Monitor the amount of fluid infused in the first hour to ensure proper fluid administration.

## MANAGING IV SITE

### Equipment

Dressing tray or
    Sterile four-by four-inch gauze dressings
    Sterile two-by two-inch gauze dressings
    Tape (Check patient for adhesive allergy.)
    Alcohol or Betadine swab
    Antimicrobial ointment
    Protective pad

### Procedure

1. Wash your hands.

2. Assemble all equipment and bring to bedside.

3. Place protective covering under IV site. **Rationale:** Protect linen from becoming soiled.

4. Remove tape and dressings, keeping pressure over IV site to prevent dislodging needle.

5. Discard dressing in container.

6. Wash your hands.

7. Observe IV site for erythema, edema, infiltration.

8. Cleanse IV site with alcohol or Betadine starting at the puncture site and moving peripherally using a circular motion.

9. Apply antimicrobial ointment over IV site, according to hospital policy.

10. Place on two- by two-inch gauze under hub of over the needle catheter.

11. Cover IV site with sterile two- by two-inch gauze.

12. Place four- by four-inch gauze doubled in half over IV site and tape securely. **Rationale:** Used for stabilizing needle at insertion site.

13. Secure arm to IV arm board if needed.

---

**Clinical Alert**

Check frequently for IV infiltration.

☐ Watch IV flow for consistency of flow rate.

☐ Check for flashback of blood when tubing is pinched or IV container lowered below IV site.

---

## CHANGING GOWN FOR PATIENT WITH IV

### Equipment

Clean gown

Bath blanket

Washing equipment if needed

### Procedure

1. Check Patient Care Plan for infusion drip rate, type of solution, and any special considerations.

2. Wash your hands.

3. Gather equipment and take to patient's room.

4. Explain to patient what you are going to do.

5. Raise bed to comfortable working height and lower side rails.

6. Untie back of gown and remove gown from unaffected arm.

7. Support arm with IV and slip gown down arm to IV tubing.

8. Remove IV bottle from hook and slip the sleeve over the bottle, keeping bottle above patient's arm. **Rationale:** This prevents backflow of blood into vein. Do not jar or pull tubing. **Rationale:** IV tubing may become dislodged and infiltrate into surrounding tissue.

9. Rehang bottle on hook and check to see that infusion is running according to ordered drip rate.

---

This procedure is applicable for a simple IV set-up. If IV pumps or controllers are used, the sleeve may be left open or a gown with snap closure used.

---

10. Place clean gown over patient's chest and abdomen.

11. Remove IV bottle from hook and pass it through sleeve of gown, remembering to hold level of bottle above patient's arm.

12. Return bottle to IV stand and guide sleeve of gown up the patient's arm to the shoulder.

13. Assist patient to put other arm through remaining sleeve.

14. Tie gown at the back.

15. Check IV infusion rate and IV tubing to determine that solution is flowing unimpeded into patient's vein. **Rationale:** Kinks in the tubing will impede solution flow.

16. Return bed to comfortable position for patient and replace side rails.

17. Remove dirty linen from room.

18. Wash your hands.

## REMOVING IV EQUIPMENT

### Equipment

Bandaid or sterile pad and two-by two-inch strip of tape

### Procedure

1. Wash your hands.

2. Gather equipment.

3. Explain procedure to patient.

4. Remove tape from tubing and wings of needle. Hold needle wings while manipulating tape. **Rationale:** This action prevents unnecessary movement that could injure the vein.

5. Remove needle quickly and smoothly. Do not press down on top of needle point while it is in the vein.

6. Quickly press sterile strips or bandage over venipuncture site and hold firmly until bleeding stops.

7. Apply sterile pad and tape in place.

8. Observe venipuncture site for redness, swelling, or formation of hematoma.

9. Check site again in 15 to 30 minutes.

### CHARTING  *for Intravenous Management*

☐ Location of insertion site

☐ Gauge of needle inserted

☐ Time of insertion

☐ Type of controller and pump

☐ Cassette or module changed

☐ IV flow rate

☐ Site care given

☐ Condition of site

☐ Time dressing changed

☐ Any unusual conditions or reactions of skin

☐ Time IV terminated

---

## CLINICAL PROBLEM SOLVING

### Potential Problems

Patient develops unexplained fever with chills and rising pulse rate.

### Suggested Solutions

☐ Unexplained fever may be associated with catheter-related sepsis. Report to physician.

☐ Check that IV solution has not been hanging for more than 24 hours.

□ Check patient's vital signs: temperature usually above 100° F when caused by IV-related sepsis.
□ Check for other symptoms of pyrogenic reactions, e.g. backache, headache, malaise, nausea and vomiting.
□ Stop the infusion.
□ Obtain blood cultures, if ordered.

IV solution does not flow properly.

□ The height of the bottle may be too low and therefore the IV fluid does not flow. Increase the height of the bottle.
□ Ensure that the control clamp is open.
□ Assess that vein is not thrombosed or erythematous.
□ Check that blood pressure readings are not taken on arm in which IV is running, as flow is impeded and a clot can form on the end of the needle.
□ Check that correct tubing was used with pump or controller. Most machines require special administration sets.
□ Check that IV tubing is not compressed in pump or controller.

Alarm sounds on pump or controller.

□ Follow protocol for checking IV systems.

IV solution appears to be infiltrating into surrounding tissue resulting in erythema and edema.

□ Decrease the flow rate and check for needle placement (follow hospital policy regarding discontinuing the infusion).
□ Lower bottle of IV solution below IV insertion site; if blood returns, needle is in the vein.
□ Check IV bottle for solution and medications being administered. If protein hydrolysates, potassium or sodium lactate are being infused, call physician immediately.

Thrombophlebitis is suspected at the infusion site.

□ Check infusion area for pain along the vein, erythema, and edema at the insertion site.
□ Check IV solution; hypertonic solution causes irritation necessitating the change in IV sites more frequently.
□ Stop infusion and apply cold compresses to site for 30 minutes followed by hot compresses.

## UNIT THREE   INTAKE AND OUTPUT

### NURSING PROCESS DATA

#### ASSESSMENT   *Data Base*

Assess patient's need for intake and output recording if the patient is not taking sufficient fluids, even if there has been no physician's request.

Assess patient's ability to keep intake and output fluid records.

Evaluate patient for any factors that might affect his intake and output, e.g., preexisting disease states, concurrent diagnosed diseases, drug therapies, and current physical status.

Determine all measurable sources of fluid intake: fluids with and between meals, liquid medications, IV fluids, and IV medications as baseline for urinary output.

Determine all measurable sources of fluid output: urine, vomitus, diarrhea, and drainage.

Determine alterations in nonmeasurable sources of fluid intake and loss: food, increased metabolism, rapid respirations, and excessive perspiration.

### PLANNING *Objectives*

To establish a written record of the patient's total fluid intake (oral, parenteral, and/or feeding tubes) and fluid output (urine, stool, GI and chest drainage, unexpected loss from a wound, diarrhea, vomiting).

To plan fluid replacement or appropriate therapy by assessing deficits and/or excesses of fluids and/or electrolytes.

To ensure a fluid intake of at least 1500 cc unless contraindicated by diagnosis, e.g., CHF, pulmonary edema.

To monitor the patient's hydration state, vital signs, and mental state to determine homeostasis.

### IMPLEMENTATION *Procedures*

Monitoring Intake and Output

Monitoring IV Intake

### EVALUATION *Expected Outcomes*

Intake and output, though not exactly equal, are within 200 cc to 300 cc of each other.

Fluid intake is at least 1500 cc unless contraindicated by diagnosis.

Patient's hydration state, vital signs, and mental status are within normal range.

## MONITORING INTAKE AND OUTPUT

### Equipment

Graduated container in patient's bathroom

Intake and output bedside record and 24 hour record in chart

Urinal/bedpan; bedside commode/underseat basin for toilet

Hourly inline urine measurement device for patients requiring frequent monitoring

Posted measurement standards for commonly used drinking and eating utensils, e.g., glasses, mugs, bowls

Posted signs, dietary slips, and other communication devices to notify hospital personnel about how patient's intake and output is to be measured

### Procedure

1. Determine if patient needs intake and output measurements by checking Kardex or patient's chart.

2. Measure intake from all sources
   a. Oral fluids.

**TABLE 3** BODY SITES FOR ASSESSMENT OF HYDRATION

| SITE | EXCESS HYDRATION | DEHYDRATION |
|---|---|---|
| **HEAD AND NECK** | | |
| Face | Eyeballs firm and/or protruding | Eyeballs soft and/or sunken |
| | Edema, especially around eyes | Poor skin turgor over forehead |
| Mucous | Excessive salivation | Dry or sticky mucosa |
| Membranes | Swollen tongue | Shrunken tongue |
| | | Crusted lips |
| Neck | Jugular vein distention | |
| **TRUNK** | | |
| Chest | Moist rales | Poor skin turgor |
| | Pulmonary congestion | Dry, flaking skin |
| Abdomen | Ascites (measure girth at umbilicus) | |
| Sacrum | Edema | Poor skin turgor |
| **EXTREMITIES** | | |
| Arms | Edema, particularly of the hands | Poor skin turgor |
| | Delayed capillary refill | Delayed capillary refill |
| | Unequal quality of radial pulses | Dry, flaking skin |
| | Pulse bounding | Pulse weak and thready |
| Legs | Edema | Poor skin turgor, especially across shins |
| | Taut shiny skin | Dry, flaky skin, especially on feet |
| | Weak pedal pulse and/or decreased capillary refill | Weak pedal pulse and/or decreased capillary refill |

**TABLE 4** OBJECTIVE DATA INDICATIVE OF THE STATE OF HYDRATION

| DATA | EXCESS HYDRATION | DEHYDRATION |
|---|---|---|
| **VITAL SIGNS** | | |
| Blood Pressure | Increased* | Decreased |
| Pulse | Increased rate | Increased rate |
| Temperature | Unchanged | Elevated |
| Respirations | Increased rate | Unchanged or increased |
| **LABORATORY FINDINGS** | | |
| Urine Specific Gravity | Decreased, approaching 1.010 | Increased, approaching 1.025 or greater |
| Blood Hematocrit | Less than three times the hemoglobin | Greater than three times the hemoglobin |
| Serum Sodium (Na) | Less than 135 mEq/L | Greater than 145 mEq/L |
| **Hourly Urine Output** | More than 60 cc/hr | Less than 30 to 60 cc/hr |
| **Weight** | A 5% or greater gain | Mild: 2% loss |
| | | Moderate: 3 – 5% loss |
| | | Severe: 6% or greater loss |

*If the heart is no longer able to pump the increased blood volume, and cardiac decompensation occurs, the blood pressure will drop.

b. IV fluids.
c. Fluids with IV meds.
d. Tube feedings and water used to clear tubing.

3. Measure output from all sources to establish a written record and plan fluid replacement.
   a. Foley/French catheters.
   b. Bedpans/urinals.

c. Nasogastric drainage.
d. Drainage tubing, e.g., T-tubes.
e. Diarrheal stools.
f. Draining wounds.
g. Vomitus.

4. Record intake and output on bedside record each time you take a measurement.

**TABLE 5**   INTAKE AND OUPUT FLOW SHEET

| DATE | TIME | IV NO. | IV AMT. STARTED | DESCRIPTION | IV INTAKE | ORAL INTAKE | URINE OUTPUT | OTHER | N/G |
|---|---|---|---|---|---|---|---|---|---|
| 1/9/85 | 9 A | | | Full liquid breakfast | | 620 | | | |
| | 9:45 A | | | Vomitus | | | | 400 | |
| | 10:30 A | #1 | 1000 | | | | | | |
| | 12 N | | | | | | 450 | | |
| | 2:30 P | | | | | | 300 | | |
| | | | | 7-3 Total | 450 | 620 | 750 | 400 | 100 |
| | 6:30 P | #2 | 1000 | | 550 | | | | |
| | 9 P | | | | | | 375 | | |
| | | | | 3-11 Total | 1050 | NPO | 375 | | 250 |
| 1/10/85 | 2:30 A | #3 | 1000 | | 450 | | | | |
| | 5 A | | | | | | 250 | | |
| | | | | 11-7 Total | 1050 | NPO | 250 | | 175 |
| | | | | 24-hr Total | 2550 | 620 | 1375 | 400 | 525 |

5. Record 24-hour totals of intake and output on bedside record and on graphic sheet in patient's chart.

6. Notify physician of any abnormality which could lead to complications. **Rationale:** Hourly urine output less that 25 to 30 cc per hour or 24-hour urine output less than 500 cc can indicate dehydration, kidney damage, or alterations in hormonal balance.

## MONITORING IV INTAKE

### Equipment

Volume control set e.g. Soluset, Metriset, Volu-Trol, etc.

Intake and output record

Graphic sheet

IV container with timed intervals

### Procedure

1. Place intake and output record at bedside.

2. Determine time interval required for monitoring IV intake.

3. Mark time intervals on IV container according to facility policy (use felt-tip pen, preprinted time strips, etc.)

4. Set IV drip rate according to physician's orders.

5. Observe volume control set or IV container and read IV solution level.

### Fluid Replacement Solutions

☐ Hypertonic solution—a solution with higher osmotic pressure than blood serum.
  a. Cell placed in solution will crenate.
  b. Used in severe salt depletion.
  c. Common types of solution: normal saline, dextrose 10% in saline, dextrose 10% in water, and dextrose 5% in saline.
  d. Should not be administered faster than 200 cc/hr.

☐ Hypotonic solution—a solution with less osmotic pressure than blood serum.
  a. Causes cells to expand or increase in size.
  b. Used in diarrhea and dehydration.
  c. Common types of solution: dextrose 5% in ½ strength (0.45%) NS, dextrose 5% in ¼ strength (0.2) NS, and dextrose 5% in water.
  d. Should not be administered faster than 400 cc/hr.

☐ Isotonic solution—a solution with the same osmotic pressure as blood serum.
  a. Cells remain unchanged.
  b. Used for replacement or maintenance.
  c. Common type of solution: lactated Ringer's solution.

6. Record amount of IV solution infused at prescribed time (eg. every hour, every shift).

7. Record total IV intake on intake and output record at end of each shift.

8. Record 24 hour IV total at midnight. Take into account all sources of IV fluid (all IV sites, IV fluid used for medications).

(For complete I and O procedure, see Chapter 18.)

### CHARTING  *for Intake and Output*

☐ Exact measurements of intake and output

☐ Approximate volume of loss when unable to measure contents, e.g., incontinent of urine in bed

☐ Dietary intake (food as well as water)

☐ Time, amount, and description of all measurable intake and output

☐ Signs and symptoms of patient's state of hydration, including vital signs, urine output and weight

---

## CLINICAL PROBLEM SOLVING

**Potential Problems**

Fluid balance is not correct as stated on intake and output record.

**Suggested Solutions**

☐ Report to charge nurse so she can determine if all nurses are keeping accurate records.
☐ Check if patient and/or family can help with keeping the I and O record.
☐ Check the addition on the I and O record to see if an error was made.

Patient does not maintain an intake of at least 1500 cc.

☐ Ensure that the diagnosis allows a 1500 cc intake.
☐ Check if the patient is able to drink fluids by himself, or if he needs assistance.
☐ Ensure that adequate fluids are available at the bedside for the patient.

IV fluids not maintained at appropriate rate to provide adequate intake.

☐ Monitor IV level hourly.
☐ Observe IV site for infiltration.
☐ Restart IV's immediately when infiltrated to ensure continuous IV fluid intake.
☐ Document IV levels at least every shift.

---

## UNIT FOUR   IV MEDICATION ADMINISTRATION

### NURSING PROCESS DATA

#### ASSESSMENT  *Data Base*

Note patient's allergies.

Note any drug and/or solution incompatibilities.

Assess patient's general condition to establish a baseline for administering medications.

Assess patency of infusion set and conditions of IV insertion site.

Assess amount of diluent needed to mix with medications.

#### PLANNING  *Objectives*

To maintain a therapeutic level of medication in the patient's bloodstream.

To administer medication in larger volumes over a longer period of time.

To prevent complications associated with bolus administration, such as speed shock and vein irritation.

### IMPLEMENTATION  *Procedures*

Adding Medications to IV

Using a Partial-Fill Additive Bottle

Using a Volume Control Set

Using a Secondary Bottle

Using a Heparin Lock

Administering by Bolus Injection

### EVALUATION  *Expected Outcomes*

Solutions from additive bottles and/or bags infuse without difficulty.

Therapeutic blood level of medication is maintained.

Complications of medication administration are prevented.

Medication is infused over appropriate time span.

## ADDING MEDICATIONS TO IV

### Equipment

IV solution bottle or bag

Syringe with medications

Alcohol swab

Label with medication, date, time and initials

### Preparation

1. Check physician's orders and Kardex.
2. Wash hands.
3. Gather equipment. Check patient ID band.

### Procedure

1. Draw up medication into syringe according to directions on medication label.
2. Wipe top of IV bottle, especially the triangle area, or port on side of IV bag with alcohol swab.
3. Inject medication into bottle or bag while maintaining aseptic technique.
4. Mix the IV solution and medication by gently shaking the bottle.
5. Affix the medication label to the IV bottle or bag.
6. Insert the IV tubing into the bottle or bag and proceed with the appropriate method of administration as ordered.

## USING A PARTIAL-FILL ADDITIVE BOTTLE

### Equipment

Primary IV set, consisting of IV solution bottle and IV administration set with injection port

Medication mixed in syringe

Partial-fill additive bottle or bag set: macrodrip administration set, 20-gauge one-inch needle, and extension hook or lowering hanger for primary bottle

Label with name of medication, date, time, and nurse's initial

### Preparation

1. Check physician's order and Kardex.
2. Wash hands.
3. Gather equipment.

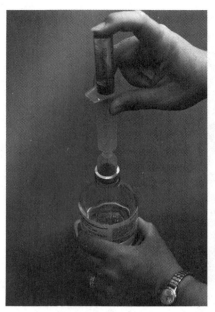 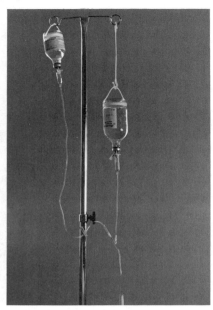

Instill medications in additive bottle before inserting IV tubing.

Hang the additive bottle higher than the primary bottle.

## Procedure

1. Prepare medication following directions on label. Add medication to partial-fill bottle using aseptic technique.

2. Spike partial-fill bottle with administration set. Affix the needle to the end of the tubing, and prime both the tubing and the needle. Close the clamp on the tubing.

3. Cleanse the injection port of the primary IV with an alcohol swab.

4. Insert the needle of the partial-fill bottle set and secure in place with tape.

5. Hang the partial-fill bottle on the IV pole. Use the extension hook to lower the primary bottle below the partial-fill bottle.

6. Open the clamp on the partial-fill bottle tubing. The solution in the partial-fill bottle should begin to flow.

7. Using the clamp on the primary IV tubing, adjust the drip rate to the desired rate of administration.

8. Make sure that the partial-fill bottle is higher than the primary IV bottle so the solution will drip until the partial-fill bottle is empty. **Rationale:** The flow continues because of an increased hydrostatic pressure. When medication is finished, a valve automatically occludes flow from the additive bottle and maintains a patent access site.

9. When the partial-fill bottle and drip chamber are empty, readjust the rate of administration in the primary solution to desired flow.

10. To hang a new partial-fill bottle, prepare the medication and add it to the new bottle aseptically. Remove the old partial-fill bottle and spike the new bottle. Close the clamp on the partial-fill bottle tubing.

11. Lower the partial-fill bottle below the injection port of the primary IV.

12. Open the clamp on the partial-fill tubing and allow the solution from the primary IV set to enter the tubing, back-filling the tubing to the drip chamber. **Rationale:** This procedure will displace any air left in the tubing.

13. Replace new partial-fill bottle on IV pole and proceed with administration.

14. Change partial-fill tubing every 48 hours.

## USING A VOLUME CONTROL SET

### Equipment

Primary IV set, consisting of IV solution bottle and IV administration set with injection port

Volume control set: Soluset®, Metriset®, VoluTrol®, or Buretrol (depending on need and/or manufacturer)

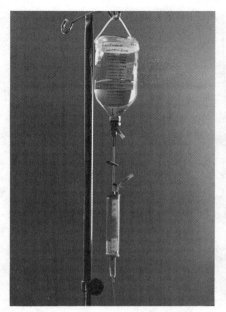

Fill volume-control set to appropriate fluid level by opening tubing clamp.

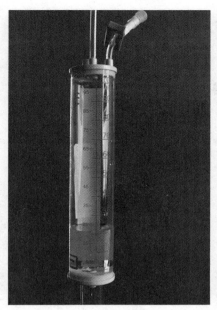

Check that the rubber diaphragm is not occluding the opening to the drip chamber.

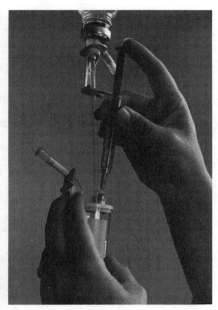

Wipe injection site; then inject medication while rotating the chamber to mix.

Medication mixed in syringe

Alcohol swab

Label with medication, date, time, and nurse's initials

### Preparation

1. Check physician's orders.
2. Wash hands.
3. Obtain volume control set, IV bottle, and IV tubing if needed.

### Procedure

1. Close clamps on volume control set, both above and below the volume chamber.
2. Open the air vent by turning the clamp located on top of volume chamber.
3. Spike IV bottle with the volume control set, and then hang the bottle. Insert the IV tubing into the volume control set.
4. Open the upper clamp (between the bottle and the volume chamber) and fill the chamber with IV solution so that the chamber is one-third full.
5. Close the upper clamp.
6. Open the lower clamp and squeeze the drip chamber (located underneath the volume chamber) until it is one-half full.
7. Allow the solution to flow down the tubing.

8. Prime the tubing and needle affixed to the end of the tubing. If the volume control set has a membrane filter instead of a floating valve filter, follow the manufacturer's instructions for priming so that you do not damage the filter.
9. Close the clamp.
10. Swab off the injection port (located on top of the volume chamber) with alcohol.
11. Inject prepared medication into chamber and agitate gently to mix medication with solution in chamber.
12. Dilute medication, if necessary, by opening the upper clamp and adding additional fluid from the IV bottle.
13. Open clamp on volume control set and adjust drip rate to desired rate of administration.
14. Place medication label on volume control set. Include patient's name, medication, dose, and time medication infusion begun.

## USING A SECONDARY BOTTLE

### Equipment

Primary IV set, consisting of IV solution bottle and IV administration set with injection port

Secondary bottle and administration set: administration set and 20-gauge one-inch needle

Label with medication, date, time, and nurse's initials

**Preparation**

1. Check physician's orders.
2. Wash hands.
3. Gather equipment.

**Procedure**

1. Prepare medication per instructions. Add medication to compatible IV solution in small IV bottle or bag.
2. Label bottle with date, time, medication, dosage, and your name.
3. With administration set, spike the bottle.
4. Hang bottle and prime the tubing.
5. Affix and prime a 20-gauge one-inch needle.
6. Close tubing clamp.
7. Swab injection port on primary IV tubing.
8. Carefully insert needle and tape securely in place.
9. Depending on physician's orders, either clamp off primary IV or run in secondary IV solution concurrently with primary IV solution. **Rationale:** A secondary solution further dilutes the medication.
10. When medication is finished, clamp off tubing, remove needle from injection port, and discard tubing, bottle, and needle.

## USING A HEPARIN LOCK

### Equipment

Heparin solution or prefilled heparin syringe

Normal saline diluent

Alcohol or iodophor swab

Normal saline prefilled syringe

Injection port [if one not available] for lock

### Preparation

1. Check physician's orders and Patient Care Plan.
2. Wash your hands.
3. Gather equipment.
4. Explain procedure to patient.
5. If patient does not have an intermittent infusion set in place, proceed with venipuncture, selecting veins that are both large enough to receive the bolus of medicine and away from areas of move-

ment, e.g., the elbows and wrists. When taping the set in place, secure the injection port away from the needle insertion site. **Rationale:** This action minimizes needle movement when the port is being used.

**Procedure**

1. Prepare medication to be administered, e.g., antibiotic, and draw it up into a syringe.
2. Fill a syringe with 2 to 2½ cc of saline.
3. Fill a third syringe with heparin solution from vial or use a prefilled heparin syringe. (Method will be determined by hospital policy.)

---

Heparin solution is usually prepared with 1 cc 1:1000 heparin added to 9 cc of normal saline to produce 100 u/cc solution.

---

4. Swab injection port with alcohol or iodophor swab. Insert saline syringe into port and flush system. Some drugs are incompatible with heparin.

---

Some protocols state that a saline syringe is used to check patency of the infusion set. If so, draw up 2 syringes with 2 to 2½ cc of saline and use one syringe at this time.

---

5. Insert medication syringe into port.
6. Pull back on syringe plunger and check for flow of blood into syringe. **Rationale:** The presence of blood indicates that the needle is placed into the vein, not into surrounding tissues.
7. Inject medication into the vein, timing the flow rate according to physician's orders or drug manufacturer's instructions.
8. Observe patient for any adverse reactions.
9. Remove medication syringe.
10. Insert syringe filled with saline.
11. Flush the catheter tubing with saline to clear the line.
12. Remove saline syringe.
13. Insert heparin syringe and inject the heparin to fill the catheter and needle lumen. **Rationale:** The heparin should prevent the catheter from clotting.
14. Remove syringe and secure the injection port with tape.

# ADMINISTERING IV MEDICATIONS BY BOLUS

## Equipment

Medication

Alcohol swab

Sterile syringe and small gauze needle

## Preparation

1. Check physician's orders.
2. Wash your hands.
3. Gather equipment.
4. Prepare medications according to directions on vial or medication insert sheet. **Rationale:** IV medications should be diluted according to drug instructions to prevent vein irritation.
5. Check the medication according to the five rights.
6. Take the medication to the patient's bedside.

## Procedure

1. Check the patient's identaband and ask him to state his name.
2. Clean the injection port closest to the needle or catheter with an alcohol swab.

3. Close the clamp on the IV tubing or pinch off the tubing.
4. Insert the needle into the port. **Rationale:** The needle should be inserted straight through the rubber end to ensure it does not pierce the plastic tubing.
5. Pull back on the plunger and observe for blood flashback. **Rationale:** This procedure ensures the needle or catheter is in the vein.
6. Inject the medication slowly or according to directions, and withdraw the needle when medication is infused.
7. Reopen the clamp and readjust the flow rate as ordered.

---

If the medication is to be injected directly into the vein, perform a veinpuncture and slowly inject the medication into the vein. Withdraw the needle and apply pressure or a bandaid to the puncture site until bleeding ceases.

---

## CHARTING  *for Medications*

☐ Type and amount of medication administered

☐ Rate medication administered

☐ Patient's response to medication

---

# CLINICAL PROBLEM SOLVING

## Potential Problems

Partial-fill bottle solution does not infuse adequately.

Solution in primary IV tubing is incompatible with medication to be administered via secondary additive set.

Unable to infuse solution through heparin lock.

## Suggested Solutions

☐ Check height of IV bottle.
☐ Check that primary IV bottle is lower than partial-fill bottle.
☐ Ensure that needle is positioned properly in the injection port.

☐ Prior to running medication into primary IV tubing, flush tubing with solution that is compatible with medication, e.g., normal saline or 5% dextrose in water. Then proceed with medication administration.
☐ If solution precipitates, discontinue the IV tubing and place new tubing on additive set. Flush the primary IV tubing with compatible solution and start the additive set infusing again.

☐ Gently push plunger on syringe. If resistance is met, do not force the plunger.
☐ Remove heparin lock and reinsert in another site.

# UNIT FIVE   BLOOD TRANSFUSIONS

## NURSING PROCESS DATA

### ASSESSMENT   *Data Base*

Assess if patient has an 18- or 19-gauge catheter or needle inserted in the vein.

Assess patient's vital signs, especially temperature, for baseline data.

Assess skin for eruptions or rashes to provide baseline data.

Assess for signs and symptoms of blood reactions during the transfusion.

Assess blood type and label before administration to ensure compatibility.

### PLANNING   *Objectives*

To provide blood or blood components, such as red blood cells, platelets, blood protein, and plasma, for patients who have a demonstrated deficiency.

To ensure compatibility between the patient's blood and the whole blood or packed red blood cells which may be transfused.

To prevent the infusion of fibrin clots and microaggregates (broken-down blood cells).

To monitor the transfusion of blood or blood components to ensure the blood infuses without complications.

To assess that the needle remains patent throughout the transfusion procedure.

To monitor for potential complications during and immediately following the blood transfusion.

### IMPLEMENTATION   *Procedures*

Administering Blood Through a Straight-Line

Administering Blood Through a Y-Set
Monitoring for Potential Complications
Administering Blood Components

### EVALUATION   *Expected Outcomes*

Transfusion of blood is performed smoothly without complications.

Needle remains patent throughout transfusion procedure.

Equipment is properly used for transfusion.

## ADMINISTERING BLOOD THROUGH A STRAIGHT-LINE

### Equipment

Blood unit

250 cc bottle of normal saline

Blood administration straight-line set

Venipuncture tray, if patient does not already have an IV in place

18- or 19-gauge needle or 18- to 20-gauge catheter

15-gauge needle if blood is to be administered rapidly

Alcohol swabs and tape

IV pole

### Preparation

1. Check physician's order for number of units and type of transfusion to be given.

2. Check that type and crossmatch has been completed and that blood is ready in the blood bank.

3. Obtain whole blood unit or packed blood cells unit from blood lab or blood bank.

4. Obtain the requisition form for the transfusion.

5. With lab technologist, check requisition form and lab blood record against the blood unit for essential data: patient's name and ID number, blood group and type (ABO and Rh), blood unit number, and expiration date of blood unit.

6. With another RN, check the requisition form and the lab blood record with the information on the patient's identification band to make sure that all data matches. Essential data includes patient's name and ID number, blood group, blood type, blood unit number, and expiration date on the blood unit.

7. Sign the form with the other RN according to hospital policy. Remember that blood must be started within 30 minutes from the time it is removed from refrigeration.

8. Check the blood bag for bubbles, cloudiness, dark color or sediment. **Rationale:** These signs indicate bacterial contamination.

9. Prime the blood administration set with normal saline. Use procedure for priming any IV tubing.

10. Ensure all air bubbles are out of tubing.

### Procedure

1. Rotate the blood unit bag gently to mix the blood cells and plasma.

2. With blood administration set ready, pull back the tabs on the blood unit bag and expose the port.

3. Carefully spike the port and hang the unit.

4. Fill the drip chamber by gently squeezing its flexible sides. Make sure the filter is submerged in the blood.

5. Open the clamp on the tubing, run the blood through the tubing, and cap the tubing.

6. If the patient needs a venipuncture, select a vein and insert an IV needle and tubing.

7. If the patient has a primary IV in place with an appropriate-sized needle, place an 18-gauge needle (or larger needle) in the end of the blood unit tubing.

8. If the primary IV solution is *not* compatible with the blood to be infused, remove the primary IV solution and cap it for sterility.

9. Spike the small bottle of normal saline and run this solution through the tubing. **Rationale:** Normal saline prevents cell hemolysis.

10. Prime the blood unit tubing.

11. Swab the injection port with alcohol.

12. Insert the needle carefully and tape it into place.

13. Shut off the primary IV and begin the blood transfusion.

14. Give blood slowly for the first 15 minutes, approximately 20 drops per minute which equates to 100 cc/hr.

15. Observe the patient closely for adverse reactions. Chilling, backache, headache, nausea or vomiting, tachycardia, tachypnea, skin rash, or hypotension are signs of complications.

---

**Clinical Alert**

Most patients can tolerate a flow rate of one unit of packed cells in one-and-a-half to two hours.

---

16. If there are no adverse effects, administer the blood unit at the prescribed rate.

17. Transfusion of the blood should be completed in

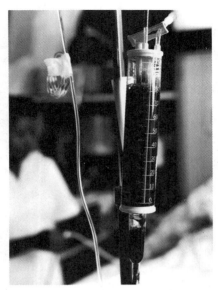

Volume-control sets, with a blood filter, can be used for administering blood.

less than four hours. **Rationale:** Blood deteriorates rapidly after a two-hour exposure to room temperature.

18. Continue to monitor the patient throughout the transfusion.

19. When you have completed the transfusion, flush the line with normal saline, inject the primary IV solution, and adjust the drip to the desired rate.

20. Remove the blood unit bag and administration set. If you are going to transfuse a second unit of blood, obtain that unit and a new administration set and repeat the procedure described above.

## ADMINISTERING BLOOD THROUGH A Y-SET

### Equipment

Blood unit

250-cc bottle of normal saline

Y-set IV tubing

### Procedure

1. Obtain and check blood as stated in Preparation for Administering Blood Through a Straight-Line.

2. Close all clamps on the Y-set.

3. Spike the small saline bottle with one port of the Y-tubing using aseptic technique; then spike the blood bag.

4. Hang both the saline bottle and blood bag on the IV pole.

5. Open the clamp to the saline bottle and squeeze the sides of the drip chamber until the filter is half covered and the drip chamber is full.

6. Open the main clamp and prime the rest of the tubing. To ensure easier flow, remove the cap that protects the end of the IV tubing.

7. When the tubing is primed, replace the cap and close the main clamp.

8. Cleanse the injection port on the primary IV.

9. Affix a large-gauge needle to the end of the tubing and prime the needle.

10. Insert the needle into the injection port and clamp off the primary IV flow.

11. Using saline solution, open the clamp to the saline bottle and turn clamp on the main tubing to begin the flow to clear primary IV tubing.

12. Clamp off the saline bottle and open the clamp to the blood bag.

13. Squeeze the sides of the Y-set drip chamber so that blood covers all the filter.

14. Follow procedure as you did with previous bottle.

15. When the blood bag is empty, clamp off the tubing to the bag, open the clamp to the normal saline bottle and flush the line.

16. Close all clamps and remove the needle from the injection port.

17. Open the clamp on the primary IV and establish the desired rate of administration.

18. Monitor the patient for signs and symptoms of blood transfusion reactions throughout procedure.

## MONITORING FOR POTENTIAL COMPLICATIONS

### Equipment

Sphygmomanometer

Stethoscope

Thermometer

### Procedure

1. Check temperature, blood pressure, pulse, and respiration before the transfusion is started.

2. Check vital signs every 5 to 15 minutes for the

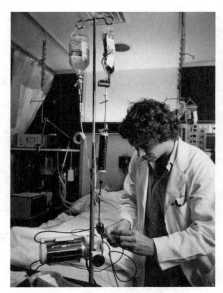

Blood should be warmed when large volumes are given over a short time period.

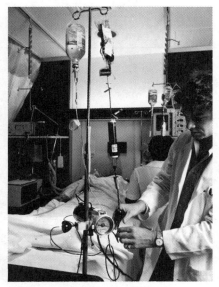

Blood should not be warmed above normal body temperature to prevent cell lysis.

first 100 cc's after the transfusion has been started. Most blood transfusion reactions occur during this time.

3. Maintain vital sign assessment throughout the blood infusion according to hospital policy.

4. Monitor the patient for possible transfusion reactions.

5. Notify the physician immediately if any unusual signs or symptoms occur during the blood infusion.

6. The registered nurse is responsible for preventing transfusion reactions by completing the following interventions:
   a. Identify patient and blood bottle or bag.
      (1) ID band number matches transfusion record number.
      (2) Name spelled correctly on transfusion record.
      (3) Blood bottle number and pilot tube number are the same.
      (4) Blood type matches on transfusion record and blood bottle.
   b. Check blood with another RN before infusing.
   c. Ask patient about allergy history and report any previous blood reactions.
   d. Establish baseline vital sign data.
   e. Start transfusion slowly to observe for severe reactions.

> ### Blood Transfusions
> Routine transfusions should not be warmed. If warming is required, as in massive transfusions, a blood warming coil is inserted into the transfusion line. Immerse coil in a 98.6°–100° F water bath. Once blood is warmed, it must be used or disposed of, as it cannot be returned to the blood bank. Hemolysis of the blood occurs at temperatures above 104° F.

   f. Maintain aseptic technique during procedure.
   g. Observe time rules (length of time blood can hang) for administering blood.
   h. Observe blood bag or bottle for bubbles, cloudiness, dark color, or black sediment, which is indicative of bacterial invasion.
   i. Do not allow blood to remain at room temperature unnecessarily.

## ADMINISTERING BLOOD COMPONENTS

### Equipment

Blood component

Appropriate IV administration set

**TABLE 6** BLOOD COMPONENT THERAPY

| TYPE | USE | ALERTS | ADMINISTRATION EQUIPMENT |
|---|---|---|---|
| Fresh Plasma | To replace deficient coagulation factors<br><br>To increase intravascular compartment | Hepatitis is a risk.<br><br>Administer as rapidly as possible.<br>Use within 6 hours. | Any straight line administration set |
| Platelets | To prevent or treat bleeding problems, especially in surgical clients<br><br>To replace platelets in clients with acquired or inherited deficiencies (thrombocytopenia, aplastic anemia)<br>To replace when platelets drop below 30,000 cu/mm (normal 150,000–350,000 cu/mm) | Administer at rate of 10 minutes a unit (usually come in multiple platelet packs). | Platelet transfusion set with special filter to allow platelets to infuse through filter |
| Granulocytes | To treat oncology clients with severe bone marrow depression and progressive infections<br><br>To treat granulocytopenic clients with infections that are unresponsive to antibiotics<br>To treat clients with gram-negative bacteremia or infections where marrow recovery does not develop | Administer slowly, over two to four hours.<br><br>Give one transfusion daily until granulocytes increase or infection clears.<br>Use within 48 hours after drawn.<br><br>Give when granulocytes are below 500.<br>Observe for shaking, fever, chills (treat with Tylenol before transfusions).<br>Observe for hives and laryngeal edema (treat with antihistamines). | Use Y-type blood filters and prime with physiological saline. A microaggregate filter is not used as it filters out platelets. |

## Procedure

1. Check physician's orders and Kardex.
2. Wash hands.
3. Obtain blood component from lab or appropriate source.
4. Obtain appropriate administration set.
5. Read directions for proper administration of the solution.
6. Identify rate at which blood component should infuse.
7. Check blood component therapy chart for appropriate rate, risk factors, and possible complications.

## CHARTING *for Blood Transfusions*

☐ Type and amount of blood administered

☐ Amount of normal saline used

☐ Size of needle inserted for administration

☐ Time transfusion began and ended

☐ Vital signs before transfusion begins; 15, 30, and 60 minutes after infusion begins; and then hourly until infusion completed

☐ Blood bank slip may have space for vital sign information as well

☐ Patient's response to procedure

☐ Any unusual clinical manifestations; any nursing interventions utilized

**TABLE 6** BLOOD COMPONENT THERAPY (continued)

| TYPE | USE | ALERTS | ADMINISTRATION EQUIPMENT |
|---|---|---|---|
| Serum Albumin | To treat shock | Available as 5% or 25% solution. | Special tubing accompanies albumin solution in individual boxes |
| | To treat hypoproteinemia | Infuse 25% solution slowly 1 ml/minute to prevent circulatory overload. | |
| | | Administer 100–200 cc (25% solution) for shock clients and 200–300 cc for hypoproteinemia. | |
| Gamma Globulin | To treat agammaglobulinemia | Pooled plasma contains antibodies to infectious agents. | Given IM |
| | To act as a prophylaxsis for hepatitis exposure | Administer 0.25 ml–0.50 ml of immune serum globulin per kg of body weight every two to four weeks. | |
| Coagulation Factors | To treat clients with von Willebrand's disease | Made from fresh-frozen plasma. | Standard syringe or component drip set only |
| Factor VIII (cryoprecipitate) | To treat clients with factor VIII, hemophilia A | Administer one unit cryoprecipitate for each 6 kg of body weight initially, followed by 1 unit/3 kg of body weight at 6- to 12-hour intervals until treatment discontinued. | |
| | | Administer one unit per five minutes. | |
| | | Observe for febrile reactions: shaking, fever, chills, and headache. | |
| Factor IX | To treat clients with factor IX, hemophilia B | Administer in 12- to 24-hour cycle. | Any straight line set |
| | | Preparation for administration is 400 to 500 u/vial. Must reconstitute in 10- to 20-cc diluent. | |
| | | One unit/lb. of body weight increases the circulating factor activity by 5%. | |
| | | Serum hepatitis can be transmitted. | |

# CLINICAL PROBLEM SOLVING

## Potential Problem

Transfusion reaction or alert conditions occur.

Blood does not flow through tubing.

## Suggested Solutions

□ Check transfusion chart for appropriate nursing intervention.
□ Complete all relevant nursing actions.

□ Check site where IV needle has been inserted to make sure it is in place.
□ Gently agitate the blood bag to mix the blood cells with the plasma.
□ Raise the blood bag to a higher location on the IV pole. Squeeze the flexible tubing to promote blood flow.

    ☐  Adjust clamp on tubing. As the blood unit passes over the filter, more blood microaggregates clog the filter and slow the drip rate.
    ☐  Replace the tubing.

Blood has been hanging for more than four hours.

    ☐  Take down blood bag and send to lab.
    ☐  Maintain IV with normal saline or ordered IV solution.
    ☐  Monitor vital signs for complications.

**TABLE 7** TRANSFUSION REACTIONS

| TYPE | CLINICAL MANIFESTATIONS | NURSING INTERVENTIONS |
|------|------------------------|----------------------|
| Bacterial | Sudden increase in temperature | Stop transfusion immediately. |
| | Hypotension | Maintain IV site; change tubing as soon as possible. |
| | Dry, flushed skin | Observe for shock. Monitor vital signs every 15 minutes until stable. |
| | Abdominal pain | Obtain urine specimen. Insert Foley if necessary. |
| | Headache | Notify physician and obtain order for broad spectrum antibiotic. |
| | Lumbar pain | Draw blood cultures before antibiotic administration. |
| | Sudden chill | Send blood tubing and bag to lab for culture and sensitivity. |
| | | Control hyperthermia. |
| Allergic | Urticaria and hives, pruritus | Stop transfusion immediately if symptoms are severe. |
| | Respiratory wheezing, laryngeal edema | Monitor vital signs for possible anaphylactic shock. |
| | Anaphylactic reaction | If symptoms are mild, slow down transfusion and obtain order for antihistamine. |
| | | Monitor for signs of progressive allergic reaction as transfusion continues. |
| Hemolytic | Severe pain in kidney region and chest | Stop transfusion immediately. |
| | Pain at needle insertion site | Change IV tubing as soon as possible, maintaining patent IV. If necessary, disconnect IV tubing from needle and run normal saline through IV tubing into emesis basin. Reconnect tubing to needle and obtain new tubing as soon as possible. |
| | Fever (may reach 105° F), chills | Administer oxygen. |
| | Dyspnea and cyanosis | Send two blood samples, from different sites, urine sample (cath if necessary), blood, and transfusion record to lab. |
| | Headache | Obtain orders for IV volume expansion and diuretic (mannitol) to ensure flushing of kidneys to prevent acute renal tubular necrosis. |
| | Hypotension | Monitor vital signs every 15 minutes for shock. |
| | Hematuria | Monitor urine output hourly for possible renal failure. Foley catheter may need to be inserted. |

# UNIT SIX   CENTRAL VENOUS PRESSURE SYSTEM

## NURSING PROCESS DATA

### ASSESSMENT  *Data Base*

Check presence of deformities that would interfere with insertion.

Determine patient's level of consciousness so full explanation of procedure can be done to allay anxiety.

Assess level of anxiety to determine need for possible premedication.

Assess skin and surrounding tissue for erythema, edema, and warmth.

**PLANNING**   *Objectives*

To assist the physician with CVP insertion.

To maintain patency of CVP line.

To change CVP dressing without complications.

To maintain the insertion site free of infection and the catheter free of clots.

To accurately measure and record the CVP reading.

**IMPLEMENTATION**   *Procedures*

Assisting with CVP Catheterization

Changing a CVP Dressing

Measuring and Monitoring a CVP

**EVALUATION**   *Expected Outcomes*

CVP line is properly placed in right atrium.

CVP manometer and line remain open, accurately reflecting pressure in the patient's right atrium.

Central venous dressing is changed without complications.

CVP reading is accomplished accurately.

Complications associated with fluid balance are detected early.

## ASSISTING WITH CVP CATHETERIZATION

### Equipment

Routine IV setup with pole

CVP catheter

Water manometer

Three-way stopcock

Tape

In-the-needle radiopaque catheter, 14- to 16-gauge needle that is 15 to 20 cm long

Sterile two- by two-inch and four- by four-inch sponges

Anesthetic, sterile syringes, and needles

Sterile gloves, drapes, and sutures

### Procedure

1. Explain procedure to patient.

> **Clinical Alert**
> Central venous pressure is a measure of the pressure of blood in the right atrium or vena cava. It is measured in centimeters of water pressure, which vary even within the normal range of values cited.

2. Place patient in Trendelenburg's position (approximately 15- to 30-degree angle). **Rationale:** This position prevents air embolism.

3. Extend patient's neck and upper chest by placing a rolled pillow or blanket under the shoulders. Make sure that the side of the patient's neck or chest where the CVP line will be inserted is closest to physician.

4. Turn patient's head away from the site of the venipuncture. **Rationale:** This facilitates filling the vessel with blood.

5. Maintaining sterility, open the glove packet and sterile drape pack. (Physician should wear sterile gloves for this procedure.)

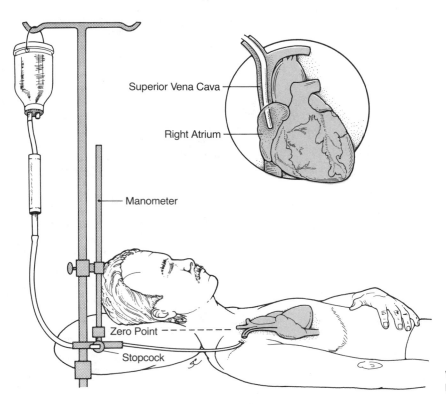

Superior Vena Cava

Right Atrium

Manometer

Zero Point

Stopcock

When a CVP reading is taken, the patient should
be lying in a horizontal position.

6. Open the povidone-iodine prep pads.

   *Physician's Actions*

   a. Physician dons sterile gloves for this procedure.

   b. The physician preps the patient's skin, drapes the area, and, using a sterile syringe and needle, draws up anesthetic to infiltrate the site.

   c. Using the large needle and syringe, the physician will insert the needle into the central vein (subclavian or internal jugular).

   d. Once the vein is entered and the needle is placed correctly, the physician will remove the syringe and advance the catheter through the needle to the desired length. (The needle and catheter must be handled as one unit. The catheter must never be pulled back through the needle as this may shear off a part of the catheter and create an embolus.)

   e. With the catheter in place, the physician will withdraw the obturator, if one is used, and pull back the needle.

   f. The physician will then attach the IV tubing to the hub of the needle or to an adapter.

   g. The physician will finally snap the needle

   guard around the needle and suture the catheter into place.

7. As the physician is working, have the patient perform Valsalva's maneuver to prevent air embolism.

   a. Instruct patient to exhale against a closed glottis.

   b. If patient is unable to do this, compress the patient's abdomen. **Rationale:** Both these procedures will help to decrease chances of air embolism.

8. When the physician has completed the catheterization, adjust the infusion drip to the desired rate of administration.

9. Cover the insertion site with povidone-iodine ointment, sterile gauze pads, and tape.

10. After the position of the radiopaque catheter has been checked with an x-ray, dress the catheter insertion site according to hospital policy. (See following intervention for dressing change.)

11. Tape all connections on the tubing.

12. Label the insertion site with the date, nurse's initials, and the time of insertion.

# CHANGING A CVP DRESSING

## Equipment

Routine IV setup with pole

CVP catheter

Water manometer

Three-way stopcock

Tape

Mask

Central catheter dressing kit or sterile gloves, mask(s), drape(s), acetone wipes, 70% alcohol pads, saline or hydrogen peroxide, povidone-iodine ointment, sterile two- by two-inch gauze pads with precut slits

Tincture of benzoin

Air-occlusive tape

Receptacle for soiled dressing, e.g., paper bag, plastic bag

## Preparation

1. Check Patient Care Plan and Kardex for last dressing change.
2. Gather equipment.
3. Check the location of the central vein catheter.
4. If located in the patient's neck or subclavian area, position the patient flat on his back. **Rationale:** This eliminates the risk of air embolism.
5. Turn the patient's head away from the insertion site and mask the patient's nose and mouth if necessary.
6. Wash your hands thoroughly.
7. Explain the procedure to the patient.
8. Make sure that all personnel don masks.

## Procedure

1. Carefully remove the old dressing and tape without pulling on the catheter or touching the soiled surfaces of the dressing.
2. Discard the old dressing in the receptacle obtained for the purpose.
3. Put on sterile gloves.
4. Using a sterile gauze pad and saline or hydrogen peroxide, clean the debris, such as dried blood or serum, from the insertion site and catheter.

> **Clinical Alert**
>
> It is important to be aware that only an RN who has had special preparation is qualified to change a central venous dressing due to the danger of air embolism during dressing change.

5. After the site is clean, check for signs of infection, inflammation, or infiltration.
6. If skin, insertion site, and catheter look normal, cleanse the skin around the catheter, working from the insertion site outward in a circular motion. Do not scrub the catheter with acetone solution. **Rationale:** Acetone will damage the plastic part of the catheter.
7. Apply an antimicrobial solution, such as povidone-iodine, working from the insertion site outward in a circular motion. **Rationale:** Working from cleanest area to least clean prevents contamination.
8. Apply the povidone-iodine ointment directly on the insertion site.
9. Place precut sterile two- by two-inch gauze pads around the insertion site. The catheter should protrude through the center of the pads.
10. Apply tincture of benzoin around the edges of the pads.
11. Change the tubing, if hospital policy requires dressing and tubing to be changed at the same time.
    a. Loosen the tubing in the catheter hub. (Policy may dictate that you wipe the hub with an alcohol swab at this time.)
    b. Tell the patient to hold his breath and bear down while you insert the new tubing into the hub of the catheter. **Rationale:** This prevents air embolism.
    c. Tape the connection.
12. Tape the dressing around the catheter site.
13. Tape the connection of the tubing on the catheter hub to the patient's skin. (If a filter is part of the central line tubing, i.e., a hyperalimentation catheter, you may secure the filter to the dressing with tape.)
14. Label the dressing with the date and your initials.
15. Change the catheter dressings every 48 hours. If the dressing becomes loose, wet, or soiled, it is contaminated and should be changed.

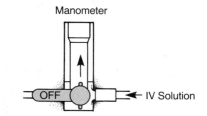

Solution to Manometer

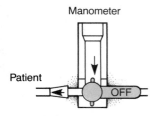

Manometer to Patient

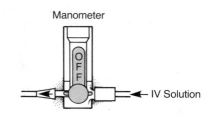

Solution to Patient

Top stopcock: Fill the manometer by turning stopcock OFF to the patient. This allows solution to flow from the bottle to the manometer. Middle stopcock: Measure CVP by turning stopcock OFF to IV solution allowing fluid to flow from manometer to patient. Bottom stopcock: Reinstitute flow from IV bottle to patient by turning stopcock OFF to the manometer.

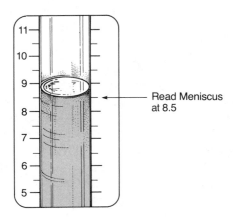

Read Meniscus at 8.5

Take CVP reading at highest level of meniscus and in response to patient's breathing.

# MEASURING AND MONITORING A CVP

## Equipment

Stopcock

Manometer

IV solution bottle

Administration set

IV pole with C arm

## Procedure

1. Determine the desired CVP parameters. Check the Patient Care Plan, physician's orders and Kardex. **Rationale:** When changes occur beyond the values established for the patient, check the CVP system and the patient's vital signs. If the CVP system is functioning correctly, report changes in values to the physician.

2. Establish a baseline by taking the patient's vital signs and by checking the patient's hydration status.

3. Spike the IV solution bottle with the IV administration set.

4. Prime the tubing with the solution, making certain that no air bubbles are present in the tubing.

5. Close the clamp on the tubing. If you are using a reusable manometer scale, affix a three-way stopcock to one end of the IV tubing.

6. Place tubing into manometer scale and snap stopcock into place below the manometer. If you are using a one-piece disposable manometer and stopcock, affix the unit to an IV pole with a C-shaped clamp.

7. Push the male end of the IV administration set into the female end of the stopcock connecting the IV set to the stopcock.

8. Turning the stopcock so that the manometer and IV solution are open to each other, open the clamp on the IV tubing and fill the manometer with IV solution to between 18 and 20 cm.

9. Close the clamp and rotate the stopcock so that the IV solution is open to the patient.

10. With IV solution, prime the rest of the IV tubing that extends from the stopcock and connect tubing to CVP catheter.

11. Place the patient flat in bed, without a pillow.

12. Locate the patient's right atrium (midaxillary at the fourth intercostal space). Mark this location on the patient's skin.

13. Adjust the level of the manometer so that zero on the manometer scale is at the same level as the patient's right atrium. (Use a yardstick and carpenter's level if this type of apparatus is not part of the manometer.)

14. Turn the stopcock to the open position for the manometer IV solution, filling the manometer with additional solution if needed.

15. Turn the stopcock to the manometer-patient position and watch the level of the solution in the manometer fall to the pressure level existing in the right atrium. **Rationale:** Normally, this pressure should be between 3 and 12 cm. It is important to remember, however, that there are no absolute values and that the trends—the rise and fall—of CVP readings are more important to the individual patient than one pressure level reading.

16. Observe the meniscus at eye level and watch the rise and fall of the fluid column in response to the patient's breathing. **Rationale:** Respiratory fluctuations reflect the changes in intrathoracic pressures during the respiratory cycle.

17. Take the reading at the highest level of the fluid column.

18. Turn off the stopcock to the manometer and adjust the rate of infusion with the clamp.

19. Return the patient to the desired position and record CVP readings.

### CHARTING  *for CVP Catheterization*

☐ Location of insertion site

☐ Type and size of needle or cannula used for insertion

☐ Time of insertion

☐ Appearance of needle insertion site

☐ Name of physician performing catheterization

☐ Types of solutions used, including all additives listed in sequence used

☐ Amount of solution infused

☐ Time x-ray was performed to check position of radiopaque catheter

☐ Time and date dressing and/or tubing changed

☐ Initials of person changing the dressing

☐ Condition of catheter insertion site when dressing changed

☐ Date and time of CVP reading (record subsequent CVP readings on appropriate forms)

☐ Condition of flow rate

☐ Patient's response to treatment

☐ Any unusual conditions or reactions

---

## CLINICAL PROBLEM SOLVING

| Potential Problems | Suggested Solutions |
|---|---|
| Air enters central vein, producing air embolism. | ☐ Inform physician immediately.<br>☐ Place patient in a head-down position with the right atrium uppermost. Monitor until physician arrives. |
| CVP system does not drip. | ☐ Check the entire line for kinks in the tubing. Change patient's position. Check to make sure the manometer stopcock is in the IV-patient position.<br>☐ Notify physician and gather equipment for catheter irrigation.<br>☐ Obtain order for placing heparin in IV bottle to prevent clotting at tip of catheter. |
| CVP readings appear to be inaccurate. | ☐ Assess patency of set-up.<br>☐ Assess patient's level of pain; pain increases the CVP reading. |

☐ Assess if position of patient has been changed; raising the head of the bed alters the reading.

☐ If patient is on a respirator take him off the respirator, instruct him to deep breathe, and repeat reading. The respirator, if not removed, causes a falsely high reading.

☐ Check that the marked area at midaxillary level is at the level of the patient's right atrium. Patients with barrel chests should be marked different from normal patients.

☐ Assess if the patient has COPD, CHF (especially right-sided), or hypovolemia, as they alter the reading.

CVP dressing is wet following dressing change.

☐ If leakage around the catheter has wet the dressing and skin, check all connections.

☐ Lower the solution and check for backflow of blood in the tubing.

☐ Describe the type of leakage to the physician.

☐ Tape the dressing securely to ensure connections do not become loosened.

## UNIT SEVEN   HICKMAN CATHETER

### NURSING PROCESS DATA

#### ASSESSMENT   *Data Base*

Assess patency of catheter.

Assess insertion site for signs of infection.

Assess the tubing for accidental breaks.

Assess injection cap at the end of catheter to ensure tightness.

#### PLANNING   *Objectives*

To provide an access for blood drawing.

To provide an access for chemotherapeutic infusions.

To provide total parenteral nutrition.

To monitor central venous pressure if a CVP catheter is not available.

#### IMPLEMENTATION   *Procedures*

Maintaining the Hickman Catheter

Changing the Dressing

Drawing Blood from the Catheter

#### EVALUATION   *Expected Outcomes*

The catheter remains patent.

The catheter site is infection free.

Blood samples are obtained without difficulty.

Infusions of medications or fluids are accomplished without difficulty.

## MAINTAINING THE HICKMAN CATHETER

### Equipment

Clamp without teeth

Cap such as Leur lock or Becton-Dickinson

Heparin 1:1000 cc solution

Normal saline

6 cc syringe and small gauge needle

3 tuberculin syringes

10 cc syringe

Betadine or alcohol swab

Nonallergic tape

### Preparation

1. Check physician's orders and Patient Care Plan.

2. Wash hands.

3. Gather equipment.

4. Prepare heparin solution. Mix 0.3 cc of heparin in 30 cc of normal saline. (Use 1:1000 cc solution of heparin.)

5. Explain procedure to patient.

6. Provide privacy for patient.

7. Raise bed to high position.

### Procedure

*For securing catheter*

1. Remove pressure dressing from catheter insertion.

2. Cleanse insertion site at entrance and exit sites according to procedure.

3. Replace cap with Becton-Dickinson at end of catheter, if desired.

4. Wrap a piece of tape around catheter (approximately 3 inches from end). **Rationale:** The clamp is placed over the taped area of the catheter to prevent a break in the tubing. Clamp without teeth is used to prevent piercing.

5. Tape the cap at the end of catheter. **Rationale:** Tape secures the cap to the catheter and prevents separation of the two parts.

6. Secure catheter to gown or tape securely to chest.

*For irrigating catheter*

1. Wipe the end of the catheter cap with Betadine or alcohol swab.

2. Insert the needle of the 6 cc syringe filled with heparin solution into cap.

3. Unclamp catheter.

4. Insert heparin solution slowly through catheter until ½ cc remains.

5. Clamp the catheter over the taped area of catheter as the plunger is moving forward. **Rationale:** This procedure promotes positive pressure in the catheter and prevents clotting by preventing backflow of blood into the catheter.

6. Withdraw the syringe.

7. Secure the catheter end to catheter tubing.

*For irrigating a nonpatent catheter*

1. Prepare three tuberculin syringes with heparin. **Rationale:** The size of this syringe increases the pressure exerted in the system.

2. Take cap off catheter. Insert syringe tip into catheter.

3. Inject the heparin from the syringes, to a total of 3 cc.

4. Place cap back on catheter. Leave heparin in catheter tubing for one hour.

5. At the end of one hour, use a 10 cc syringe to aspirate the solution from the catheter by placing the tip of the syringe securely into catheter and gently pulling back on plunger.

6. If aspiration is successful, follow with an irrigation of 5 to 10 cc of heparinized solution. Use same dilution factor for irrigation solution as with the maintenance solution.

7. The procedure may be repeated once. If unsuccessful, notify the physician.

## CHANGING THE DRESSING

### Equipment

Betadine solution

Alcohol swab

Cleansing solution, e.g., hydrogen peroxide

2″ × 2″ dressings

Nonallergic tape

Sterile cotton-tipped swabs

### Procedure

1. Remove old dressing.

2. Observe for signs and symptoms of infection at insertion site. **Rationale:** Signs most frequently observed are erythema, edema, and drainage.

3. Clean the exit site with cleansing solution and sterile applicators. Starting from the inner aspect, move toward the periphery. **Rationale:** Clean from cleanest to least clean area to prevent contamination at the insertion site.

4. Clean the catheter tubing starting from the exit site down toward the cap using an alcohol swab.

5. Apply antibacterial ointment around exit site.

6. Place clean 2″ × 2″ gauze over site and tape securely.

7. Secure catheter to prevent dislodging.

---

**Clinical Alert**

The dressing should be changed daily when the patient is immunosuppressed. Sterile dressings should be used when infection could be life-threatening.

---

## DRAWING BLOOD FROM THE CATHETER

### Equipment

6 cc syringe

6 cc syringe filled with heparinized saline

10 cc syringe (or larger size if needed) for drawing blood

Blood tubes appropriate for tests ordered

Receptacle (e.g., plastic cup) for discarded blood

### Procedure

1. Remove cap from catheter end.

2. Place 6 cc syringe into catheter and unclamp catheter.

3. Withdraw 6 cc of blood from catheter and clamp catheter.

4. Discard blood into receptacle.

5. Attach 10 cc syringe to catheter and withdraw required amount of blood for lab tests. **Rationale:** Each lab test requires a specific number of cc's of blood for the test. Check the lab manual for exact amount needed for each test.

6. Clamp catheter and withdraw syringe. Inject blood into the lab blood tubes by taking the cap off tubes and gently filling the tubes with blood. **Rationale:** Blood cells are easily damaged if put through needles into the lab tubes, which causes hemolysis and abnormal lab results.

7. Attach 6 cc syringe filled with heparin solution into catheter.

8. Unclamp catheter and gently infuse solution.

9. Clamp catheter according to procedure and withdraw syringe.

10. Replace cap at end of catheter.

11. Secure catheter.

---

**Clinical Alert**

If solutions or medications are to be infused through the catheter, use the same procedure as for infusing any IV. Use a small gauge needle for infusing fluid through the cap. If fluid viscosity allows, attach extension IV tubing to catheter and infuse solution.

---

### CHARTING  *for Hickman Catheter*

☐ Irrigation performed with heparinized solution

☐ Dressings changed with type of ointment applied

☐ Patency of catheter

☐ Amount of blood withdrawn for testing

☐ Color of blood withdrawn

☐ Exit site condition

☐ Any medications or solutions administered through the catheter

## CLINICAL PROBLEM SOLVING

| Potential Problems | Suggested Solutions |
|---|---|
| Unable to aspirate blood even though solution flows through the catheter. | ☐ Since tip of catheter is probably lodged against the wall of the right atrium, perform the following actions:<br>    Use less pressure on barrel of syringe when aspirating blood.<br>    Have patient raise arms above head. This can alter position of catheter.<br>    Have patient perform Valsalva's maneuver. |
| Clotting of catheter occurs. | ☐ Use irrigating procedure.<br>    If catheter is clotted only a brief time you can attempt to instill 1 cc of 1:1000 cc heparin solution followed by 1 cc normal saline. Allow 15 minutes of clamping to see if declotting occurs. You may need to repeat this procedure several times. |
| Catheter breaks or is pierced by clamp. | ☐ Immediately clamp catheter above break site.<br>☐ Place a blunt-ended needle or intracatheter into catheter. Number 14 usually works best.<br>☐ Tape catheter and needle together securely.<br>☐ Notify physician immediately. |

## TERMINOLOGY

**Anaphylaxis:** a hypersensitive state of the body to a foreign protein or drug.

**Antiarrhythmic:** an agent used to regulate heart rhythm.

**Antidiuretic:** a drug which decreases urine secretion.

**Antimicrobic:** preventing the development or pathogenic action of microbes.

**Ascites:** the excessive accumulation of serous fluid in the peritoneal cavity.

**Aspirate:** to remove material by suction.

**Cardio:** pertaining to the heart.

**Cardiovascular:** pertaining to the heart and blood vessels.

**Cyanosis:** slightly bluish, grayish, slatelike, or dark-purple discoloration.

**Diarrhea:** frequent passage of watery bowel movements.

**Diffusion:** spreading or dispersing of molecules in solution, as a gas or liquid.

**Diuretic:** a chemical agent that increases the secretion of urine.

**Dyspnea:** air hunger resulting in labored or difficult breathing.

**Edema:** body tissues containing an excessive amount of fluid.

**Electrolyte:** a solution that is a conductor of electricity; minerals are common electrolytes.

**Evaporation:** change from liquid to vapor.

**Extracellular:** outside the cell.

**Girth:** the distance around something; circumference, as in measuring abdominal circumference.

**Granulocytes:** a granular leukocyte.

**Hematoma:** a collection of clotted blood confined in a space.

**Hematuria:** blood in the urine.

**Hemo-:** prefix meaning blood.

**Hemolytic:** pertinent to the breaking down of red blood cells.

**Homeostasis:** state of equilibrium of the internal environment.

**Hydration:** the chemical combination of a substance with water.

**Hydrostatic:** pertaining to the pressure of liquids in equilibrium and the pressure exerted on liquids.

**Hypersecretion:** Abnormally large amount of secretion.

**Hypovolemia:** diminished circulating fluid volume.

**Infusion:** a liquid substance introduced into the body via a vein for therapeutic purposes.

**Intracellular:** inside the cell.

**Intravascular:** within blood vessels.

**Metabolism:** the sum of all physical and chemical changes that take place within an organism.

**Nephro:** prefix meaning kidney.

**Nephrotoxic:** a toxin that destroys renal cells.

**Osmosis:** the passage of solvent through a partition separating solutions of different concentrations.

**Palpate:** to examine by touch; to feel.

**Pruritis:** severe itching.

**Purulent:** containing pus.

**Skin turgor:** the tension or fullness of the cells.

**Specific gravity:** weight of a substance compared with an equal volume of water.

**Transfusion:** injection of the blood or a blood component of one person into the blood vessels of another.

**Urticaria:** a vascular reaction of the skin characterized by the eruption of pale raised wheals, which are associated with severe itching.

**Valsalva's maneuver:** attempt to forcibly exhale with the nose and mouth closed.

**Venipuncture:** puncture of a vein with a needle.

**Viscosity:** resistance offered by a fluid; property of a substance that is dependent on the friction of its component molecules as they slide by each other.

# Chapter 27

# *Orthopedic Measures*

## LEARNING OBJECTIVES

Define the mnemonic ICE.

Differentiate between four types of fractures.

Compare and contrast skeletal and skin traction.

Write three nursing diagnoses which would be appropriate for patients requiring special orthopedic procedures.

Demonstrate the application of a circular and figure-eight bandage.

Demonstrate the procedure of applying an air splint.

Compare and contrast plaster and synthetic casts.

Describe the steps in assessing a casted extremity.

Complete a patient teaching guide for patients requiring a synthetic cast.

Outline the procedure for monitoring a patient in traction.

Discuss the nursing care necessary for patients in a halo traction.

List the relevant charting data for halo traction.

Explain the rationale for applying a shrink bandage to an amputated limb.

Demonstrate the various bed positions for the Nelson bed.

Demonstrate a patient turn on a CircOlectric bed.

State one potential problem of turning a patient on a Stryker frame and describe at least two suggested solutions.

Discuss the nursing care for patients on special beds.

**RESTORING FUNCTION**

Orthopedic nursing involves the prevention and correction of alterations in the musculoskeletal system. To help patients achieve and maintain optimal mobility, nurses use preventative, restorative, and rehabilitative methods. Preventative and restorative measures include the use of bandages, splints, traction, and casts. Rehabilitative treatments include the use of special beds and halo traction.

Bandages are used for applying pressure over an area; immobilizing a body part; preventing or reducing edema; correcting a deformity; and securing splints in place. Several types of material are used as bandages. Woven cotton, elastic webbing, and gauze are the most common materials.

When sprains, strains, contusions, or dislocations occur, remember the mnemonic ICE. ICE will assist you in recalling the initial interventions for these injuries. "I" refers to immobilization, usually with a bandage or by splinting. "C" stands for application of cold treatments, such as ice packs. Cold is applied for 24 to 48 hours. "E" refers to elevation of the affected extremity. These interventions will prevent edema formation and other complications.

**Fractures**   The long bone, the most common type involved in fractures, is composed of the shaft, or diaphysis, and the flared end of the bone, termed the metaphysis. In children there are two important segments—the physis, which is the growth region, and the epiphysis, which is directly adjacent to joints. The epiphysis fuses to the metaphysis at the end of the growth period. Injuries to long bones in childhood can result in growth retardation or arrest in the longitudinal growth of the limb.

When a bone is fractured, a specific repair process takes place. This process begins with the formation of a blood clot at the site of the fracture. Once this clot is formed, osteoblasts and fibroblasts converge on the site and start laying down the organic matrix. Together, the fibrin net, the osteoblasts, and the organic matrix form a callus into which calcium salts are deposited. This callus evolves into regular bone tissue, which connects the pieces of original bone. In the final stage of the repair process, osteoblasts and osteoclasts remodel the callus area into a permanent and strong bone.

Fractures are classified in a variety of ways. One classification is by the type of injury to the bone or surrounding tissue. Examples of these fractures include a transverse fracture, which proceeds directly across the bone; an oblique fracture, which proceeds at an angle across the bone; and, a comminuted fracture, which results in more than two fragments of bone being displaced.

Fractures can also be classified as open or closed. An open fracture is one in which the skin has been broken due to penetration of a bone fragment or external trauma. An open fracture requires additional treatment to prevent infection as a result of the skin puncture. Surgical debridement and irrigation must be completed within hours of the fracture. A closed fracture indicates that the fracture is contained under the skin surface.

Soft tissue injury is also a probability with fractures. Immediate splinting and elevation of the extremity can prevent complications.

## TYPES OF FRACTURE

| | |
|---|---|
| A crack; the bending of a bone with incomplete fracture. Only affects one side of the periosteum. Common in skull fractures or in young children when bones are pliable. | *Greenstick* |
| Bone completely broken in a transverse, spiral, or oblique direction (indicates the direction of the fracture in relation to the long axis of the fracture bone). Bone broken into several fragments. | *Comminuted* |
| Bone is exposed to the air through a break in the skin. Can be associated with soft tissue injury as well. Infection is common complication due to exposure to bacterial invasion. | *Open, or compound* |
| Skin remains intact. Chances are greatly decreased for infection. | *Closed, or simple* |
| Frequently seen with vertebral fractures. Fractured bone has been compressed by other bones. | *Compression* |
| Bone is broken with a disruption of both sides of the periosteum. | *Complete* |

| *Impacted* | One part of fractured bone is driven into another. |
| --- | --- |
| *Depressed fracture* | Usually seen in skull or facial fractures. Bone or fragments of bone are driven inward. |
| *Pathological* | Break caused by disease process. |

Fractures are treated by simple reduction. This results in manipulating broken bones to return to their normal anatomical position. Closed fractures are treated in this manner. Casts are generally applied to maintain the reduced fracture in proper alignment. Casts are made from plaster of Paris or synthetic materials, such as polyester, cotton, fiberglass, or plastic. The synthetic casts dry faster, weigh less, and can get wet without fear of cracking or disintegration. One major disadvantage of synthetic casts is the cost. Another disadvantage is the inability to mold easily which prevents their use for immobilizing severely displaced bones or unstable fractures. Casted extremities need to be observed frequently during the drying process. When assessing the patient in a cast, remember to check for pulse, distal to the cast, pain, pallor, and paresthesia (the four P's).

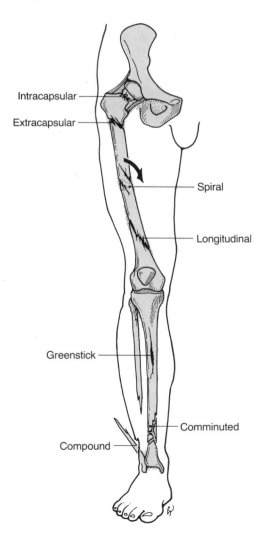

Types of fractures.

**Traction** Traction is another measure used to treat fractures. It is most effective and useful when reduction of the bone fracture is required. Two types of traction are used: skin traction and skeletal traction. Skeletal traction is usually more reliable and effective for it maintains the reduction of the fractured limb. To provide the traction, a steel pin or wire is inserted through the distal fragment and attached to the traction apparatus. The usual types of skeletal traction are Russell's and the Thomas splint with Pearson attachment. With skeletal traction, the affected limb is maintained in an elevated position, which decreases edema and promotes healing.

Skeletal traction can pose problems by causing infection at the pin site and promoting neurovascular complications. Much of the nurse's responsibility centers on the assessment and prevention of these complications. Manipulating and altering traction are not a nursing responsibility; however, ensuring that ropes go through pulleys and that weights hang freely are part of the nursing responsibility.

Many types of skin traction are seen in hospital settings. The oldest and simplest type is Buck's traction. This type of traction is usually applied for short periods of time on young patients with knee injuries. Elderly patients may require Buck's traction prior to surgical repair for a fractured hip. With skin traction, a skin prep is placed on the leg before applying strips of moleskin to either side of the leg. An ace bandage wrapped around the extremity holds the traction in place. Circulatory compromise and skin allergies or abrasions are two of the complications that can occur with this type of traction.

Bryant's traction, another type of skin traction, is used primarily for children under 3 years of age who have sustained a fractured femur. Neck halters and pelvic traction are also forms of skin traction. Neurovascular and skin complications can occur with each of these modalities of treatment; therefore, frequent observations by the nurse are required.

Patients who require the more sophisticated orthopedic procedures may be immobilized by the use of several pieces of equipment. The halo traction, the Jewett-Taylor brace, and the Stryker frame are used to immobilize patients with spinal cord injury.

Patients with spinal cord injury are immobilized to prevent further complications and to promote healing. Cervical traction can be maintained most easily with the Stryker frame. Skeletal traction may be necessary and is applied by placing tongs through burr holes in the outer layer of the skull. Weights are applied to ropes connected to the tongs to provide constant hyperextension of the head.

Following surgical immobilization of the spinal cord with Harrington rods, patients are usually placed on the Stryker frame or in a regular hospital bed. When placed in the hospital bed, patients are turned in log-roll fashion to prevent torsion of the spine. Generally, a Jewett-Taylor brace is applied before getting the patient out of bed. The brace maintains spinal cord alignment.

Halo traction is becoming more popular because this form of immobilization allows early mobility of patients. When the patient is able to be up in the wheelchair, physical complications such as pneumonia and circulatory impairment can be avoided. Some spinal cord fractures can be immobilized with the halo while others require surgical intervention. Application of the halo follows surgery and functions as a stabilizing modality.

**Special Beds** The Nelson bed is used when movement of a body part could result in a complication. Following total hip replacement surgery, patients are often placed in this bed to prevent hip flexion when getting out of bed.

The CircOlectric bed can be helpful in the treatment of immobility when the patient requires turning and positioning. To facilitate positioning and dressing changes, burn patients are sometimes placed on these beds. This bed also provides optimal care for immobilized patients.

Patients on long-term bed rest are prone to the following complications: respiratory problems, especially pneumonia; thrombophlebitis or embolus due to stasis in circulation; muscle atrophy and contractures; skin breakdown; urinary retention and calculi; constipation; and altered body image. Nursing measures to prevent complications are a major factor in providing care for orthopedic patients.

## NURSING DIAGNOSES

The following nursing diagnoses may be appropriate to include in a Patient Care Plan when the components relate to a patient who requires special orthopedic procedures.

| Nursing Diagnosis (Potential) | Defining Characteristic; Etiology (Examples) |
| --- | --- |
| □ Comfort, Alteration in: Pain, *related to* | Improper position, alignment, or application of equipment, e.g., cast, sling, Stryker frame. |
| | Improper alignment, e.g., position on Stryker frame or in traction. |
| □ Mobility, Impaired Physical, *related to* | Decreased motor function or interruption of central nervous system, e.g., physical injury, disease process (spinal cord injury or surgical intervention). |
| | Joint contractures, e.g., inappropriate or inadequately performed range-of-motion exercises. |
| □ Self-Care Deficit, *related to* | Physical limitations, e.g., immobilized body or limb. |
| □ Self-Concept, Disturbance in: Body Image, *related to* | Change in body capability, e.g., spinal cord injury or long-term immobilization. |
| □ Skin Integrity, Impairment of, *related to* | Pressure points, e.g., improper application of cast, sling, or traction. |
| □ Social Isolation, *related to* | Decreased opportunity for communication or interaction with peers, e.g., long-term confinement in traction, on Stryker frame or CircOlectric bed. |

# UNIT ONE   BANDAGE APPLICATION

## NURSING PROCESS DATA

### ASSESSMENT   *Data Base*

Assess need for bandages.

Identify appropriate type of bandage required.

Assess surrounding area of bandage to ensure it is not restrictive.

Evaluate bandage for tightness and evenness of pressure.

Evaluate the affected extremity for circulation, sensation and movement.

### PLANNING  *Objectives*

To immobilize a joint or extremity.

To provide support to an injured extremity or surgical site.

To prevent edema to injured extremity.

To secure a dressing in place.

### IMPLEMENTATION  *Procedures*

Applying a Sling

Applying a Circular Bandage

Applying a Spiral Bandage

Applying a Figure Eight Bandage

### EVALUATION  *Expected Outcomes*

Affected joint or extremity is immobilized.

Edema is decreased in affected extremity.

Dressings are held securely in place.

## APPLYING A SLING

### Equipment

Sling or

Triangular bandage

Safety pin

### Procedure

1. Check physician's order for sling.
2. If commercial slings are not available, obtain a triangular cloth or bandage.
3. Explain use of sling to patient.
4. Place one end of triangular cloth over the shoulder on the unaffected arm.
5. Place cloth against the body and under the affected arm.
6. Place the apex, or point, of the triangle toward the elbow.

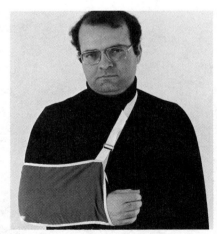

The purpose of this type sling is to support the entire arm and hand.

7. Bring the opposite end of the triangle around the affected arm and over the affected shoulder.
8. Tie the sling at the side of the neck.

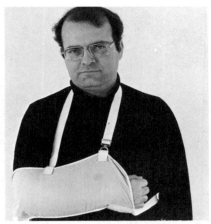

This type of sling supports the arm and hand and immobilizes the shoulder.

9. Fold the apex of the triangle over the elbow in the front and secure with a safety pin.

10. Assess patient for comfort and for support of the affected arm.

11. Monitor for adequate circulation every two hours.

---

**If Using Commercial Sling**

Check directions on package for proper application.

---

## APPLYING A CIRCULAR BANDAGE

### Equipment

Roller bandages

Metal clip or safety pin

### Procedure

1. Gather necessary roller bandages. The number and size of the bandages are dependent on the extent and area of the extremity to be bandaged.

2. Explain the use of the bandage to the patient.

3. Elevate the extremity. **Rationale:** This position prevents the bandage from becoming too tight after wrapping.

4. Begin to wrap the extremity at the distal end. Anchor the bandage with at least two circular turns. A moderate amount of tension should be maintained on the bandage during the application.

5. Continue to unroll the bandage and overlap the previous circle until the designated area is covered.

6. Secure the bandage with tape, safety pin, or metal clip.

7. Observe for even, tight fit of the bandage and ensure the bandage is not occluding circulation.

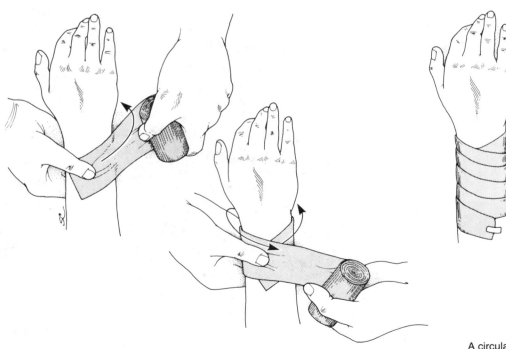

A circular turn is used for anchoring and securing a bandage.

**Rationale:** Uneven wrapping can result in circulatory impairment and skin disruption.

8. Assess extremity every two hours for circulation, and ensure that the bandage is wrinkle-free.

9. Rewrap bandage at least every eight hours.

## APPLYING A SPIRAL BANDAGE

### Equipment

Roller bandages

Metal clip or safety pin

### Procedure

1. Gather necessary roller bandages.

2. Explain necessity for bandage to patient.

3. Elevate the extremity to be bandaged.

4. Anchor the bandage with two circular turns at the distal end of the extremity.

5. After anchoring the bandage, begin the spiral turns by moving up the extremity on the first turn, then straight around the extremity toward the back and then down the extremity. Complete the turn by encircling extremity.

6. With each turn of the bandage, overlap the preceding turn by at least one-half the bandage width.

7. After wrapping the extremity, assess for adequate circulation, evenness of pressure, and comfort of patient. **Rationale:** Uneven or too much pressure can impede circulation; therefore, pulses should be monitored.

8. Secure bandage with tape, safety pin, or metal clip.

9. Assess patient for circulation, fit of bandage, and comfort every two to four hours.

10. Rewrap bandage every eight hours.

## APPLYING A FIGURE EIGHT BANDAGE

### Equipment

Roller bandage

Metal clip or safety pin

### Procedure

1. Gather necessary bandages.

2. Explain necessity for bandage to patient.

3. Anchor bandage around the distal end of the extremity using circular turns.

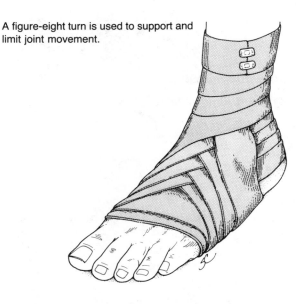

A figure-eight turn is used to support and limit joint movement.

---

**Clinical Alert**

For all bandages assess extremity for circulation after the first 20 minutes and then every two hours. Ensure that the bandage is wrinkle-free. **Rationale:** Partial occlusion of the vessels can occur within 20 minutes of application.

---

4. Make a circular turn around the foot and ankle.

5. Make a spiral turn down over the ankle and around the foot.

6. Continue to make alternate turns around the ankle and foot. Overlap the preceding bandage by at least one-half or two-thirds of the bandage.

7. Wrap the entire area below and above the involved point. **Rationale:** This will immobilize the affected area.

8. Assess extremity for circulation and evenness of pressure as well as comfort of patient.

9. Assess extremity at least every four hours and rewrap every eight hours.

### CHARTING  *for Bandage Application*

☐  Type of bandage applied

☐  Condition of extremity following application, skin color and temperature

☐  Note drainage, if any, from wound

☐  Effectiveness of bandage

☐  Patient's tolerance of bandage

## CLINICAL PROBLEM SOLVING

| **Potential Problems** | **Suggested Solutions** |
|---|---|

Affected joint or extremity is not immobilized with bandage.

- ☐ Assess if type of bandage is effective or if an alternate type of bandage would provide more support.
- ☐ Assess the need for a possible cast or immobilizer in place of the bandage.
- ☐ Evaluate if the bandage is applied tightly enough to immobilize the extremity.

Edema is noted in the area surrounding the bandage.

- ☐ Take bandage off and check circulation and skin condition.
- ☐ Keep extremity elevated.
- ☐ Rewrap bandage after edema has subsided.
- ☐ If edema persists, notify physician for orders.

Distal pulses are diminished or absent.

- ☐ Take off bandages immediately and reassess pulses. If pulses are present, rewrap bandage, keeping pressure even and bandage loose.
- ☐ If pulses remain diminished or absent, notify physician immediately.

## UNIT TWO   SPLINTING A FRACTURE

### NURSING PROCESS DATA

#### ASSESSMENT   *Data Base*

Note location of fracture.

Determine whether the fracture is open or closed.

Note presence and amount of hemorrhage.

Assess for deformities of fractured extremity.

Assess for signs of fat emboli.

- ☐ Classical sign is petechiae deposits across chest, shoulders, and axilla.
- ☐ Pulmonary signs: dyspnea, pallor, cyanosis.
- ☐ Cardiac signs: tachycardia, shock.
- ☐ Neurological signs: restlessness, change in level of consciousness, confusion.

#### PLANNING   *Objectives*

To immobilize a fractured limb and maintain good alignment.

To minimize pain and injury to soft tissue.

To prevent complications associated with a fracture (hemorrhage, edema, shock, emboli, etc.)

To monitor circulation and neurological status of the affected extremity.

**IMPLEMENTATION** *Procedures*

Applying a Splint

Applying an Air Splint

**EVALUATION** *Expected Outcomes*

Patient experiences minimal pain and injury to soft tissues.

Complications associated with a fractured limb are minimized.

Circulation and neurological status are maintained.

## APPLYING A SPLINT

### Equipment

Splint materials: pieces of wood and/or pillows, magazines, blankets

Padding materials: pieces of cloth and/or towels, blankets

Strapping materials: strips of cloth, rope, tape

### Procedure

1. If the patient's life is in danger, move the patient to a safe place.

> **Clinical Alert**
> Splinting, using these materials, is usually done in a pre-hospital setting.

2. Control hemorrhage by applying direct pressure and by using pressure dressings.

3. Explain the rationale for the intervention to patient.

4. Move the affected extremity as little as possible.
   a. Splint legs in an extended position.
   b. Splint arms in a flexed or extended position.

5. Pad joints, bony prominences, and skin areas as much as possible. **Rationale:** This prevents skin damage. Also make sure that the padding does not affect the patient's circulation, e.g., don't put padding in the axilla.

6. If splint material is not available, use the patient's body for support.
   a. Splint the legs together.
   b. Splint an arm to the torso.
   c. Splint toes or fingers together.

7. Reinforce soft splint materials (pillows, blankets) with something to make them more firm, such as magazines.

8. Strap the splint and extremity together tightly so that the extremity is immobile. Try to include the proximal and distal joints in the splint.

9. Check the patient's circulation by assessing pulse, capillary refill, color, and temperature.

10. Get the patient to medical facility as soon as possible.

## APPLYING AN AIR SPLINT

### Equipment

Appropriate size air splint

Dressings for wound if necessary

### Procedure

1. Cover compound fracture with absorbent dressings.

2. Place air splint over fractured extremity. **Rationale:** This splint is used most often to splint the forearm or lower leg.

3. Inflate splint by blowing into mouth piece. Pressure should be about 30 mm Hg in the splint.

4. Check the tension in the splint. Press a finger into the splint; it should dimple to the depth of ½ inch.

> **Clinical Alert**
> Once inflated, do not deflate splint. Only physicians may deflate air splints.

## CHARTING  *for Splinting*

☐ Location of the fracture

☐ Time splint applied

☐ Materials used in splinting

☐ Circulatory and neurological status of the extremity

☐ Any change in patient's condition

☐ Patient's comfort and reactions to the fracture

☐ Presence and treatment of open wound

---

## CLINICAL PROBLEM SOLVING

**Potential Problems**

Patient complains of pain or numbness in splinted extremity.

Extremity still moves in the splint.

**Suggested Solutions**

☐ Elevate extremity above level of heart to decrease edema.

☐ Check for padding, straps, or splint material that is impinging on a major nerve or blood vessel. Correct the problem.

☐ Apply more padding if possible.

☐ Tighten straps slightly. Observe condition of patient's extremity: color, temperature, and sensation.

---

# UNIT THREE   CAST CARE

## NURSING PROCESS DATA

### ASSESSMENT   *Data Base*

Identify type of cast applied.

Note condition for which the cast was applied.

Observe condition of the cast.

Assess for neurovascular complications.

### PLANNING   *Objectives*

To increase the patient's level of activity after injury or disease.

To maintain normal sensation, movement, and circulation in a casted extremity.

To improve muscle tone and joint flexibility.

To strengthen muscles weakened by immobility, trauma, or surgery.

To increase patient's psychological sense of freedom.

### IMPLEMENTATION   *Procedures*

Caring for a Wet Cast

Assessing a Casted Extremity

Instructing in Care of Synthetic Casts

**EVALUATION** *Expected Outcomes*

Complications are prevented during the casting procedure.

Cast dries without cracking or indentation areas on the cast.

The patient experiences minimal discomfort from pain or swelling.

**TABLE 1**  COMPARISON OF CASTS

|  | **PLASTER** | **SYNTHETIC** |
|---|---|---|
| MATERIAL | Plaster of Paris, comprised of powdered calcium sulfate crystals impregnated into the bandages. | Polyester and cotton, fiberglass or plastic. Polyester and cotton is impregnated with water-activated polyurethane resin. |
| DRYING TIME | 24 to 48 hours | 7 to 15 minutes for setting 15 to 30 minutes for weight-bearing |
| ADVANTAGES | Less costly More effective for immobilizing severely displaced bones Smooth surface Doesn't require expensive equipment for application | Less likely to indent into skin Lighter in weight Less restrictive Doesn't crumble Nonabsorbent; can be immersed in water |

## CARING FOR A WET CAST

### Equipment

Bedboard

Pillows covered with plastic

### Procedure

1. Explain to the patient that the cast will feel warm as the plaster dries.
2. Use ONLY the palms of your hands on the cast when turning and positioning for the first 24 hours. **Rationale:** Fingers can cause dents in the cast, which may create pressure areas on the inside of the cast.
3. Support the cast with pillows as necessary.
   a. Keep the casted extremity above the level of the heart. **Rationale:** This position decreases venous pooling and edema.
   b. Maintain the angles that were built into the cast.
   c. Prevent cracking from undue pressure.
   d. Prevent flat spots in the cast caused by pressure on the bed. For example, when the pa-

**Clinical Alert**

If patient is wearing a spica or body cast, place a bedboard under the mattress to provide firm support.

tient has a long leg cast, place pillows under knees to maintain the angle of the cast and under lower leg to prevent pressure and flattening of heel area.

4. Keep the cast uncovered. **Rationale:** This allows heat and moisture to dissipate and air to circulate.
5. If the cast is near the patient's groin, protect this area with plastic to avoid soiling the edges of the cast.
6. If edges of cast are rough or crumbling, pull stockinette over edge of cast and tape down.
7. "Petal" edges of cast with tape if stockinette is used.
   a. Cut tape into 4 inch strips.
   b. Place half the tape on the inside of the cast and pull it over the top of the cast.
   c. Anchor the remaining tape to the outside of the cast.

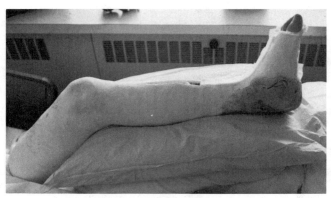

Position casted extremity above level of heart to prevent edema.

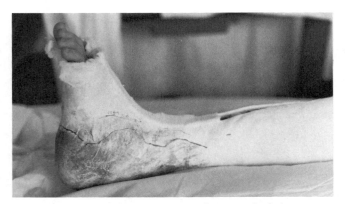

Circle and time stained areas to assess increases in drainage.

## ASSESSING A CASTED EXTREMITY

### Equipment

Pen to mark drainage on cast

### Procedure

1. Explain the rationale for the procedure to the patient.

2. Encourage the patient to notify you if he feels any unusual sensations or changes in sensations in the casted extremity.

3. Check the patient's fingers or toes to make sure they are pink in color.

4. Feel the patient's fingers or toes to make sure they are warm.

5. Ask what the patient feels when you touch his toes. The patient should have normal sensation and be able to identify which digit you are touching. He should not have a "pins-and-needles" sensation. **Rationale:** Changes in color, temperature and sensation might indicate inadequate blood supply or nerve damage.

6. Assess for capillary refill by applying pressure to one of the patient's toenails or fingernails. After you stop the pressure, observe the nail to see how rapidly the color returns. **Rationale:** Comparing one of your nails to the patient's nail is a check on how quickly color should return.

7. Ask the patient to move the fingers or toes that are affected by the cast. The patient should be able to move them without difficulty.

8. Ask the patient to identify the exact location of any pain. Assess for adequate blood supply or nerve paralysis.

> **Clinical Alert**
> Casted extremity should be assessed every ½ hour for two hours, then every hour for 24 hours, then every four hours for 48 hours.

9. Check for any drainage from a wound under the cast. Note the color and amount of drainage. Mark the circumference of the stain on the cast as a gauge for any increases in the amount of drainage.

10. Report any unusual odor or increase in drainage.

## INSTRUCTING IN SYNTHETIC CAST CARE

### Equipment

Pamphlet on cast care

### Procedure

1. Explain necessity for neurovascular check:
   a. Check temperature, color, and blanching of extremity.
   b. Observe for edema, numbness or tingling sensations.

2. Check cast daily for:
   a. Odor or drainage.
   b. Cracks or position change.

3. Instruct avoidance of overly rigorous activities. **Rationale:** This will prevent dislodging or maligning of the fracture.

4. Instruct in bathing procedures when cast can be wet.
   a. Use only mild soap and water when bathing.

b. Avoid getting soap on cast.

c. Flush cast with water following bathing. **Rationale:** This prevents skin irritation and maceration from soap.

d. Place non-slip mat on floor to prevent slipping when getting out of shower or tub.

5. Instruct on drying cast.

a. Remove excess water by blotting with towel.

b. Set blow dryer on cool setting and dry cast by moving dryer along all aspects of cast. **Rationale:** If cast remains wet the patient will feel a cold, clammy sensation.

6. Explain necessity for keeping particles and dirt out of cast. Cast can be flushed with water to remove debris. Dry cast thoroughly.

### CHARTING  *for Cast Care*

☐ Type of cast applied

☐ Positioning of cast

☐ Patient's complaints and nursing responses

☐ Color, warmth, movement, and sensation in casted extremity

☐ Presence, location, and amount of drainage from wound

☐ Patient's acceptance of the cast

---

## CLINICAL PROBLEM SOLVING

**Potential Problems**

Patient complains of numbness, discomfort, and/or pain.

Cast cracks from improper drying procedure or stress.

Synthetic cast has rough edges.

**Suggested Solutions**

☐ Notify physician immediately.

☐ Reevaluate condition of casted extremity every fifteen minutes.

☐ Reassess circulation, movement, and sensation (CMS).

☐ Notify physician immediately.

☐ Reassure patient.

☐ Do not reposition patient until physician assesses.

☐ Smooth edges by filing with nail file.

☐ Make sure furniture and clothing are protected from scratches and snags by covering cast with a cloth.

---

# UNIT FOUR   TRACTION

## NURSING PROCESS DATA

### ASSESSMENT  *Data Base*

Determine type of traction used.

Note the amount of weight ordered.

Note any conditions requiring special treatment.

Assess for circulation, movement and sensation of affected extremity.

### PLANNING  *Objectives*

To maintain correct alignment of bone ends.

To prevent unnecessary injury to soft tissue.

To prevent ischemia and necrosis which can be caused by continued pressure on the soft tissues.

### IMPLEMENTATION  *Procedures*

Monitoring Skin Traction

Monitoring Skeletal Traction

### EVALUATION  *Expected Outcomes*

Extremity is maintained in correct alignment.

Bone ends are approximated and do not override.

Skin of affected extremity remains intact.

Patient maintains correct position while in bed.

## MONITORING SKIN TRACTION

### Procedure

1. Examine the material (tape, foam rubber, or plastic) that attaches the weights to the extremity.
   a. Material should be held in place, not slipping.
   b. Material should fit comfortably, neither too loose nor too tight.
2. Examine all bony prominences of the involved extremity for abrasions or pressure areas.
   a. Traction should be removed every 4 hours.
   b. Wash, dry thoroughly and powder skin before reapplying traction.
3. Examine the extremity distal to the traction.
   a. Note any presence of edema.

b. Take and record peripheral pulses.
   c. Check temperature and color to see if both are normal.
4. Observe for possible neurological impediment from traction slings encroaching on popliteal space or axilla. **Rationale:** Numbness or tingling if present, indicates neurological problems have occurred.
5. Ask the patient to move the extremity that is distal to the traction.
   a. Note if full range of motion is present.
   b. Ask the patient if he has any decreased or unusual sensations.
6. Examine the rope and weights to see that the pull goes directly through the long axis of the fractured bone.

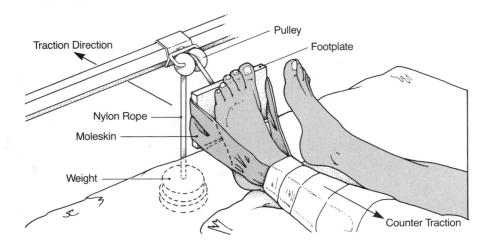

Traction Direction

Pulley

Footplate

Nylon Rope

Moleskin

Weight

Counter Traction

Buck's extension, a type of skin traction, is used to maintain bones in correct alignment.

7. Check the traction mechanism.
   a. Weights should hang freely, off the floor and bed.
   b. Knots should be secure in all ropes.
   c. Ropes should move freely through pulleys.
   d. Pulleys should not be constrained by knots.

8. Make sure the patient is positioned correctly in bed. **Rationale:** The patient should not be pulled down to the end of the bed since this would negate the traction.

9. Place sheepskin or an alternative material under the affected extremity. **Rationale:** This will help to prevent pressure areas.

10. Provide foot plates for the affected side to prevent footdrop.

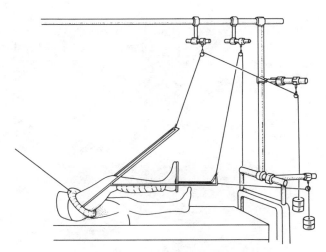

Weights must hang freely and rope must move through pulleys with ease to ensure proper traction.

---

**Types of Skin Traction**

| | |
|---|---|
| Buck's | Pelvic |
| Russell's | Cervical |
| Bryant's | |

---

## MONITORING SKELETAL TRACTION

### Equipment

Sterile cotton-tipped applicators

Normal saline or

Hydrogen peroxide

Sterile water

Antibacterial ointment

### Procedure

1. Check the pin and the wound area surrounding the pin.
   a. Pin should be immobile.
   b. Wound should be clean and dry.

2. Assess for infection at the pin site. Note any local pain, redness, heat, or drainage.

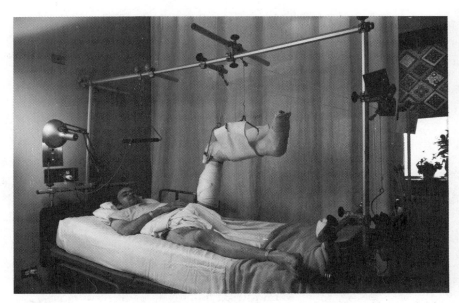

Skeletal traction, such as the Thomas splint with Pearson attachment, provides traction by the insertion of a pin through a bone.

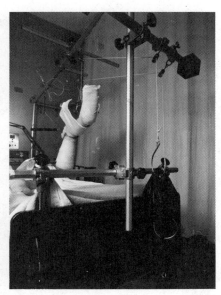

Weights are counterbalanced by the patient. Weights must be freehanging to exert force.

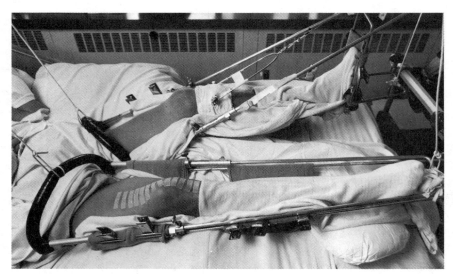

Patients in skeletal traction must be kept in alignment to promote proper healing.

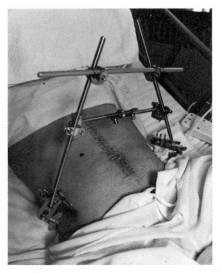

Hoffman Colles Frame for alignment.

3. Provide pin site care if ordered:
   a. Clean area with normal saline or hydrogen peroxide soaked cotton-tipped applicators.
   b. Rinse with sterile water or normal saline.
   c. Apply antibacterial ointment to site as ordered.

4. Examine all bony prominences for pressure areas or abrasions.

5. Assess distal extremity for pulses, temperature, color, and edema.

6. Check for normal range of motion and sensation in the affected extremity.

7. Check the ropes and weights to make sure the pull goes directly through the long axis of the fractured bone. **Rationale:** This pull maintains the fracture in alignment.

8. Check the traction mechanism.
   a. Weights should hang freely, off the floor and bed.
   b. Knots should be secure in all ropes.
   c. Rope should move freely through pulleys.
   d. Pulleys should not be constrained by knots.

9. Make sure the patient is positioned correctly in bed. The patient should not be pulled down to the foot of the bed since this would negate traction.

10. Check placement of the foot rest. The patient's foot should be correctly positioned to prevent footdrop.

### CHARTING   *for Traction*

☐ Type of traction

☐ Alignment of traction

☐ Integrity of the skin

☐ Temperature, color, pulse, and range of motion in extremity

☐ Specific complaints by patient and nursing actions taken to solve problems

☐ Patient's comfort and overall feelings

---

## CLINICAL PROBLEM SOLVING

**Potential Problems**

There is a change in the temperature, color, or pulses of the extremity.

**Suggested Solutions**

☐ Notify physician at once.
☐ If the patient has a fractured femur, measure the size of the thigh with a tape measure every 15 to 30 minutes. Look for areas of ecchymosis. (It is possible to sequester several units of blood in the thigh if a vessel has been torn.)
☐ Assess for circulatory shock.

# UNIT FIVE  HALO TRACTION AND BACK BRACE

## NURSING PROCESS DATA

### ASSESSMENT  *Data Base*

Assess for respiratory impairment: absence of breath sounds or adventitious sounds.

Assess for orthostatic hypotension while placing patient in sitting position.

Assess pin sites for infection.

Assess skin under vest for erythema or skin breakdown.

Assess alignment of vest and position of traction.

### PLANNING  *Objectives*

To promote adequate respiratory function.

To prevent orthostatic hypotension.

To maintain pin site free of infection.

To maintain skin integrity.

### IMPLEMENTATION  *Procedures*

Placing a Jewett-Taylor Back Brace

Monitoring Halo Traction

### EVALUATION  *Expected Outcomes*

Complications are prevented or identified early

Immobilization and proper alignment are maintained

## PLACING A JEWETT-TAYLOR BACK BRACE

### Equipment

Front and back brace with Velcro straps

T-shirt

ABD dressings

### Procedure

1. Wash your hands.

2. Explain procedure to patient.

3. Provide privacy.

4. Put T-shirt on patient. **Rationale:** This will protect the skin from the brace rubbing on bare skin. This brace is used frequently with spinal cord injured patients who already have potential skin problems.

5. Place the bed in a flat position. Keep side rail in UP position on side of bed opposite from you.

6. Log roll or ask patient to turn to side farthest away from you. **Rationale:** This position prevents torque on the spinal cord.

7. Position brace on back so that struts fit on either side of the spinal cord and fits the natural lumbar curve of the back. **Rationale:** The struts provide an open space along the spinal cord so pressure is not exerted on a surgical site or on the vertebrae.

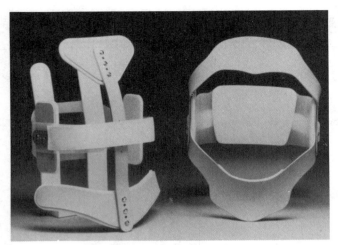

Jewett-Taylor Braces are used to provide back support without exerting pressure following spinal cord surgery.

8. Log roll the patient to a supine position.

9. Place the front section of the brace by positioning the iliac wings (made of plastic material) over the iliac crest. Adjust the triangular sternum piece, the metal struts will fall into place.

10. Secure the brace with the Velcro straps.

11. Observe under the brace for pressure areas. If pressure areas are present, pad the area under the brace with ABD pads until the brace can be readjusted. **Rationale:** The physician should be notified immediately so the brace can be adjusted before complications occur.

## MONITORING HALO TRACTION

### Equipment

Allen wrench

Tracheostomy tray

Hydrogen peroxide

Antibacterial ointment e.g. Neosporin, Bacitracin

Normal saline

Sterile cotton-tipped applicators

Antiembolic stockings, if needed

Abdominal binder, if needed

Wheelchair, if needed

### Procedure

1. Evaluate patient's psychological status and knowledge base. Explain procedure at patient's level of understanding.

2. Evaluate respiratory status.
   a. Check respiratory rate and rhythm at least every 2 to 4 hours.
   b. Observe respiratory excursion.
   c. Monitor breath sounds every shift for presence of adventitious sounds or absence of breath sounds. **Rationale:** Pulmonary embolus is a common complication associated with spinal cord injury patients. Due to sensory loss, the patient is unable to feel the pain associated with an embolus.
   d. Keep Allen wrench and tracheostomy tray at bedside. **Rationale:** The Allen wrench is used to remove screws from the vest in order to perform CPR in the advent of respiratory or cardiac arrest. Endotracheal intubation is contraindicated in these patients, so a tracheostomy would be required.

3. Monitor alignment of cast and vest. If traction is intact the neck should not be flexed or extended. **Rationale:** Traction is maintained by anterior metal bars. Do not pull on anterior bars; use posterior bars for positioning patients.

4. Prevent orthostatic hypotension when placing patient in sitting position.
   a. Apply antiembolic stockings. **Rationale:** Stockings promote venous return to heart.
   b. Apply abdominal binder. **Rationale:** Binders increase venous return to the heart.
   c. Raise patient to 90 degree sitting position over period of 20 to 30 minutes. Take vital signs with each increment.
   d. Administer medications such as Ephedrine, 30 minutes before patient is scheduled to move to a wheelchair. **Rationale:** Medication will prevent hypotension.
   e. If hypotension persists, keep patient in bed for one hour and attempt procedure again.

5. Prevent skin breakdown under vest.
   a. Open vest at both sides during bath.
   b. Wash skin and dry thoroughly.
   c. Check skin for reddened area or skin breakdown. Treat skin problems immediately. **Rationale:** With poor vasomotor action, skin breakdown is difficult to treat.
   d. Remove sheepskin lining once a week for cleaning.

6. Prevent pin site infection.
   a. Observe pin sites for drainage, edema or erythema. If present, take culture and send to lab. **Rationale:** Clinical signs of infection should be treated immediately, as brain abscess can occur from pin site infections.

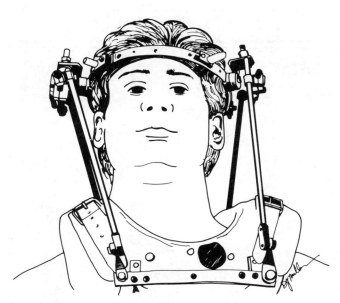

Halo traction is used to provide support to the neck and prevent flexion or extension following cervical spinal cord injury.

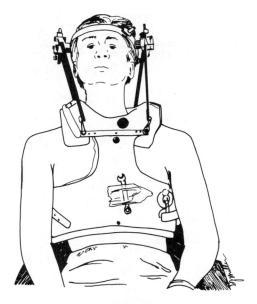

Allen wrench is taped to vest for emergency removal of screws when CPR is required.

---

**Clinical Alert**

If pins are loose, notify physician immediately; keep patient immobilized until physician arrives.

---

b. Cleanse pin sites with sterile cotton-tipped applicators and hydrogen peroxide or normal saline. **Rationale:** Hydrogen peroxide has a tendency to remove tissue and loosen pins; therefore, check with hospital procedure for cleaning policy.
c. Rinse sites with sterile saline if hydrogen peroxide is used.
d. Apply light covering of antibacterial ointment to site. **Rationale:** Betadine or iodine-based ointments tend to corrode the pins so they should not be used.
e. Hair should be shaved around the pin sites to allow easy observation and cleaning.

**CHARTING**  *for Halo Traction*

☐ Pin site assessment
☐ Pin site care
☐ Skin condition under vest
☐ Presence of signs or symptoms of orthostatic hypotension
☐ Nursing measures used to prevent orthostatic hypotension
☐ Respiratory status

---

## CLINICAL PROBLEM SOLVING

**Potential Problems**

Infection at pin site.

**Suggested Solutions**

☐ Monitor neuro signs closely, as brain abscess is a major complication.
☐ Obtain culture of drainage.
☐ Call physician for systemic antibiotic order.
☐ Cleanse sites more frequently.
☐ Apply dressing over pin site to absorb drainage.

Pins are loose.

☐ Immobilize patient immediately.
☐ Contact physician.
☐ Have Allen wrench available for physician.

## UNIT SIX   PATIENTS WITH AMPUTATED LIMBS

### NURSING PROCESS DATA

**ASSESSMENT**   *Data Base*

Assess incision for intactness.

Assess range of motion and muscle strength.

Note condition of patient's skin: pressure areas, edema, etc.

Assess for phantom limb pain.

Assess for signs of hemorrhage or infection.

**PLANNING**   *Objectives*

To provide the stump with full range of motion.

To ensure adequate muscle strength in both extremities for optimal use of the prosthesis.

To promote a smooth conical stump that fits into a prosthesis comfortably.

To assist the patient in accepting the disability.

To decrease the incidence of phantom limb pain.

To prevent edema and pressure areas.

**IMPLEMENTATION**   *Procedures*

Positioning and Exercising

Applying a Shrink Bandage

**EVALUATION**   *Expected Outcomes*

Stump exhibits full range of motion and adequate muscle strength.

A smooth conical stump that fits into a prosthesis comfortably.

Stump incision is kept clean, dry and free of infection.

## POSITIONING AND EXERCISING

### Equipment

Bedboard

### Procedure

1. Explain the rationale for the intervention to patient.

2. Place a bedboard under mattress, preferably at the time of surgery. **Rationale:** The patient will not sag into the mattress and develop contractures.

3. For the first 24 hours, elevate foot of bed. **Rationale:** Do not place pillow under stump as this leads to hip contracture.

4. Place patient in prone position every shift for at least one hour.

5. Explain the importance of the exercises to the patient. Tell patient that because the flexor muscles are stronger than the extensors, the stump will be permanently flexed and abducted unless the patient practices the range-of-motion exercises. **Rationale:** Range-of-motion exercises increase muscle strength and improve mobility of amputated extremity.

6. If ordered, assist the patient with quadriceps setting exercises with a below-the-knee amputation.

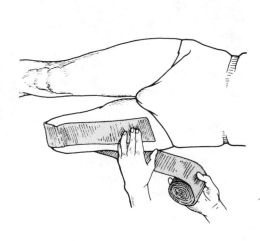

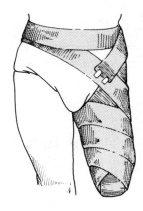

Shrink bandages applied to an amputated limb mold the stump in preparation for a prosthesis.

a. Extend leg and try to push the popliteal area of the knee into the bed; try to move the patella proximally.
b. Contract quadriceps and hold the contraction for ten seconds.
c. Repeat this procedure four or five times.
d. Repeat the exercise at least four times a day.

7. Teach stump extension exercises.
a. Lie in a prone position with foot hanging over the end of the bed.
b. Keep stump next to intact leg to extend stump and to contract gluteal muscles.
c. Hold the contraction for ten seconds.
d. Repeat this exercise at least four times a day.

8. Teach adduction exercise.
a. Place a pillow between the patient's thighs.
b. Squeeze the pillow for ten seconds and then relax for ten seconds.
c. Repeat this exercise at least four times a day.

9. Have the patient keep track of time spent with the stump flexed and then spend an equal amount of time with the stump extended.

## APPLYING A SHRINK BANDAGE

### Equipment

Elastic bandages: two or three 4- to 6-inch bandages, sewn together if possible for lower extremity

Elastic bandages: one or two 3- to 4-inch bandages for upper extremity

### Procedure

1. Explain the rationale for the intervention to patient.

2. For amputations above the knee, apply 3- to 4-inch shrink bandages as illustrated.
a. Ask the patient to hold the loops of bandage at the top of the thigh.
b. Apply pressure evenly. **Rationale:** This allows tissues to be shaped properly.
c. Apply the bandage smoothly, making sure there are no wrinkles to cause pressure areas.
d. Extend the bandage as high as possible into the groin. **Rationale:** This prevents formation of an abrasion or loose roll of tissue which can hamper the fit and use of a prosthesis.
e. If you use spica turns, make sure that the stump is not pulled into a flexed position by the bandages.

3. For amputations below the knee, apply a shrink bandage using same principles, anchoring bandage on thigh.

4. Carefully observe the bandages you have applied to ensure proper tension and molding of the stump.

5. Rewrap bandages three to four times a day.

### CHARTING  *for Shrink Bandaging*

☐ When bandage was changed

☐ Condition of patient's skin and incision

☐ Extent of range of motion

☐ Any changes in how the bandage has been applied

☐ Patient's response to seeing the stump and assisting with the care

---

## CLINICAL PROBLEM SOLVING

| Potential Problems | Suggested Solutions |
|---|---|
| Stump edema occurs even with application of shrink bandage. | ☐ When on bed rest, elevate foot of bed to increase venous blood flow and decrease edema.<br>☐ Assess for possible complications of infection or obstruction in blood flow.<br>☐ Evaluate wrapping procedure. Ensure bandages are properly applied. |
| Shrinkage of stump is delayed or doesn't occur as expected. | ☐ Continue treatment as ordered.<br>☐ Observe carefully for signs of infection or edema. |
| Stump is unable to be put through full range of motion. | ☐ Observe the patient to see which positions he uses most often. Assess stump for continued flexion and/or abduction.<br>☐ Explain why the patient should practice full range-of-motion exercises and demonstrate exercises again if necessary.<br>☐ Show the patient how to position the stump to attain optimal stump movement. Help the patient assume these positions several times a day.<br>☐ Notify the physician. |

---

# UNIT SEVEN   THE NELSON BED

## NURSING PROCESS DATA

### ASSESSMENT  *Data Base*

Assess patient's vital signs, including peripheral pulses and circulation.

Determine if symptoms of orthostatic hypotension are present.

Determine patient's ability to maintain balance.

Assess patient's knowledge of the bed and its function.

Ascertain patient's previous experience with the bed.

### PLANNING  *Objectives*

To maintain optimal functioning of body systems by putting patient's body in positions of normal activity.

To assist the patient with total hip replacement in ambulation without flexion of the affected hip.

To allow patients with spinal surgery to ambulate without torsion of the spine.

To provide a vertical position at intervals to maintain stress on bone. This prevents loss of calcium.

To change a patient on bed rest from a horizontal to a vertical position without symptoms of orthostatic hypotension.

To maintain or attain normal movement of ankles, knees, and hips while patients are on bed rest.

**IMPLEMENTATION**   *Procedures*

Using a Nelson Bed

Moving to Chair Position

Moving to Contour Position

Tilting Bed to Vertical Position

Tilting Bed to Trendelenburg's Position

**EVALUATION**   *Expected Outcomes*

Total hip replacement patients ambulate without flexion of the affected hip.

Spinal surgery patients ambulate without torsion of the spine.

Patients are able to change from horizontal to vertical position without symptoms of orthostatic hypotension.

Patient maintains normal movement of ankles, knees, and hips.

## USING A NELSON BED

### Equipment

Nelson bed

Safety restraining straps

### Procedure

1. Explain the function of bed to patient.

2. Adjust seat section of the bed to the height of the individual patient. This is most easily done before the patient is put into bed, but it may be done afterward.
   a. Unscrew knobs at each side of the bed at the area marked "To adjust for patient height."
   b. Slide head section until knob position corresponds to the height of the patient as printed on the side of the bed.
   c. Tighten knobs securely.

3. Place patient on the bed.

4. Familiarize patient with the bed controls for section changes.

   a. Tilt: whole bed goes up at head end.
   b. Head.
   c. Knee.
   d. Foot: whole bed goes up at foot end.

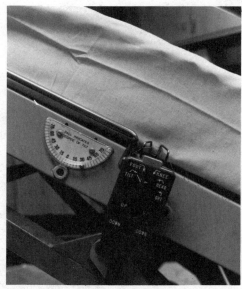

The Nelson bed provides position variation. Control knobs allow patients to maintain mobility.

5. Instruct patient how to change height position of bed.

6. Instruct patient how to control UP and DOWN for each section and height of bed.

7. Place safety straps across patient when tilting bed.

## MOVING TO CHAIR POSITION

### Equipment

Nelson bed

Safety restraining straps

### Procedure

1. Explain the procedure to patient.

2. Put the side rails in UP position.

3. Adjust the footboard to patient's need.
   a. To move toward patient, push the footboard forward by holding the middle of the supporting legs.
   b. To move away from patient, tilt the footboard slightly forward and then pull downward to the desired position. **Rationale:** The patient's weight will lock the footboard in position.

4. Adjust the casters at the foot of the bed so they are parallel to the bed and locked in place.

5. Put safety straps around patient if necessary.

6. Put head section up to vertical position.

7. Put knee section down until the foot of the bed is vertical.

8. Lower the bed by choosing HEIGHT and DOWN until the footboard is on the floor.

9. To return the bed to a horizontal position, reverse the procedure.

## MOVING TO CONTOUR POSITION

### Procedure

1. Explain the procedure to patient.

2. Put the side rails up.

3. Put the head of bed up to a comfortable position.

4. Put knee section down as desired.

5. Use the FOOT control to tilt the whole bed back (head end down).

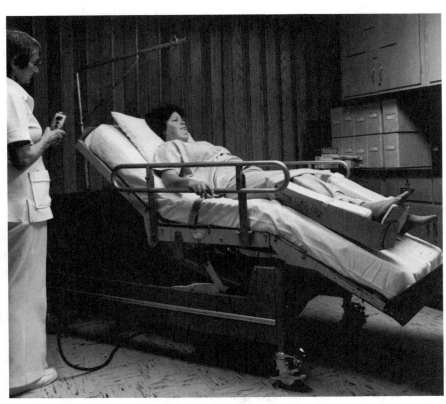

Facilitate self-care by positioning Nelson bed in a sitting position.

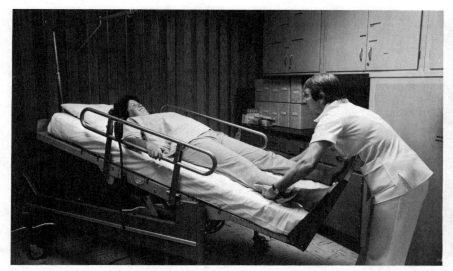

Step one in assisting a patient out of bed is to pull patient down toward footboard.

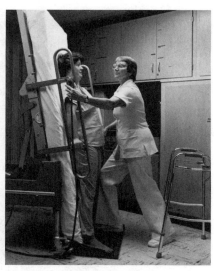

Step three is to place bed in vertical position.

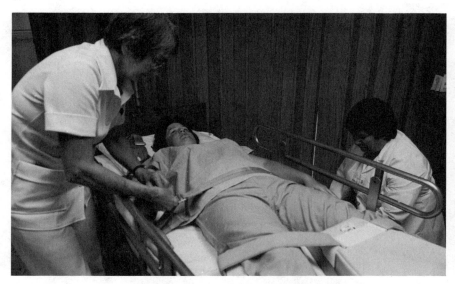

Step two is to place straps across abdomen and legs to prevent sliding down.

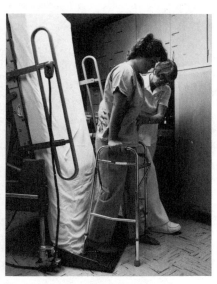

Step four is to assist patient to walk.

6. Adjust all parts as necessary for comfort.

7. To return to a flat position, reverse the procedure.

## TILTING BED TO VERTICAL POSITION

### Procedure

1. Explain the procedure to patient.

2. Align and lock the foot casters parallel to the bed frame.

3. Place the bed in the flat position.

4. Put height up to highest position.

5. Put the footboard down to farthest position.

6. Slide patient down until patient's feet are on the footboard.

7. Apply safety restraining straps around the patient as needed.

8. Put the side rails up.

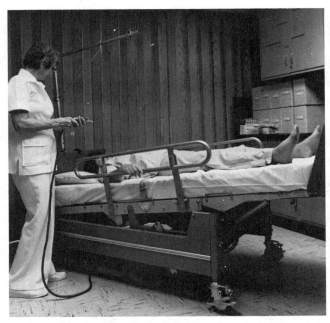

Nelson bed can be placed in Trendelenburg's position with control.

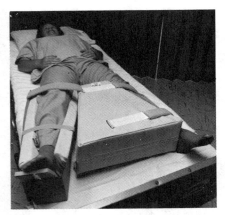

Charnley pillow maintains abduction and external rotation of the hips.

9. Select TILT and put the bed up to full tilt (82 degrees) or to a level the patient can tolerate.

10. When bed is in vertical position, support patient with your knee to prevent fall.

11. Assist patient to step from bed with support of walker.

12. To place the patient back to a horizontal position, reverse the procedure.

## TILTING BED TO TRENDELENBURG'S POSITION

### Procedure

1. Explain the procedure to the patient.
2. Place the mattress flat.

3. Set the controls to FOOT, and press UP button.

4. To place patient back to a flat position, set controls to FOOT and press DOWN button.

### CHARTING   *for Nelson Bed*

☐  Bed position used

☐  Degree of tilt

☐  Time patient was in a specific position

☐  Vital signs

☐  Emotional reaction of patient

☐  Signs and symptoms of untoward reactions

☐  Straps used, if any

## CLINICAL PROBLEM SOLVING

### Potential Problems

The patient experiences syncope when the body's position is made more vertical.

### Suggested Solutions

☐  Lower the head of the bed at once.

☐  Check blood pressure and pulse every 5 to 10 minutes until stable.

☐  When raising bed next time, raise patient to a lower degree of tilt and keep patient in that position for a longer time period before continuing to raise bed.

□ Increase degree of tilt in small increments, checking blood pressure and pulse with each increment.

The patient is not strapped in and falls from the bed.

□ Have patient checked by physician.
□ Obtain x-rays if ordered.
□ Complete incident report.
□ Assess patient's ability to maintain his balance while tilting the bed.
□ Use safety straps until sure of patient's ability to maintain balance.
□ Strap patient's legs if they are weak before changing bed's position.

The patient is fearful of the movement of the bed.

□ Fully explain the reasons for using the bed.
□ Answer all the patient's questions.
□ Let the patient control movement of the bed.
□ Stay while the patient moves the bed.
□ Strap patient in place while moving the bed.
□ Change bed positions slowly.

# UNIT EIGHT   STRYKER FRAME

## NURSING PROCESS DATA

### ASSESSMENT   *Data Base*

Determine patient's level of movement and sensation.

Evaluate patient's ability to understand explanation of turning procedure.

Assess condition of traction apparatus.

Evaluate ability of patient to assist with turning.

### PLANNING   *Objectives*

To assist the patient in turning horizontally from supine to prone to supine without torsion or abnormal flexion/extension of the spinal column.

To provide optimal skin care for patients who require immobility.

To prevent pressure areas and decubitus ulcers.

To provide optimal nursing care to patients with skin grafts or other conditions that require minimum patient movement.

### IMPLEMENTATION   *Procedures*

Using a Stryker Wedge Turning Frame

Turning Supine to Prone

Using a Stryker Parallel Frame

Assisting Patient with Bedpan

Attaching Fixed Traction

Attaching Skeletal Traction

---

**EVALUATION**  *Expected Outcomes*

Patient turns horizontally without torsion or abnormal flexion/extension of the spinal column.

Patient receives optimal skin care without developing decubiti.

Patient receives optimal nursing care for skin grafts or similar conditions.

---

## USING A STRYKER WEDGE TURNING FRAME

### Equipment

Stryker wedge turning frame

Arm rests and footboard

Software: mattress, canvases, linen, straps

Safety straps

Pillows and sheepskins

### Procedure

1. Explain procedure to patient.
2. Show patient the Stryker frame before placing on the frame.
3. Position the posterior frame at the bottom of the turning circle.
4. Place patient supine on the posterior frame using the three-man carry transfer method.
5. If patient is on a back board, place patient and board on the posterior frame.
6. Attach the anterior frame.
7. Turn patient and remove the back board.
8. Reverse the procedure and turn patient to his back.

## TURNING FROM SUPINE TO PRONE

### Procedure

1. Explain procedure to patient. This procedure requires only one person; however, it is advisable to have two people when possible.
2. Position sheepskin, pillows, or comfort aids on top of patient.
3. With patient on the posterior frame, open the turning circle and put the head end of the anterior frame on the securing bolt and fasten it with the nut.

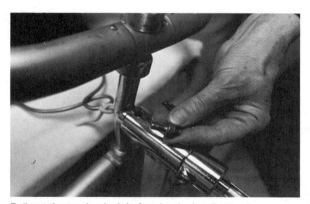

Before turning, fasten nut securely at head and foot of frame.

Pull out the turning lock before beginning the turning process.

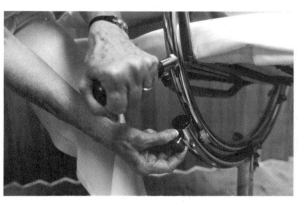

Hold handle while pulling knob and begin turn.

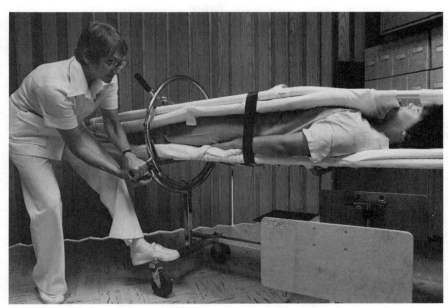

Strap in patient before turning on Stryker frame.

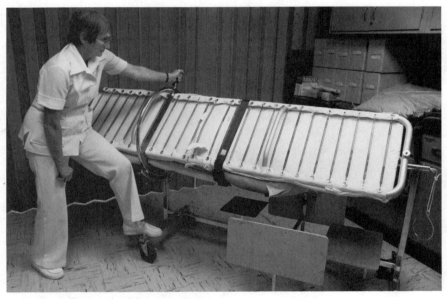

Patients can be turned safely by one person.

4. Fasten the foot end of the anterior frame with the nut, making sure that patient's legs and feet are correctly positioned.

5. Have patient clasp hands around the anterior frame. If patient is unable to do this, put a safety strap around the whole frame at elbow level to keep arms contained.

6. Close the turning circle until it locks.

7. Move the arm rests down out of the way of the turn.

8. Pull out the bed-turning lock.

9. Turn the frame toward the patient's right until it locks automatically. The narrow side of the wedge (at the patient's right) will always turn down. The frame will automatically lock when the bottom frame is horizontal.

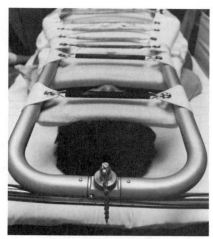

Unscrew nut and lift frame to remove.

10. Open the turning circle, unscrew the nuts, and remove the upper posterior frame. Relock the turning circle for safety.

11. To turn the patient on the Stryker wedge from prone to supine, reverse procedure for turning from supine to prone. Remember that the narrow side of the wedge (on patient's right) always turns down so patient cannot slip out.

## USING A STRYKER PARALLEL FRAME

### Equipment

Stryker parallel frame

Arm rests and footboard

Software: mattress, canvases, linen, straps

Safety straps

Pillows and sheepskins

### Procedure

1. Place a pillow lengthwise over the patient's legs to prevent moving during turning.

2. Attach the anterior frame to the main frame using the two nuts on the turning circle. Make sure the patient is held firmly between the frames.

3. Put three safety straps around the frame at level of knees, waist, and elbows. Tighten securely.

4. With a person at each end of the frame, pull out the locking pins at the center of each end, turn the frame slightly to hold the lock open, and then

quickly finish turning the patient. The bed will automatically lock when the bottom frame is horizontal.

5. Remove the top frame and reposition the patient for comfort.

## ASSISTING PATIENT WITH BEDPAN

### Equipment

Special bedpan

Plastic drape

Towels

### Procedure

1. Explain procedure to patient.

2. Place patient in a supine position.

3. Drop the center section of the posterior frame by releasing the hooks/rubber bands from the sides of the frame.

4. Protect the linen by putting plastic or towels around the edges.

5. Insert the bedpan into the opening and hold securely with hands or with the arm supports.

6. Remove the bedpan, clean the patient, and reattach the center section of the frame.

## ATTACHING FIXED TRACTION

### Equipment

Traction halter

Weights

Pulleys

Rope

### Procedure

1. Explain procedure to patient.

2. Attach the rope to the frame of the Stryker through the hole in the center pin of the disc.

3. Apply a traction halter or belt to the patient. (Patient's body forms counterweight.)

4. Attach the rope from the frame to the halter or belt.

5. Determine the number of centimeters the end of the frame must be elevated to provide for sufficient traction. Determine the patient's weight, and use the table provided in the operating instructions to obtain the number of centimeters.

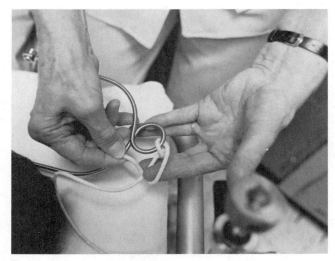

Tie knot through the loop in tongs to prevent rope from slipping.

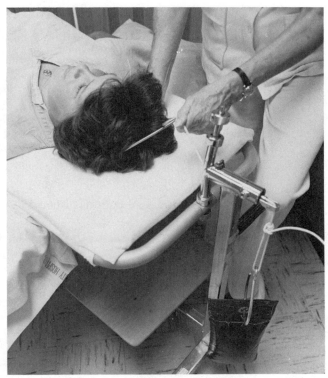

Ensure that weights hang freely and do not touch bed or floor.

6. Lift up the head or foot of the Stryker, depending on the type of traction. Put the stop pins into the holes corresponding to the elevation needed.

7. Check that the patient's body is positioned so the feet or head is free to maintain traction.

## ATTACHING SKELETAL TRACTION

### Equipment

Weights

Rope

Pulley

### Procedure

1. Explain procedure to patient.

2. Attach the rope to weights by placing it through the hole in the center of the disc and laying it over the pulley.

3. Attach the rope to the skeletal traction and tape all knots. Traction is applied to head or lower extremities.

4. Assess that weights are clear of frame and remain above the floor.

### CHARTING   *for Stryker Frame*

☐  Length of time spent on each side

☐  How patient tolerates turning procedure

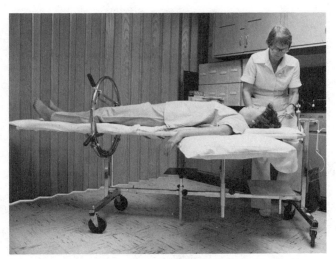

Cervical spine immobilization is accomplished through use of tongs.

☐  Complaints of physical discomfort despite frequent position changes

☐  Status of the traction apparatus

☐  Vital signs

## CLINICAL PROBLEM SOLVING

| Potential Problems | Suggested Solutions |
|---|---|
| The patient expresses fear of being turned. | □ Encourage patient to lie on the frame and be turned before being placed on it after surgery.<br>□ Carefully explain each step of the turning process and the use of each piece of equipment.<br>□ Allow the patient to express fears and concerns.<br>□ Carefully answer all questions in a way that the patient can understand your explanation. |
| The patient experiences unusual pain or discomfort when turned. | □ Have the patient describe details of pain.<br>□ Assess the patient's neurological status and compare it to the patient's status before turning.<br>□ Ensure that the traction apparatus is intact.<br>□ Assess for psychological component of pain.<br>□ Notify physician if pain persists or if there is a change in neurological status. |

# UNIT NINE    CIRCOLECTRIC BED

## NURSING PROCESS DATA

### ASSESSMENT    *Data Base*

Determine patient's level of movement and sensation.

Evaluate patient's ability to understand the procedure.

Assess the ability of patient to control his own turning.

### PLANNING    *Objectives*

To turn from supine to prone to supine without excess patient movement.

To provide optimal skin care for immobilized patients.

To maintain good skin condition for patients on long-term bed rest.

### IMPLEMENTATION    *Procedures*

Preparing to Operate Bed

Placing Ambulatory Patient on Bed

Placing Nonambulatory Patient on Bed

Turning from Supine to Prone

Assisting Patient with Bedpan

### EVALUATION    *Expected Outcomes*

Patient turns from supine to prone to supine without excess movement.

Patient receives optimal skin care.

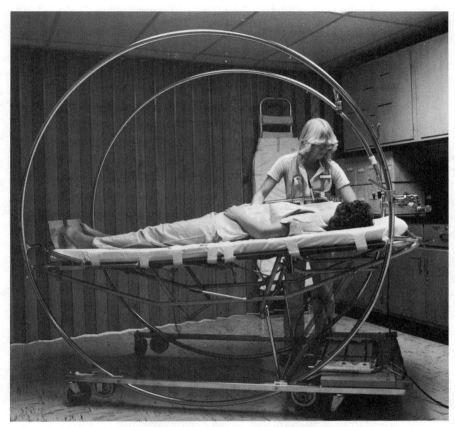

The CircOlectric bed provides position change for patients with restricted mobility.

## PREPARING TO OPERATE BED

### Equipment

CircOlectric bed

Hand control unit

### Procedure

1. Learn the mechanical aspects of operating the CircOlectric bed.

2. Hand control unit has two parts: a toggle switch designated FACE or BACK and a push-button switch for actual movement.

3. Bed is operated by selecting FACE or BACK position and pressing button until bed is in desired position.

4. A crank is stored in a tray at the head of the bed to adjust the bed if the electricity is off.

5. Two wheel locks are located on opposite corners of the bed.

6. Two automatic stops are on the bottom rail of the bed. They should be set whenever the anterior frame is not in use.

   a. The sitting stop, on the patient's right side, prevents rotation beyond an upright sitting position.
   b. The standing stop, the patient's left side, prevents rotation beyond a semi-erect position.

7. The gatch lever, at the patient's right hip, changes the posterior frame from a flat to a semi-sitting position.

## PLACING AMBULATORY PATIENT ON BED

### Equipment

CircOlectric bed

Hand control unit

### Procedure

1. Explain procedure to patient.

2. Demonstrate bed movement by using the controls.

3. Place bed in a vertical position.

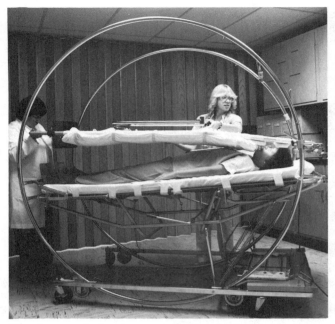

Place frame on bed and secure bolt at head of bed first.

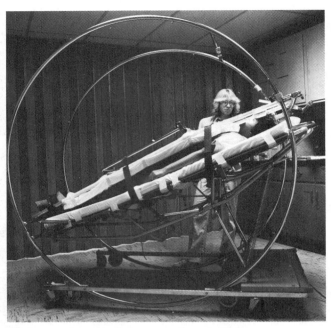

The first step in turning is to secure the anterior frame.

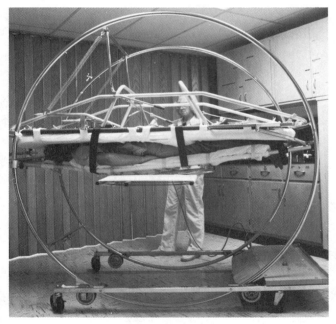

Stop turn with patient in prone position with head slightly down.

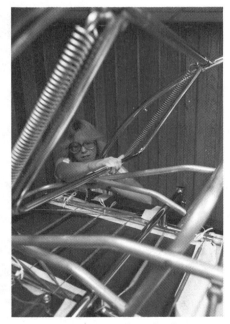

Pull support bar outward to raise frame.

4. Have patient step backward onto the footboard with his back toward the posterior frame.

5. Rotate the bed backward to the desired position.

6. Adjust patient's position so that hips are at level of gatch.

## PLACING NONAMBULATORY PATIENT ON BED

### Equipment

CircOlectric bed

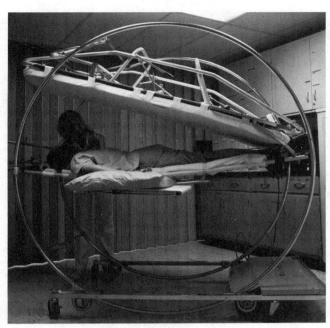

Lock frame with support bar to complete turn.

## Procedure

1. Explain transfer to patient.
2. Demonstrate bed movement to patient if patient is alert.
3. Position bed/guerney parallel to CircOlectric bed.
4. Alert patient when you are ready to move him to the CirOlectric bed.
5. Transfer patient using a standard sheet or the three-man carry method.

## TURNING FROM SUPINE TO PRONE

### Equipment

CircOlectric bed

Bed linen

### Procedure

1. Explain procedure to patient.
2. Move the footboard from the patient's feet to the foot of the bed.
3. Place the anterior frame through the large rings one end at a time.
4. Attach the anterior frame on bolt at the head of the patient and secure it with a nut.
5. Adjust the footboard of the anterior frame to the patient.
6. Attach the anterior frame to the foot of the bed with a bolt and nut as at the head of the bed.
7. Adjust the support bar (at the head of the anterior frame) at the level of the chest to hold patient firmly but comfortably.
8. Adjust the security collar knobs against the support bar.
9. Adjust the headbands to patient's forehead and chin.
10. Put patient's arms into the slings attached to the anterior frame.
11. Double-check all attachments and release all stops.
12. Turn patient to slightly head-down position.
13. Raise the posterior frame by removing the nut, pulling the support bar in the frame outward, and lifting the frame until it locks with the support bar.
14. Gatch the posterior frame to remove pressure from the patient's feet.
15. Rotate bed backward to a prone or a slightly upright position.
16. To turn the patient from a prone to a supine position, reverse the procedure.

## ASSISTING WITH BEDPAN

### Equipment

CircOlectric bed

Absorbent pads

Stryker bedpan

### Procedure

1. Explain procedure to patient.
2. Provide privacy for patient.
3. Place patient on the posterior frame in a flat or semi-sitting position.
4. Pull apart the elastic cords under the posterior frame and remove the round mattress insert.
5. Insert the bedpan into the opening and hold it there with the elastic cord.
6. Place absorbent pads at the edges of the opening to prevent soiling linen (optional).
7. Remove the bedpan when the patient is finished and replace the mattress insert.
8. Wash hands.

**CHARTING** *for CircOlectric Bed*

☐ Length of time patient spends on each side

☐ How patient tolerates the turning procedure

☐ If applicable, how patient tolerates being in a relatively vertical position

☐ Complaints of physical discomfort despite frequent position changes

☐ Status of condition for which patient is on the CircOlectric bed

☐ Vital signs

---

## CLINICAL PROBLEM SOLVING

**Potential Problems**

The patient expresses a fear of turning.

The patient experiences unusual pain or discomfort when turned.

**Suggested Solutions**

☐ If possible, ensure that patient has preoperative teaching. Encourage the patient to lie on the bed and be turned.

☐ Carefully explain each step of the turning process and the use of each piece of equipment.

☐ Allow patient to express his fears and concerns.

☐ Carefully answer all the patient's questions in a way that the patient can understand.

☐ Change positions slowly to allow the patient to adjust to the turning position.

☐ Have patient describe details of the pain.

☐ Assess the patient's neurological status and compare it to the patient's status before turning.

☐ Assess for psychological component of pain. Notify the physician if pain persists or if there is a change in neurological status.

---

## TERMINOLOGY

**Abduction:**  movement of a bone away from the midline of the body or body part, as in raising the arm or spreading the fingers.

**Adduction:**  movement of a bone toward the midline of the body or part.

**Alignment:**  arranged in a straight line.

**Ambulate:**  walking; able to walk.

**Amputation:**  surgical removal of a diseased limb, part, or organ.

**Bryant's traction:**  a type of skin traction used to treat small children with fractures of the femur.

**Buck's traction:**  a type of skin traction used occasionally in the elderly patient with a hip fracture prior to surgery.

**Callus:**  localized hyperplasia of the horny layer of the epidermis usually due to pressure or friction.

**Cardiovascular:**  pertaining to heart and blood vessels.

**Circulation:**  movement in a circular course, as the movement of blood.

**Comminuted:**  broken in pieces.

**Contusion:**  soft tissue injury as a result of a blow.

**Diaphysis:**  the part of the long bone between the ends, also known as the shaft.

**Edema:**  a condition in which body tissues contain an excessive amount of fluid.

**Embolus:**  a mass of undissolved matter present in a blood or lymphatic vessel brought there by the blood or lymph current.

**Epiphysis:**  the end of a long bone.

**Evisceration:**  protrusion of the viscera; removal of the viscera.

**Extension:**  a movement that increases the angle between two bones, straightening a joint.

**Fibroblasts:**  an immature fiber-producing cell of connective tissue.

**Flexion:** a movement that decreases the angle between two bones; the act of bending a joint.

**Hyperextension:** continuation of extension beyond the anatomical position, as in bending the head backward.

**Metaphysis:** wide part of bone at end of shaft adjacent to the epiphyseal disk.

**Mobility:** state or quality of being mobile; facility of movement.

**Musculo:** pertaining to muscles.

**Musculoskeletal:** pertaining to the muscles and bones.

**Osteoblasts:** immature cell which on maturation plays a role in bone production.

**Orthostatic:** concerning an erect or standing position.

**Orthostatic hypotension:** low blood pressure in a standing or upright position.

**Paralysis:** temporary or permanent loss of function, especially loss of sensation or voluntary motion.

**Paresthesis:** pertains to an abnormal sensation.

**Pearson attachment:** an attachment to skeletal traction that allows continuous traction in line of the femur by the use of cords and weights.

**Prosthesis:** replacement of a missing part by an artificial substitute.

**Restorative:** promoting a return to health.

**Russell's traction:** type of skeletal traction to treat fractures of the shaft of the femur.

**Sprain:** injury caused by wrenching or twisting of a joint that results in tearing or stretching of the associated ligaments.

**Strain:** injury caused by excessive force or stretching of muscles or tendons around the joint.

**Stryker frame:** a special bed used to treat spinal cord injured patients.

**Syncope:** a transient loss of consciousness due to inadequate blood flow to the brain.

**Thomas splint:** skeletal traction used for long-term immobilization of fractures.

**Torque:** a rotary force.

**Traction:** process of drawing or pulling, often by weights to keep the body or parts in proper alignment.

Chapter **28**

# Pain Management

## LEARNING OBJECTIVES

Discuss what is meant by the experience of pain.

Explain the use of endorphins for pain control.

Describe the body's physiological response to pain.

Identify the most important information elicited from the patient regarding pain.

Describe the four types of pain.

Discuss the Gate Control Theory.

Outline the main points of one noninvasive method of relieving pain.

Describe the pain relief method known as TENS.

List and discuss five of the main parameters of pain assessment.

Summarize at least two methods of relieving pain.

Describe three potential problems for pain control and at least one suggested solution for each problem.

Define the term referred pain.

Write two nursing diagnoses appropriate for patients experiencing pain.

## COPING WITH PAIN

The experience of pain is direct and personal. In this culture we tend to view pain as a negative condition and often will go to any lengths to avoid the sensation. The positive aspect of pain is that it is an early warning system; its presence triggers an awareness that something is wrong in our body. Without the sensation of pain we could not survive, for we would have no cues with which to modify our reactions and direct our behavior. One perspective of pain is that it is a message to our conscious self to check out any pain sensation before it gets worse, for that is the nature of pain. Without intervention it may well get worse.

McCaffery, a nurse-author who writes about managing the patient in pain, defines pain as "whatever the patient experiencing pain says it is, existing whenever he says it does." The nurse is totally dependent on the patient to describe the sensation of pain, identify the location, and tell about what kind of pain is being experienced.

The most important information in pain assessment, then, is the patient's report. The pain experience is totally subjective. The onset of acute pain stimulates the sympathetic nervous system "fight or flight" response that results in certain signs or symptoms. While observation of these symptoms provides objective data, it cannot be considered conclusive evidence to the indentification of pain—that must come from the patient.

The sensation of physical pain arouses some specific responses in the patient. The sympathetic nervous system response is usually stimulated by superficial pain, and the parasympathetic nervous system response is usually stimulated by deeper pain and results in the slowing down of all the systems to conserve energy.

**Gate Control Theory**   The neurophysiological basis of pain can be explained by several theories, none of which is mutually exclusive nor totally comprehensive. One of the most popular and credible concepts is the gate control theory. The first premise of the gate control theory is that the actual existence and intensity of the pain experience is dependent upon the particular transmission of neurological impulses. Secondly, gate mechanisms along the nervous system control the transmission of pain. Finally, if the gate is open, the impulses that result in the sensation of pain are able to reach the conscious level. If the gate is closed, the impulses do not reach the level of consciousness and the sensation of pain is not experienced.

Three primary types of neurological involvement affect whether the gate is open or closed. The first type involves activity in the large and small nerve fibers that affect the sensation of pain. Pain impulses travel along small diameter fibers. The large diameter nerve fibers close the gate to the impulses that travel along the small fibers. The technique of using cutaneous stimulation on the skin, which has many large diameter fibers, may help to close the gate to the transmission of painful impulses, thereby relieving the sensation of pain. Interventions that apply this theory to practice include massage, hot and cold applications, touch, acupressure, and transcutaneous electric nerve stimulation. These interventions are described in detail later in this chapter.

The second form of neurological involvement is the impulses from the brainstem that affect the sensation of pain. The reticular formation monitors in the brainstem regulate sensory input. If the person receives adequate or excessive amounts of sensory stimulation, the brainstem transmits impulses that close the gate and inhibit pain impulses from being transmitted. If on the other hand, the patient experiences a lack of sensory input, the brainstem would not inhibit the pain impulses, the gate would be open, and the pain impulses would be transmitted. Interventions that apply to this part of the gate control theory are those related in some way to sensory input, such as techniques of distraction, guided imagery, and visualization.

The third type of neurological involvement is the neurological activities or impulses in the cerebral cortex and thalamus. A person's thoughts, emotions, and memories may activate certain impulses in the cortex that trigger pain impulses, which are transmitted to the conscious level. Past experiences relating to pain affect how the patient responds to current pain. For this reason, it is important to explore the patient's previous experiences and teach the patient what to expect from the present situation. Interventions that apply to this part of the gate control theory include utilizing and teaching various relaxation techniques, teaching the patient about what expectations to have about pain as related to a specific illness, allowing the patient to feel he or she has some control over the taking of medication for pain relief, and giving medications properly, i.e., preventively, before the pain is so severe that the patient fears he or she will receive no relief.

**The Discovery of Endorphins**   A recent and exciting theory of pain relief was developed when Avron Goldstein, looking for morphine and heroin receptors, discovered that receptors in the brain fit only morphine or morphine-like molecules. He asked himself why these receptors were located in the brain, when MS is not naturally found in this area. The answer, learned through diligent research, is that the brain produces natural brain opiates. These substances are hormones, chemicals produced by different parts of the body to regulate certain biological processes. At the present time, five of

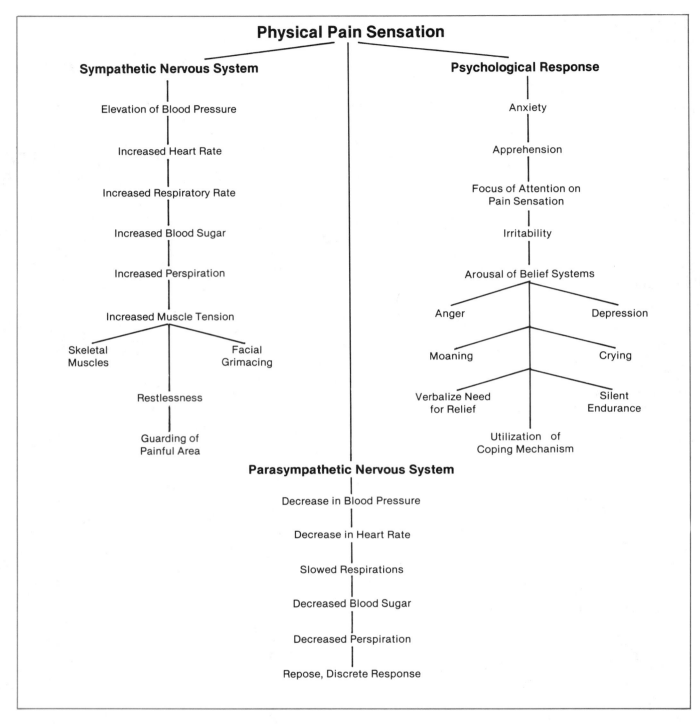

these natural opiates have been found. Three are called endorphins, one dynorphin, and one enkephalin. Endorphins fit into special cells, called receptors, in order to activate their regulating powers. In addition to endorphin "keys" and receptor "locks," researchers have found anti-locks, called antagonists, that keep endorphins from working. Endorphin receptors and anti-locks have been found throughout the body—in the stomach, intestines, pancreas, spinal cord, and bloodstream as well as the brain.

A beta-endorphin is 50 times stronger than morphine, and a dynorphin is 190 times stronger than morphine. In one test, fourteen men and women suffering from extreme pain from cancer were given tiny injections of an endorphin. *All* felt relief within minutes, and the relief lasted from one to three days.

Endorphins are now being produced synthetically, but they are very expensive and at this time used only for research. Researchers must discover how the body makes and releases endorphins before a method is developed to encourage the body to produce more of its own endorphins to control pain.

The pain experience is a mixture of physical sensations, physiologic changes, and psychosocial factors. The patient's interpretation of the physical sensation is influenced by the patient's culture, previous experiences with and without pain, beliefs about self, interpretation of the future, present environment, and the persons in that environment. The intensity of pain is influenced by what the sensation means to the patient, the patient's level of anxiety, degree of fatigue, and the number of stressors in the patient's environment.

---

### CHARACTERISTICS OF PAIN

| *Location* | *Factors Associated with Pain* | *Aggravating Factors* |
|---|---|---|
| Area of the body | Nausea | Position changes |
| Diffuse or localized | Vomiting | Environmental stressors |
| Radiates and area involved | Bradycardia/tachycardia | Fatigue |
| | Hypotension/hypertension | Inadequate pain relief |
| *Quality* | Profuse perspiration | measures |
| | Apprehension or anxiety | |
| Stabbing, knife-like | | *Alleviating Factors* |
| Throbbing | *Precipitating Factors* | |
| Cramping | | Position change |
| Vise-like, suffocating | Motion affecting incision area | Medications |
| Searing, burning | (e.g., coughing, turning, | Biofeedback |
| Superficial, deep | deep breathing) | Visualization |
| | Fear and emotional distress | Relaxation techniques |
| *Intensity* | Inflammation or infection | TENS |
| | Trauma | Massage |
| Rate on scale of zero to ten | Disease state | |
| (zero = no pain, ten = most pain ever experienced) | | |

---

**Pain Pathways**    The pathway to pain is a complicated, wondrous expression of how our amazing bodies work. First there is the source of pain, a direct causative factor. Stimulation of a pain receptor may be mechanical, chemical, thermal, electrical, or ischemic. The sensation travels along the sensory pathways and ascends the spinal cord to the thalamus. The autonomic nervous system is activated, and sensations travel to the sensory area of the cerebral cortex. Pain reception occurs in the thalamus, where awareness and integration take place, and pain interpretation occurs in the cerebral cortex. Once awareness of pain takes place and it has been interpreted by the cerebral cortex, the person becomes aware and the response patterns are activated.

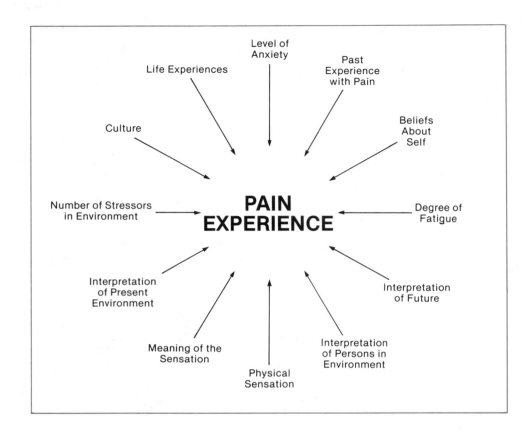

## NONINVASIVE PAIN RELIEF

When a method to relieve pain is noninvasive, it is both safer and results in less potential side effects for the patient. Such measures will probably become the pain control choice of the future.

**TENS** Transcutaneous electric nerve stimulation is a noninvasive method to relieve pain that has gained credibility and popularity in the past few years. The procedure involves stimulation to the skin via a mild electrical current. The stimulator is a solid-state battery-powered unit that has two to four electrodes attached by lead wires. These electrodes are placed on the skin, and the patient experiences a buzzing, tingling, or vibrating sensation. This method relieves pain, but just exactly how this phenomenon occurs is not clear. What is apparent through clinical research is that this method offers relief from chronic pain. In fact, the most common use today is for relief of chronic pain in adults.

Is TENS effective for acute pain? This is a question the medical world is asking, for the traditional method of controlling pain through analgesics has never been a perfect solution. Research indicates that ten to twenty percent of the patients who receive narcotics following major surgery do not receive adequate pain relief. Recent studies on the use of TENS for postoperative patients reveal that this method proved to be significantly more effective. There was also less depression and a higher level of activity in the patients receiving TENS versus those receiving narcotics. The conclusion appears to be that TENS is a viable alternative to the more traditional methods of administering medication for pain control. It is infinitely more appealing because it is: non-invasive; safer; results in more pain relief; has less depressive side-effects; results in a higher activity level in post-surgery patients; and finally it gives the staff the confidence that they can do something concrete to relieve a patient's pain.

Exactly how or why this form of electrical stimulation works to relieve pain is not clear. There are, however, several theories that attempt to explain how TENS works.

Increased production of endorphins.

Fatigue of peripheral nerve fibers by high frequency electrical stimulation.

Blockade of primary afferent fibers.

Stimulation of afferent nerve fibers, which masks or modifies perception of pain.

Gate theory (large cutaneous nerve fibers close the gate to the transmission of pain impulses).

**Biofeedback**    Biofeedback is a second noninvasive method to relieve pain. It is also used to reduce stress. The biofeedback system is based on three principles: individuals can be taught to regulate any biological function that can be monitored by electrical instruments; changes in physiology in the body will be accompanied by changes in one's mental-emotional state and vice versa; and biofeedback training can assist people to enter a relaxed state that is fundamental to consciously controlling internal functions.

The first phase of biofeedback training involves teaching the learner, who is hooked up to an electrical monitoring instrument (EEG, ECG, EMG, GSR), to experience how behavior affects internal processes. The second phase involves imagining or visualization. The trainee experiences that thinking pleasant or happy thoughts slows down heart rate while unhappy thoughts speed up the heart rate. The third and last phase teaches the trainee to imagine heaviness and warmth in his or her arms and hands or around the heart. At the same time the trainee is instructed to notice that the heart beat decelerates. Conversely, when constriction is felt, the heart beat increases. This last phase establishes a link between internal sensations (warmth around the heart) and the effect on a body system (slowing of heart rate).

When the trainee understands that he or she can duplicate the sensation through visualization and affect his or her body processes, an important principle has been learned; once these connections have been made, the biofeedback equipment is no longer necessary and the trainee can manipulate certain internal functions on demand.

**Pain Relief**    There are many pain-reduction techniques and medications. The physical sensation of pain itself is usually a small factor in the pain experience. Indeed, the physiologic response of muscle tension alone may increase pain. Rarely is pain relief successfully achieved with only one method. Two or more methods have an additive effect. Also, massive doses of narcotics do not always control pain because pain has been allowed to escalate. Relief of pain by prescribing small, frequent doses of medication and preventing escalation of pain can provide the patient with a comfortable and speedy recovery.

The most significant aspect of pain relief is the relationship that exists between the nurse and the patient. The patient knows that the nurse has the power to relieve pain or to withhold pain relief. This knowledge creates anticipatory anxiety. The patient who has a nurse who is supportive and caring and who will assist the patient with pain management will need and ask for less medication. On the other hand, the clock watcher craves pain relief. This raises the patient's anxiety and pain escalates with each moment that the patient realizes his or her needs are of little concern to the nurse.

Nursing interventions that provide the best pain relief are those that elicit behaviors incompatible with the behaviors of pain. For example, when the patient is talking about something of great interest or pleasure, he or she is not talking about pain. If distracted, the patient is not focusing on pain. Relaxation is as incompatible with muscle tension and anxiety as breathing slowly and deeply is incompatible wih rapid, shallow respirations. The nurse should teach pain-relief techniques when there is no experience of pain, preferably before surgery, so that the patient can practice. The nurse should also encourage the patient to use techniques that the patient has already found effective, no matter how "unscientific" they may be.

## NURSING DIAGNOSES

The following nursing diagnoses may be appropriate to include in a Patient Care Plan when the components are related to alleviating pain in a patient.

| Nursing Diagnosis (Potential) | Defining Characteristic; Etiology (Examples) |
|---|---|
| ☐ Anxiety, *related to* | Increased stress or pain, e.g., illness, trauma, or loss. |
| ☐ Comfort, Alteration in: Pain, *related to* | Tissue damage or decreased endorphins, e.g., recent surgical intervention or disease state, inadequate pain control. |
| ☐ Fear, *related to* | Increased or intractable pain, e.g., terminal disease states, knowledge deficit, or perceived inability to control pain. |

## UNIT ONE    PAIN RELIEF

### NURSING PROCESS DATA

**ASSESSMENT**    *Data Base*

Assess type of pain.

Acute pain: short duration of a few seconds to six months.

Chronic pain: longer duration of six months to years.

Intractable pain: severe and constant and resistant to relief measures.

Assess nonverbal indications of pain.

Assess patient's behavioral responses to pain.

Depression, withdrawal, or crying.

Stoicism or expressive.

Assess location, quality, intensity, onset, aggravating factors, associated factors and alleviating factors. (See Pain Chart)

### PLANNING    *Objectives*

To prevent pain from retarding recovery.

To prevent pain from causing nausea and vomiting, a decrease in fluid intake which would result in fluid and electrolyte imbalance.

To prevent pain from causing undue fatigue.

To prevent pain from inhibiting moving, ambulating, turning and coughing. Pain increases the possibilities of secondary problems from inactivity e.g., pneumonia, emboli.

To relieve pain or prevent pain from escalating by relaxing muscles; muscle tension increases the pain.

To decrease patient's anxiety that present and future pain relief will not be achieved.

To bring pain relief to a level acceptable to the patient.

### IMPLEMENTATION  *Procedures*

Achieving Pain Relief Using Medication

Alleviating Pain Through Touch

Alleviating Pain Using Heat or Cold

Achieving Pain Relief Using Relaxation Techniques Following a Written Plan

Achieving Pain Relief Using Transcutaneous Electric Nerve Stimulation (TENS)

### EVALUATION  *Expected Outcomes*

Pain is controlled to the patient's satisfaction.

Pain is relieved and does not interfere with ambulation or sitting in a chair.

Patient is free from nausea and vomiting due to pain.

Patient's anxiety level is low.

---

## ACHIEVING PAIN RELIEF USING MEDICATION

### Procedure

1. Check physician's orders.
2. Use a preventive approach to pain management. **Rationale:** Giving medication before pain becomes severe will result in more effective pain control.
3. Follow steps outlined in assessment to determine the nature, quality, and extent of pain.
4. Start with p.o. medications. If ineffective or only mildly effective, give IM medications, or combine p.o. and IM medications.
5. Evaluate result of pain medication. Was it effective? How long did the effect last? What was the extent of relief?
6. Evaluate patient for possible side effects of the medication.
7. Discuss with physician the effects of medication and whether a change of prescription is needed.

## ALLEVIATING PAIN THROUGH TOUCH

### Equipment

Cream or talcum powder

Massage oil

### Procedure

1. Determine whether patient achieves more relief from pain with massage over painful area, near painful area, or from foot rub, back rub, or hand rub.
2. Warm your hands by rubbing them together or rinsing in warm water.

3. Warm lotion to be used by holding closed bottle under warm running water.

4. Massage area of patient's choice with slow and steady motion.

5. Use deep pressure or light stroking motion, whichever is more comfortable for the patient. **Rationale:** Relaxed muscles result in a decreased pain level.

## ALLEVIATING PAIN USING HEAT OR COLD

### Equipment

Aquathermic pad

Gel pack

Ice bag or collar

### Procedure

1. Determine whether heat, which increases circulation, or cold, which impairs circulation, brings more relief to patient.

2. Obtain order from physician for heat application. Obtain a temperature-regulated device. (Example: aquathermic pad.)

3. Obtain order from physician for cold application. Obtain a gel pack or ice bag.

4. Cover devices with towel or special cover. **Rationale:** A soft cover will prevent skin irritation.

5. Apply treatment for 20–30 minutes only.

## ACHIEVING PAIN RELIEF USING RELAXATION TECHNIQUES FOLLOWING A WRITTEN PLAN

### Equipment

A printed relaxation technique (the nurse can read slowly to patient until patient learns technique)

A cassette recorder and tape

### Procedure

1. Help patient assume a comfortable position.
   a. If lying, place support under knees, lower legs, and under head. Be sure body is in good alignment.
   b. If sitting, sit comfortably positioned with both feet on the floor, hands on knees, back straight, and head balanced comfortably straight.

2. Instruct patient to inhale deeply, hold breath for a moment, then exhale deeply. Repeat several times.

3. Give the following instructions to patient, using a slow soothing voice.
   a. Continue to breathe in and out slowly. Concentrate on my voice and follow my words.
   b. Find a point of tension in your body.
   c. As you identify the tension, tense the area up even more.
   d. Then relax the area, letting all the tension drain out.

4. Continue with these instructions until the patient has had time to relax all points of tension.

5. To end the process, instruct the patient to open eyes slowly and say, "I feel relaxed and awake."

## ACHIEVING PAIN RELIEF USING TRANSCUTANEOUS ELECTRIC NERVE STIMULATION (TENS)

### Equipment

Cutaneous stimulator with lead wires and leads

Cream for lead placement

### Procedure

1. Obtain physician's order (may be intermittent or continuous).

2. Follow directions for electrode placement. (Check electrode placement chart provided by manufacturer of TENS unit.)
   a. Place electrode on skin over or near the area of pain.
   b. Identify trigger points (specific points which are extremely sensitive when stimulated ) and place electrode.
   c. Identify acupressure point, and place electrode.
   d. Place electrode on peripheral nerves, enervating area of pain. (Patient adjusts each pair of electrodes to produce a sensation that is pleasant and to relieve pain.)

3. Apply electrodes.
   a. Some electrodes are water conductive: moisten with water.
   b. Some electrodes require a conductive gel: place gel on electrode before attaching to skin.

4. Instruct patient to adjust intensity of skin stimulation until it creates a pleasant sensation that relieves the pain.

**CHARTING** *for Pain Relief*

☐ Describe the patient's pain, including location, quality, intensity, precipitating factors, associated factors, and aggravating factors

☐ Describe alleviating factors, including what the patient does to relieve pain as well as nursing assistance

☐ Describe behavioral changes due to pain relief or the absence of objective changes in response to the medication and/or nursing interventions

☐ If there is a poor response to therapy, state what other measures will be attempted and chart results

☐ Continue to document attempts to relieve pain until relief occurs and the patient is satisfied

---

## CLINICAL PROBLEM SOLVING

**Potential Problems**

Patient achieves no relief from relaxation, visualization, or massage.

**Suggested Solutions**

☐ Try combining methods with use of medications, i.e., use these methods while waiting for the medication to take effect.

☐ Patient has to trust the technique before it will be effective. Have patient talk to another person who has found technique helpful.

Patient achieves little or no relief from TENS.

☐ Use another brand or type of stimulator as ordered.

☐ If using continuous cutaneous stimulation, try using intermittent stimulation and vice versa.

Patient develops skin irritation at electrode sites.

☐ Use hypoallergic tape to secure electrodes.

☐ Discontinue tape. Use velcro or elastic bandage to hold electrodes in place.

☐ If rash appears to be caused by gel, mix cortisone gel with the electrode cream. Change gel. Cleanse skin and electrodes with soap and water frequently.

Patient develops constipation from regularly administered narcotic preparations.

☐ Obtain order for and administer stool softener and peristaltic stimulant.

☐ Encourage intake of high-fiber diet, if not contraindicated.

☐ Encourage adequate fluid intake.

---

## TERMINOLOGY

**Acupressure:** Chinese method of treatment that involves compression of certain areas of the body by following a system of meridians or energy flow.

**Adaptive reaction:** a response by which the person attempts to improve or alter his or her condition in relation to the environment.

**Alleviate:** to make more bearable; reduce (pain, grief, or suffering).

**Angina:** a sense of suffocation with symptoms of severe, steady pain and feeling of pressure in region of the heart.

**Arrhythmia:** irregular rhythm.

**Arthritis:** inflammation of a joint, usually accompanied by pain and frequently, deformity.

**Autogenic training:** a method of deep muscle relaxation that enables one to reduce the stress response, regain homeostasis, and prepare to handle additional stress.

**Autoimmunization:** immunity produced by an attack of the disease or by processes occurring within the body.

**Autonomic nervous system:** the part of the nervous system that regulates the functioning of internal organs and glands; it controls such functions as digestion, respiration, and cardiovascular activity.

**Behavior:** the manner in which one acts.

**Biofeedback:** a training technique that utilizes monitoring instruments to assist people to control stress-related disorders through self-regulation of internal functions.

**Brady:** prefix indicating slow.

**Bradycardia:** slowed heart action, below 60 beats/minute.

**Cardio:** prefix pertaining to the heart.

**Cardiovascular:** pertaining to the heart and blood vessels.

**Cerebral cortex:** the extensive outer layer of grey tissue of the cerebral hemispheres (brain), responsible for higher nervous functions.

**Coping mechanisms:** means by which an individual adjusts or adapts to a threat or a challenge; actions that assist in maintaining homeostasis.

**Diaphoresis:** profuse sweating.

**Dynamics of homeostasis:** danger or its symbols, whether internal or external, resulting in the activation of the sympathetic nervous system and the adrenal medulla. The organism prepares for fight or flight.

**Emotional:** affected by strong feelings, as of joy and sorrow.

**Endorphins:** a naturally occurring body chemical similar to morphine but many times stronger.

**Fight or flight:** one's immediate response to stress that is, although archaic and often inappropriate, part of our central nervous system biological heritage.

**Gastro:** term that denotes the stomach.

**Gastrointestinal:** pertaining to the stomach and the intestine.

**General adaptation syndrome:** a general theory of stress response formulated by Dr. Hans Selye; describes the action of stress response in three stages—the alarm reaction, the stage of resistance, and the stage of exhaustion.

**-Genic:** suffix indicating generation or production.

**Health:** the state of physical, psychological, and sociological well-being.

**Hypertension:** a condition in which the patient has a higher blood pressure than judged to be normal.

**Illness:** a state characterized by the malfunction of the biopsychosocial organism.

**Insomnia:** inability to sleep.

**Ischemic:** local and temporary anemia due to obstruction of the circulation to a part.

**Meditation:** the act of reflecting upon or pondering; contemplation.

**Musculo:** pertaining to the muscles.

**Musculoskeletal:** pertaining to the muscles and the skeleton.

**Nausea:** inclination to vomit, usually preceding emesis.

**Neuro:** prefix pertaining to nerves.

**Pain:** a sensation in which a person experiences discomfort, distress, or suffering.

**Parasympathetic nervous system:** a division of the autonomic nervous system that regulates acetylcholine and conserves energy expenditure; it slows down the system.

**Physiological:** concerning body function.

**Psychogenic:** of mental origin.

**Referred pain:** pain felt in a part removed from its point of origin.

**Regression:** a turning back or return to a former state.

**Relaxation:** a lessening of tension or activity in a part.

**Resistance:** opposition to or the ability to oppose.

**Rheumatism:** a term applied to conditions of acute and chronic, characterized by soreness and stiffness of muscles and pain in joints.

**Stamina:** constitutional energy; strength; endurance.

**Stress:** a nonspecific response of the body to any internal or external event or change that impinges on a person's system and creates a demand.

**Stressor:** a specific demand that gives rise to a coping response.

**Sympathetic nervous system:** a division of the autonomic nervous system that controls energy expenditure and mobilizes for action when confronted with a threat.

**Tachy:** prefix meaning fast.

**Tachycardia:** abnormal rapidity of heart action; above 100 beats/minute.

**TENS:** a noninvasive method to relieve pain that involves stimulation to the skin via a mild electric current.

**Touch:** a tactile sense.

**Visceral:** pertaining to internal organs.

**Wellness:** a state of physical, psychological and sociological well-being of a whole person.

# Chapter **29**

# *Diagnostic Tests*

**Unit One   Dye Injection Studies**
Preparing for Oral Cholecystogram
Preparing for Intravenous Cholangiogram
Preparing for Intravenous Pyelogram
Preparing for Myelogram
Preparing for Arteriogram
Preparing for Computerized Axial Tomography (CAT Scan)
Preparing for Cardiac Catheterization

**Unit Two   Radioactive Studies**
Preparing for Bone Scan
Preparing for Lung Scan
Preparing for Brain Scan

**Unit Three   Air Contrast Studies**
Preparing for Pneumoencephalogram
Preparing for Ventriculogram

**Unit Four   Barium Studies**
Preparing for Barium Enema
Preparing for Upper Gastrointestinal Study

**Unit Five   Diagnostic Procedures**
Assisting with Lumbar Puncture
Assisting with Liver Biopsy
Assisting with Thoracentesis
Assisting with Paracentesis
Assisting with Bone Marrow Aspiration
Assisting with Vaginal Examination and Papanicolaou
   Smear
Assisting with Proctoscopy
Assisting with Gastroscopy/Endoscopy
Assisting with Cystoscopy
Assisting with Amniocentesis

## LEARNING OBJECTIVES

Describe the major components of patient teaching for diagnostic studies.

List at least three preparatory functions for patients undergoing diagnostic studies.

Explain the importance of determining allergic responses to shellfish before patients undergo contrast media studies.

List the signs and symptoms that occur when the patient experiences an allergic reaction.

Explain the reason for giving blocking agents before administering radioisotopes to patients.

Outline the nursing care responsibilities when a patient returns from a myelogram.

Discuss the nursing care responsibilities when a patient returns from an arteriogram.

Describe the post-heart-catheterization care that is carried out to prevent post-procedural complications.

List at least two safety precautions for staff members who are working with patients undergoing studies using radioactive material.

Outline the essential steps in preparing a patient for a pneumoencephalogram.

Identify at least two potential problems for patients undergoing air contrast studies and state two suggested solutions for each problem.

Explain the steps you would take if a patient was given medications prior to a GI series.

Describe patient positions for at least four diagnostic procedures commonly performed at the bedside.

Compare and contrast post-procedure nursing observations for patients undergoing liver biopsy, paracentesis, and thoracentesis.

Describe the data that should be included in the charting for patients undergoing diagnostic procedures.

**PREPARATION**

The responsibility of the nurse begins with the initial scheduling of the test and continues after the results of the test are explained to the patient. The physician explains the results of the test, but the nurse answers questions, interprets terminology, and listens to the patient express his feelings or apprehensions.

The preparation of patients for diagnostic tests must be done on an individual basis. Some patients are well informed about the test they are scheduled to take. They know about diet and fluid restrictions, what to expect during the procedure, whether or not there is any discomfort with the test, and how long the procedure will take. Others need a great deal of explanation. There are also patients who prefer not to be given any explanation about the test. Nurses need to respect the patient's preferences and provide only information requested, unless it in some way is a danger to the patient.

Many patients who are frightened are unable to communicate. Communication involves an active, verbal interchange of ideas as well as paying attention to the patient's nonverbal cues. One effective way to allow patients time to think about questions is to provide a printed form explaining the diagnostic test. The form may cover such information as how long a test takes, equipment used for the test, and any sensations experienced during the test. Leaving the form at the bedside can stimulate interest and prompt the shy, reserved patient to ask questions when you return later.

Another important aspect of teaching involves the way in which you approach the patient. Avoid giving the impression that you are in a hurry and that you have no time to answer any questions. On the other hand, be aware of the patient's ability to pay attention to what you have to say. If the patient seems distracted, he or she may be worried about finances, about who is watching the children, or whether or not the job will be waiting after discharge from the hospital. This preoccupation may prevent assimilation of knowledge and the patient will be unprepared for the events that follow.

Remember, the patient probably does not know medical jargon; therefore, explain procedures in terms the patient can understand. If the patient looks puzzled and does not ask any questions, evaluate how you presented the information.

Feedback is the only way in which you can evaluate the learner's knowledge. Feedback can be in the form of direct questioning about certain aspects of the test. Feedback can also be determined through direct observation of facial expressions, posturing, and activities.

**Dye Injection Studies**    Many x-rays utilize the normal contrasts of the body, such as air, water in soft tissues, and bone; however, for some tests a contrast media is required. Several types of contrast media are used routinely. Barium sulfate, helium, carbon dioxide, and organic iodides are some substances that are commonly used.

One of the major problems with the use of some contrast media is the adverse reaction or sensitivity that can occur. This is more common when iodine preparations are used. The degree of reaction varies from mild, such as nausea, to severe, such as cardiovascular collapse. The usual symptoms include: urticaria, hives, nausea, vomiting and decreased blood pressure.

Patients allergic to food, especially shellfish, or drugs are often allergic to some dyes used in diagnostic studies, particularly those that are iodine based. Following injections of iodine dye, many tests are abnormal for varying lengths of time. Urine sodium, specific gravity, protein, and osmolality are abnormal for 16 hours. Urine catecholamines are abnormal for 16 hours.

Barium can cause some uncomfortable feelings and problems with the gastrointestinal tract, but with proper postprocedure care this condition can be greatly reduced.

**Ultrasound Studies**    Ultrasound is a relatively new procedure used to study alterations in soft tissue images. Many organs are now studied through this procedure: the gallbladder, reproductive organs, liver, spleen and thyroid gland. Ultrasound utilizes a high frequency sound wave to display an echo pattern on an oscilloscope.

Ultrasound is painless, requiring only that the patient lie quietly during the fifteen or thirty minute procedure. These procedures need to precede barium studies as barium impedes the transmission of sound waves.

When ultrasound is used to study the pelvic organs the patient is instructed to drink four glasses of water to promote a full bladder. The full bladder enhances the transmission of sound waves and thus improves visualization of the organs.

Echocardiography and echoencephalography procedures are similar to those of ultrasound. They are painless, noninvasive techniques which utilize transducers and oscilloscopes similar to the ultrasound procedures. The echocardiogram records heart motion, not heart outline. The echoencephalogram measures, by spikes produced from the echo, the midline structures of the brain. There is no preparation or postprocedure alteration in activity for these procedures.

**Radioactive Material Studies**  Radioisotopes distribute uniformly through normal tissue but unevenly in pathologically involved or diseased tissue. The radioisotopes emit radiation and gamma rays and can be picked up by scanning devices.

Radioisotopes tend to concentrate in specific organ tissues and thus are more effective when administered for scanning a particular organ. For example, hippuran ($^{131}$I) is specifically used for thyroid scanning while thallium 201 ($^{201}$Tl) is used for scanning heart tissue. Scanning allows visualization of organs that are unobservable by x-ray alone. Tumors present as areas of reduced radioisotopic activity. Radioisotope studies are contraindicated with pregnancy, breast-feeding mothers, or persons who are allergic to the radioisotopes.

The radioactive isotopes are administered intravenously or orally to the patient. A specified time elapses before the scanning is done. This allows time for the radioactive material to reach the specific tissue under study. Then, a scanning device is used to record the concentration of radiation that emerges from the radioisotope.

Some patients are given blocking agents before the administration of the radioisotope. This prevents the radioactive material from entering organs other than those being studied. A common blocking agent is Lugol's solution. This is given to a patient who is having a study done on any organ but the thyroid gland.

**Air Contrast Studies**  Two of the most common air contrast studies are the pneumoencephalogram and the ventriculogram.

Visualization of the cerebral ventricular system is accomplished by injecting small increments of sterile gas through lumbar or cisternal burr holes. The different densities of the gas and cerebral spinal fluid provide the necessary contrast for the x-ray films.

These studies are very difficult for patients because the patients are positioned in a somersaulting chair and rotated 360 degrees throughout the procedure, which can lead to severe nausea and vomiting. The patient often submits to this test knowing that an immediate craniotomy may be necessary. This knowledge therefore compounds the patient's anxiety and fear. In addition, the patient experiences an excruciating headache. The headache will decrease in intensity following the test and will not be completely eradicated for several days.

**Assisting The Physician During Tests**  Nurses are frequently called upon to assist the physician with procedures at the bedside as well as in the treatment room. The procedures presented in this chapter are the most common ones performed in the hospital unit. It is important that the nurse be aware of the correct patient positioning in order to facilitate the procedure, decrease complications, and decrease the time it takes to complete the procedure.

Some diagnostic tests frequently used in the past have limited use today. One such procedure is the lumbar puncture. Removal of fluid from the spinal tract may cause the brain, because of edema, to herniate down through the tentorium. Because of this complication, a lumbar puncture is not done on a patient with head trauma or potential increased intracranial pressure. The CAT scan is now frequently used to dertermine intracranial bleeding.

The following nursing diagnoses may be appropriate to include in a Patient Care Plan when the components are related to patients undergoing diagnostic procedures.

**NURSING DIAGNOSES**

| Nursing Diagnosis (Potential) | Defining Characteristic; Etiology (Examples) |
|---|---|
| ☐ Anxiety, *related to* | Apprehension related to test or procedure outcome, e.g., procedure, pain, diagnosis. |
| ☐ Fear, *related to* | Pain and/or complications, e.g., diagnostic test. |
| ☐ Fluid Volume Deficit, *related to* | Anaphylactic shock, e.g., reaction to dye used for contrast studies. |
| ☐ Knowledge Deficit, *related to* | Misunderstanding of instructions or information, e.g., inadequate data and/or explanation of procedure (maintaining position after spinal tap, liver biopsy). |

## UNIT ONE  DYE INJECTION STUDIES

### NURSING PROCESS DATA

#### ASSESSMENT  *Data Base*

Assess patient's knowledge of procedure to be done.

Identify any history of drug or food allergies.

Evaluate patient's ability to follow directions before and during the test.

Assess vital signs and document for baseline data.

#### PLANNING  *Objectives*

To determine if the patient is physically prepared for the test.

To determine if the patient is psychologically prepared for the test.

To determine if the patient is a candidate for an allergic reaction.

To determine if the patient is able to cooperate with the preparation and completion of the test.

#### IMPLEMENTATION  *Procedures*

Preparing for Oral Cholecystogram

Preparing for Intravenous Cholangiogram

Preparing for Intravenous Pyelogram

Preparing for Myelogram

Preparing for Arteriogram

Preparing for Computerized Axial Tomography (CAT Scan)

Preparing for Cardiac Catheterization

> EVALUATION *Expected Outcomes*
>
> Patient is able to complete the test without untoward effects.
>
> Patient understands procedure and has anxiety level under control.
>
> Patient is properly prepared for diagnostic test.

## DYE INJECTION STUDIES

### Diagnostic Test

Oral Cholecystogram:

Intravenous Cholangiogram:
Intravenous Pyelogram:
Myelogram:
Arteriogram:

Computerized Axial Tomography:

Cardiac Catheterization:

### Rationale

To visualize shape and position of the gallbladder and to identify the presence of stones.
To visualize the biliary tract.
To visualize structures of the urinary tract.
To visualize distortions of the spinal cord.
To visualize abnormalities or obstructions to specific blood vessels.
To visualize a cross-section of the brain to precisely localize intracranial lesions.
To measure oxygen concentration, provide blood samples, determine cardiac output and visualize coronary arteries.

### Equipment

Signed permit

Pajama bottoms and hospital gown

Allergy identaband, if needed

Wheelchair

### Preparation

1. Identify the specific diagnostic test that will be performed.

2. Determine if any tests must precede others in order to schedule test appropriately.

---

**Clinical Alert**

After injection of iodine dye the following tests will be abnormal for at least 16 hours:

☐ Urine sodium, specific gravity, protein, and osmolality

☐ 24-hour urine collection for 17-hydroxyketosteroids, 17-hydroxycorticoids, and catecholamines

☐ PBI (may be affected for three to six months)

---

3. Obtain patient's history to determine allergies to food or drugs and note these on the chart. Notify physician of findings.

4. Identify specific preparations that need to be carried out before the studies.

5. Monitor food and fluid restrictions that need to be altered for the studies.

6. Obtain special consent forms for all invasive diagnostic studies after the physician has explained the study to the patient.

7. Provide patient teaching regarding the purpose of the study, including any special preparation required and restrictions imposed by the study.

8. Provide psychological support and reassurance to the patient.

9. Obtain orders regarding medications or nutrition for patients with special problems, such as diabetes or seizure disorders.

10. Carry out safety precautions immediately prior to the study:

    a. Check identaband for accuracy.

    b. Have patient void if necessary.

    c. Remove patient's hairpins, jewelry, and dentures if necessary.

    d. Chart premedication given.

    e. Monitor safe transfer from the bed to guerney or wheelchair.

    f. Accompany patient to x-ray department if needed. (Usually nurses accompany critically ill patients.)

---

**Clinical Alert:**

Symptoms of dye reactions:

☐ Urticaria, hives

☐ Nausea, vomiting

☐ Respiratory distress

☐ Decreased blood pressure

Patients allergic to food or drugs generally are allergic to some dyes used for diagnostic studies.

---

## Procedure

### for Oral Cholecystogram

1. Explain purpose for procedure to patient.
2. Identify allergies to shellfish or iodine.
3. Administer iodine radiopaque medication after dinner.
   a. Number of tablets administered is based on weight of patient.
   b. Tablets are given five minutes apart with 8 oz. of water for each tablet.
4. Patient is n.p.o. after midnight. **Rationale:** This prevents contraction of gallbladder and expulsion of radiopaque dye.
5. Patient is taken to x-ray department.
6. Explain details of procedure to patient.
   a. Patient will be x-rayed in standing and lying positions for good visualization of gallbladder and common bile duct.
   b. Patient will be fed a fatty meal to test ability of the gallbladder to contract.
   c. If visualization does not occur, additional medications may be given and the test repeated the following day, or an IV cholangiogram may be done.

## Procedure

### for Intravenous Cholangiogram

1. Follow steps as appropriate in Preparation for Dye Injection Studies.
   a. Keep patient n.p.o. for at least three hours pretest.
   b. Identify allergies to shellfish or iodine.
   c. Patient is taken to x-ray department.
2. Explain procedure to patient.
   a. Procedure will involve dye injection given over a 15- to 30-minute period.
   b. X-rays will be taken every 15 to 30 minutes until the common bile duct tree is visualized.
   c. The procedure may take one to three hours.

3. Patient is returned to room.
4. Encourage fluids and offer diet.
5. Have patient resume previous activity orders.
6. Monitor patient for allergic response to dye.

## Procedure

### for Intravenous Pyelogram

1. Follow steps as appropriate in Preparation for Dye Injection Studies.
   a. Give patient clear liquids the evening before the IVP. Usual order is four to six glasses of fluid from 6 p.m. to midnight, then place patient on n.p.o.
   b. Give laxative or enema as ordered.
   c. Identify allergies to shellfish or iodine.
   d. Obtain permit.
   e. Take patient to x-ray department when notified.
2. Explain details of procedure to patient.
   a. Dye will be injected as a large single dose.
   b. X-rays are taken over period of one hour to determine extent to which dye is filtered through the kidneys.
3. Warn patient that dye can cause feelings of nausea, shortness of breath, and a hot, flushed effect.
4. Return patient to room and have patient resume ordered activity level.
5. Encourage fluids and offer diet.
6. Observe signs and symptoms for reactions to dye such as oliguria, nausea, and vomiting.

## Procedure

### for Myelogram

1. Follow steps as appropriate in Preparation for Dye Injection Studies.
   a. Identify allergies to shellfish, iodine, or other contrast media.
   b. Keep patient n.p.o. for four to six hours.
   c. Obtain baseline levels of motor and sensory function.
   d. Obtain permit.
   e. Take patient on guerney to x-ray department.
2. Explain details of procedure to patient.
   a. Patient is placed in prone position with pillow under abdomen. **Rationale:** This position allows physician to visualize ruptured disc or neoplasms.
   b. A lumbar puncture needle is inserted between the vertebrae into the subarachnoid space.

c. A small amount of cerebrospinal fluid is sent to lab for study.

d. Contrast media is injected, and patient is tilted on table to allow flow of dye to designated areas of spine to allow visualization by x-rays.

e. Contrast media (Pantopaque) is removed through aspiration. Explain to patient that sudden pain in legs may occur.

f. Procedure lasts about one hour.

g. Patient is returned on guerney to room.

3. Keep patient in supine position 8 to 12 hours without a pillow. **Rationale:** This position prevents a headache. Position patient in Sim's position if ordered.

4. Monitor vital signs and motor and sensory function.

a. Cervical myelogram: check upper and lower extremities and bladder function.

b. Lumbar myelogram: check lower extremities and bladder function.

5. Medicate for pain as ordered.

6. Increase fluids to at least 2500 cc per day. **Rationale:** Fluids replace cerebrospinal fluid and may prevent headache following procedure. Offer diet.

7. Monitor output and observe for distention.

8. Utilize comfort measures and relaxation techniques when needed.

## Procedure

*for Arteriogram*

1. Explain purpose of procedure to patient.

2. Identify allergies to shellfish, iodine, or any contrast media.

3. Obtain permit.

4. Shave and scrub puncture site when ordered.

5. Place patient on n.p.o. if ordered.

6. Have patient void before procedure.

7. Administer preprocedure medications if ordered and transport patient to x-ray department.

8. Explain details of procedure to patient.

a. Puncture site will be scrubbed and a local anesthetic administered.

b. Contrast media will be injected to visualize abnormalities or obstruction to specific vessels.

c. Patient may be instructed to hold breath for

x-rays. Procedure takes about one hour if an automatic film changer is used.

9. Patient is returned on guerney to room.

10. Monitor vital signs, pulses, and puncture site, as with surgical patients.

11. Observe for signs of shock and presence of pain, which indicate hemorrhage or thrombosis.

12. Apply ice pack to puncture site if ordered. Do not flex the involved extremity.

13. Maintain bed rest with head elevated slightly for 12 hours.

14. Offer fluids and diet as ordered and tolerated.

15. Provide comfort measures as needed.

## Procedure

*for Computerized Axial Tomography (CAT Scan)*

1. Explain purpose for procedure to patient.

2. Identify allergies to shellfish or iodine.

3. Obtain permit.

4. Place patient on n.p.o. as dye can cause nausea.

5. Administer preprocedure medication if ordered.

6. Patient is taken on guerney to x-ray department.

7. Explain equipment and need for patient's head to be placed in rubber cap. Face will not be covered.

8. Patient will have IV injection of contrast material if enhanced study is to be done. Explain that a warm, flushed feeling or nausea can occur.

9. Instruct patient to lie very still during the procedure. Length of procedure, usually 30 to 60 minutes, depends on number of radiographs taken.

10. Return patient to room.

11. Provide diet and force fluids to 3000 cc as ordered.

12. Medicate for headache if needed.

## Procedure

*for Cardiac Catheterization*

1. Explain purpose for procedure to patient.

2. Obtain permit.

3. Identify allergies to drugs, iodine, shellfish, or any other contrast media.

4. Complete prep and shave of groin and/or brachial area.

5. Establish baseline data for vital signs, peripheral pulses, coagulation studies (PTT, Protime), ECG pattern.

6. Place patient on n.p.o. after midnight.

7. In morning, obtain vital signs, take weight, have the patient void, and administer preprocedure medication.

8. Take patient on guerney to cardiac catheterization lab.

9. Explain equipment and details of procedure to patient.
   a. Patient is strapped onto a table. ECG leads and blood pressure equipment are applied.
   b. Groin or brachial area is scrubbed and injected with Xylocaine.
   c. Arterial and venous catheters are placed in femoral or brachial sites.
   d. When dye is injected for coronary artery visualization, explain to patient that a warm, flushed feeling, shortness of breath, or nausea can occur.
   e. Patient is asked to hold breath about ten seconds during dye injection.
   f. Reinforce that patient will not fall off table as patient may be turned on side for cineangiography. Total procedure takes one to one-and-a-half hours.
   g. Following catheterization, pressure is applied to puncture site for 10 to 15 minutes.

10. Transport patient on guerney to room.

11. Provide post-cardiac-catheterization care.
    a. Monitor vital signs, puncture site, heart and lung sounds, and peripheral pulses as with a surgical patient.
    b. Elevate extremity used for catheterization site. Keep extremity extended. **Rationale:** Position promotes blood supply back to heart and prevents thrombus formation.
    c. Apply pressure dressing or sandbags to puncture site if bleeding continues.
    d. Encourage fluids and diet when vital signs are stable and no evidence of nausea or drowsiness is present.
    e. Monitor for signs and symptoms of allergic response.

12. Position patient for comfort. Place on back for several hours postprocedure, then turn from side to side.

## CHARTING  *for Dye Injection Studies*

☐ Preparation completed, e.g., n.p.o., clear liquid dinner

☐ Patient teaching completed

☐ Medication administered

☐ Allergies noted

☐ Unusual anxiety or fears of patient

☐ How patient transported to test

☐ Time sent and returned from test

☐ Postprocedure care

☐ Appearance of dressing or puncture sites

## CLINICAL PROBLEM SOLVING

### Potential Problems

Patient has allergic reaction.

### Suggested Solutions

☐ Follow protocol and/or standing orders for allergic reactions.

☐ Start $O_2$ at 6L/min unless otherwise contraindicated. Use nasal cannula.

☐ Place in semi or high Fowler's position if not contraindicated.

☐ Administer medications as outlined in protocol or according to physician's orders.

☐ Provide reassurance and encouragement.

☐ Have patient take slow, deep breaths.

☐ If nausea or vomiting occur, obtain an order for an antiemetic from the physician.

Patient is given meal when on n.p.o. status.

- ☐ Call x-ray and change time of test. If possible, arrange for test to be done later in the day to avoid additional hospitalization.
- ☐ Instruct patient on what n.p.o. means.
- ☐ Ensure that diet Rand has appropriate information on n.p.o. status.

Patient very apprehensive and refuses test at last minute.

- ☐ Identify reasons for anxiety and attempt to allay fears.
- ☐ Notify physician and ask if he wants to cancel or postpone test to later time. Do not attempt to "talk patient into it."

Bleeding or hemorrhage occurs from arteriogram puncture site.

- ☐ Notify physician.
- ☐ Apply direct pressure until pressure dressing can be applied.
- ☐ Monitor amount of blood loss and possible signs and symptoms of shock.
- ☐ Elevate and keep extremity in extension position.

Patient develops irregular pulse following cardiac catheterization.

- ☐ Notify physician immediately.
- ☐ Prepare for possible Code and IV administration.
- ☐ Monitor vital signs frequently.

Bleeding occurs at catheter insertion site following cardiac catheterization.

- ☐ Apply pressure dressing.
- ☐ Elevate extremity.
- ☐ Monitor peripheral pulse and vital signs.
- ☐ If bleeding does not subside, notify physician.

Peripheral vessels occluded or diminished circulation occurs following cannula or catheter insertion.

- ☐ Elevate extremity above level of heart.
- ☐ Observe puncture site for signs/symptoms of hematoma or bleeding.
- ☐ Apply direct pressure if bleeding occurs at puncture site.
- ☐ Monitor peripheral pulses.
- ☐ Observe color and temperature of extremity.

# UNIT TWO   RADIOACTIVE STUDIES

## NURSING PROCESS DATA

### ASSESSMENT   *Data Base*

Assess patient's understanding of diagnostic test.

Evaluate patient's ability to tolerate procedure.

Identify need for staff to accompany patient to procedure.

Identify allergies to radioactive materials.

Assess vital signs and document for baseline data.

### PLANNING   *Objectives*

To prepare the patient physically to ensure that diagnostic test results in visualization of appropriate organ and regions within the organ.

To prepare the patient psychologically to prevent undue stress.

To complete patient teaching to ensure the patient has an understanding of the procedure.

### IMPLEMENTATION *Procedures*

Preparing for Bone Scan

Preparing for Lung Scan

Preparing for Brain Scan

### EVALUATION *Expected Outcomes*

Patient is physically prepared for the diagnostic study.

Patient is psychologically prepared for the diagnostic study.

Patient expresses an understanding of the diagnostic test.

## RADIOACTIVE STUDIES

| Diagnostic Test | Rationale |
|---|---|
| Bone Scan: | To determine presence of bone cancer. |
| Lung Scan: | To determine presence of pulmonary emboli or pneumothorax. |
| Brain Scan: | To determine presence of cerebral infarctions, abscess, neoplasms or contusions. |

### Equipment

Signed permit

IV equipment (optional)

Hospital gown and pajama bottoms

### Preparation

1. Identify the specific diagnostic test that will be performed.

2. Determine if any tests must precede others in order to schedule test appropriately.

3. Identify specific preparations that need to be carried out before the studies.

4. Monitor fluid alterations that need to precede the studies.

5. Obtain special consent forms if required by facility after the physician has explained the study to the patient.

6. Provide patient teaching regarding the study, including any special preparation required for the study.

7. Provide psychological support and reassurance to the patient.

8. Carry out safety precautions immediately prior to the study:
   a. Check identaband for accuracy.
   b. Chart premedication if given.
   c. Monitor safe transfer from the bed to guerney or wheelchair.
   d. Accompany patient to nuclear medicine department if needed. (Usually nurses accompany critically ill patients.)

### Procedure

*for Bone Scan*

1. Follow steps as appropriate for Preparation for Radioactive Studies.
   a. Explain purpose for procedure to patient. **Rationale:** If patient is of child-bearing age, determine whether she is pregnant. If so, test cannot be done.
   b. Have patient ready for injection of tracer

amount of radioactive material two hours before scan.
c. Force fluids for one hour.
d. Take patient to nuclear medicine department.

2. Explain procedure.
a. Patient is positioned under scintillation camera.
b. Instruct patient to remain very still for 20 minutes to ensure observation of bone abnormalities.
c. Return patient to room.

3. Instruct patient to resume activities.

## Procedure

### for Lung Scan

1. Follow steps as appropriate in Preparation for Radioactive Studies.
a. Explain purpose for procedure.
b. Obtain permit if required.
c. Transport to nuclear medicine department.

2. Explain details of procedure.
a. Explain equipment to patient.
   Closed-breathing system.
   Scintillation camera.
b. Patient is injected intravenously with a tracer amount of radioactive material.
c. Patient is positioned in several ways to obtain clear images.
d. Patient is instructed to breathe through a closed system until all radioactive gas is cleared from the system.
e. Instruct in use of mouthpiece or nose clips if used.
f. Patient is instructed to lie quietly for 30 minutes as radiography is completed.

3. Transport patient on guerney to room.

4. Instruct to resume pre-study activities.

## Procedure

### for Brain Scan

1. Follow steps as appropriate in Preparation for Radioactive Studies.
a. Explain purpose for procedure.
b. Obtain permit, if required.
c. Transport to nuclear medicine department.

2. Explain details of procedure.
a. IV injection of radioactive material will be administered.
b. Patient's head will be placed under scintillation camera and patient is to remain still for five minutes.
c. Patient will be kept comfortable and monitored carefully for 90 minutes.
d. Patient is placed in several different positions to assist distribution of radioisotopes.
e. Patient is instructed to remain still for 20 minutes.

3. Return patient to room.

4. Instruct patient to resume pre-study activities.

## CHARTING  *for Radioactive Material Studies*

☐ Patient teaching completed

☐ Patient's emotional state

☐ Any radioisotopes given on the unit

☐ Preprocedural preparation completed, i.e., enema or laxative

☐ Means by which patient transported to nuclear medicine department

☐ Time sent and returned from scan

---

## CLINICAL PROBLEM SOLVING

**Potential Problems**

Patient appears not to understand purpose of diagnostic test.

**Suggested Solutions**

☐ Observe for nonverbal cues or misunderstandings in order to clarify.
☐ Provide alternative teaching aids.
☐ Show patient the equipment if necessary.
☐ Ask patient to repeat explanation to you.

Patient is unable to cooperate during the procedure.

☐ If not contraindicated by condition, ask physician for sedation order.

- □ Nursing staff members may be asked to help patient remain quiet. If so, wear lead apron shield.

Patient is uncomfortable during procedure

- □ Reposition patient for comfort if possible. (It may not be possible depending on area of body to be scanned.)
- □ Provide support by propping patient in position needed for scanning.
- □ Assist patient to focus on other things, e.g., the ball game, weather, or something pleasant.

## UNIT THREE   AIR CONTRAST STUDIES

### NURSING PROCESS DATA

#### ASSESSMENT   *Data Base*

Assess ability of patient to tolerate procedure. Usually patients will experience a very severe headache during the air contrast study.

Assess patient's knowledge of the procedure.

Assess vital signs and neurological signs for baseline data.

Monitor and compare pre- and post-test vital signs and symptoms.

#### PLANNING   *Objectives*

To prepare patient psychologically and physically for the test.

To provide adequate baseline data to determine post-test complications.

To determine if patient is able to understand and follow directions during the test.

To minimize post-test side effects and complications.

#### IMPLEMENTATION   *Procedures*

Preparing for Pneumoencephalogram

Preparing for Ventriculogram

#### EVALUATION   *Expected Outcomes*

Patient is able to cooperate during test.

Patient's headache is controlled.

Patient does not experience hypotension during or following test.

Patient's motor and sensory status remains unchanged.

# AIR CONTRAST STUDIES

**Diagnostic Test**
Pneumoencephalogram or Ventriculogram:

**Rationale**
To visualize ventricular system and subarachnoid space in order to determine presence of lesions or masses or diagnose degenerative cerebral diseases.

## Equipment

Signed permit

Pajama bottoms and gown

Lumbar or cisternal puncture tray

Guerney

## Preparation

1. Identify the specific diagnostic test that will be performed.

2. Determine if any tests must precede the air contrast study in order to schedule test appropriately.

3. Identify specific preparations that need to be carried out before the studies.

4. Monitor food and fluid restrictions that need to be altered for the studies.

5. Obtain special consent forms after the physician has explained the study to the patient.

6. Provide patient teaching regarding the study, including any special preparation required and restrictions imposed by the study.

7. Provide psychological support and reassurance to the patient.

8. Obtain orders regarding medications or nutrition for patients with special problems, such as diabetes or seizure disorders.

9. Carry out safety precautions immediately prior to the study:
   a. Check identaband for accuracy.
   b. Have patient void.
   c. Remove hairpins, jewelry, and dentures if necessary.
   d. Chart premedication given.
   e. Monitor safe transfer from the bed to guerney.
   f. Accompany patients to x-ray department if needed.

## Procedure

*for Pneumoencephalogram*

1. Explain purpose for procedure to patient.

2. Obtain permit. Check if possible craniotomy may need to be included on permit.

3. Place patient on n.p.o. after midnight.

4. Obtain baseline vital signs, neurological signs, and motor and sensory function.

5. Have patient void.

6. Remove dentures.

7. Administer preprocedure medication.

8. Transport to special procedures department or operating room via guerney.

9. Explain steps of procedure.

10. Position patient in lateral or seated position (check position with physician).

11. Explain to patient that during a pneumoencephalogram a small amount of cerebral spinal fluid will be obtained and then a small amount of air will be injected through the lumbar puncture needle.
    a. X-rays will be taken to check placement of air.
    b. Injection of additional air.
    c. Positioning of patient prone, supine, and upright during radiography.

12. Instruct patient that when air is injected he might experience a severe headache, vertigo, nausea, diaphoresis, and chills.

13. Explain the procedure visualizes a patency of the ventricular system and identifies any abnormalities. The procedure takes about one hour.

14. Following the procedure, apply dressing to puncture site.

15. Transport patient on guerney to room.

16. Monitor vital signs, neurological signs, and motor and sensory functions as with a surgical patient.

17. Provide comfort measures for headache, nausea, and generalized discomfort.

18. Keep patient flat until headache has dissipated or decreased in intensity.

## Procedure

*for Ventriculogram*

1. Explain purpose for procedure to patient.

2. Obtain permit. Check if possible craniotomy may need to be included on permit.

3. Place patient on n.p.o. after midnight.

4. Obtain baseline vital signs, neurological signs, and motor and sensory function.

5. Have patient void.

6. Remove dentures.

7. Administer preprocedure medication.

8. Transport to special procedures department or operating room via guerney.

9. Explain steps of procedure.

10. Position patient in lateral or seated position (check position with physician).

11. Explain to patient that during a ventriculogram, air is injected directly into the ventricles through a small scalp incision in the frontal region. Explain to patient that a hole is drilled in the skull and a spinal needle is inserted in the ventricle.

12. Explain to patient that a ventriculogram takes about one hour and is done if patient has increased intracranial pressure.

13. Following the procedure, apply dressing to puncture site.

14. Transport patient on guerney to room.

15. Monitor vital signs, neurological signs, and motor and sensory functions as with a surgical patient.

16. Provide comfort measures for headache, nausea, and generalized discomfort.

17. Keep patient flat until headache has dissipated or decreased in intensity.

18. Provide quiet environment.

19. Encourage fluids unless contraindicated.

20. Offer diet.

## CHARTING  *for Air Contrast Studies*

☐ Patient teaching completed

☐ Baseline vital signs, neurological checks, motor and sensory findings

☐ Patient's emotional status

☐ Premedication

☐ Post-test vital signs, neurological signs, motor and sensory findings

☐ Any evidence of severe headaches, nausea, vomiting, increased temperature

☐ Condition of puncture site and dressing

---

## CLINICAL PROBLEM SOLVING

### Potential Problems

Patient's temperature increases and he or she complains of nausea and severe headaches.

Patient experiences shortness of breath.

### Suggested Solutions

☐ Notify physician immediately. Patient has experienced the most common complications following this procedure.
☐ Obtain orders for and administer antiemetics.
☐ Obtain blood cultures if ordered to determine if the patient has infection.

☐ Use relaxation techniques with patient.
☐ Administer oxygen.
☐ Instruct to breathe slowly.

# UNIT FOUR  BARIUM STUDIES

## NURSING PROCESS DATA

### ASSESSMENT  *Data Base*

Assess results of laxative and enema administration to ensure a clean colon for the study. Notify physician if patient is unable to "hold" enema solution.

Evaluate patient's ability to cooperate with test.

Evaluate patient's knowledge of test.

### PLANNING  *Objectives*

To identify the patient's ability to understand the preparatory process.

To clean out colon in order to ensure visualization of colon.

To prepare the patient psychologically for the test.

### IMPLEMENTATION  *Procedures*

Preparing for Barium Enema

Preparing for Upper Gastrointestinal Study

### EVALUATION  *Expected Outcomes*

Patient is able to cooperate with test.

Patient's colon is clear of stool.

Barium is expelled following test.

## BARIUM STUDIES

| Diagnostic Test | Rationale |
| --- | --- |
| Barium Enema: | To visualize the lower GI tract for presence of lesions or obstructions. |
| Upper Gastrointestinal Study: | To visualize the upper GI tract for presence of lesions or obstructions. |

### Equipment

Enema tube and bag

Ordered solution for enema

Laxative

Wheelchair

### Preparation

1. Identify the specific diagnostic test that will be performed.
2. Provide patient teaching including any special preparation required.
3. Provide psychological support and reassurance to the patient.

**Clinical Alert:**
Barium studies should follow IVPs, ultrasound exams, and arteriograms as barium interferes with visualization of other structures.

4. Carry out safety precautions immediately prior to the study:
   a. Check identaband for accuracy.
   b. Monitor safe transfer from the bed to guerney or wheelchair.

## Procedure

*for Barium Enema*

1. Explain purpose for procedure to patient.
2. Give clear liquid meal evening before procedure.
3. Place on n.p.o. after midnight.
4. Administer laxative as ordered in early evening before procedure.
5. Administer enema as ordered morning of study.
6. Transport patient to x-ray usually via wheelchair.
7. Explain details of procedure to patient.
   a. An enema tube is inserted and barium solution is administered into the large bowel in order to detect lesions, obstructions, or abnormalities.
   b. X-rays are taken as the patient is positioned several ways.
   c. Patient is asked to retain barium while x-ray is processed.
   d. Patient is allowed to expel barium in x-ray department.
   e. Entire procedure takes one hour.

**Clinical Alert:**
Obtain specific orders for enemas when patient has severe abdominal pain, ulcerative colitis, or history of megacolon. Do not follow general preprocedural orders.

8. Transport patient to room.
9. Force fluids unless contraindicated.
10. Administer laxative and/or enema as ordered.
11. Ensure patient has bowel movement within two to three days.

## Procedure

*for Upper Gastrointestinal Study*

1. Explain purpose of procedure to patient.
2. Place patient on n.p.o. after midnight.
3. Administer laxative and/or enema particularly if this test follows barium enema study.
4. Instruct patient not to smoke. **Rationale:** Smoking causes an increase in flow of digestive juices.
5. Transport to x-ray department.
6. Explain details of procedure to patient.
   a. Patient will be instructed to drink a cup of flavored barium.
   b. Patient is instructed to turn to several positions while x-rays are obtained.
   c. X-rays will be taken every 30 minutes until barium advances through small bowel. This usually takes about two hours.
7. Transport patient to room.
8. Force fluids unless contraindicated.
9. Administer laxative.
10. Ensure bowel movement within two to three days. Enema may need to be administered.

### CHARTING *for Barium Studies*

□ Laxative administered
□ Type, amount of fluid, number of enemas administered
□ Enema results, consistency of stool, color of returning enema solution
□ Unusual symptoms such as pain, bleeding, or nausea associated with enemas
□ Color of stool following test

## CLINICAL PROBLEM SOLVING

**Potential Problems**

Barium is unable to be expelled even following administrations of laxatives and enemas.

**Suggested Solutions**

Obtain order for and administer oil retention enema.

Laxatives and/or enemas are ordered for patients with ulcerative colitis or severe abdominal pain.

☐ Administer tap water enema following oil retention enema.

☐ Continue to administer laxatives until barium is expelled.

☐ Do not administer either the laxative or enema without checking with the physician.

☐ If physician confirms order, administer small amount of enema fluid carefully and observe and document effects on patient.

☐ Chart the type of pain if any, characteristics of stool, and any symptoms noted while enema is administered.

☐ If patient complains of excruciating pain, stop procedure and notify the physician.

Patient's medications are administered in error.

☐ Notify x-ray department and ask for specific orders as to what action needs to be taken regarding the test.

☐ Inform physician, complete a medication error form and send to nursing office. An incident form may need to be completed as well.

☐ If this is a frequent problem on the unit or in the hospital, an in-service education program should be given which includes a discussion of when medications should be given and when held.

## UNIT FIVE   DIAGNOSTIC PROCEDURES

### NURSING PROCESS DATA

#### ASSESSMENT   *Data Base*

Assess vital signs prior to, during, and following the procedure.

Assess patient's ability to maintain position necessary for procedure.

Assess patient's knowledge of the procedure to be performed.

Review pertinent laboratory tests prior to procedure.

Evaluate signs and symptoms which indicate a potential problem could exist if test performed.

#### PLANNING   *Objectives*

To provide reassurance for patients undergoing diagnostic tests.

To position the patient in a manner that facilitates the introduction of a needle through the skin surface to obtain a tissue sample.

To position patient in a manner for ease in passing an instrument in order to visualize a body cavity.

To position the patient in as comfortable a position as possible.

## IMPLEMENTATION  *Procedures*

Assisting with Lumbar Puncture

Assisting with Liver Biopsy

Assisting with Thoracentesis

Assisting with Paracentesis

Assisting with Bone Marrow Aspiration

Assisting with Vaginal Examination and Papanicolaou Smear

Assisting with Proctoscopy

Assisting with Gastroscopy/Endoscopy

Assisting with Cystoscopy

Assisting with Amniocentesis

## EVALUATION  *Expected Outcomes*

Patient is prepared psychologically and physically for procedure.

Diagnostic tests performed with minimal discomfort.

Vital signs remain within normal range.

Specimens sent to lab in appropriate container and in a timely manner.

## DIAGNOSTIC PROCEDURES

| **Diagnostic Test** | **Rationale** |
| --- | --- |
| Lumbar Puncture: | To obtain a specimen to determine presence of microorganisms, RBC's or WBC's. |
| Liver Biopsy: | To obtain a specimen to determine presence of tumor or disease. |
| Thoracentesis: | To remove fluid from the thoracic cavity; to obtain a specimen for cell study. |
| Paracentesis: | To remove fluid from the abdominal cavity; to obtain a specimen for cell study. |
| Bone Marrow Aspiration: | To study cells obtained from the specimen. |
| Vaginal Examination and Papanicolaou Smear: | To determine cell changes through a smear; to obtain a specimen for veneral disease identification. |
| Proctoscopy: | To determine alterations in tissue; to determine if active bleeding is present. |
| Gastroscopy/Endoscopy: | To visualize areas of bleeding in upper GI tract; to obtain specimen for cell studies. |
| Cystoscopy: | To visualize the bladder and lower urinary tract. |
| Amniocentesis: | To remove amniotic fluid for studies of fetal maturity and genetic abnormalities. |

## ASSISTING WITH LUMBAR PUNCTURE

### Equipment

Diagnostic tray or equipment specific for procedure

Bath blanket

Sterile collection bottles if indicated and not on tray

Sterile gloves

Xylocaine injection, if not on tray

Examining light

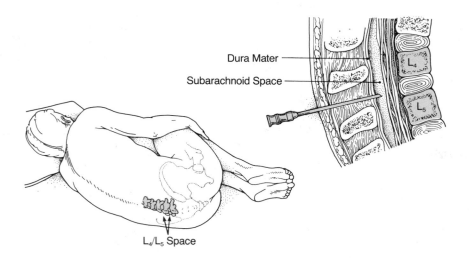

Dura Mater

Subarachnoid Space

L₄

L₅

L₄/L₅ Space

Place patient in Sims' position to facilitate needle insertion for lumbar puncture.

## Procedure

1. Explain purpose.

2. Explain procedure.

3. Obtain permit.

4. Obtain tray and any additional equipment needed, such as sterile gloves, bath blanket.

5. Open sterile tray if requested by physician. Pour antiseptic solution into sterile medicine cup if needed.

6. Position patient in lateral recumbent position with his back at the edge of the examining table. Cover with bath blanket, exposing only patient's back.

7. Pull knees up to abdomen and flex chin on chest. (This position widens the space between the spinous processes of the lower lumbar vertebrae for ease of needle insertion.)

8. Assist patient in relaxation exercises or instruct in deep, slow breathing through the mouth.

9. Assist physician with the Queckenstedt's test when requested. After opening pressure is obtained, apply compression to neck veins with your fingers.

---

**Clinical Alert**

Queckenstedt's test is used to identify blockage of CSF flow in the spinal subarachnoid space. Generally when neck pressure is applied, there is a rapid rise in pressure level on the manometer with a return to normal within seconds when pressure is released.

---

10. Label cerebral spinal fluid samples with number on each specimen container.

11. After removal of needle, apply bandaid to puncture site.

12. Fill out lab slips for appropriate test, i.e., cell count, serology.

13. Instruct patient to lie flat for 4 to 24 hours, depending on hospital policy. Head is to remain flat and even with position of body.

14. Encourage fluids if not contraindicated by patient's condition.

15. Observe for spinal fluid leak from puncture site.

16. Check for headaches or alterations in neurological status.

## ASSISTING WITH LIVER BIOPSY

### Equipment

Same as for lumbar puncture

### Preparation

1. Obtain lab values such as prothrombin time, bleeding time, and platelet count if ordered.

2. Determine if a blood typing and cross-matching is needed.

3. Determine if patient is to be n.p.o.

### Procedure

1. Explain purpose.

2. Explain procedure.

3. Obtain permit.

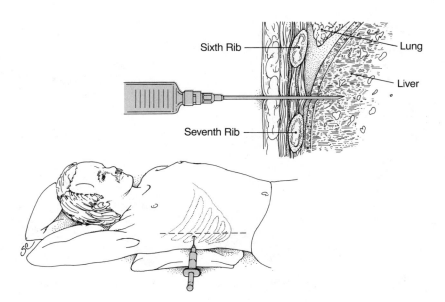

Instruct patient to raise arm over head to facilitate needle insertion for liver biopsy.

4. Obtain tray and any additional equipment needed such as sterile gloves, sandbag, bath blanket.

5. Open sterile tray.

6. Place patient in supine position at the right edge of the bed. Raise right arm and extend it over the left shoulder behind the head. Turn head to left. **Rationale:** This position provides maximal exposure of right intercostal space.

7. Instruct patient to take a deep breath and hold it on expiration after the local anesthetic has been given. After physician obtains specimen, instruct patient to breathe normally. **Rationale:** Holding the breath prevents the needle from tearing the diaphragm.

8. Place bandaid over puncture site.

9. Position patient on right side for one hour. Sandbags may be placed under patient's right side to provide hemostasis.

10. Instruct patient to remain on bed rest for 24 hours.

11. Assess for signs of hemorrhage at least every hour for 12 hours.

12. Monitor vital signs as you would for a surgical patient every fifteen minutes for one hour, etc.

## ASSISTING WITH THORACENTESIS

### Equipment

Same as for lumbar puncture

### Procedure

1. Explain purpose.

2. Explain procedure.

3. Obtain permit.

4. Position patient on edge of bed with arms crossed and resting on the overbed table. **Rationale:** This position provides good access to the intercostal spaces.

5. Provide adequate warmth and covering for patient using bath blanket.

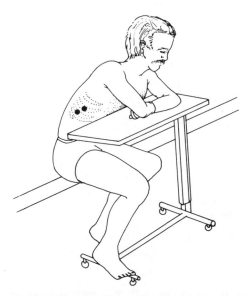

Place patient in a leaning forward position to expose intercostal space for thoracentesis.

6. Obtain baseline vital signs and breath sounds.

7. Place unwrapped sterile tray on bedside stand. Open sterile gloves as indicated.

8. Assist physician as needed with skin prep.

9. Instruct patient not to cough during placement of needle by the physician. **Rationale:** Pleural perforations can occur.

10. Following insertion of needle, observe patient for pallor, dyspnea, tachycardia, chest pain, or vertigo. Report these findings immediately to the physician. **Rationale:** These symptoms occur with a pneumothorax.

11. Apply bandaid or pressure dressing (as determined by policy) after fluid is removed.

12. Observe patient for pulmonary edema (blood-tinged sputum), cardiac distress (changes in respirations, pulse, or color) or a shift in the mediastinum.

13. Place patient on unaffected side with head elevated 30 degrees for at least one hour.

14. Monitor vital signs and breath sounds as with postoperative patients for two hours.

15. Obtain chest x-ray following procedure to check for pneumothorax.

16. Record color, amount, consistency, and samples of fluid obtained.

## ASSISTING WITH PARACENTESIS

### Equipment

Same as for lumbar puncture

### Procedure

1. Explain purpose.
2. Explain procedure.
3. Obtain permit.
4. Have patient empty bladder. **Rationale:** This will prevent accidental puncture of the bladder.
5. Position patient in chair or on edge of bed with legs spread apart.
6. Provide adequate warmth and covering for patient with a bath blanket.
7. Obtain baseline vital signs.
8. Position and open tray on overbed table.
9. Open sterile gloves if needed.

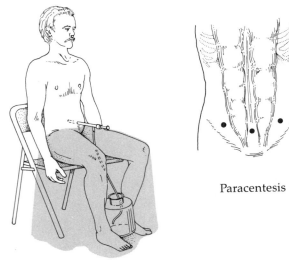

Paracentesis

Place patient in chair for ease in trocar insertion and drainage.

10. Assist physician as needed.

11. Obtain vital signs and observe patient for pallor and vertigo during procedures. **Rationale:** These symptoms are indicative of shock.

12. Apply pressure dressing following removal of needle. **Rationale:** To prevent bleeding from puncture site.

13. Position patient in bed. Semi-Fowler's to high-Fowler's position is usually most comfortable for patient.

14. Monitor vital signs, urine output, and dressing for at least two hours.

15. Reinforce or change dressings as needed.

16. Record color, amount, consistency, and samples obtained for paracentesis.

## ASSISTING WITH BONE MARROW ASPIRATION

### Equipment

Same as for lumbar puncture

### Procedure

1. Explain purpose.
2. Explain procedure. **Rationale:** Patient will experience discomfort of pressure when needle is inserted.
3. Obtain permit.

4. Obtain tray and provide any additional equipment needed such as specimen container or gloves.

5. Premedicate with prescribed drugs.

6. Position patient in supine position if sternum or anterior iliac crest is the biopsy site, or on abdomen if posterior iliac crest is the biopsy site. Place a sandbag under iliac crest area if physician requires.

7. Open tray on overbed table.

8. Assist physician as needed.

9. Apply direct pressure for 5 to 15 minutes following removal of needle. **Rationale:** To prevent bleeding.

10. Cover puncture site with small dressing or band-aid.

11. Monitor vital signs and observe puncture site for drainage, edema, or pain, as with surgical patient.

12. Position the patient for comfort.

13. Properly label specimens and send to laboratory.

## ASSISTING WITH VAGINAL EXAMINATION AND PAPANICOLAOU SMEAR

### Equipment

Two slides

Cytology container

Vaginal speculum, several sizes

Gloves

Water-soluble lubricant jelly

Examining light

### Procedure

1. Explain purpose of procedure.

2. Explain procedure.

3. Instruct patient not to douche before exam.

4. Assist patient to examination room. Patient may walk if not contraindicated.

5. Position in lithotomy position using stirrups.

6. Provide adequate coverings to preserve modesty and prevent chilling.

7. Open speculum package, gloves, and lubricant. Place on tray. Place cytology slides and container on tray.

8. Label two slides with patient's name and area where smear obtained.

9. Position light for good exposure.

10. Stay with patient if patient is a child or physician is a male.

11. Assist physician as needed.

12. Place slides in cytology container and send to the lab. Complete all cytology forms.

12. Assist patient in perineal care.

13. Assist patient to room.

## ASSISTING WITH PROCTOSCOPY

### Equipment

Rigid endoscope with light source, anoscope, and obturator

Suction set up

Air insufflator

Biopsy forceps

### Preparation

1. Give clear liquid diet 24 hours before examination.

2. Administer laxative and enema as ordered the evening before exam.

3. Allow clear liquids after midnight as ordered.

4. Give tap water enema morning of examination.

### Procedure

1. Explain purpose.

2. Explain procedure.

3. Obtain permit.

4. Have patient void before exam.

5. Transport patient in wheelchair or on guerney to treatment room. Place on Proctoscopy table.

6. Position in a knee-chest position if using examining table. Drape patient.

7. Position light for good exposure. Open tray and gloves and place lubricant on tray.

8. Explain equipment and details of procedure to patient.
   a. Physician will digitally examine the rectum.
   b. Proctoscope is lubricated and passed through anus into the rectum to visualize any abnormality of rectum, sigmoid colon, and large bowel.

c. Air may be introduced to increase visualization of bowel wall.

d. Biopsy may be obtained by passing a snare through scope.

9. Return patient in wheelchair or on guerney to room, and instruct to resume preexam activities.

10. Monitor stools for bleeding.

11. Encourage fluids, offer diet.

## ASSISTING WITH GASTROSCOPY/ ENDOSCOPY

### Equipment

Fiber-optic endoscope for specific area to be studied or universal endoscope

Light source

Local anesthetic preparation

Specimen containers

### Procedure

1. Explain purpose.

2. Obtain permit.

3. Keep n.p.o.

4. Remove dentures.

5. Transport to special procedures room on guerney. (May be done at bedside for critically ill patients).

6. Explain details of procedure:
   a. Throat will be anesthetized by swabbing with local anesthetic.
   b. Sedated with intravenous medication (usually Valium).
   c. Placed in left lateral recumbent position.
   d. Endoscope passed through esophagus.
   e. Specimens may be taken and sent to lab.

7. Transport to room on guerney.

8. Monitor vital signs as for surgical patient.

9. Check for signs and symptoms of bleeding and/ or perforation. **Rationale:** Sharp, intense pain in stomach or chest and cool, pale skin indicate perforation.

10. Check gag reflex. **Rationale:** May take two to three hours before gag reflex returns.

11. Keep side rails up until effects of medications have subsided.

12. Provide ice chips or throat lozenges for sore throat.

## ASSISTING WITH CYSTOSCOPY

### Procedure

1. Explain purpose of procedure to patient.

2. Obtain permit.

3. Premedicate as for surgical patient.

4. Keep patient n.p.o.

5. Transport patient on guerney to cystoscopy room.

6. Place patient in lithotomy position. Provide covering to preserve modesty and prevent chilling.

7. Prep external genitalia with povidone-iodine solution.

8. Explain equipment and details of procedure to patient.
   a. Cystoscope is inserted through the urethra to inspect bladder and urethral wall and facilitate a biopsy.
   b. Bladder is filled with sterile water to assist in visualization of bladder wall.
   c. Biopsy forcep may be passed through cystoscope to obtain tissue.
   d. Bladder is emptied and scope removed.

9. Return patient on guerney to room.

10. Observe closely for signs of septicemia, i.e., chills, fever, flushed feeling.

11. Force fluids unless contraindicated.

12. Monitor urine for persistent bright red color.

13. Assess patient for severe pain (colicky pain is normal with urethral catheterization), continual burning, and frequency.

14. Monitor vital signs.

## ASSISTING WITH AN AMNIOCENTESIS

### Procedure

1. Explain purpose for procedure to patient.

2. Obtain permit.

3. Have patient void prior to test. **Rationale:** This prevents injury to the bladder.

4. Transport patient to treatment room.

5. Instruct patient to lie quietly in supine position for 30 minutes.

6. Obtain fetal heart tones.

7. Open amniocentesis tray and gloves. Place Xylocaine nearby if not included on tray. **Rationale:**

Procedure is performed under sterile conditions to prevent infection.

8. Explain details of procedure to patient.
   a. Physician preps abdomen with Betadine and/or alcohol.
   b. Xylocaine injection will provide local anesthesia for needle insertion area.
   c. Needle is inserted and amniotic fluid is withdrawn.
   d. Amniotic fluid is placed in specimen container and labeled with patient's name. Appropriate lab slips are completed.
   e. Procedure takes about ten minutes.
9. Place small dressing or bandaid over needle site.
10. Monitor fetal heart tones and observe for signs of labor.
11. Instruct patient to notify physician of any unusual occurrences, signs of labor, or signs of infection.

## CHARTING  *for Diagnostic Procedures*

☐ Preparation completed for test

☐ Patient teaching completed

☐ How patient tolerated procedure

☐ Fluid or specimens sent to lab for analysis

☐ Preprocedure and postprocedure vital signs if required

☐ Record color and amount of fluid withdrawn from paracentesis, thoracentesis or lumbar puncture

☐ Type of dressing applied

☐ Specific position assumed postprocedure

---

## CLINICAL PROBLEM SOLVING

### Potential Problems

Patient has spinal fluid leak following lumbar puncture.

### Suggested Solutions

☐ Keep patient in supine position.
☐ Notify physician.
☐ Keep sterile dressing over puncture site. Do not allow dressing to become wet.
☐ If leak persists, physician may place patient in Trendelenburg's position to prevent headache. This position is contraindicated in patients with increased intracranial pressure or following a craniotomy.

Patient complains of shortness of breath or expectorates blood-tinged sputum following a thoracentesis.

☐ Place patient in Fowler's position.
☐ Assess vital signs.
☐ Administer oxygen.
☐ Monitor breath sounds.
☐ Notify physician and check on order for chest x-ray.
☐ Have chest tube insertion tray available.
☐ Allay patient's fears and provide emotional support.

Urine output is blood-tinged following paracentesis.

☐ Notify physician at once; bladder may have been punctured during procedure.
☐ Monitor vital signs for shock.
☐ Maintain patient on bed rest.
☐ Observe for urine output.

Lower gastrointestinal tract not clear and proctoscopy not completed.

☐ Repeat laxative and enemas per physician orders.
☐ Observe results of enema; if solution not clear, notify physician.

Vertigo occurs while maintaining knee-chest position during proctoscopy.

Upper gastrointestinal bleeding begins when scope inserted.

☐ Have patient lie in supine position for few minutes.
☐ Have patient assume standing position slowly.
☐ Insert nasogastric tube and apply suction.
☐ Monitor vital signs for evidence of shock.

## TERMINOLOGY

**Abscess:** a localized collection of pus in any part of the body.

**Allergy:** an altered reaction of body tissues to a specific substance; essentially an antibody-antigen reaction and may be due to the release of histamine.

**Amniocentesis:** puncturing the amniotic sac, usually by using a needle and syringe, in order to remove amniotic fluid for assessment of fetal maturity.

**Antiemetic:** an agent that will prevent or arrest vomiting.

**Arteriogram:** radiopaque dye injected into an artery to study arteries.

**Barium:** a radiopaque compound used in roentgenography of the gastrointestinal tract.

**Catheterization:** use or passage of a catheter, a tube for evacuating or injecting fluids.

**Centesis:** perforation or puncture through the skin to obtain fluid.

**Cholangiography:** X-ray examination of the bile ducts.

**Cholecystogram:** X-ray picture of the gallbladder.

**Cinecystourethrogram:** motion picture record of radiological investigation of the urethra and urinary bladder when they are filled and during emptying.

**Contrast media:** a radiopaque substance used during x-ray examination to provide a contrast in density between the tissue being filmed and the media.

**Contusion:** an injury in which the skin is not broken.

**Cranio:** prefix pertaining to the skull.

**Craniotomy:** incision involving the skull.

**Diagnosis:** method or art of identifying the disease or condition a person has or is believed to have.

**Diaphoresis:** profuse sweating.

**Dissipate:** to scatter, disperse, dispel, disintegrate.

**Dyspnea:** shortness of breath.

**Enema:** introduction of a solution through a tube into the rectum or colon.

**Fluoroscopy:** type of examination using a screen to view shadows with the aid of x-rays.

**Lithotomy:** incision into the bladder for removing a stone.

**Lumbar:** pertaining to the loins and lower vertebrae in the back.

**Myelogram:** X-ray inspection of the spinal cord by the use of radiopaque medium.

**Neoplasm:** a new and abnormal formation of tissue, as a tumor or growth.

**n.p.o.:** nothing by mouth.

**Oliguria:** diminished amount of urine formation.

**Paracentesis:** puncture of the abdominal cavity with the removal of fluid.

**Peripheral:** outer part or surface of a body.

**Pneumo:** pertaining to air, gas, and respiration.

**Pneumoencephalogram:** X-ray examination of the ventricles and subarachnoid spaces of the brain following withdrawal of cerebrospinal fluid (CSF) and injection of air via a lumbar puncture.

**Pyelo:** pertaining to the pelvis of the kidney.

**Pyelogram:** X-ray study of the renal pelvis and ureter.

**Scintillation:** the emissions from radiographic substances; a subjective sensation of seeing sparks.

**Septicemia:** blood poisoning; septic products in blood and tissue.

**Tachycardia:** fast pulse above 100 beats per minute.

**Thoracentesis:** surgical puncture of the chest wall for the removal of fluid.

**Tumor:** new growth or tissue forming an abnormal mass which performs no physiologic function.

**Urticaria:** a vascular reaction of the skin characterized by the eruption of pale elevated wheals, which are associated with severe itching.

**Ventriculogram:** an x-ray process to visualize the size and shape of the cerebral ventricles.

**Ventro:** denoting the abdomen or ventral (anterior) surface of the body.

**Vertigo:** sensation of moving or having objects move when they are actually still.

# Chapter *30*

# *Operative Care*

## LEARNING OBJECTIVES

Define the word perioperative.

Discuss the nursing care focus in each of the three stages of the perioperative period.

Identify at least three factors that influence the surgical patient's degree of stress.

Explain why postoperative complications are reduced by decreasing the stress level.

Describe at least one potential problem and the suggested solution for patients demonstrating high stress levels in the preoperative period.

State the primary purpose of providing preoperative care for patients.

Discuss how preoperative teaching can reduce the surgical patient's stress.

Describe the information contained in the surgical permit.

Demonstrate the steps for completing a surgical scrub.

Outline the essential steps in physically preparing a patient for surgery.

Explain the purpose for administering the three classifications of drugs used for preoperative medications.

Outline the essential postoperative nursing interventions completed in the surgical unit.

Summarize the major categories of post-operative pain medications and describe the general side effects of each category.

Discuss at least three major postoperative complications and the nursing interventions to prevent and treat the complications.

**NURSE'S ROLE**

Nurses are taking a more active role in the psychological and physiological preparation of the surgical patient. In many areas of the country, nurses are instructing the preoperative patient in stress-reduction techniques, expectations for the postoperative period, and use of special postoperative equipment. In fact, many hospitals provide time for the operating room nurse to make postoperative visits to patients to assess the patient's evaluation of the surgical intervention.

**PERIOPERATIVE STAGES**

The first stage of the perioperative period is the *preoperative stage.* During this stage a thorough physical assessment of the patient is completed. The nurse records all baseline data and reports any alteration from normal to the surgeon and/or anesthesiologist. Patient teaching and interviewing are also completed during this period. The physical preparation of the patient includes the preoperative shave, identifying the correct patient in the operating room, and the preoperative scrub.

The *intraoperative stage* is the period of time from when the patient undergoes the surgical procedure until the patient is admitted to the recovery room. During the intraoperative stage, nursing interventions are focused on the surgical scrub, positioning, and safety measures.

The *postoperative stage* can be divided into three segments. The immediate postoperative period includes the care given to the patient in the recovery room and in the first few hours on the surgical floor. The intermediate period usually involves the care given during the course of surgical convalescence to the time of discharge. The third segment in the postoperative stage is discharge planning, teaching, and referral.

Besides nursing care, nursing management during the postoperative period centers around assessing the patient's postoperative condition and monitoring for complications. It also includes patient teaching, pain control, and psychological support of both the patient and family.

In each phase of the patient's perioperative experience—preoperative, intraoperative and postoperative—physiological elements will be affected by the threat of the surgical trauma, the actual trauma, and the response to the trauma. The predominance of each element varies in each operative phase.

Admission to the hospital and anticipation of surgery result in some degree of anxiety and/or stress. Stress is a physiological and psychological response to a stressor—a demand to adapt. Anxiety is a stress response to an existing stressor. The degree of anxiety and stress is dependent on many factors.

## PREOPERATIVE ANXIETY

- The patient's proneness to react to anticipated stressors with high anxiety.

- The number of stress-producing events that have occurred recently in the patient's life or within the patient's family.

- The patient's perceptions of the hospitalization and surgical experience.

- The significance of the surgery to the patient.

- The number of unknowns that confront the patient on admission.

- The patient's degree of self-esteem and self-image.

- The patient's belief system and religious conviction.

The body responds physiologically to an actual or perceived threat. The hypothalamus controls a neurohormonal response. The heart rate is increased, and the heart contracts more forcefully. Blood volume is redistributed by vasoconstriction of the vessels in the skin, stomach, mesentery, and kidneys. Increased blood volume increases cardiac output. Increased blood flow to the skeletal muscles results in the muscles becoming tensed for action. The bronchi dilate, and the increased respiratory rate increases oxygenation. Mechanisms that provide energy include increased glucose release and decreased insulin production.

Behavioral responses to stress or anxiety can be adaptive or maladaptive. Adaptive behaviors are purposeful. The patient adapts to a stressful situation by preparing to face it or by removing the threat. Maladaptive behaviors result from the inability to adapt to a stressful situation.

One of the objectives of providing preoperative care is to identify the level of stress present in the patient. If nursing interventions can be planned that will reduce high anxiety levels, a safer intraoperative period will result. High levels of anxiety can prevent successful preoperative adaptation and can negatively influence postoperative recovery. Mild anxiety, on the other hand, increases alertness, increases the ability to learn, and increases the ability to assess and to adjust to one's environment. Mild anxiety also increases the ability to adjust to several simultaneous stressors. In the preoperative patient this level of anxiety is adaptive in nature, while a high level is maladaptive. When levels of anxiety or stress become intolerably high, defense mechanisms are unconsciously implemented to reduce the distress by concealing, falsifying, or distorting reality.

**TABLE 1**

RESPONSES TO ANXIETY STATES

| Low Anxiety | High Anxiety |
| --- | --- |
| Less prone to react with high anxiety to stressors | Prone to react with high anxiety to stressors |
| Few changes in personal situation in recent past | Many changes in personal situation in recent past |
| Perceives hospital and surgical experience as beneficial | Perceives hospital and surgical experience as threatening |
| Believes surgery will end chronic problem | Fears that surgery may lead to pain, disability, and possibly death |
| Regards admission procedures as friendly and supportive | Regards admission procedures as strange and frightening |
| Finds hospital conditions comfortable and the nursing staff supportive and informative | Finds hospital conditions unbearable and the nursing staff nonsupportive |

Preoperative anxiety is increased by ambiguity, conflicting perceptions, misconceptions, fears of the unknown, and bombardment by many simultaneous stressors. Ambiguity occurs from uncertainty or vagueness concerning the hospital environment, preoperative procedures, intraoperative procedures, and/or postoperative events.

Conflicting perceptions occur when preconceived notions about the operative experience are different from those actually encountered. The patient who thought that a herniorrhaphy would be a quick, safe cure can become quite anxious after the anesthesiologist informs him of potential complications.

Misconceptions arise when inaccurate information is given, when terminology used is not understood, and when events are not explained clearly. A patient who is scheduled for a bronchoscopy in the morning, and whose nurse silently places an n.p.o. sign over the bed, may believe that he is destined for the same hospital regimen as his roommate, who had a gastrectomy.

**TABLE 2**

MANAGING SURGICAL PATIENTS

Conscientious preoperative care of patients prevents postoperative complications.

□ Preparing the patient psychologically reduces the patient's stress level and helps to prevent postoperative complications.

□ Teaching coughing and deep breathing exercises, procedures for getting out of bed, and uses of specialized equipment enhance the patient's cooperation and prevents postoperative complications.

□ Completing the surgical scrub reduces microorganisms on the body surface and the possibility of wound infections postoperatively.

Scrupulous asepsis throughout the perioperative period reduces complications.

□ Maintaining strict asepsis reduces cross contamination.

□ Identifying breaks in sterile technique and taking appropriate action decrease the risk of postoperative complications.

The stress responses are additive. An increasing number of stressors can eventually drain adaptive energy. The newly admitted surgical patient who has been confronted with many stressors before admission will have increased vulnerability and is likely to respond with a higher level of stress as each new stressor is encountered.

Psychological preparation includes preoperative teaching of the patient and the family as well as the administration of preoperative medications. Preoperative teaching prepares the patient by explaining the events that will occur preoperatively and postoperatively. Preoperative teaching reduces stress by minimizing the patient's fears—fears of the unknown, pain, anesthesia, and loss of control. Many hospitals have teaching programs developed for the surgical patient. Group teaching sessions are valuable ways of disseminating information.

Postoperative complications can also be decreased by reducing stress levels. Prolonged high stress levels are associated with deficient immune systems, stress ulcers, hypertension, life-threatening arrhythmias, sodium and water retention, and congestive heart failure.

The need for frequent and high doses of analgesia is reduced when stress levels are low and when patients are assured of pain relief when needed. Levels of stress closely correlate with levels of perceived pain. Reduction of stress reduces perceived pain. Anxiety levels are increased when the patient envisions having to endure pain without relief. Assurance that medication is available and encouragement to utilize the medication for relief reduces anxiety significantly.

The degree of patient participation in recovery affects the complication rate. Effective pulmonary care significantly curtails the most frequent postoperative complications—atelectasis and pneumonia. The patient's active and willing participation in deep breathing, coughing, use of incentive spirometers, and early ambulation will enhance a rapid recovery and thus shorten hospitalization.

The influence of the family can also affect the patient's recovery. In many cases, the patient's strongest support system is the family. To be an effective support system, the family must be informed. Also, the anxiety and/or stress of each family member must be within tolerable limits. Knowledge of the patient's problems, type of surgery proposed, and recovery rate will allow the family to provide support. The knowledgeable family can reinforce preoperative teaching for each other and the patient.

## NURSING DIAGNOSES

The following nursing diagnoses are appropriate to utilize on Patient Care Plans when the components are related to perioperative care.

| Nursing Diagnosis (Potential) | Defining Characteristic; Etiology (Examples) |
|---|---|
| ☐ Airway Clearance, Ineffective, *related to* | Improper aeration and/or ventilation, e.g., inappropriate deep breathing exercises. |
| ☐ Anxiety, *related to* | Potential loss of body function, e.g., surgical procedure. |
| | Fear of unknown outcome of surgical procedure, e.g., lack of definitive data. |
| ☐ Comfort, Alteration in: Pain, *related to* | Restrictive movement or incisional area, pain, e.g., recent surgery, immobility. |

□ Coping, Ineffective Individual, *related to* — Intense stressor or diminished capacity to handle stress, e.g., prolonged pain, altered body image.

□ Fluid Volume Deficit, *related to* — Excessive fluid and/or blood loss, e.g., operative procedure, hemorrhage.

## UNIT ONE   STRESS IN PREOPERATIVE PATIENTS

### NURSING PROCESS DATA

#### ASSESSMENT   *Data Base*

Identify if high level of stress exists.

Assess exaggerated anxiety and/or stress behaviors.

Evaluate defensive behaviors.

Assess vulnerability of patient due to number and significance of changes in life before admission.

Evaluate level of patient knowledge and perceptions of the impending surgery and perioperative period.

#### PLANNING   *Objectives*

To identify the level of stress and/or anxiety present in preoperative patients.

To provide interventions that decrease stress levels and promote optimal preoperative behavioral and physiological responses.

To observe for use of defensive behaviors that mask a failure to adapt appropriately in stressful situations.

To prepare the patient for a smooth preoperative and postoperative period.

To prevent postoperative complications.

#### IMPLEMENTATION   *Procedures*

Preventing Anxiety and Stress

Reducing Anxiety and Stress

Assisting the Patient Who Uses Denial

#### EVALUATION   *Expected Outcomes*

Patient's level of stress and/or anxiety is identified.

Nursing interventions are provided that decrease stress levels and promote optimal preoperative responses.

Denial, as a defense mechanism, is identified in the patient.

## PREVENTING ANXIETY AND STRESS

### Procedure

1. Establish a trusting relationship.

2. Encourage verbalization of feelings.

3. Listen attentively.

4. Communicate acceptance of the patient as an individual.

5. Identify the needs of the patient and keep the charge nurse informed of the patient's needs.

6. Give adequate information regarding hospital procedures.

a. Hospital environment, including sights, sounds, and equipment.

b. Hospital personnel and routine procedures: mealtimes, telephone usage, call light.

c. Ordered preoperative procedures: lab tests, diagnostic procedures (explain the sensory experiences that will be encountered).

d. Scheduled time of surgery.

e. Hospital regulations: visiting hours, smoking.

f. Preoperative procedures: shave, n.p.o., medications, side rails, dentures, nail polish.

g. Anticipated postoperative events: recovery room, pain and pain medications, coughing and deep breathing exercises, dressings, IVs.

**TABLE 3**   PREOPERATIVE STRESS ASSESSMENT

| Physiological Responses | Emotional/Defensive Responses | Anxiety/Activity Responses |
|---|---|---|
| Heart rate: rate increases 10 beats per minute over baseline during three observations. Presence of palpitations. Blood pressure: increases more than 10 mm Hg over baseline during three observations. Respiratory rate: increases more than five per minute over baseline during three observations. Vasoconstriction of blood vessels near the skin: cool, pale fingers and toes; increased capillary filling time of more than 3 seconds. Vasoconstriction of renal vessels: decreased urine output compared to baseline and fluid intake. Vasoconstriction of gastric and mesenteric vessels: anorexia, nausea, vomiting, abdominal distention with flatus, decreased bowel sounds, hyperactivity, diarrhea. | Withdrawal: daydreaming, increased time in sleep, unwillingness to talk, disinterest. Anger: resentment, aggressiveness, noncompliance, swearing, boasting, attempts to gain control and independence. Denial: joking, carefree attitude, inappropriate laughter, refusal to discuss impending surgery. | Hyperactivity: pacing, hand-wringing, lip or nail biting, finger-tapping, impatience, irritability, insomnia. Disorganization of thought: repetitive speech, constant conversation, difficulty concentrating. Increased sensitivity to environmental noise, light, temperature, activity. Increased muscle tensing: furrowed eyebrows, facial tics, clenched jaws, loud or high-pitched voice, stammering, rapid speech, elevated shoulders, clenched fists, urinary frequency. Patient complains of tension or inability to relax. Increased energy and preparedness: restlessness, easily startled, increased activity level. |

# REDUCING ANXIETY AND STRESS

## Equipment

Cassette tape player

Appropriate relaxation tape

## Procedure

1. Establish a trusting relationship.
2. Encourage verbalization of feelings.
3. Use touch to communicate caring and genuine interest.
4. Avoid reassurance.
5. Utilize realistic outcomes.
6. Assist patient in exploring effective coping methods to reduce anxiety and/or stress.
   a. Ask the patient or the family what method the patient normally uses to successfully reduce stress.
   b. Provide activity: walking, range of motion.
   c. Provide a back rub to loosen tense muscles. **Rationale:** Physical relaxation will often lead to mental relaxation.
   d. Teach patient relaxation techniques. One technique is to ask the patient to picture a blue sky that is clear except for one white, fluffy cloud. Tell patient to concentrate on this scene for ten minutes. This technique will often relax the mind and the body.
   e. An alternative is to ask the patient to picture a favorite place, e.g., a warm, sunny beach with sand and gentle surf.
7. As the patient begins to relax, reinforce success. Assist patient in recognizing patient's strengths and progress.
8. Encourage self-awareness of increasing tension and immediate reversal of escalation.

# ASSISTING THE PATIENT WHO USES DENIAL

## Procedure

1. Establish a trusting relationship.
2. Encourage verbalization of feelings.
3. Use touch to communicate caring and genuine interest.
4. Do not attempt to enforce reality. The patient is denying reality to prevent outright panic. Allow use of this defense.
5. Utilize techniques to reduce anxiety and/or stress to manageable proportions.
6. Attempt to determine the cause of the need for denial.
7. Listen for cues that indicate readiness to discuss the stressors causing the need for denial.
8. Notify physician of your findings.

## CHARTING   *for Preoperative Stress*

☐ Observed and subjective indications of anxiety and/or stress levels

☐ Nursing interventions used to decrease stress and the results of the intervention

☐ Changes which occurred as a result of the nursing interventions

☐ Specific fears verbalized by the patient

☐ Nonverbal indications of stress and/or anxiety

---

## CLINICAL PROBLEM SOLVING

### Potential Problems

Anxiety level increases rapidly.

### Suggested Solutions

☐ Maintain calm composure and speak in a soft, caring manner.

☐ Use touch to communicate caring and peacefulness.

☐ Reinforce patient self-acceptance as an individual.

☐ If unable to achieve success with stress-reducing techniques, notify physician.

| | |
|---|---|
| Patient becomes angry or hostile. | ☐ Maintain calm composure. |
| | ☐ Accept anger but place limits on how it may be expressed, e.g., destructive behavior. Understand that anger is usually the result of feeling helpless and powerless to change an intolerable situation. |
| | ☐ Do not reward this behavior but explore other means of meeting patient's needs. |
| | ☐ Do not isolate patient but continue to respond to needs. |
| | ☐ Notify physician of patient's behaviors and your actions which were used to decrease anger or hostility. |
| Patient becomes depressed because of overwhelming anxiety and feelings of helplessness or hopelessness. | ☐ Convey respect and belief that the patient is worthwhile. Question the patient's appraisal of reality and provide support while the patient works through his feelings. |
| | ☐ Provide positive feedback and recognition of strengths, progress, and improved self-esteem. |
| | ☐ Spend additional time with the patient to allow him time to verbalize fears. |

# UNIT TWO   PREOPERATIVE CARE

## NURSING PROCESS DATA

### ASSESSMENT   *Data Base*

Assess type of surgical procedure to be carried out and extent of data base needed.

Evaluate the ability of the patient to provide accurate data base information.

Assess level of anxiety present that may interfere in the transmission of information at that moment.

Identify the appropriate physical care needed for the specific surgical intervention.

Assess special needs for the surgical shave.

Check if a special permit is needed for shaving, such as the head for neurosurgical patients, extremities for orthopedic patients, or children.

Check for need for special soap or antiseptic scrub prior to shave.

Check if sterile drape is required following shave.

Check if a policy exists in the hospital for disposing or handling of scalp hair.

Assess area before shaving for unusual cuts, abrasions, or markings and report findings to charge nurse.

Assess patient's learning needs.

**PLANNING** *Objectives*

To assist with monitoring the patient's progress through the operative experience.

To assist in identifying deviations from the patient's usual baseline data that may occur as a result of anxiety or stress of admission, preoperative events, diagnostic procedures, the surgical trauma, postoperative complications, responses to and side effects of drugs.

To provide appropriate preoperative physical care to enable the patient to have a safe intraoperative and postoperative period.

To report patient's statements about allergies or chronic problems which could affect postoperative nursing care.

To complete a surgical scrub correctly and without cuts.

To provide appropriate preoperative teaching.

**IMPLEMENTATION** *Procedures*

Obtaining Baseline Data

Providing Preoperative Teaching

Shaving the Surgical Patient

Preparing the Patient for Surgery

Administering Preoperative Medications

**EVALUATION** *Expected Outcomes*

The patient's physical and/or emotional deviations from normal are identified preoperatively.

Preoperative baseline data is obtained.

Explicit preoperative care is provided to ensure a safe intraoperative and postoperative course.

Surgical shave is completed correctly and without cuts.

Patient is psychologically prepared for surgery.

## OBTAINING BASELINE DATA

### Equipment

Thermometer

Sphygmomanometer and stethoscope

Chart for documenting findings

### Procedure

1. Establish rapport with the patient.
2. Ask about allergies to drugs or food.
3. Take and record vital signs and weight of patient.
4. Check if patient wears dentures, hearing aid, or glasses, or has an artificial eye.
5. Record any unusual stress or anxiety exhibited by the patient.
6. Complete a physical assessment and health history. Report unusual findings to physician.
7. Evaluate lab values for abnormalities (EKG, x-rays, blood work and urinalysis).
8. Identify areas requiring patient teaching.

## PROVIDING PREOPERATIVE TEACHING

### Equipment

Prepared teaching aids when available—audio-visual, filmstrips, pamphlets, pictures, posters, programmed learning, slides, cassette tapes, overhead transparencies

Quiet room for patient and family where there will be no interruptions during the teaching program

Equipment that may be used postoperatively by the patient, e.g., IV bottle and tubing, Stryker frame, nasogastric tube, cardiac monitor and electrodes

### Procedure

*Provide preoperative information*

1. Blood work, EKG, urinalysis, chest x-ray.
2. Preoperative skin preparation.
3. Placement of nasogastric tube, Foley catheter, as indicated.
4. Enema or special bowel preparation as ordered.
5. Use of medications preoperatively and postoperatively.
6. Deep breathing and coughing exercises (use of spirometer or IPPB if indicated).
7. Leg exercises and antiembolic stockings.
8. Turning and moving in bed.
9. Reason for n.p.o. and when it begins.
10. Alterations in diet preoperatively or postoperatively.
11. Activities and preparation the morning of surgery.
12. Need for quiet environment after medications have been given.
13. Information usually provided by anesthesiologist and surgeon.
14. Tour and explanation of monitoring devices and special equipment in ICU if patient is to be transferred there postoperatively.

*Provide intraoperative information*

1. Mode of transportation to operating room.
2. Discussion of procedure in preinduction room or operating room suite in relationship to anesthesia.
3. Reinforce physician's explanation of surgery.

4. Description of dressings, tubes, or equipment that will be used postoperatively.
5. Recovery room physical environment and procedures.

*Provide postoperative information*

1. Assessment procedures.
2. Routine procedures of vital signs.
3. Deep breathing, turning, and coughing exercises.
4. IV therapy if indicated.
5. Irrigation of tubes when directed.
6. Catheter care.
7. Dietary alterations.
8. Observation and changes of dressing.
9. Ambulation and/or restrictions in ambulation.
10. Medications.

*Provide Family Teaching*

1. Include family in teaching provided to patient.
2. Instructions to family members should include:
   a. Visiting hours.
   b. Where to wait during surgery.
   c. Where the surgeon will meet with them, and when.
   d. Where they can find bathrooms, telephones, and food and beverage service.
   e. When they can see the patient after surgery.
3. How to contact a spiritual/religious resource person.
4. How they can best get information regarding the patient's condition while they are at home or in the hospital.
5. Whether they will be called if there is a change in the patient's condition.
6. What to expect: patient's behavior, which may be regressive; attitude which may be depressed and/or angry; physical condition, which may appear worse than it is, and post recovery period.

## SHAVING THE SURGICAL PATIENT

### Equipment

Absorbent pad

Bath blanket or drape

Scissors

Disposable prep kit (if available)

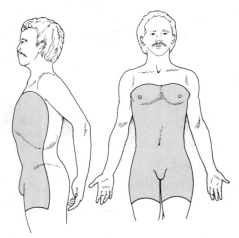

The area shaved for abdominal surgeries.

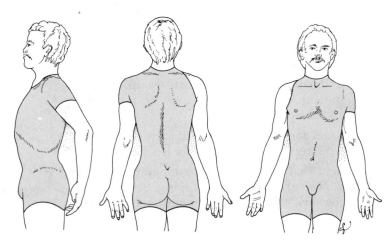

Areas shaved for thoracotomy and upper abdominal surgeries.

If kit not available:
   Sterile safety razor and blades
   Two sterile bowls
   4 × 4 gauze pads
   Emesis basin
   Applicator sticks
   Cleansing solution
   Sterile water
   Sterile gloves

### Procedure

1. Refer to physician's orders for specific operative site or area to be shaved. If orders do not state preference for site, refer to procedure manual for appropriate area to be shaved, based on surgical procedure.

2. Gather equipment.

3. Explain procedure to patient and provide privacy.

4. Adjust light to ensure good visualization.

5. Wash your hands.

6. Position patient for maximum comfort and prep site exposure.

7. Drape patient for comfort and to prevent undue exposure.

8. Protect bed with absorbent pad.

9. Arrange shaving equipment for your convenience.

10. Cut long hair with scissors for craniotomy.

11. Dispose of cut hair.

12. Put on sterile gloves.

13. Apply cleansing solution with 4 × 4 gauze pads.

14. Begin at incision site and, with light friction, make ever-widening circles, moving outward from the center to the most distant line of prep area. **Rationale:** Working from most clean to least clean area prevents contamination.

15. Discard soiled sponges frequently.

16. Using sharp razor, shave hair moving away from incision site. With free hand, stretch skin taut and shave, following the hair growth pattern and using firm, steady strokes. **Rationale:** Shave will be closer and nicks prevented.

17. Change blade as often as necessary. Avoid nicking the skin. Report if skin is nicked. **Rationale:** Nicks, if severe, can cause infection because of the bacteria normally found on the skin.

18. When all hair has been removed, re-scrub area as above. Scrub area for at least two to five minutes. Orthopedic surgery may require a ten-minute scrub.

19. Rinse shaved area with warm water and blot dry with 4 × 4 gauze pads.

20. Assist patient to put on clean gown.

21. Remove and dispose of equipment.

22. Position the patient for comfort.

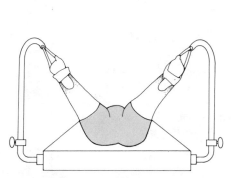

Shaved area for gynecological surgery.

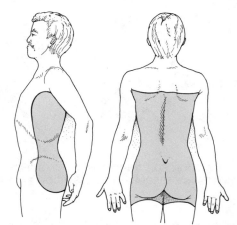

Shaved areas for laminectomy and renal surgery.

## PREPARING THE PATIENT FOR SURGERY

### Equipment

Preoperative check list

Specific equipment needed to provide physical care as ordered, such as enema equipment, nasogastric tube, Foley catheter

Operative permit

### Procedure

1. Obtain patient's signature on preoperative permit.

2. Administer enema if ordered.

3. Complete skin prep and shave if ordered.

4. Observe for signs of cold or upper respiratory infection.

5. Explain need for patient to be n.p.o. for 8 to 10 hours preoperatively.

6. Remove lipstick and nail polish.

7. Provide preoperative showers with bacteriostatic soap.

8. Insert Foley catheter if ordered.

9. Take and record vital signs.

10. Remove earrings, necklaces, medals, watch, rings (ring may be taped to finger in some facilities).

11. Remove contact lenses, glasses, hair pieces and dentures.

12. Assist patient to void and record time and amount.

13. Place surgical cap on patient's head.

14. Administer preoperative medications.

15. Place side rails in UP position following administration of medications.

16. Darken room and provide quiet environment following administration of medications.

17. Check patient 15 minutes after medication administered to observe for side effects.

---

**Patients at risk for postoperative infection:**
Uncontrolled diabetes
Renal failure
Obesity
Receiving corticosteroids
Receiving immunosuppressive agents
Prolonged antibiotic therapy
Protein and/or ascorbic acid deficiencies
Marked dehydration and hypovolemia
Decreased cardiac output
Edema and fluid and electrolyte imbalances
Anemia
Preoperative infection

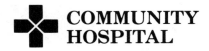

# COMMUNITY HOSPITAL

Client Information

## AUTHORIZATION FOR AND CONSENT TO SURGERY, ADMINISTRATION OF ANESTHETICS, SPECIAL DIAGNOSTIC OR THERAPEUTIC PROCEDURES

Date _____   Time _____

Your admitting physician is _____, M. D.

Your surgeon is _____, M. D.

1.  The hospital staff and facilities assist your physicians and surgeons in the performance of various surgical operations and other diagnostic and therapeutic procedures. These surgical operations and special diagnostic or therapeutic procedures all may involve calculated risks of complications, injury or even death, from both known and unknown causes and no warranty or guarantee has been made as to result or cure. Except in a case of emergency or exceptional circumstances, these operations and procedures are not performed upon clients unless and until the client has had an opportunity to discuss them with his/her physician. Each client has the right to consent to or refuse any proposed operation or special procedure (based upon the description or explanation received).

2.  Your physicians and surgeons have determined that the operations or special procedures listed below may be beneficial in the diagnosis or treatment of your condition. Upon your authorization and consent, the operations or special procedures will be performed by your physicians and surgeons and their staff. The persons in attendance for the purpose of administering anesthesia or performing other specialized professional services, such as radiology, pathology and the like, are not the agents, servants or employees of the hospital or your physician or surgeon, but are independent contractors performing specialized services on your behalf and, as such, are your agents, servants, or employees. Any tissue or member severed in any operation will be disposed of in the discretion of the pathologist, except _____ and those body parts specified as donor organs.

3.  Your signature opposite the operations or special procedures listed below constitutes your acknowledgement (a) that you have read and agreed to the foregoing, (b) that the operations or special procedures have been adequately explained to you by your attending physicians or surgeons and that you have all of the information that you desire, and (c) that you authorize and consent to the performance of the operations or special procedures.

*Operation or Procedure*

_____

_____

Signature _____   Signature _____
                      Client                                              Witness

(If client is a minor or unable to sign, complete the following): Client is a minor, is unable to sign because

_____

_____         _____
            Father                                              Guardian

_____         _____
            Mother                                  Other person and relationship

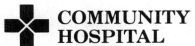

## COMMUNITY HOSPITAL

Client Information

### SURGICAL CHECK LIST

Unit Check List

PLEASE PRINT

1. Surgical Procedure scheduled: _____

_____ Rt.     Lt.
                                            (circle)

2. Consent for surgery _____
   Yes or No

3. Consent for Sterilization or Special Procedure _____
   Yes or No

4. Consultation _____
   Yes or No

5. Surgical Prep done by _____
   (Signature)

6. History and Physical _____
   Yes or No

7. Urinalysis _____ CBC _____ Type & Xmatch _____
   Yes or No        Yes or No                Yes or No

8. Chest X-ray_____ EKG _____
   Yes or No                      Yes or No

9. List allergies (if none, state "none")_____

10. Allergy Band _____
    Yes or No

11. TPR _____ BP _____

12. Voided _____ Time _____ Retention Cath. _____
    Yes or No

13. Pre-op medication and times _____

14. Condition after pre-op medication: _____ awake   asleep   drowsy
    (circle)

| 15. Prosthesis: | None | Removed | Disposition | Left In |
|-----------------|------|---------|-------------|---------|
| a. Bridge | | | | |
| b. Partial | | | | |
| c. Plates | | | | |
| d. Artificial limbs | | | | |
| e. Artificial eyes | | | | |
| f. Contact lenses | | | | |
| g. Hearing aid | | | | |
| h. Pacemaker | | | | |
| i. Hairpieces, Hairpins, Eyelashes | | | | |

| 16. Valuables | Removed Yes or No | Disposition, if yes |
|---------------|-------------------|---------------------|
| a. Rings | | |
| b. Watch | | |
| c. Medal and chain | | |
| d. Glasses | | |
| e. Radio | | |
| f. Wallet | | |
| g. Other | | |

17. Identification band checked with chart _____
    Yes or No

    Signature _____ R.N.

### Operating Room Check List

Check                          Comment

1. _____
2. _____
3. _____
4. _____
5. _____
6. _____
7. _____
8. _____
9. _____
10. _____
11. _____
12. _____
13. _____
14. _____
15. _____
  a. _____
  b. _____
  c. _____
  d. _____
  e. _____
  f. _____
  g. _____
  h. _____
  i. _____
16. _____
17. _____

Signature _____
                        Circulating Nurse

### POSTOPERATIVE

Sponge Count _____

Needle Count _____

Drains Left In _____

Catheter In _____

Scrub Nurse _____

Signature _____
                        Circulating Nurse

## ADMINISTERING PREOPERATIVE MEDICATIONS

### Equipment

Preoperative check list

Preoperative medications

### Procedure

1. Complete preoperative check list.

2. Check orders for medication, dosage, route and time.

3. Check history for allergy to ordered medication.

4. Explain the purpose of the medication to the patient.

5. Warn the patient that the injection may sting or burn.

6. Follow procedure for administration of intramuscular injections.

7. Administer medication.

8. Raise side rails to UP position.

9. Explain why the patient should not get out of bed after the medications have been given. **Rationale:** Medication will make the patient drowsy and his equilibrium will be affected.

10. Place the call light within reach and encourage the patient to use it.

11. Ask if there are any questions or assistance you can offer before leaving the room. Darken the room or close curtains.

12. Give the patient the estimated time of surgery.

---

**Preoperative Medications: Type and Action**

Hypnotic or opiate—given night before surgery
  Decreases anxiety
  Promotes good night's sleep
Hypnotic or opiate—preoperative medication
  Decreases anxiety
  Allows smooth anesthetic induction
  Provides amnesia for immediate perioperative period
Anticholinergic—preoperative medication
  Decreases secretions
  Counteracts vagal effects during anesthesia

---

### CHARTING  *for Preoperative Care*

☐ Safety measures carried out preoperatively

☐ Completion of preoperative shave and area involved

☐ Solution used and length of time of scrub

☐ Operative checklist completed

☐ Review physician's explanation of potential surgical complications

☐ Physical care completed prior to surgery

☐ Preoperative medications given and effects of medications

☐ Time and method of transportation to operating room

☐ Preoperative teaching completed

---

## CLINICAL PROBLEM SOLVING

### Potential Problems

Factors that can affect the postoperative course are identified during the preoperative care, e.g., arthritic changes in patient's back, history of thrombophlebitis, etc.

Patient refuses to go to operating room without dentures.

### Suggested Solutions

☐ Place information on patient's care plan and inform charge nurse about findings.

☐ Write a note on patient's chart and alert the operating room and recovery room staff of the findings so that they can assess for the problems.

☐ Explain to patient that dentures are likely to be lost, broken, or inadvertently pushed to back of mouth if not removed.

☐ If patient refuses to remove dentures, alert anesthesiologist that dentures are in place.

| | |
|---|---|
| Patient unable to void before surgery. | ☐ Run water so patient can hear trickling sound to stimulate voiding.<br>☐ Run warm water over perineum.<br>☐ Place ammonia or oil of wintergreen on a cotton ball in urinal or bedpan. |
| Patient appears to be abnormally stressed. | ☐ Explore feelings and reasons for patient's and/or family's stressed behaviors.<br>☐ Explore more effective methods to reduce stress for patient and family.<br>☐ Provide additional stress reduction exercises.<br>☐ Clarify misconceptions and inappropriate perceptions.<br>☐ Introduce patient to another patient who has had similar surgery.<br>☐ Have physician speak to patient and answer questions. |
| Patient is not adequately prepared for surgery. | ☐ Ascertain where data is insufficient or unclear and provide additional teaching in this area.<br>☐ Use a different approach or vocabulary to explain content.<br>☐ Use additional audio-visual equipment if available. |
| Patient's preoperative laboratory findings are abnormal. | ☐ Check with laboratory to have them reevaluate if lab results are accurate.<br>☐ Have laboratory rerun tests if extremely abnormal.<br>☐ Notify physician of abnormal findings. |

## UNIT THREE  POSTOPERATIVE CARE

### NURSING PROCESS DATA

#### ASSESSMENT  *Data Base*

Assess for patent airway.

Check if oxygen is ordered.

Check gag reflex especially in recovery room.

Observe for adverse signs of general anesthesia or spinal anesthesia.

Take vital signs.

Check patient's temperature for heat control.

Observe dressings and surgical drains.

Check IVs for type and amount of fluid to be infused.

Observe color and amount of urine.

Observe patient's overall condition.

### PLANNING *Objectives*

To ensure that the patient experiences an uneventful postoperative course.

To provide safe, effective nursing care in the immediate postoperative period.

To ensure that postoperative pain is relieved promptly.

To be aware of the common postoperative drugs for pain control.

### IMPLEMENTATION *Procedures*

Providing Postoperative Care

Administering Postoperative Medications

### EVALUATION *Expected Outcomes*

Patient experiences an uneventful postoperative course.

Postoperative pain is relieved promptly.

Postoperative nursing interventions are carried out effectively and in a timely manner.

Action of the major postoperative medications is understood.
  Opiate drugs.
  Synthetic opiate-like drugs.
  Nonnarcotic pain relievers.
  Narcotic antagonists.
  Antiemetics.

## PROVIDING POSTOPERATIVE CARE

### Equipment

Surgical bed

Absorbent pads

Warm blankets

IV pole

Oxygen source, tubing, and equipment

Emesis basin and tissues

Sphygmomanometer and stethoscope

Thermometer (rectal or oral)

Nurses' notes

Intake and output record

Special equipment depending on type of surgery

### Procedure

1. Assess for patent airway and level of consciousness; administer oxygen if ordered.

2. Take vital signs: usual orders are q15 minutes until stable; then q½ hour × 2; qhour × 4; then q4 hours for 24–48 hours.

3. Check IV site and patency frequently.

4. Observe and record urine output.

5. Measure intake and output.

6. Observe skin color and moisture.

7. Position patient for comfort and maximum airway ventilation according to orders.

8. Turn every two hours and p.r.n.

9. Give back care at least every four hours.

10. Encourage coughing and deep breathing every two hours (may use IPPB or blow bottles if ordered).

11. Keep patient comfortable with medications.

12. Check dressings and drainage tubes every two to four hours; if abnormal amount of drainage, check more frequently.

13. Give oral hygiene at least every four hours; if

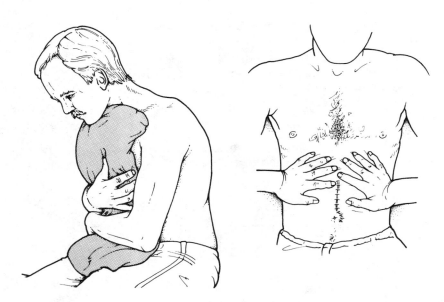

Teach deep breathing and coughing preoperatively to enhance lung expansion post-operatively.

nasogastric tube, nasal oxygen, or endotracheal tube is inserted, give oral hygiene every two hours.

14. Bathe patient when temperature can be maintained. **Rationale**: Bathing removes the antiseptic solution and stimulates circulation.

15. Keep patient warm and avoid chilling, but do not increase temperature above normal. **Rationale**: Increased temperature increases metabolic rate and need for oxygen. Excessive perspiration causes fluid and electrolyte loss.

16. Irrigate nasogastric tube every two hours and p.r.n., as ordered, with normal saline to keep patent and to prevent electrolyte imbalance.

17. Maintain dietary intake: type of diet depends on type and extent of surgical procedure.
    a. Minor surgical conditions: patient may drink or eat as soon as he is awake, desires food or drink, and has gag reflex present.
    b. Major surgical conditions:
       n.p.o. until bowel sounds return.
       Clear liquid advanced to full liquid as tolerated.
       Soft diet advanced to full diet within three to five days (depending on type of surgery and physician's preference).

18. Place patient on bedpan two to four hours postoperatively if catheter not inserted.

19. Check physician's orders when to begin the patient's postoperative activity. Most patients are dangled within first 24 hours.

20. Observe for signs and symptoms of possible postoperative complications. See Postoperative Complications chart.

## ADMINISTERING POSTOPERATIVE MEDICATIONS

### Equipment

Medication as ordered

Appropriate syringe and needle for parenteral medications

### Procedure

1. Evaluate patient's need for pain relief.

2. Provide nonmedication measures for relief of pain such as relaxation techniques, back care, positioning.

3. Identify the pharmacological action of the medication.

4. Review the general side effects of the medication.
   a. Drowsiness.
   b. Euphoria.
   c. Sleep.
   d. Respiratory depression.
   e. Nausea and vomiting.

5. Administer medications as ordered, usually at three to four hour intervals for first 24 to 48 hours for better action and pain relief. Assess for pain relief.

6. Know the action of the following drugs.
   a. Opiates.
   b. Synthetic opiate-like drugs.
   c. Nonnarcotic pain relievers.
   d. Narcotic antagonists.
   e. Antiemetics.

## CHARTING  *for Postoperative Care*

☐ Postoperative nursing interventions

☐ Fluid replacement—type and amount of solution

☐ Condition of dressings and drains

☐ Urine output, intake and output

☐ Vital signs

☐ Signs and symptoms of potential complications

☐ Preventive nursing measures

☐ Patient's activity level

☐ Clinical manifestations indicating pain

☐ Type, time and amount of pain medication administered

☐ Site of injection

☐ Any side effects of medications observed

☐ Whether or not pain relieved

---

## CLINICAL PROBLEM SOLVING

Postoperative complications are presented in chart format on the following pages.

---

## TERMINOLOGY

**Adaptation:**  ability of an organism to adjust to a change in environment.

**Analgesia:**  absence of the normal sense of pain.

**Analgesic:**  a drug that relieves pain without altering the conscious state.

**Anesthesia:**  partial or complete loss of sensation by administration of a drug or gas.

**Anxiety:**  a troubled feeling; experiencing a sense of dread or fear without a stimulus. A condition associated with physiological changes.

**Arthritis:**  inflammation of a joint, usually accompanied by pain and sometimes by change in structure.

**Asepsis:**  sterile, a condition free from germs.

**Atelectasis:**  a collapsed or airless condition of the lungs.

**Bronchitis:**  inflammation of the bronchial mucous membrane.

**Bronchoscopy:**  examination of the bronchi with a scope.

---

### TABLE 4  POSTOPERATIVE COMPLICATIONS

| POTENTIAL COMPLICATION | PATIENTS AT RISK | INDICATIVE FINDINGS |
|---|---|---|
| **Atelectasis:** collapse of alveoli; may be diffuse and involve a segment or lobe, or lung<br><br>*Potential Onset:*<br>First 48 hours | All with general anesthesia<br>*Special risk clients:*<br>Smokers<br>Chronic bronchitis<br>Emphysema<br>Obesity<br>Elderly<br>Upper abdominal surgery<br>Chest surgery<br>Abdominal distention | Fever to 102° F<br>Tachycardia<br>Restlessness<br>Tachypnea 24–30 min<br>Altered breath sounds<br>    Dullness to percussion<br>    Diminished or absent breath sounds<br>    Rales<br>ABGs: decreased $PaO_2$ |

**Contamination:** the introduction of disease, germs, or infectious materials into or on normally sterile objects.

**Dehydration:** to deprive the body or tissues of water.

**Diplopia:** double vision.

**Egophony:** a nasal sound heard while auscultating the lungs of a person as he speaks; a sound heard in pleural effusion.

**Emesis:** vomiting.

**Emphysema:** a condition in which the alveoli of the lungs become distended or ruptured.

**Enema:** injection of water or fluid into rectum and colon to empty the lower intestine or to introduce medicine or food for therapeutic purposes.

**Euphoria:** an exaggerated feeling of well-being.

**Exudate:** accumulation of fluid in a cavity.

**Hernia:** the protrusion or projection of an organ or part of an organ through the wall of the cavity that normally contains it.

**Hypertension:** higher blood pressure than normal; usually over 140 mm/Hg/90 mm/hg.

**Hypnotic:** drugs that cause insensibility to pain or partial to complete unconsciousness; includes sedatives, analgesics, anesthetics, and intoxicants.

**Hypothermia:** the state of low body temperature.

**Hypovolemia:** diminished blood supply.

**Immunosuppressive:** acting to suppress the body's natural immune response to an antigen.

**Induction:** the process of causing or producing; in anesthesia, the period from the initial inhalation or injection until optimum level of anesthesia is reached.

**Intervention:** the act of coming in or between so as to modify.

**Lethargy:** a condition of sluggishness; stupor.

**Maladaptive:** poorly adjusted; inability to adapt.

**Mesentery:** a peritoneal fold connecting the intestine with the postabdominal wall.

**Narcotic:** producing stupor or sleep; a drug that depresses the central nervous system.

**Neurohormonal:** concerning the interaction between nerves and hormones.

**Orthopedic:** concerning the prevention or correction of deformities of the musculo-skeletal system.

**Palpitation:** rapid, violent, or throbbing pulsation, as an abnormally rapid, throbbing, or fluttering heart.

**Peritonitis:** inflammation of the peritoneum.

**Pneumonia:** inflammation of the lungs caused primarily by bacteria, viruses, and chemical agents; can be characterized by chills, high fever, pain in the chest, cough, and purulent and often bloody sputum.

**Stress:** a mentally or emotionally disruptive or disquieting influence; distress.

**Therapeutic:** having medicinal or healing properties.

**Thrombophlebitis:** inflammation of a vein associated with thrombus.

**Topical:** pertinent to a particular area; local.

**Trauma:** a physical injury or wound caused by external force or violence; an emotional or psychological shock that may produce disordered feelings to behavior.

**Vaso:** a word part meaning vessel, as a blood vessel.

**Vasoconstriction:** constriction of a blood vessel.

| PREVENTION | INTERVENTION | CHARTING |
|---|---|---|
| *Preoperative:* have client practice turning, coughing, and deep breathing | Increase effectiveness of pulmonary toilet | Signs and symptoms noted |
| Discuss importance of exercises | Administer supplemental oxygen as ordered | Location of abnormal chest findings |
| *Postoperative clients at risk:* | Monitor response to treatment | Frequency of nursing treatment |
| Turn q30 min. | Monitor for onset of pneumonia | Client's response to treatment |
| Deep breathe and cough | If entire lobe of lung is involved, prepare for bronchoscopy to remove plug | Oxygen: method of administration in liters per min. |
| *Other clients:* | | Sputum: character, color, and amount in teaspoons or cc |
| Initiate turning and deep breathing exercises q1–2 hrs. | | Changes in chest findings in response to treatment |
| Ambulate as soon as possible | | |
| Medicate to reduce pain, splinting, and resistance to treatment | | |

**TABLE 4** POSTOPERATIVE COMPLICATIONS (continued)

| POTENTIAL COMPLICATION | PATIENTS AT RISK | INDICATIVE FINDINGS |
| --- | --- | --- |
| **Gastric distension:** accumulation of swallowed air and gastric juices in presence of ileus<br><br>*Potential onset:*<br>First 24 to 36 hours | All surgical clients | Increased abdominal circumference (measured)<br>Client's complaining of fullness and/or "gas pains"<br>Tympanic abdominal percussion sounds |
| **Ileus:** failure of peristalsis<br><br>*Potential onset:*<br>First 24 to 36 hours | All surgical clients<br>Stress response to surgical trauma | No bowel sounds or fewer than 5/min. (normal: 5–35 clicks or gurgles/min.) |
| **Intestinal obstruction:** adhesions, trap or kink in segment of intestine<br><br>*Potential onset:*<br>Third to fifth day | Abdominal surgery | No postoperative bowel movement<br>Abdominal distention<br>Client complains of periodic sharp, colicky pains<br>Hyperactive bowel sounds<br>Abdominal tenderness<br>Nasogastric drainage: dark brown or black<br>The lower the obstruction the more gradual the onset |
| **Paralytic ileus:** paralysis of intestinal peristalsis<br><br>*Potential onset:*<br>First three to four days | Intraperitoneal surgery<br>Peritonitis<br>Kidney surgery<br>Decreased cardiac output<br>Pneumonia<br>Electrolyte imbalance<br>Wound infection | No bowel sounds<br>Abdominal distention<br>No passage of flatus<br>Nasogastric drainage green to yellow, 1–2 liters in 24 hrs. |
| **Pneumonia:** inflammatory process in which alveoli are filled with exudate<br><br>*Potential onset:*<br>First 36 to 48 hours | Clients with unresolved atelectasis<br>Following aspiration<br>Smoker<br>Elderly<br>Chronic bronchitis<br>Emphysema<br>Heart failure<br>Debilitated<br>Alcoholic<br>Immobile<br>Cough suppressant medications<br>Respiratory depressant medications | Client complains of dyspnea; tachycardia; increasing temperature; productive cough and increasing amount of sputum becoming tenacious, rusty, or purulent<br>Tactile fremitus<br>Dullness to percussion<br>Bronchial breath sounds<br>Increased wet rales or rhonchi<br>Voice sounds present<br>  Bronchophony<br>   Egophony<br>    Whispered pectoriloquy<br>ABGs: decreased $PaO_2$ |

| PREVENTION | INTERVENTION | CHARTING |
|---|---|---|
| Encourage client to avoid air swallowing | Provide frequent turning to move air and secretions<br>Have client sit up in chair or ambulate if appropriate<br>Insert nasogastric tube and connect to low suction<br>Monitor abdominal circumference by measuring q1 hr.<br>Monitor for return of bowel sounds<br>Monitor for passage of flatus<br>Insert rectal tube | Measurement of changes in abdominal girth<br>Client's complaints<br>Presence/absence of bowel sounds<br>Presence/absence of flatus<br>Nursing treatment<br>Client's response to treatment |
| None | Monitor for return of normal bowel sounds<br>Offer only sips of water until return of bowel sounds<br>Monitor for distention<br>Monitor for passage of flatus signaling return of peristalsis | Presence/absence of bowel sounds<br>Presence/absence of distention<br>Results obtained from client's ingestion of water<br>Presence/absence of nausea or vomiting<br>Presence/absence of flatus |
| None | Identify condition early<br>Report to physician immediately<br>Reduce client anxiety<br>Maintain patent nasogastric tube<br>Never give laxative or purgative if obstruction is suspected<br>Prepare for insertion of intestinal tube (Miller-Abbott, Canton, or Harris)<br>Prepare for surgery if necessary | Signs and symptoms that led to physician notification<br>Actions for client support and anxiety reduction<br>Client's response to nursing intervention |
| None<br>Maintain electrolyte balance<br>Maintain cardiac output<br>Prevent pneumonia<br>Prevent wound infection<br>Provide early ambulation | Same as for gastric distention<br>Maintain nasogastric suction until peristalsis returns<br>Monitor for intestinal obstruction | Character, color and quantity of nasogastric drainage<br>Measurement of changes in abdominal girth<br>Client's complaints<br>Presence/absence of bowel sounds<br>Presence/absence of flatus<br>Nursing treatment<br>Client's response to treatment |
| Provide vigorous treatment of atelectasis<br>Prevent aspiration | Turn, cough, and deep breathe q1 hr.<br>May need to stimulate cough with nasotracheal suctioning<br>Send sputum for culture and sensitivity<br>Administer antibiotic as ordered<br>Frequent mouth care for comfort<br>Administer oxygen as ordered<br>Increase fluid intake<br>Administer antipyretic as ordered<br>Monitor for response to treatment | Frequency of nursing treatment<br>Client's response to treatment<br>Resolution or lack of resolution of auscultated findings<br>Sputum character and amount<br>Fluid intake<br>Frequency of spontaneous cough |

**TABLE 4** POSTOPERATIVE COMPLICATIONS (continued)

| POTENTIAL COMPLICATION | PATIENTS AT RISK | INDICATIVE FINDINGS |
|---|---|---|
| **Pulmonary embolism:** foreign object has migrated to branch of pulmonary artery<br><br>*Potential onset:*<br>Seventh to tenth day<br><br>*Massive embolism:*<br>Pulmonary hypertension, dyspnea, right heart failure, shock, ABGs: decreased $PaO_2$, increased $PaCO_2$ | Superficial vein thrombosis: rare<br>Deep vein thrombosis: 40 to 60 percent<br>Air emboli: intraperitoneal surgery<br>Fat emboli: long bone fracture, split sternum | Only 10 percent recognized clinically<br>Pain sharp and stabbing, occurs with breathing; localized (right lower lobe most frequent)<br>Increased respiratory rate<br>Increased heart rate<br>Restlessness |
| **Pulmonary infarction:** necrosis of lung tissue due to occlusion of blood supply (less than 10 percent develop)<br><br>*Potential onset:*<br>2 to 72 hrs. after arterial obstruction | Pulmonary embolism | Hemoptysis<br>Cough<br>Fever 101° to 102°F<br>Pleural friction rub<br>Pleuritic pain |
| **Thrombophlebitis:** inflammation of vein with clot formation<br><br>*Potential onset:*<br>Seventh to fourteenth day | *Abnormal vein walls:*<br>Varicose veins<br>Previous thrombophlebitis<br>Trauma to vein wall<br>Tight strap on operating room table<br>Surgery on hips or in pelvis<br>Age more than 60 (arteriosclerosis)<br><br>*Venous stasis:*<br>Immobility<br>Casts, restrictive dressings<br>Constant Fowler's position<br>Prolonged dependent lower extremities<br>Knee-gatch elevated<br>Pillows under knees<br>Pillows under calves<br>Obesity<br>Abdominal distention<br>Shock<br>Heart failure<br><br>*Hypercoagulability:*<br>Surgical stress response<br>Stress and anxiety<br>Infection<br>Anesthesia<br>Decreased circulation<br>Hypovolemia<br>Malignant neoplasms<br>Postpartum<br>Oral contraceptives | *Superficial vein thrombophlebitis:*<br>Pain, redness, tenderness, and induration along course of vein<br>Palpable "cord" corresponding to course of vein<br>History of trauma including IV site<br><br>*Deep small-vein thrombophlebitis:*<br>Increased muscle turgor and tenderness over affected vein<br>Deep muscle tenderness<br>Most frequent site: vessels at calf<br>Affected limb warm to touch with occasional swelling<br>Client complains of tightness or stiffness in affected leg<br>Positive Homan's sign (dorsiflexion of foot leads to calf pain)<br>Fever rarely more than 101°F<br><br>*Major deep-vein thrombophlebitis:*<br>No superficial signs of inflammation<br>Homan's sign unreliable<br><br>*Femoral vein thrombosis:*<br>Pain and tenderness in distal thigh and popliteal region. Swelling extends to level of knee<br><br>*Iliofemoral vein:*<br>Often massive swelling, pain and tenderness of entire lower extremity<br>Cyanosis of extremity when dependent<br>Superficial veins sometimes visibly dilated<br>Circumference differential more than 15 mm in males and more than 12 mm in females; most reliable for diagnosis |

| PREVENTION | INTERVENTION | CHARTING |
|---|---|---|
| Provide range of motion<br>Encourage early ambulation<br>Prevent thrombophlebitis<br>Do not massage a potential or suspected thrombophlebitic area | Administer oxygen to relieve hypoxia<br>Reduce anxiety<br>Position client on left side with head dependent to prevent air embolus<br>Prevent recurrent embolization; prepare for fibrinolysis; prepare for anticoagulation<br>Prepare for x-ray, angiography, and/or ventilation/perfusion scan | Signs and symptoms that led to physician notification<br>Nursing actions<br>Client's response to therapy |
| None | Describe indicative findings to physician<br>Institute relaxation techniques to decrease client's anxiety<br>Administer oxygen<br>Support and comfort client | Signs and symptoms that led to physician notification<br>Nursing interventions<br>Client's response to treatment |
| *Avoid injury to vein wall:*<br>Use care when strapping to operating room table<br>Avoid IVs in lower extremities<br>Pad side rails for restless, convulsive, and/or combative client<br>Avoid restraints<br><br>*Avoid venous stasis:*<br>Encourage early ambulation<br>Provide feet and leg exercises: 10 min. q1–2 hr. while in bed<br>Increase frequency of exercise for client at risk<br>Prevent client's sitting with legs in dependent position<br>Place pillow between legs while client is lying on side to prevent pressure from upper leg on lower<br>Provide deep breathing exercise<br>Provide active and passive range of motion<br>Prevent restrictive dressings, casts, and positions<br>Increase velocity of blood flow:<br>  No standing<br>  Steady IV flow<br>  Antiembolic stockings (controversial)<br>Decrease hypercoagulability:<br>  Provide adequate hydration<br>  Prevent infections<br>  Maintain circulation<br>  Decrease stress/anxiety | *Superficial vein thrombophlebitis:*<br>Treat symptoms<br>Analgesic<br>Local heat<br>Continue ambulation unless accompanied by deep venous involvement<br>Monitor for progression toward saphenafemoral junction (may need ligation)<br><br>*Deep vein thrombophlebitis:*<br>Provide adequate bed rest<br>Elevate foot of bed with 6–8″ blocks<br>Administer warm moist compresses to relieve venospasm and help resolve inflammation<br>Administer and monitor:<br>  Heparin therapy<br>  Fibrinolytic therapy<br>Monitor for pulmonary embolism | Signs and symptoms that led to physician notification<br>Nursing actions<br>Client's response to therapy |

**TABLE 4** POSTOPERATIVE COMPLICATIONS (continued)

| POTENTIAL COMPLICATION | PATIENTS AT RISK | INDICATIVE FINDINGS |
|---|---|---|
| **Urinary tract infection**<br><br>*Potential onset:*<br>Third to fifth day or 48 hrs. after removal of catheter | *Decreased resistance:*<br>History of bladder distention<br>History of urinary retention<br>Previous urinary tract infection<br>History of prostatic hypertrophy<br>History of catheterization<br>Diabetic<br>Debilitated<br>Immobile | Dysuria<br>Frequency<br>Urgency<br>High fever: up to 104° F with fewer systemic toxic symptoms than would be expected<br>Change in urine odor<br>Pus in urine<br>Sediment<br>May be asymptomatic |
| **Wound infection**<br><br>*Potential onset:*<br>Streptococcal: 24 to 48 hrs. after contamination<br>Staphylococcus gram-negative rods, etc.: five to seven days postoperatively | *Slow to heal:*<br>Obese<br>Diabetic<br><br>*Poor nutrition:*<br>Debilitated<br>Elderly<br>Ulcerative colitis<br><br>*Poor circulation:*<br>Elderly<br>Hypovolemic<br>Heart failure<br><br>*Lack of oxygen to wound:*<br>Vasoconstriction<br>Severe anemia<br>Depressed immunity<br>Cancer<br>Renal failure<br>Preoperative steroid therapy<br>Prolonged complex surgery (stress response leading to increased ACTH)<br>Malnutrition<br>Elderly<br>At risk for transmission<br>Proximity of another client with infection<br>Transmission by hands of personnel | Initial inflammation: 36–48 hrs.<br>Wound tender, swollen, warm, increased redness<br>Increasing heart rate<br>Increasing temperature<br>Increasing or recurring serous drainage<br>There may be no local signs if infection is deep |

| PREVENTION | INTERVENTION | CHARTING |
|---|---|---|
| Maintain sterile technique with catheterization and catheter removal<br>Provide competent indwelling catheter care<br>Encourage early ambulation to decrease retention and stasis | Encourage fluid intake; cranberry juice to decrease urine pH<br>Increase activity to enhance bladder emptying<br>Encourage voiding q2 hrs. while awake<br>Send specimen for culture and sensitivity<br>Administer antibiotic as ordered<br>Monitor for residual urine of more than 100 cc | Signs and symptoms that led to notification of physician<br>Nursing interventions<br>Client's response to nursing intervention and medical therapy |
| Maintain nutrition<br>Maintain good circulation<br>Maintain normal blood volume<br>Provide nonrestrictive dressings, casts, etc.<br>Provide frequent turning<br>Have client sit up in chair or ambulate as soon as possible<br>Maintain PaO$_2$<br>Treat atelectasis<br>Prevent pulmonary complications<br>Monitor ABGs if necessary<br>Prevent severe anemia: replace lost RBCs<br>Increase attention to prevention for clients with depressed immunity<br><br>*Prevent transmission:*<br>Practice effective handwashing<br>Practice aseptic technique in wound care<br>Separate postoperative from infected clients<br>Maintain dry dressings<br>Use special caution for a new wound, easily contaminated | Maintain nutrition<br>Maintain oxygenation<br>Maintain circulation and blood volume<br>Maintain pulmonary toilet<br>Send wound drainage specimen for culture and sensitivity<br>Administer antibiotics as ordered<br>Cleanse wound or irrigate as ordered<br>Monitor for systemic response to infection, fever, malaise, headache, anorexia, nausea<br>Treat symptoms | Description of appearance of wound in measurable terms: define redness in cm squared; define drainage in cc's<br>Description of tissue surrounding wound<br>Condition of dressing<br>Client's complaints of wound discomfort<br>Type of dressing used<br>Nursing interventions<br>Cleansing and dressing of wound<br>Method of irrigation and fluid used<br>Client comfort measures<br>Presence/absence of systemic signs and symptoms<br>Client's response to therapy |

# Chapter 31

# Crisis and the Dying Patient

## LEARNING OBJECTIVES

Define the term crisis and describe the precipitant factors.

Describe several behavioral responses to crises.

Outline the main characteristics of a crisis.

Identify the specific stages in the development of a crisis.

Discuss assessment techniques to identify a person in crisis.

List two objectives of intervention into a crisis situation.

Outline the steps necessary to assist the patient to manage a crisis.

Describe the priorities of care for a patient hospitalized following a suicide attempt.

Discuss the stages of the grief process.

State the main characteristics observed in a person experiencing grief.

Identify the factors that influence the outcome of the grieving process.

Explain three assessment parameters for observing psychological and somatic symptoms that accompany the grief process.

Discuss at least two nursing interventions for each stage of grief.

Describe the phases of dying outlined by Elisabeth Kübler-Ross.

Explain what is meant by providing emotional care for the dying patient.

Discuss at least four nursing interventions that would assist the dying patient.

Describe the steps of providing postmortem care.

## CRISIS SITUATIONS

The word *crisis* originates from the Greek word *krisis* meaning "turning point." The contemporary definition of crisis is a crucial situation, or turning point. Such a juncture in one's life cycle immediately affects the total being. When methods of dealing with stressful situations are not adequate, and the normal coping modes are not sufficient to resolve the situation, the individual is plunged into the chaos of conflict and indecision. Successful resolution of this crisis will occur with either a return to the precrisis state of being, a level of functioning below that of the crisis period, or psychological growth evidenced by increased competence and ability to cope. When an adult individual is in a crisis, it often precipitates such total involvement of the person that therapeutic intervention is required to sustain and assist the person to cope.

Crises can occur from any external or inner source, such as loss of a loved one or a relationship, impoverishment, disaster, unemployment, marriage, birth of a child, return of a loved one, adolescence, etc. A crisis can develop from stress, and stress can develop from any untoward or even a desirable event. Any change from normal living patterns can create stress. Stress develops into a crisis situation when the person is unable to cope with the stressful situation.

Individual responses to a crisis may vary, but a central theme of this state is a loss of control and an inability to cope. There may be a panic episode that engenders a high level of anxiety, distortion of thought or perceptions, or even personality disorganization. If the latter occurs, you would observe increased motor activity, reduced sensory perception, and reduced ability to communicate, leading to complete withdrawal and even loss of higher psychic functions. In addition to panic, there may be a reaction to acute grief that results in psychological and somatic symptoms, leading to an inability to cope with activities of daily living.

We as individuals are typically in a state of balance, or homeostasis. This state is maintained by behavioral patterns involving interchange between the person and his or her environment. When problems or stress are encountered, the person employs learned coping mechanisms to deal with the stress. If the coping mechanisms work, a crisis does not develop. If, however, the problem becomes too great to be handled, a crisis situation emerges. The result is a major disorganization in functioning.

The major precipitating factors in a crisis are:

- Threat to individual security: loss or threat of loss.

- Situational crisis: actual or potential loss of job, relationship, etc.

- Developmental crisis: any change, positive or negative.

- Two or more severe problems arising concurrently.

**Characteristics**   The main characteristics of a crisis situation are that it is initiated by a triggering event, and the usual coping mechanisms are inadequate for dealing with the situation. The crisis is self-limiting, acute, and will last from a few days to a period of six weeks. The person is totally involved and hurts all over. This is a very dangerous situation for the person, and intervention is essential.

There are specific stages in the development of a crisis situation. First, there is the initial perception of the problem, which causes a rise in tension and anxiety. The usual coping mechanisms are tried, and the usual situational supports are explored. The known methods prove unsuccessful and tension increases. The problem or stress remains and the person's functioning becomes disorganized. As anxiety increases, perception narrows, and the coping ability is further reduced. Resolution of the crisis occurs within six weeks with or without intervention.

It is important to remember that the main goal is simply to resolve the immediate crisis so that the individual can continue to function. Thus, the first principle is to be reality-oriented. This entails giving the necessary support, clarifying the problem, and providing adequate anticipatory guidance.

Anticipatory guidance involves being there and listening to the patient. It includes providing the necessary information to assist the patient to make decisions. This is the moment that a person is most open for intervention; therefore, if appropriate intervention occurs, major changes can take place so that the crisis can be a turning point for the person and the individual emerges from the crisis situation functioning at a higher level than previously. This is the most positive result. An alternative outcome of intervention would be that the person survived the crisis period still able to cope with life and has accepted suggestions for future support.

## LOSS: GRIEVING AND DYING

Grief is an emotion experienced in relation to loss; it can also be viewed as a behavioral response to death and dying. Human beings experience loss as the emotion of grief and must withdraw from the painful stimulus to recuperate. Emotions allow us to experience our environment—they are the means of cognition. When we are grieving, we experience the emotion of grief; this experience is accompanied by a definite syndrome with somatic and psychological symptoms.

**Stages of Grief**    George Engle describes the classic progression of the grief process in stages. These stages may occur in order, or an individual may skip a stage, become locked in a particular stage, or even return to an earlier stage already worked through.

The first stage is *shock and disbelief,* denial and numbness. The first response upon learning of a death is shock and a refusal to accept or comprehend the fact. This reaction is followed by a stunned, numb feeling and does not allow the person to acknowledge the reality of death. This initial phase is characterized by attempts to protect oneself against severe stress by blocking recognition of the death.

*Developing awareness* is the second stage. Within minutes or hours the individual becomes acutely and increasingly aware of the anguish of loss. Anger may be present during this time and may be directed toward persons or circumstances held to be responsible for the death. Behavior that frequently accompanies this stage is crying and a regression to a more helpless and childlike state. The crying and regression appear to acknowledge the loss so conscious awareness is now present.

The third stage is *restitution,* where the various rituals of the culture, such as the funeral, attire, wake, particular folkways, and mores, help to initiate the recovery process. These rituals serve the function of emphasizing the reality of death and the very act of experiencing them assists the mourner to face the loss.

As the reality of death becomes accepted, the *resolution* of the loss begins. This stage involves a number of steps. First, the mourner attempts to deal with the painful void created by the loss of a loved one. At this time the thoughts of the mourner are occupied almost exclusively with the deceased. Then the mourner becomes more aware of his or her own body and bodily sensations. Finally, the mourner begins to talk about the dead person, recalling the dead person's attributes and personality and reminiscing about the memories they shared. Resolving the loss is a long and painful phase that continues until the mourner remembers the positive aspects of the dead person.

The next stage that is frequently experienced is that of *idealization.* All hostile and negative feelings toward the dead person are repressed. As the process proceeds, two important changes are taking place: The recurring thoughts about the dead person bring a distinct image of the loss to mind and these memories serve to bring out the more positive aspects of the lost relationship. At the same time the mourner begins to assume certain admired qualities of the dead person through the mechanisms of identification or incorporation. The mourner may begin to dress, speak, or develop mannerisms or beliefs similar to the person who was lost. Often, many months are required for this process to be experienced, and as it dissipates, the mourner's preoccupation with the dead person lessens. It may be at this point that the person begins to reinvest intimate feelings toward other love objects.

The outcome of the mourning process usually takes a year or more. The clearest evidence of healing is the ability to remember the deceased comfortably and realistically, with both the pleasures and disappointments of the relationship. At this stage the obsession with the loss is ended and the person accepts the responsibility of living his or her own life.

Each individual who experiences loss will move through at least some of these stages as he or she attempts to cope with loss. The stages of grief are the means human beings have of moving through the loss to resolution.

**Stages of Dying**    Elisabeth Kübler-Ross has beautifully described the phases of dying, which mirror those of the grieving process. As a person learns of his or her own impending death, he or she will experience grief in relation to his or her own loss.

The first stage, as Dr. Ross views this process, is that of *denial*. The denial may be partial or complete and may occur not only during the first stages of illness or confrontation but later on from time to time. This initial denial is usually a temporary defense and is used as a buffer until such time as the person is able to collect him or herself, mobilize his or her defenses, and face the inevitability of death.

The second stage is often *anger*. The person feels violent anger at having to give up life. This emotion may be directed toward persons in the environment or even projected into the environment at random. Dr. Ross explains this reaction and the difficulty in handling it for those close to the person: "The problem here is that few people place themselves in the patient's position and wonder where this anger might originate. Maybe we too would be angry if all our life activities were interrupted so prematurely."

The third stage is *bargaining*. The person attempts to strike a bargain for more time to live or more time to be without pain in return for doing something for God. Often during this stage the person turns or returns to religion.

*Depression* is the fourth stage. Usually, when people have completed the processes of denial, anger, and bargaining, they move into depression. Dr. Ross writes about two kinds of depression. One is preparatory depression; this is a tool for dealing with the impending loss. The second type is reactive depression. In this form of depression, the person is reacting against the impending loss of life and grieves for himself.

The final stage of dying is that of *acceptance*. This is when the person has worked through the previous stages and accepts his own inevitable death. With full acceptance of impending death comes the preparation for it; however, even with acceptance, hope is still present and needs to be supported realistically.

Many factors influence how individuals accept death. Personal values and beliefs about life; views of personal successes, both financial and emotional; the way they look physically when experiencing the dying process; their family and friends and their families' attitudes and reactions; their past experiences in coping with difficult or traumatic situations; and, finally, the health care staff who are caring for them during this process—all affect an individual's attitude toward dying.

The following nursing diagnoses may be appropriate to include in a Patient Care Plan when a patient is admitted for a crisis, or is in the process of grieving or dying.

## NURSING DIAGNOSES

| Nursing Diagnosis (Potential) | Defining Characteristic; Etiology (Examples) |
| --- | --- |
| ☐ Coping, Ineffective Individual, *related to* | Fear and anxiety, e.g., terminal illness, loss of body part and/or function. |
| ☐ Grieving, Anticipatory, *related to* | Loss of significant other, e.g., death, suicide. |

|  | Loss of body part and/or function, e.g., trauma or disease state. |
|---|---|
| ☐ Health Maintenance Deficit, *related to* | Inability to manage own disease treatment or health promotion activities, e.g., cognitive impairment, depression, immobility. |
| ☐ Spiritual Distress, *related to* | Anxiety, worry or depression, e.g., terminal illness, unstable religious beliefs. |

# UNIT ONE  CRISIS INTERVENTION

## NURSING PROCESS DATA

### ASSESSMENT  *Data Base*

Observe the patient's psychological state and specific behaviors.

Observe for potential loss of control.

Observe level of anxiety manifested.

Determine degree of personality disorganization.

Observe behavior indicating patient is experiencing a crisis:
Increased motor activity.
Reduced sensory perception.
Reduced ability to communicate.
Withdrawal or depression.
Symptoms of panic.

Check for presence of somatic symptoms.

Determine ability to go through activities of daily living.

Assess potential for suicide.

Assess need for hospitalization (either from lack of ability to function or danger of suicide).

### PLANNING  *Objectives*

To identify a patient who is in crisis.

To assist patient to experience relief of symptoms.

To prevent patient from committing suicide during crisis period.

To assist patient to continue to function.

To assist patient to manage anxiety.

To suggest that patient seek professional support to cope with crisis.

### IMPLEMENTATION  *Procedure*

Assisting the Patient in Crisis

**EVALUATION**  *Expected Outcomes*

Identification of patient in crisis is completed.

Patient continues to function during crisis period.

Patient experiences relief of symptoms.

Resolution of crisis occurs.

## ASSISTING THE PATIENT IN CRISIS

### Procedure

1. Establish a rapid working relationship by listening and attending to patient cues.

2. Remain with patient in a crisis or have significant persons available.

3. Encourage the patient to express feelings; avoid intellectual explanations or rationalizations.

4. Set firm limits and keep interaction goal-oriented.

5. Assist patient to clarify the problem.

6. Deal with target symptoms, such as anxiety, depression, withdrawal.

7. Remain reality-oriented, dealing with the "here and now."

8. Do not focus on weakness, pathology, or past crisis situations.

9. Assist patient to look at new social networks and support systems or alternate responses that will provide support to the patient.

10. Suggest follow-up procedures so that patient may continue therapy and avoid subsequent crisis periods.

### CHARTING  *for Crisis Intervention*

☐ Identification of crisis patient is experiencing

☐ Behavioral and somatic symptoms patient is manifesting

☐ Coping mechanisms patient is utilizing

☐ Supports available to patient

☐ Interventions utilized to assist patient

## CLINICAL PROBLEM SOLVING

### Potential Problems

Patient attempts suicide as a means of coping with crisis.

### Suggested Solutions

☐ Be aware of symptoms of possible suicidal behavior.

☐ Recognize level of depression and potential for suicide (when depression begins to lift).

☐ Determine presence of suicide ideation: Ask questions such as "Do you wish you were dead?" "Do you think you might do something about it?" "What?" "Have you taken any steps to prepare?" "What are they?"

☐ Observe behavior closely for cues to potential suicide.

☐ Observe physical status so you can intervene if necessary (if patient is not eating, sleeping, etc.).

Patient is hospitalized following suicide attempt.

☐ Provide safe environment to protect patient from self-destruction.

- ☐ Observe patient closely at all times, especially when depression is lifting.
- ☐ Establish supportive relationship, letting patient know you are concerned for his welfare.
- ☐ Encourage expression of feelings, especially anger.
- ☐ Focus on patient's strengths and successful experiences to increase self-esteem.
- ☐ Provide a structured schedule and involve the patient in activities with others.
- ☐ Structure a plan for the patient to use as a means of coping when next confronted with suicide ideation.
- ☐ Help the patient plan for continued professional support after discharge.

## UNIT TWO   THE GRIEF PROCESS

### NURSING PROCESS DATA

**ASSESSMENT** *Data Base*

Observe for presence of psychological symptoms.
  Weeping.
  Guilt.
  Anger and irritability toward others and the deceased.
  Depression.
  Inability to initiate meaningful activity.

Observe for somatic symptoms.
  Physical exhaustion.
  Insomnia.
  Restlessness and agitation.
  Digestive disturbance.
  Anorexia.

Determine patient's complaints.
  Sense of unreality.
  Sense of detachment.
  Lack of strength.

Observe stage of grief response patient is experiencing.
  Shock and disbelief.
  Developing awareness.
  Restitution.
  Resolution.
  Idealization.
  Outcome of grieving process—positive or negative.

Observe for morbid reaction to grief.
  Delay of reaction.
  Distorted reaction: acquisition of symptoms that belonged to deceased, psychosomatic illness, or disease, etc.

Atypical grief syndrome manifested by distorted pictures of grief.

**PLANNING**  *Objectives*

To assist the patient who is experiencing the grief process.

To intervene therapeutically and provide support.

To allow the patient to express feelings of loss openly.

To understand and tolerate patient's behavior that is related to loss.

To assist the patient to move successfully through stages of the grief process.

**IMPLEMENTATION**  *Procedures*

Understanding Grief

Assisting with Grief

**EVALUATION**  *Expected Outcomes*

The patient's experience of the grieving process is therapeutic.

Patient moves through grieving process.

Patient accepts loss, and outcome of grieving process is positive.

## UNDERSTANDING GRIEF

### Procedure

1. Understand the importance of the person lost as a source of support.

2. Observe the degree of dependency of the relationship. **Rationale:** The more dependent, the more difficult is the task of resolution.

3. Identify the degree of ambivalence felt toward the deceased. **Rationale:** When there are persistent hostile feelings, guilt may interfere with the work of mourning.

4. Check on the number and nature of other relationships the mourner has to depend on. **Rationale:** Few meaningful relationships makes the willingness to give up the attachment to the deceased more difficult.

5. Check on the number and nature of previous grief experiences. **Rationale:** Losses tend to be cumulative in their effects, and if previous losses have not been successfully worked through, they will only aggravate the current loss.

6. Determine the degree of preparation for the loss. **Rationale:** In terminal illness grief work may have begun long before the actual death of the person.

7. Determine the capacity to cope with loss. The more inner resources the patient has available, the better coping ability. **Rationale:** The physical and psychological health of the mourner at the time of the loss determines capacity.

## ASSISTING WITH GRIEF

### Procedure

1. Become familiar with the grief process, the stages of grief, and natural responses to grief so you can provide patient with optimal support.

2. Denial stage:
   a. Allow patient denial of grief to give patient time to move through shock and to mobilize defenses.
   b. Encourage patient to talk when he or she is ready to do so.
   c. Understand that shock and disbelief may be first response, and anticipate that behavior may be inappropriate or disturbed.
   d. Accept patient's inability to face reality, and allow mood swings and expressions of happier times (which may seem inappropriate at this time).

3. Anger stage:
   a. Allow "acting-out" of feelings and verbalization of anger.

b. Anticipate expression of anger toward others, loved ones, and the environment.

c. Understand that unreasonable, insatiable demands are an expression of this stage of grief and attempt to meet the demands. Anticipate patient's needs before demanded.

d. Encourage patient to take as much control as possible over care and environment. Avoid criticism and negative feedback at this time.

e. Avoid false reassurance and false cheerfulness, which lead to distrust. Also, avoid diversion by introducing cheerful activities or stories. These actions lead patient to believe you do not care about feelings.

f. Explain and clarify all procedures and treatments to decrease misinterpretation and expansion of fears.

4. Bargaining stage:
   a. Allow patient to move through bargaining stage; listen to verbal expressions without judgment or pointing out reality.
   b. Encourage patient to talk about bargaining with God. This may assist patient to cope with guilt and not lose faith.

5. Reactive depression stage:
   a. Encourage verbalizations about loss, its meaning in patient's life, and feelings about the loss.
   b. Support patient's self-esteem and understand that it will be affected with awareness of the loss.
   c. Encourage and reassure as appropriate; do not give false reassurance at this stage but assist patient to be realistic.
   d. Be aware of own feelings of sadness and loss so that they do not interfere with therapy.

6. Preparatory depression:
   a. Allow patient to be quiet and silent in order to internalize feelings.

b. Remain with patient and share on a nonverbal level.

c. Verbalize feelings to patient when they are appropriate; do not deny yourself expressions of sadness or empathy (crying) when appropriate.

d. Limit association with cheerful, insincere staff, friends, or family.

7. Resolution-acceptance stage:
   a. Allow patient to express whatever feelings are present, knowing that patient has moved through the above stages and may now be feeling totally empty of emotion.
   b. Spend quiet time with patient, interacting on a nonverbal, nondemanding level.
   c. Encourage patient to make preparations for impending death by supporting requests to finish tasks and discussing options for plans to complete areas in his or her life.
   d. Honor patient's requests to be alone and do not overload with external information. Patient may need a lot of quiet contemplation to prepare for death.

8. Show respect for cultural, religious, and social customs throughout stages of mourning.

9. Offer support and reassurance to family.

### CHARTING  *for The Grief Process*

☐ Stage of grief the patient is experiencing and patient's ability to cope

☐ Behavioral manifestations of grief

☐ Support systems available to patient

☐ Measures nurse has taken to assist patient to cope with grief

☐ Patient response to psychosocial interventions

---

## CLINICAL PROBLEM SOLVING

**Potential Problems**

The patient experiences a morbid reaction to grief.

Family cannot support grief of patient or handle their own grief.

**Suggested Solutions**

☐ Recognize distorted symptoms and be accepting but firm with patient.

☐ Request further assistance from the staff.

☐ Know the general response to death by recognizing the stages of the grief process.

&#9633; Understand that the behavior of the mourner may be unstable and disturbed.

&#9633; Request assistance from nursing staff to cope with the family.

---

# UNIT THREE   THE DYING PATIENT

## NURSING PROCESS DATA

### ASSESSMENT   *Data Base*

Observe the physical symptoms:
>Evidence of circulatory collapse.
>Variations in blood pressure and pulse.
>Disequilibrium of body mechanisms.
>Deterioration of physical and mental capabilities.
>Absence of corneal reflex.

Observe the patient's ability to fulfill basic needs without complete assistance.

Assess the nature and degree of pain the patient is experiencing.

Observe for impending crisis or emergency situation.

Observe for psychosocial condition:
>Need to establish a relationship for support.
>Grief pattern and stage of grief the patient is experiencing.
>Need to express feelings and verbalize fears, concerns, etc.

Determine anxiety level, which may be expressed in physical or emotional behavior.
>Sleep disturbance.
>Palpitations.
>Digestive complaints.
>Anger or hostility.
>Withdrawal.

Determine depression level that patient may be experiencing.
>High fatigue level or lethargy.
>Poor appetite, nausea, or vomiting.
>Inability to concentrate.
>Expressions of sadness, hopelessness, or uselessness.

### PLANNING   *Objectives*

To assist the dying patient to cope with the dying process.

To handle own feelings of loss and sadness that arise when caring for a patient who is dying.

To provide support for the patient and the patient's family during the dying process.

To complete the actions necessary to care for the patient who has died.

### IMPLEMENTATION   *Procedure*

Assisting the Dying Patient

**EVALUATION** *Expected Outcomes*

Patient finds internal resources to accept death.

Patient is able to verbalize feelings and needs.

Physical discomfort is minimized.

---

**TO MY FAMILY, MY PHYSICIAN, MY LAWYER, MY CLERGYMAN
TO ANY MEDICAL FACILITY IN WHOSE CARE I HAPPEN TO BE
TO ANY INDIVIDUAL WHO MAY BECOME RESPONSIBLE FOR MY HEALTH, WELFARE OR AFFAIRS**

Death is as much a reality as birth, growth, maturity and old age—it is the one certainty of life. If the time comes when I, _____ can no longer take part in decisions for my own future, let this statement stand as an expression of my wishes, while I am still of sound mind.

If the situation should arise in which there is no reasonable expectation of my recovery from physical or mental disability, I request that I be allowed to die and not be kept alive by artificial means or "heroic measures". I do not fear death itself as much as the indignities of deterioration, dependence and hopeless pain. I, therefore, ask that medication be mercifully administered to me to alleviate suffering even though this may hasten the moment of death.

This request is made after careful consideration. I hope you who care for me will feel morally bound to follow its mandate. I recognize that this appears to place a heavy responsibility upon you, but it is with the intention of relieving you of such responsibility and of placing it upon myself in accordance with my strong convictions, that this statement is made.

Signed _____

Date _____

Witness _____

Witness _____

Copies of this request have been given to _____

_____

_____

_____

In case of terminal illness, Euthenasia Council's "Living Will" can clarify your wishes. (Copies can be obtained by writing the Council at 250 W. 57 St., New York 10019.)

---

## ASSISTING THE DYING PATIENT

### Procedure

1. Minimize the patient's discomfort as much as possible.
   a. Provide warmth.
   b. Provide assistance in moving, and position patient frequently.
   c. Provide assistance in bathing and personal hygiene.
   d. Administer the appropriate medications before the pain becomes severe.

2. Recognize the symptoms of urgency and/or emergency conditions and seek immediate assistance.

3. Notify the charge nurse if there is an impending crisis and perform emergency actions until help arrives.

4. Encourage the patient to do as much as he can

for himself so that patient does not just give up— a state that only reinforces low self-esteem.

5. Provide emotional nursing care for the patient.
   a. Form a relationship with the dying patient. Be willing to be involved, to care, and to be committed to caring for a dying patient.
   b. Allocate time to spend with the patient so that not only physical care is administered.
   c. Recognize the grief pattern and support the patient as he moves through it.
   d. Recognize that your physical presence is comforting by staying physically close to the patient if he is frightened. Use touch if appropriate and nonverbal communication.
   e. Respect the patient's need for privacy and withdraw if the patient has a need to be alone or to disengage from personal relationships.
   f. Be tuned into patient's cues that he wants to talk and express feelings, cry, or even intellectually discuss the dying process.
   g. Accept the patient at the level on which he is functioning without making judgments.

6. Provide the level of care that will encourage the patient to retain confidence in the health care team.

7. Assist the patient as he lives through the experience of dying in whatever way you are able to do so.

8. Support the family of the dying patient.
   a. Understand that the family may be going through anticipatory grief before the actual event of dying.
   b. Understand that different family members will react differently to the impending death and support the different reactions.
   c. Be aware that demonstrating your concern and caring will assist the family to cope with the grief process.

9. Be aware of your own personal orientation toward the dying process.
   a. Explore your own feelings about death and dying with the understanding that until you have faced the subject of death you will be inadequate to support the patient or the family as they experience the dying process.
   b. Share your feelings about dying with the staff and others; actively work through them so that negativity does not get transferred to the patient.

### CHARTING *for The Dying Patient*

☐ Physical symptoms that the patient is experiencing

☐ Stage of dying and acceptance of patient

☐ Support systems available to patient

☐ Nursing care measures that make the patient the most comfortable

☐ Family acceptance and interaction with patient

## CLINICAL PROBLEM SOLVING

**Potential Problems**

Nurse is unable to care for the dying patient due to her own emotional reaction.

**Suggested Solutions**

☐ Request that other staff members take over, as the objective is to be able to give good nursing care.

☐ Request assistance from skilled professional to work through own feelings about death so that you will be able to cope with the next death experience.

Patient loses confidence in the health care team.

☐ Attempt to ascertain exactly what occurred to cause patient to lose confidence in the team.

☐ Report to charge nurse so that staff caring for patient may be changed. Be sure to choose experienced personnel who are equipped to cope with a dying patient.

Patient lingers on and does not fulfill expectation that death would occur in the near future.

Pain cannot be controlled adequately with ordered medication.

☐ Report status to staff so arrangements may be made for respite-supportive care for family who is having a difficult time coping.
☐ Discuss hospice care with the patient's family.

☐ Report to physician so alternative pain relief methods may be used.
☐ Assist the patient to cope by spending additional time and meeting physical needs.

## UNIT FOUR    POSTMORTEM CARE

### NURSING PROCESS DATA

#### ASSESSMENT    *Data Base*

Verify that patient has been pronounced dead by the physician.

Complete your own observations that patient has no observable responses to stimuli.

Identify patient by name and his belongings for labeling.

#### PLANNING    *Objectives*

To prepare body for removal from clinical unit.

To protect the condition of the body for the purpose of respect for the deceased and his or her family during final viewing.

To document facts and time relating to death.

To identify and label patient and patient's belongings.

#### IMPLEMENTATION    *Procedure*

Providing Postmortem Care

#### EVALUATION    *Expected Outcomes*

Postmortem care is completed by assigned staff member.

Patient's personal items have been identified and labeled properly.

Family is supported through grief process by staff.

## PROVIDING POSTMORTEM CARE

### Equipment

Bathing supplies

Shroud or morgue bag

Identification tags

Protective pads, if necessary

Rolls of gauze and abdominal pads, if necessary to secure limbs together

Paper bags or plastic bags for personal belongings

Guerney or specialized morgue cart

### Procedure

1. If there are other patients or visitors in the room, carefully explain the situation and ask them to temporarily leave the room if possible.

To ensure that your organs are donated appropriately, fill out and keep donor card with you at all times.

2. Collect necessary equipment.

3. Follow hospital procedure regarding notification of various departments and personnel.

4. Maintain proper alignment of the body. Raise the head of the bed slightly to prevent pooling of fluids in the head or face.

5. If possible, place dentures in mouth to maintain original shape of face and mouth.

6. Remove any external objects causing pressure or injury to the skin, e.g., oxygen mask.

7. Following hospital policy, remove, cut, or secure any tubes, drains, or monitoring lines.

8. Following hospital policy, secure or replace dressings.

9. Cleanse the body as needed. A partial bath may be required to remove secretions, wound drainage, stains, etc.

10. Close the eyes. If necessary, use paper tape or gauze pads. You may do this after the family has visited the deceased.

11. Place protective incontinent pad under buttocks and between legs diaper fashion.

12. If family is to visit the deceased, provide clean linen and gown for patient.

13. Remove equipment used for cleansing patient.

14. If previously determined or requested by patient or family, notify the appropriate clergy or religious support person.

15. After family and clergy have visited, label the body, attaching ID tags to the big toe, wrist, and morgue bag or as determined by standard procedure.

16. Tie limbs loosely together, using padding and gauze roll. Attach wrist and ankles, using proper alignment.

17. Place the body in the shroud or in morgue bag.

18. Label all personal belongings and place them in a bag.

19. Close doors to patient's room and clear hallways in preparation to transfer the body to the morgue.

20. Transfer the body to the morgue on a guerney or a special morgue cart.

21. Place patient's personal belongings in the appropriate place determined by hospital policy.

### CHARTING  *for Postmortem Care*

☐ The events leading to the actual death, i.e., termination of vital signs, etc.

☐ The exact time the physician was informed and death was pronounced

☐ When family members or significant others were notified

☐ Consent forms signed

☐ Condition of the body and postmortem care delivered

☐ Time the body and belongings were sent to the morgue

---

## CLINICAL PROBLEM SOLVING

**Potential Problems**

Patient is not identified properly when sent to the morgue.

Donated organs are needed.

**Suggested Solutions**

☐ Check identaband and shroud label before releasing patient to mortician.
☐ Request another nurse to check labels.

☐ Provide support to family and give an opportunity for questions.

☐ Obtain signatures for consent form. (Kidneys should be removed within one hour after death. Eyes should be removed within 6 to 24 hours after death.)

☐ Examine reverse side of driver's license, or remind the charge nurse to call mortician if burial plans have been made previously, to check on permission for organ donation through a living will.

## TERMINOLOGY

**Agitation:**  excessive restlessness; increased mental and physical activity.

**Anger:**  a feeling of extreme displeasure, hostility, indignation, or exasperation toward someone or something.

**Anorexia:**  loss of appetite occurring from a variety of possible reasons.

**Anxiety:**  a troubled or apprehensive feeling; experiencing a sense of dread or fear.

**Cope:**  to contend with, strive, or handle.

**Corneal reflex:**  closure of eyelids resulting from direct corneal irritation or touch.

**Counseling:**  giving assistance to or guidance.

**Crisis:**  a crucial point or situation in the course of anything; turning point.

**Denial:**  refusal to grant the truth of a statement or allegation.

**Depression:**  being dispirited, saddened; low in mood.

**Empathy:**  objective awareness of and insight into the feelings, emotions, and behavior of another person.

**Esteem:**  regard, respect.

**Grief:**  intense mental anguish, deep remorse, sorrow, or the like.

**Homeostasis:**  an internal state of equilibrium or balance.

**Idealization:**  to regard as ideal; to make or regard someone or something as absolute perfection.

**Insomnia:**  inability to sleep; difficulty with sleeping.

**Pain:**  suffering, distress, or discomfort.

**Psychosomatic:**  pertaining to phenomena that are both physiological and psychological in origin.

**Resolution:**  the state of having made a firm determination; a course decided upon.

**Restitution:**  a return to a former status.

**Shock:**  term used to designate a clinical syndrome with varying degrees of disturbances of oxygen supply to the tissues.

**Somatic:**  referring to the body.

**Stress:**  a mentally or emotionally disruptive or disquieting influence; distress.

**Therapeutic:**  having medicinal or healing properties.

**Withdrawal:**  to pull back or away.

# *Bibliography*

Abels, Linda. *Mosby's Manual of Critical Care.* St. Louis: The C. V. Mosby Company, 1979.

Abrams, Anne Collins. *Clinical Drug Therapy.* Philadelphia: J. B. Lippincott Company, 1983.

Adams, Catherine, and Alberta R. Macione, eds. *Handbook of Psychiatric Mental Health Nursing.* New York: John Wiley & Sons, Inc., 1983.

Adams, Nancy. "The Nurse's Role in Systematic Weaning from a Ventilator." *Nursing 79,* August 1979.

Agee, Barbara L., and Christine Herman. "Cervical Logrolling on a Standard Bed." *American Journal of Nursing,* Vol. 84, No. 3, March 1984.

Aguilera, Donna. *Crises Intervention: Theory and Methodology.* St. Louis: The C. V. Mosby Company, 1978.

Allardyce, D. B., and A. C. Groves. "A Comparison of Nutritional Gains Resulting from Intravenous and Enteral Feeding." *Surg. Gyn. and Obst.* August 1974.

Altemeier, Wm. A., et al. *Manual on Control of Infection in Surgical Patients,* 2nd ed. Philadelphia: J. B. Lippincott Company, 1984.

Amas, George. *The Rights of the Hospital Patients.* ACLU Handbook. Avon Books, 1975.

American College of Chest Physicians and American Thoracic Society Joint Committee on Pulmonary Nomenclature. "Pulmonary Terms and Symbols." *Chest,* 67:583–593, 1975.

American Heart Association and National Academy of Sciences–National Research Council. "Standards and Guidelines for Cardiopulmonary Resuscitation (CPR) and Emergency Cardiac Care (ECC)." *JAMA,* 244(5):453–509, 1980.

*American Journal of Nursing.* "Fetal and Maternal Monitoring." December 1978.

*American Journal of Nursing.* "How to Work with Chest-Tubes." Vol. 80, No. 4, April 1980.

Anderson, Betty Anne, et al. *The Childbearing Family,* Vol. II, *Pregnancy and Family Health.* New York: McGraw-Hill Book Company, 1979.

Anderson, Marjorie A., et al. "The Double-Lumen Hickman Catheter." *American Journal of Nursing,* February 1982.

Andreoli, Kathleen, et al. *Comprehensive Cardiac Care: A Textbook for Nurses, Physicians, and Other Health Practitioners.* 5th ed. St. Louis: The C. V. Mosby Company, 1983.

Arieti, Silvano, ed. *American Handbook of Psychiatry,* Vols. I, II, and III. New York: Basic Books, Inc., Publishers, 1974.

Armstrong, Margaret, et al. *McGraw-Hill Handbook of Clinical Nursing.* New York: McGraw-Hill Book Company, 1979.

Ayres, Stephen. "Pulmonary Physiology at the Bedside: Oxygen and Carbon Dioxide Abnormalities." *Cardiovascular Nursing,* January-February 1973.

Babson, S. G., et al. *Diagnosis and Management of the Fetus and Neonate at Risk.* St. Louis: The C. V. Mosby Company, 1980.

Bachm, Frank. "FHR Variability: Key to Fetal Well-Being." *Contemporary OB/GYN,* Volume 9, May 1977.

Banyard, Sandra G. "New Drug-Free Technique Cuts Postop Pain." *RN Magazine,* April 1982.

Baranowski, Karen, et al. "Vital Hepatitis—How to Reduce Its Threat to the Patient and Others." *Nursing 76,* May 1976.

Barber, Janet, and Susan Budassi. *Mosby's Manual of Emergency Care.* St. Louis: The C. V. Mosby Company, 1984.

Barnard, Martha U., et al. *Human Sexuality for Health Professionals.* Philadelphia: W. B. Saunders Company, 1978.

Barry, Jean. *Emergency Nursing.* New York: McGraw-Hill Book Company, 1978.

Bates, Barbara. *A Guide to Physical Examination.* 3rd ed. Philadelphia: J. B. Lippincott Company, 1984.

Beland, Irene, and Joyce Passos. *Clinical Nursing.* 4th ed. New York: Macmillan Publishing Company, Inc., 1981.

Bellack, Janis P., and Penny A. Bamford. *Nursing Assessment: A Multidimensional Approach.* Monterey: Wadsworth Health Sciences Division, 1984.

Bergersen, Betty S. *Pharmacology in Nursing.* 14 ed. St. Louis: The C. V. Mosby Company, 1979.

Bernheim, C. H., et al. "Fever: pathogenesis, pathophysiology and purpose." *Annals of Internal Medicine,* 1979.

Binkley, Lowanna S. "Keeping Up with Peritoneal Dialysis." *American Journal of Nursing,* Vol. 84, No. 6, June 1984.

Birchenall, Joan, and Mary Eileen Streight. *Care of the Older Adult.* Philadelphia: J. B. Lippincott Company, 1982.

Bishop, B. "How to cool a feverish child." *Pediatric Nursing,* January/February, 1978.

Bistrain, B. R., and G. L. Blackburn. "Prevalence of Malnutrition in General Medical Patients." *JAMA,* 235:1567–1570, 1976.

Bloom, B. S., ed. *Taxonomy of Educational Objectives, Handbook I: Cognitive Domain.* New York: David McKay Co., 1956.

Bordick, Katherine. *Patterns of Shock: Implications for Nursing Care.* New York: Macmillan Publishing Company, Inc., 1980.

Borg, Nan, et al. *Core Curriculum for Critical Care Nursing.* Philadelphia: W. B. Saunders Company, 1981.

Borgen, Linda. "Total Parenteral Nutrition in Adults." *American Journal of Nursing,* February 1978.

Bradshaw, Troy Wayne. "Making Male Catheterization Easier for Both of You." *RN Magazine,* December 1983.

Brink, Pamela J., ed. *Transcultural Nursing.* Englewood Cliffs, NJ: Prentice-Hall, Inc., 1976.

Britt, Michael, et al. "Severity of Underlying Disease as a Predictor of Nosocomial Infection." *JAMA,* March 13, 1978.

Brooks, Stewart. *Basic Facts of Body Water and Ions*. New York: Springer Publishing Company, Inc., 1973

Brown, B. *New Mind, New Body*. New York: Harper and Row, 1982.

Brown, B. *Stress and the Art of Biofeedback*. New York: Harper and Row, 1977.

Broughton, Joseph O. "Chest Physical Diagnosis for Nurses and Respiratory Therapists." *Heart and Lung*, March-April 1972.

Broughton, Joseph O. "Understanding Blood Gases." Ohio Medical Products Article Reprint Library, August 1971.

Brubacher, Lynda, and Patricia Beard. "A Helpful New Handout for Your Ostomy Patients." *RN Magazine*, Vol. 46, No. 8, August 1983.

Brunner, Lillian Sholtis, and Doris Smith Suddarth. *Textbook of Medical Surgical Nursing*. 5th ed. Philadelphia: J. B. Lippincott Company, 1984.

Brunner, Lillian Sholtis, and Doris Smith Suddarth. *The Lippincott Manual of Nursing Practice*. 3rd ed. Philadelphia: J. B. Lippincott Company, 1982.

Budassi, Susan. "An Emergency Nurse's Guide to Drawing Arterial Blood Gases." *Journal of Emergency Nursing*, January-February 1977.

Budassi, Susan, and Janet Barber. *Emergency Nursing: Principles and Practice*. St. Louis: The C. V. Mosby Company, 1981.

Bullough, Bonnie. *The Law and the Expanding Nursing Role*. 2nd ed. New York: Appleton-Century-Croft, 1980.

Burgess, Ann Wolbert, and Aaron Lazare. *Psychiatric Nursing in the Hospital and the Community*. 3rd ed. Englewood Cliffs, NJ: Prentice-Hall, Inc., 1981.

Burnside, Irene Mortenson. *Nursing and the Aged*. 2nd ed. New York: McGraw-Hill Book Company, 1976.

Burrow, G. N., and T. F. Ferris. *Medical Complications During Pregnancy*. 2nd ed. Philadelphia: W. B. Saunders Company, 1982.

Bushnell, Sharon Spaeth. *Respiratory Intensive Care Nursing*. Boston: Little, Brown & Company, 1973.

Butterworth, C. E. "The Skeleton in the Closet." *Nutrition Today*, March-April 1974.

Byrne, Judith. "Liver Function Studies, Part IV: Using Metabolism Tests to Investigate Liver Function." *Nursing 77*, December 1977.

Byrne, Nancy. "Overcoming the Red Menace: Preventing and Treating Decubitus Ulcers." *Nursing 84*, Vol. 14, No. 4, April 1984.

Cannon, Christine. "Hands-On Guide to Palpation and Auscultation." *RN Magazine*, 43 (3): 20–24, 1980.

Cannon, W. B. *Bodily Changes in Pain, Hunger, Fear and Rage: An Account of Recent Researches into the Function of Emotional Excitement*. New York: D. Appleton and Co., 1929.

Cannon, W. B. *The Wisdom of the Body*. New York: Norton, 1942.

Carnevali, Doris, and Maxine Patrick. *Nursing Management for the Elderly*. Philadelphia: The J. B. Lippincott Company, 1983.

Carpenito, Lynda Jual. *Nursing Diagnosis: Application to Clinical Practice*. Philadelphia: J. B. Lippincott Company, 1983.

Cataldo, C. B., and L. Smith. "Tube Feedings: Clinical Applications." Ross Laboratories, 1980.

Cazalas, Mary W. *Nursing and the Law*. Germantown, MD: Aspen Systems Corporation, 1978.

Chaffee, Ellen, and Ivan Lytle. *Basic Physiology and Anatomy*. 4th ed. Philadelphia: J. B. Lippincott Company, 1980.

Cherniack, R. M., et al. *Respiration in Health and Disease*. Philadelphia: W. B. Saunders Company, 1972.

Chinn, Peggy L. *Child Health Maintenance: Concepts in Family Centered Care*. St. Louis: The C. V. Mosby Company, 1979.

Ciuca, Rudy, et al. "Passive Range-of-Motion Exercises." *Nursing 78*, July 1978.

Clark, Ann, and Dyanne Affonso. *Childbearing: A Nursing Perspective*. 2nd ed. Philadelphia: F. A. Davis, 1979.

Cohen, Stephen. "Nursing Care of a Patient in Traction." *American Journal of Nursing*, October 1979.

Colley, Rita, and Jeanne Wilson. "Meeting Patients' Nutritional Needs with Hyperalimentation." *Nursing 79*, May, June, August, and September 1979.

Comoss, Patricia M., et al. *Cardiac Rehabilitation: A Comprehensive Nursing Approach*. Philadelphia: J. B. Lippincott Company, 1979.

Conway, Barbara. *Carini and Owens' Neurological and Neurosurgical Nursing*. 8th ed. St. Louis: The C. V. Mosby Company, 1982.

Craib, Alice, and Margaret Perry. *EEG Handbook*. 2nd ed. Schiller Park, Ill.: Beckman Instruments, Inc., 1975.

Croushore, Theresa. "Postoperative Assessment: the Key to Avoiding the Most Common Nursing Mistakes." *Nursing 79*, April 1979.

Daily, Elaine Kiess, and John Speer Schroeder. *Techniques in Bedside Hemodynamic Monitoring*. St. Louis: The C. V. Mosby Company, 1981.

Dickason, Elizabeth J., and Martha Olsen Schultz. *Maternal and Infant Care*. 2nd ed. New York: McGraw-Hill Book Company, 1979.

Dison, Norma. *Clinical Nursing Techniques*. 4th ed. St. Louis: The C. V. Mosby Company, 1979.

Doenges, Marilynn E., et al. *Nursing Care Plans: Nursing Diagnoses in Planning Patient Care*. Philadelphia: F. A. Davis Company, 1984.

Dossey, Barbara. "A Wonderful Prerequisite—Relaxation." *Nursing 84*, Vol. 14, No. 1, January 1984.

Dossey, Barbara. "Perfecting Your Skills for Systematic Patient Assessment." *Nursing 79*, February 1979.

Doyle, Jeanne. "If Your Patient's Legs Hurt, the Reason May be Arterial Insufficiency." *Nursing 81*, April 1981.

Drauss, P. et al. "The Other Side of Death—Good Memories and the Strength to Go On." *Nursing 78*, December 1978.

Duke University Hospital Nursing Services. *Guidelines for Nursing Care: Process and Outcome*. Philadelphia: J. B. Lippincott Company, 1983.

Dunphy, J. Englebert, and Lawrence L. Way. *Current Surgical Diagnosis and Treatment*. 5th ed. Los Altos, CA: Lange Medical Publications, 1983.

Dyer, Claire. "Burn Care in the Emergent Period." *Journal of Emergency Nursing*, 6(1): 9–16, 1980.

Engle, George L. "Grief and Grieving." *American Journal of Nursing*, September 1964. [a classic]

Erickson, Roberta. "Chest tubes: They're Really Not That Complicated." *Nursing 81*, Vol. 11, No. 5, May 1981.

Erickson, Roberta. "Solving Chest Tube Problems." *Nursing 81*, June 1981.

Erikson, Erik H. *Childhood and Society*. New York: W. W. Norton and Company, Inc., 1963. [a classic]

Ettinger, Bruce, and Dorothy McCort. "Effects of Drugs on the Fetal Heart Rate During Labor." *JOGN*, Volume 5, No. 5, Sept./Oct. 1976.

Euland, K. "Cardiovascular Diseases Complicating Pregnancy." *Clinical Obstetrics and Gynecology*. Vol. 21, pp. 426–441, 1978.

Fadden, Teresa Curtis, and Geraldine Kacerovsky Seiser. "Nursing Diagnosis—A Matter of Form." *American Journal of Nursing*, Vol. 84, No. 4, April 1984.

Fagerhough, Shizuko Y., and Anselm Strauss. "How to Manage Your Patient's Pain...and How Not To." *Nursing 80*, February 1980. From *Politics of Pain Management: Staff-Patient Interaction*. Shizuko Y. Fagerhough and Anselm Strauss. Addison-Wesley. 1977.

Farrell, Jane. *Illustrated Guide to Orthopedic Nursing*. Philadelphia: J. B. Lippincott Company, 1977.

Ferholt, Deborah. *Clinical Assessment of Children: A Comprehensive Approach to Primary Pediatric Care.* Philadelphia: J. B. Lippincott Company, 1980.

Fischbach, Frances. *A Manual of Laboratory Diagnostic Tests.* 2nd ed. Philadelphia: J. B. Lippincott Company, 1984.

Fischer, Ruth. "Measuring Central Venous Pressure." *Nursing 79,* October 1979.

Fisher, Ruth E. "Measuring Central Venous Pressure: How to Do It Accurately...and Safely." *Nursing 79,* October 1979.

Fishman, Mark C., et al. *Medicine.* Philadelphia: J. B. Lippincott Company, 1981.

Fleming, Linda M., and Jacquelyn Kone RN. "Step-by-Step Guide to Safe Peritoneal Dialysis." *RN Magazine,* February 1984.

Folk-Lightly, Marie. "Solving the Puzzles of Patients' Fluid Imbalances." *Nursing 84,* Vol. 14, No. 2, February 1984.

Food and Nutrition Board, National Research Council–National Academy of Sciences. *Recommended Dietary Allowances.* Washington, DC: 1979.

French, Ruth. *Guide to Diagnostic Procedures.* 5th ed. New York: McGraw-Hill Book Company, 1980.

Fuchs, Patricia. "Understanding Continous Mechanical Ventilation." *Nursing 79,* December 1979.

Fuchs, Patricia. "Getting the Best out of Oxygen Delivery Systems." *Nursing 80,* December 1980.

Fuchs, Patricia L. "Streamlining Your Suctioning Techniques, Part 1: Nasotracheal Suctioning." *Nursing 84,* Vol. 14, No. 5, May 1984.

Furman, Seymour. "Recent Developments in Cardiac Pacing." *Heart and Lung,* September-October 1978.

Galli, Nicholas. *Foundations and Principles of Health Education.* Santa Barbara: John Wiley & Sons, Inc., 1978.

Gardner, Ernest, et al. *Anatomy: A Regional Study of Human Structure.* 4th ed. Philadelphia: W. B. Saunders Company, 1975.

Garrity, Eileen M. "Emergency! When Intubation is Up to You." *RN Magazine,* October 1983.

Garvey, Judith. "Infant Respiratory Distress Syndrome." *American Journal of Nursing,* April 1975.

Gassner, Charles, and William Ledger. "The Relationship of Hospital Acquired Maternal Infections to Invasive Intrapartum Monitoring Techniques." *American Journal of Obstetrics and Gynecology.* Volume 126, No. 1, September 1, 1976.

Gildea, Joan H. "Pre- and Postoperative Nursing Care." *American Journal of Nursing,* February 1978.

Goodlin, Robert. "History of Fetal Monitoring." *American Journal of Obstetrics and Gynecology,* Volume 133, No. 3, February 1, 1979.

Gordon, Marjory. *Manual of Nursing Diagnosis.* St. Louis: The C. V. Mosby Company, 1984.

Grant, Harvey, and Robert Murray. *Emergency Care.* 3rd ed. Bowie, MD: Robert J. Brady Company, 1982.

Greenberg, Diane. "Hyperbaric Oxygen: Exciting New Clinical Results." *RN Magazine,* September 1979.

Griggs, B. A., et al. "Enteral Nutrition for Hospitalized Patients." *A.S.P.E.N. Monograph,* 1980.

Griggs, Barbara, and Mary C. Hoppe. "Nasogastric Tube Feeding." *American Journal of Nursing,* March 1979.

Guthrie, Helen Andrews. *Introductory Nutrition.* 5th ed. St. Louis: The C. V. Mosby Company, 1983.

Guyton, Arthur C. *Textbook of Medical Physiology.* 6th ed. Philadelphia: W. B. Saunders Company, 1981.

Haber, Judith, et al. *Comprehensive Psychiatric Nursing.* New York: McGraw-Hill Book Company, 1982.

Hall, Joanne E., and Barbara Weaver. *Nursing of Families in Crisis.* Philadelphia: J. B. Lippincott Company, 1974.

Hammond, Cecile. "ECG Made Easier than Ever." *RN Magazine,* October 1979.

Hammond, Cecile. "Plain Talk about Cardiac Monitors." *RN Magazine,* September 1979.

Hammond, Cecile. "Protecting Patients with Temporary Transvenous Pacemakers." *Nursing 78,* November 1978.

Hanlon, K. "Description and Uses of Intracranial Pressure Monitoring." *Heart and Lung.* 5:2, 1976.

Harvey, Brenda L. "Your Patient's Discharge Plan." *Nursing 81,* July 1981.

Hathaway, Rebecca. "The Swan-Ganz Catheter: A Review." *Nursing Clinics of North America.* 13:3, September 1978.

Haughey, Brenda. "CVP Lines: Monitoring and Maintaining." *American Journal of Nursing,* April 1978.

Haverkamp, Albert, et al. "The Evaluation of Continuous Fetal Heart Rate Monitoring in High Risk Pregnancy." *American Journal of Obstetrics and Gynecology,* Volume 125, No. 3, June 1, 1976.

Hays, J. S., and K. Larson. *Interacting with Patients.* New York: Macmillan Publishing Company, 1965. [a classic]

Hemelt, Mary Dolores, and Mary Ellen Mackert. *Dynamics of Law in Nursing and Health Care.* Reston, VA: Reston Publishing Company, 1978.

Henderson, Virginia, and Gladys Nite. *Principles and Practice of Nursing.* New York: Macmillan Publishing Company, Inc., 1978.

Hersen, Michel, ed. *The Clinical Psychology Handbook.* New York: Pergamon Press, 1983.

Heymsfield, S. B., et al. "Enteral Hyperalimentation: An Alternative to Central Venous Hyperalimentation." *Ann. Int. Med.* 90: 63–71, 1979.

Holderby, Robert A. "Conscious Suggestion: Using Talk to Manage Pain." *Nursing 81,* May 1981.

Holloway, Nancy M. *Nursing the Critically Ill Adult.* Menlo Park, CA: Addison-Wesley Publishing Company, 1984.

Holmes, T. H., and R. H. Rahe. "Social Readjustment Rating Scale." *Journal of Psychosomatic Research* 11:213, 1967. [a classic]

Hoppe, Mary. "The New Tube Feeding Sets or Your Patients Are What You Feed Them." *Nursing 80,* March 1980.

Howe, Jeanne, ed. *The Handbook of Nursing.* New York: John Wiley & Sons, Inc., 1984.

Hudak, Carolyn M., et al. *Critical Care Nursing.* 3rd ed. Philadelphia: J. B. Lippincott Company, 1982.

Huxley, Valerie. "Heparin Lock: How, What, Why." *RN Magazine,* October 1979.

Irwin, Betty. "Hemodialysis Means Vascular Access...and the Right Kind of Nursing Care." *Nursing 79,* October 1979.

Isacson, Laurey, and Klaus Schulz. "Treating Pulmonary Edema." *Nursing 78,* February 1978.

Jacox, Ada K. "Assessing Pain." *American Journal of Nursing,* May 1979.

Jensen, Margaret, et al. *Maternity Care: The Nurse and the Family.* 2nd ed. St. Louis: The C. V. Mosby Company, 1981.

Johnson, Marion, and Judith Quinn. "The Subarachnoid Screw." *American Journal of Nursing,* March 1977

Jones, Cathy. "Glasgow Coma Scale." *American Journal of Nursing,* September 1979.

Jones, Sande. "The Use and Misuse of Hypothermia Blankets." *RN Magazine,* March 1984.

Jones, Sande. "Simpler and Safer Tube-feeding Techniques." *RN Magazine,* October 1984.

Juliani, Louise M. "Acute Glomerulonephritis." *Nursing 79,* September 1979.

Kalkman, Marion, and Ann Davis. *New Dimensions in Mental-Health Psychiatric Nursing.* 5th ed. New York: McGraw-Hill Book Company, 1979.

Karones, Shelton B. *High-Risk Newborn Infants.* St. Louis: The C. V. Mosby Company, 1981.

Keithley, Joyce. "Proper Nutritional Assessment Can Prevent Hospital Malnutrition." *Nursing 79,* February 1979.

Kelso, I. M., et al. "An Assessment of Continous Fetal Heart Rate Monitoring in Labor: A Radomize Trial." *American Journal of Obstetrics and Gynecology,* Volume 131, No. 1, 1978.

Kessler, Diana. "The 12 Lead Electrocardiogram." *Journal of Emergency Nursing,* December 1979.

Kim, Mi Ja, et al., eds. *Classification of Nursing Diagnosis.* St. Louis: The C. V. Mosby Company, 1984.

Kim, Mi Ja, et al., eds. *Pocket Guide to Nursing Diagnosis.* St. Louis: The C. V. Mosby Company, 1984.

King, Eunice, et al. *Quick Reference to Adult Nursing Procedures.* Philadelphia: J. B. Lippincott Company, 1982.

Kinney, M. R., et al. AACN's *Clinical Reference for Critical-Care Nursing.* New York: McGraw-Hill Book Company, 1981.

Kintzel, Kay Carmen. *Advanced Concepts in Clinical Nursing.* 2nd ed. Phildelphia: J. B. Lippincott Company, 1977.

Korczowski, Marian M. "Strengthen the Nurse's Role in Nutritional Counseling." *Nursing and Health Care,* April 1981.

Koretz, R. L., and T. H. Meyer. "Elemental Diets—Facts and Fantasies." *Gastroenterolgy* 78: 393–410, 1980.

Koszuta, Laurie Einstein. "Choosing the Right Infusion Control Device for Your Patient." *Nursing 84,* Vol. 14, No. 3, March 1984.

Kozier, Barbara, and Glenora L. Erb. *Fundamentals of Nursing: Concepts and Procedures.* 2nd ed. Menlo Park, CA: Addison-Wesley Publishing Company, 1983.

Krebs, H. B., et al. "Intrapartum Fetal Heart Rate Monitoring." *American Journal of Obstetrics and Gynecology,* Volume 133, No. 7, April 1, 1979.

Krizinofski, Marian T. "Human Sexuality and Nursing Practice." *Nursing Clinics of North America,* December 1973.

Krueger, Judith A., and Janis C. Ray. *Endocrine Problems in Nursing.* St. Louis: The C. V. Mosby Company, 1976.

Krupp, Marcus A., and Milton J. Chatton. *Current Medical Diagnosis and Treatment.* Los Altos, CA: Lange Medical Publications, 1980.

Krupp, Marcus, et al. *Physician's Handbook.* 19th ed. Los Altos, CA: Lange Medical Publications, 1979.

Kübler-Ross, Elisabeth. *On Death and Dying.* New York: Macmillan Publishing Company, Inc., 1969. [a classic]

Langley, L. L. et al. *Dynamic Anatomy and Physiology.* 5th ed. New York: McGraw-Hill Book Company, 1980.

Lewis, Sharan Mentik, and Idolia Cox Collier. *Medical-Surgical Nursing: Assessment and Management of Critical Problems.* New York: McGraw-Hill Book Company, 1983.

Lipkin, Gladys B. *Psychosocial Aspects of Maternal-Child Nursing.* 2nd ed. St. Louis: The C. V. Mosby Company, 1978.

Long, Gail D. "Managing the Patient with Abdominal Aortic Aneurysm." *Nursing 78,* August 1978.

Luckmann, Joan, and Karen Creason Sorensen. *Medical-Surgical Nursing: A Psychophysiologic Approach.* 3rd ed. Philadelphia: W. B. Saunders Company, 1984.

MacKinnan, Roger, and Robert Michels. *The Psychiatric Interview in Clinical Practice.* Philadelphia: W. B. Saunders Company, 1971.

Malasanos, Lois, et al. *Health Assessment.* 2nd ed. St. Louis: The C. V. Mosby Company, 1981.

Manzi, Catherine Ciaverelli. "Cardiac Emergency! How to Use Drugs and CPR to Save Lives." *Nursing 78,* Vol. 8, No. 3, March 1978.

Marchiondo, Kathleen. "The Very Fine Art of Collecting Culture Specimens." *Nursing 79,* April 1979.

Marinelli-Miller, Donna. "What the Patient May Not Ask About Angiography." *RN Magazine,* November 1983.

Marlow, D. R. *Textbook of Pediatric Nursing.* Phildelphia: W. B. Saunders Company, 1979.

Masoorli, Susan Thomas. "Tips for Trouble-free Subclavian Lines." *RN Magazine,* February 1984.

Matheny, Leona G. "Defibrillation: When and How to Use it." *Nursing 81,* June 1981.

McCaffery, Margo. *Nursing Management of the Patient with Pain.* 2nd ed. Philadelphia: J. B. Lippincott Company, 1979.

McCaffery, Margo. "Relieving Pain with Noninvasive Techniques." *Nursing 80,* December 1980.

McCalister, Donald, et al. *Readings in Family Planning.* St. Louis: The C. V. Mosby Company, 1973.

McConnell, Edwina. "Ensuring Safer Stomach Suctioning with the Salem Sump Tube." *Nursing 77,* September 1977.

McConnell, Edwina. "Ten Problems with Nasogastric Tubes—and How to Solve Them." *Nursing 79,* April 1979.

McFarland, Mary Brambilla, and Marcia Moeller Grant. *Nursing Implications of Laboratory Tests.* New York: John Wiley & Sons, Inc., 1982.

McGuire, Lora. "A Short, Simple Tool for Assessing Your Patient's Pain." *Nursing 81,* March 1981.

Mead, Johnson. *Dialogues in Nutrition. Nutritional Care of the Critically Ill Patient: Selection of Appropriate Feeding Modalities.* Vol. 3, No. 2, 1979.

Meador, Billie. "If Your 'Continuous' Tube Feeding Stops." *RN Magazine,* Vol. 46, No. 7, July 1983.

Meissner, Judith. "Measuring Patient Stress with the Hospital Stress Rating Scale." *Nursing 80,* August 1980.

Meltzer, Lawrence E., et al. *Intensive Coronary Care: A Manual for Nurses.* 4th ed. Bowie, MD: The Charles Press, 1983.

Mendels, Joseph. *Concepts of Depression.* New York: John Wiley & Sons, Inc., 1970.

Mereness, Dorothy, and Cecelia Taylor. *Essentials of Psychiatric Nursing.* 10th ed. St. Louis: The C. V. Mosby Company, 1978.

Metheny, Norma M., and W. D. Snively. *Nurses' Handbook of Fluid Balance.* 4th ed. Philadelphia: J. B. Lippincott Company, 1983.

Meyers, F. H., et al. *Review of Medical Pharmacology.* 5th ed. Los Altos, CA: Lange Medical Publications, 1976.

Michael, Sharon. "Home IV Therapy." *American Journal of Nursing,* July 1978.

Millar, Sally. *Methods in Critical Care: The AACN Manual.* Philadelphia: W. B. Saunders Company, 1980.

Miller, Emmett, M.D. Relaxation Tapes, P. O. Box W, Stanford, California 94305.

Monk, Heather Boyd, "Screening for Glaucoma." *Nursing 79,* August 1979.

Moree, Nancy A., and Julia S. Garner. "New infection control guideline." *American Journal of Nursing,* Vol. 84, No. 2, February 1984.

Morrissey, Barbara G. *Quick Reference to Therapeutic Nutrition.* Philadelphia: J. B. Lippincott Company, 1984.

Mowinski, Bonnie. "Improving Your Management of DIC." *Nursing 79,* May 1979.

Munro-Black, Janet. "The ABC's of Total Parenteral Nutrition." *Nursing 84,* Vol. 14, No. 2, February 1984.

Murphy, Patricia and Barbara L. Schere. "Timely Techniques in Caring for the Patient with an Endotracheal Tube." Part 1 and Part 2. *Nursing 81,* September 1981 and October 1981.

Narrow, Barbara W. *Patient Teaching in Nursing Practice, A Patient and Family-Centered Approach*. New York: John Wiley & Sons, Inc., 1979.

Neeson, Jean D., and Stockdale, Connie R. *The Practitioner's Handbook of Ambulatory Obstetrics and Gynecology*. New York: Wiley, 1981.

Norris, Debra L. "What all Those Pressures Mean...and Why." *RN Magazine*, October 1981.

*Nursing 80*. "Giving Medication Through a Nasogastric Tube." May 1980.

*Nursing 81*. "The Ins and Outs of Administering I.V. Bolus Injections." November 1981. Adapted from *Nursing Photobook: Managing IV Therapy*.

*Nursing 84*. "NursingUpdate: Antilipemics." Vol. 14, No. 3, March 1984.

Nursing Grand Rounds. "The Nursing Care Plan: A Communiction System that Really Works." *Nursing 78*, August 1978.

Nursing Photobook. *Dealing with Emergencies*. Horsham, PA: *Nursing 80* Books, Intermed Communications, Inc., 1980.

Nursing Photobook. *Giving Medication*. Horsham, PA: *Nursing 80* Books, Intermed Communications, Inc., 1980.

Nursing Photobook. *Preventing and Correcting Tube and Cuff Problems in Artificial Airways*. Horsham, PA: *Nursing 80* Books, Intermed Communications, Inc., 1980.

Nursing Photobook. *Providing Early Mobility*. Horsham, PA: *Nursing 80* Books, Intermed Communications, Inc., 1980.

Nursing Photobook. *Assessing Your Patients*. Horsham, PA: *Nursing 81* Books, Intermed Communications, Inc., 1981.

Nursing Photobook. *Giving Cardiac Care*. Horsham, PA: *Nursing 81* Books, Intermed Communications, Inc., 1981.

Nursing Photobook. *Managing IV Therapy*. Horsham, PA: *Nursing 81* Books, Intermed Communications, Inc., 1981.

Nursing Photobook. *Using Monitors*. Horsham, PA: *Nursing 81* Books, Inc., Intermed Communications, Inc., 1981.

Nurse's Reference Library. *Diseases*. Horsham, PA: *Nursing 81* Books, Intermed Communications, Inc., 1981.

Nurse's Reference Library. *Drugs*. Horsham, PA: *Nursing 80* Books, Springhouse Corp., 1982.

Nursing Skillbook. *Helping Cancer Patients—Effectively*. Horsham, PA: *Nursing 78* Books, Intermed Communications, Inc., 1978.

Nursing Skillbook. *Monitoring Fluid and Electrolytes Precisely*. Horsham, PA: *Nursing 79* Books, Intermed Communications, Inc., 1979.

O'Donnell, Bridgett. "How to Change Tracheotomy Ties—Easily and Safely." *Nursing 78*, March 1978.

Orthopedic Nurses Association, Inc. *Manual of Orthopedic Nursing Care Plans*. Atlanta, GA: May 1975.

Owen, Patricia M. "Defibrillating Pacemaker Patients." *American Journal of Nursing*, Vol. 84, No. 9, September 1984.

Page, C. P., et al. "Continual Catheter Administration of an Elemental Diet." *Surg. Gyn. and Obst.* 142: 184–188, 1976.

Parent, Bea. "Are In-line IV Filters Really Worthwhile?" *Nursing 81*, August 1981.

Payne, Dorris B. *Psychiatric Mental Health Nursing*. 2nd ed. Nursing Outline Series. Flushing, NY: Medical Examination Publishing Company, Inc., 1977.

Pellitteri, Adele. *Nursing Care of the Growing Family: A Child Health Text*. Boston: Little, Brown & Company, 1977.

Peplau, Hildegarde. "Talking With Patients." *American Journal of Nursing*, 1960. [a classic]

Perez, R. H. *Protocol for Perinatal Nursing Practice*. St. Louis: The C. V. Mosby Company, 1981.

Petrillo, M., and S. Sanger. *Emotional Care of Hospitalized Children*. 2nd ed. Philadelphia: J. B. Lippincott Company, 1980.

Petty, Thomas L. *Intensive and Rehabilitative Respiratory Care*. Philadelphia: Lea and Febiger, 1974.

Phipps, Marion, et al. "Staging Decubitus Care." *American Journal of Nursing*, Vol. 84, No. 8, August 1984.

*Physician's Desk Reference to Pharmaceutical Specialties and Biologicals*. Oradell, NJ: Medical Economics, Inc., 1984.

Pierce, Michael E. "Reporting and Following-up on Medication Errors." *Nursing 84*, Vol. 14, No. 1, January 1984.

Polk, Hiram, Jr. "Prevention of Surgical Wound Infection." *Annals of Internal Medicine*, 89 (Part 2), 1978.

Pritchard, Jack A., and Paul C. MacDonald. *Williams Obstetrics*. 17th ed. New York: Appleton-Century-Crofts, 1984.

Proctor, Diane, et al. "Temporary Cardiac Pacing: Causes, Recognition, Management of Failure to Pace." *Nursing Clinics of North America*. Vol. 13, No. 3, September 1978.

Promisloff, Robert A. "Administering Oxygen Safely: When, Why, How." *Nursing 80*, October 1980.

Pumphrey, John B. "Recognizing Your Patients' Spiritual Needs." *Nursing 77*, December 1977.

Querin, Janice Johnson, and Linda Dixon Stahl. "Twelve Simple, Sensible Steps for Successful Blood Transfusions." *Nursing 83*, Vol. 13, No. 11, November 1983.

Rambeau, J. L., and R. Miller. "Nasoenteric Tube Feeding." *Practical Aspects*, Hedeco, 1979.

Rau, Joseph and Mary. "To Breathe or Be Breathed: Understanding IPPB." *American Journal of Nursing*, April 1977.

Redman, Barbara Klug. *The Process of Patient Teaching in Nursing*. 5th ed. St. Louis: The C. V. Mosby Company, 1984.

Reeder, Sharon, et al. *Maternity Nursing*. 15th ed. Philadelphia: J. B. Lippincott Company, 1983.

Rettig, Fannie M. "Appraisal of Intracardiac Monitoring." *AORN*, April 1979.

Reusch, Jurgen. *Therapeutic Communication*. New York: W. W. Norton & Company, Inc., 1961. [a classic]

Reynolds, Janis I., and Jann B. Logsdon. "Assessing Your Patient's Mental Status." *Nursing 79*, August 1979.

Rodman, Morton J., and Dorothy Smith. *Pharmacology and Drug Therapy in Nursing*. 3rd ed. Philadelphia: J. B. Lippincott Company, 1984.

Rosen, Ted, and Julie Mills. "Tattletale Lesions: What Nails Can Tell." *RN Magazine*, Vol. 45, No. 6, June 1982.

Rosenberg, Jack. "New Sophistication in Assessment: Finding the Therapeutic Window." *RN Magazine*, July 1980.

Rutecki, Barbara, and David Seligson. "Caring for the Patient in a Halo Apparatus." *Nursing 80*, October 1980.

Sager, Diane, and Suzanne Bomar. *Intravenous Medications: A Guide to Preparation, Administration and Nursing Management*. Philadelphia: J. B. Lippincott, 1982.

Sanderson, Richard. *The Cardiac Patient, a Comprehensive Approach*. 3rd ed. Philadelphia: W. B. Saunders Company, 1983.

Satir, Virginia. *Conjoint Family Therapy*. Palo Alto, CA: Science & Behavior Books, Inc., 1967. [a classic]

Saul, Lauren. "For CE Credit: Heart Sounds and Common Murmurs." *American Journal of Nursing*, Vol. 83, No. 12, December 1983.

Saxton, Dolores, and Patricia Hyland. *Planning and Implementing Nursing Intervention*. St. Louis: The C. V. Mosby Company, 1979.

Scherer, Jeanne C. *Introductory Clinical Pharmacology*. 2nd ed. Philadelphia: J. B. Lippincott Company, 1982.

Schessl, Eileen. "Learning The Basics of Cardiac Monitors." *Nursing 84*, Vol. 14, No. 10, October 1984.

Schroeder, J., and E. Darly, *Techniques in Bedside Hemodynamic Monitoring.* St. Louis: The C. V. Mosby Company, 1980.

Schumann, Lorna. "Commonsense Guide to Topical Burn Therapy." *Nursing 79*, March 1979.

Scipien, Gladys, et al. *Comprehensive Pediatric Nursing.* New York: McGraw-Hill Book Company, 1983.

Selye, Hans. *The Stress of Life.* New York: McGraw-Hill Book Company, 1965. [a classic]

Shafer, Kathleen Newton, et al. *Medical Surgical Nursing.* 6th ed. St. Louis: The C. V. Mosby Company, 1979.

Shannon, Mary L. "Five Famous Fallacies about Pressure Sores." *Nursing 84*, Vol. 14, No. 10, October 1984.

Shepherd, Mary Jane, and Pamela L. Swearington. "Z-track Injection." *Nursing 84*, Vol. 14, No. 10, October 1984.

Shields, Donna. "Maternal Reactions to Fetal Monitoring." *American Journal of Nursing*, Volume 78, December 1978.

Shils, M. E. *Defined Formula Diets for Medical Purposes.* Chicago: American Medical Association, 1977.

Shils, M. E. "Enteral Nutrition by Tube." *Cancer Research.* 37: 2432–2439, 1977.

Shils, M. E., Bloch, A. S., and R. Chernoff. *Liquid Formula for Oral and Tube Feeding.* 2nd ed. New York: Memorial Sloan Kettering Cancer Center, 1979.

Shils, M. E., and D. Coiro. *Nutrition Assessment of the Cancer Patient: Report of a Pilot Study.* New York: Memorial Sloan Kettering Cancer Center.

Shipley, Susan. "Pitfalls and Perils of Intracardiac Monitoring." *AORN*, April 1979.

Shoemaker, William C., et al. *Textbook of Critical Care.* Philadelphia: W. B. Saunders Company, 1984.

Shrake, Keven. "The ABC's of ABG's or How to Interpret a Blood Gas Value." *Nursing 79*, September 1979.

Silver, H. K., et al. *Handbook of Pediatrics.* 14th ed. Los Altos, CA: Lange Medical Publications, 1983.

Smith, Carol. "Abdominal Assessment: A Blending of Science and Art." *Nursing 81*, 11(2): 42–49, 1981.

Smith, Laurel. "Reactions to Transfusions." *American Journal of Nursing*, Vol. 84, No. 9, September 1984.

Smith, Rae. "Invasive Pressure Monitoring." *American Journal of Nursing*, September 1978.

Smith, Sandra. *Sandra Smith's Review of Nursing for State Board Examinations.* 3rd ed. Los Altos, CA: National Nursing Review, Inc., 1985.

Smith, Sandra Fucci, and Donna J. Duell. *Foundation Skills for Nursing and Allied Health Professionals.* Los Altos, CA: National Nursing Review, 1982.

Solnick, Robert L., ed. *Sexuality and Aging.* Los Angeles: Ethel Percy Andrus Gerontology Center, 1978.

Sorenson, Karen Creason, and Joan Luckmann. *Basic Nursing: A Psychophysiologic Approach.* Philadelphia: W. B. Saunders Co., 1979.

Spitz, Phyllis, and Hannelore Sweetwood. "Kids in Crisis." *Nursing 78*, March 1978.

Storlie, Frances. "Pointers for Assessing Pain." *Nursing 78*, May 1978.

Stroot, Violet R., et al. *Fluids and Electrolytes: A Practical Approach.* Philadelphia: F. A. Davis Company, 1977.

Suitor, Carol W., and Merilly F. Hunter. *Nutrition: Principles and Application in Health Promotion.* 2nd ed. Philadelphia: J. B. Lippincott Company, 1984.

Sumner, Sara. "Refining Your Technique for Drawing Arterial Blood Gases." *Nursing 80*, April 1980.

Sumner, Sara M. "Guidelines for Using Artificial Breathing Devices." *Nursing 84*, Vol. 13, No. 10, October 1983.

Swearingen, Pamela L., ed. *Photo-Atlas of Nursing Procedures.* Menlo Park, CA: Addison-Wesley Publishing Company Nursing Division, 1984.

Swift, Nancy. "Why the MS Patient Needs Your Help." *Nursing 79*, September 1979.

Tecklin, Jan S. "Positioning, Percussing, and Vibrating Patients for Bronchial Drainage." *Nursing 79*, March 1979.

Timmons, Joan. "Breath Sounds." *J. Emergency Nursing*, 6(6): 16–19, 1980.

Torosian, M. E., and J. L. Rambeau. "Feeding by Tube Enterostomy. *Surg. Gyn. and Obst.* 150: 918–924, 1980.

Travelbee, Joyce. *Intervention in Psychiatric Nursing. Process in the One-to-One Relationship.* 2nd ed. Philadelphia: F. A. Davis Company, 1979.

Traver, Gayle. "Assessment of Thorax and Lungs." *American Journal of Nursing*, March 1973.

Traver, Gayle. "Symposium on Care in Respiratory Disease." *Nursing Clinics of North America*, March 1974.

Tucker, Susan Martin et al. *Patient Care Standards.* 3rd ed. St. Louis: The C. V. Mosby Company, 1983.

Turner, Jeffrey S., and Donald B. Helms. *Contemporary Adulthood.* Philadelphia: W. B. Saunders Company, 1979.

U.S. Department of Agriculture. *A Daily Food Guide: The Basic Four.* Rev. ed. Washington, DC: Government Printing Office, 1979.

Urdang, Laurence, ed. *Mosby's Medical and Nursing Dictionary.* St. Louis: The C. V. Mosby Company, 1983.

Van Meter, Margaret. "Keeping Cool in a Code." *RN Magazine*, 44(3): 29–35, 1981.

Vasey, Ellen. "Writing Your Patient's Care Plan...Efficiently." *Nursing 79*, April 1979.

Vaughan, Victor C. R., et al. *Nelson Textbook of Pediatrics.* 11th ed. Philadelphia: W. B. Saunders Company, 1979.

Wade, Jacqueline. *Respiratory Nursing Care: Physiology and Techniques.* 3rd ed. St. Louis: The C. V. Mosby Company, 1982.

Waechter, Eugenia, et al. *Nursing Care of Children.* Philadelphia: J. B. Lippincott Company, 1976.

Walker, J. Ingram. *Psychiatric Emergencies: Intervention & Resolution.* Philadelphia: J. B. Lippincott Company, 1983.

Wasserman, Edward, and Laurence B. Slobody. *Survey of Clinical Pediatrics.* 7th ed. New York: McGraw-Hill Book Company, 1981.

Waterson, Marian. "Teaching Your Patients Postural Drainage." *Nursing 78*, March 1978.

Wells, Marcia I. "Discharge Planning: Closing the Gaps in Continuity of Care." *Nursing 83*, Vol. 13, No. 11, November 1983.

Wells, Ruthann, and Kathy Trostle. "Creative Hairwashing Techniques for Immobilized Patients." *Nursing 84*, Vol. 14, No. 1, January 1984.

West, B. Anne. "Understanding Endorphins: Our Natural Pain Relief System." *Nursing 81*, February 1981.

West, John. *Respiratory Physiology—The Essentials.* Baltimore: Williams & Wilkins Company, 1979.

White, Sara. "Fluids and Electrolytes: Heading Off the Risks." *RN Magazine*, November 1979.

Widmann, Frances. *Clinical Interpretation of Laboratory Tests.* 9th ed. Philadelphia: F. A. Davis Company, 1983.

Wiener, Matthew B., et al. *Clinical Pharmacology and Therapeutics in Nursing.* New York: McGraw-Hill Book Company, 1979.

Williams, Emily. "Food for Enough: Meeting the Nutritional Needs of the Elderly." *Nursing 80*, September 1980.

Williams, Robert H., ed. *Textbook of Endocrinology.* 6th ed. Philadelphia: W. B. Saunders Company, 1981.

Williams, Sue Rodwell. *Essentials of Nutrition and Diet Therapy.* 3rd ed. St. Louis: The C. V. Mosby Company, 1982.

Wills, Sheryle L., and Sharyn F. Tremblay. *Critical Care Review for Nurses.* Monterey, CA: Wadsworth Health Sciences Division, 1984.

Wilson, Holly Skodal, and Carol Ren Kneisl. *Psychiatric Nursing.* Menlo Park, CA: Addison-Wesley Publishing Company, 1983.

Wing, Kenneth. *The Law and The Public's Health.* St. Louis: The C. V. Mosby Company, 1976.

Wood, Lucile A., ed. *Nursing Skills for Allied Health Services.* Philadelphia: W. B. Saunders Company, 1980.

Woods, Nancy Fugate, *Human Sexuality in Health and Illness.* St. Louis: The C. V. Mosby Company, 1983.

Worthington, Laura. "What Those Blood Gases Can Tell You." *RN Magazine*, October 1979.

Yarborough, Mary G. "Training Needs of the Infection Control Nurse." *Annals of Internal Medicine*, November 1978.

Young, Shelley. "Understanding Intracranial Pressure." *Nursing 81*, February 1981.

Yura, Helen, and Mary B. Walsh. *The Nursing Process: Assessing, Planning, Implementing, Evaluating.* 4th ed. New York: Appleton-Century-Crofts, 1983.

Ziegel, Erna, and Mecca Cranley. *Obstetric Nursing.* 8th ed. New York: Macmillan Publishing Company, Inc., 1984.

# *Index*